Understanding Nursing Research

BUILDING AN EVIDENCE-BASED PRACTICE

5th EDITION

Understanding Nursing Research

BUILDING AN EVIDENCE-BASED PRACTICE

Nancy Burns, PhD, RN, FCN, FAAN
Professor Emeritus
College of Nursing
The University of Texas at Arlington
Arlington, Texas;
Faith Community Nurse
St. Matthew Cumberland Presbyterian Church
Burleson, Texas

Susan K. Grove, PhD, RN, ANP-BC, GNP-BC
Professor
College of Nursing
The University of Texas at Arlington
Arlington, Texas;
Adult Nurse Practitioner
Family Practice
Grand Prairie, Texas

With Special Contributions By:
Jennifer Gray, PhD, RN
George W. and Hazel M. Jay Professor, College of
   Nursing
Associate Dean, PhD in Nursing Program
The University of Texas at Arlington
Arlington, Texas

ELSEVIER
SAUNDERS

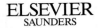

3251 Riverport Lane
Maryland Heights, MO 63043

UNDERSTANDING NURSING RESEARCH, 5ᵀᴴ EDITION
Copyright © 2011 by Saunders, an imprint of Elsevier Inc.

ISBN: 978-1-4377-0750-2

Notice

Knowledge and best practice in this field are constantly changing. As new research and experience broaden our understanding, changes in research methods, professional practices, or medical treatment may become necessary.

Practitioners and researchers must always rely on their own experience and knowledge in evaluating and using any information, methods, compounds, or experiments described herein. In using such information or methods they should be mindful of their own safety and the safety of others, including parties for whom they have a professional responsibility.

With respect to any drug or pharmaceutical products identified, readers are advised to check the most current information provided (i) on procedures featured or (ii) by the manufacturer of each product to be administered, to verify the recommended dose or formula, the method and duration of administration, and contraindications. It is the responsibility of practitioners, relying on their own experience and knowledge of their patients, to make diagnoses, to determine dosages and the best treatment for each individual patient, and to take all appropriate safety precautions.

To the fullest extent of the law, neither the Publisher nor the authors, contributors, or editors, assume any liability for any injury and/or damage to persons or property as a matter of products liability, negligence or otherwise, or from any use or operation of any methods, products, instructions, or ideas contained in the material herein.

The Publisher

Previous editions copyrighted 1995, 1999, 2003, 2007

Library of Congress Cataloging-in-Publication Data
Burns, Nancy, Ph. D.
   Understanding nursing research : building an evidence-based practice / Nancy Burns, Susan K. Grove ; with special contributions by Jennifer Gray.—5th ed.
       p. ; cm.
   Includes bibliographical references and index.
   ISBN 978-1-4377-0750-2 (pbk. : alk. paper)   1. Nursing–Research–Methodology.   2. Evidence-based nursing.   I. Grove, Susan K.   II. Gray, Jennifer, 1955-   III. Title.
   [DNLM: 1. Nursing Research—methods.   2. Evidence-Based Nursing.   WY 20.5 B967u 2011]
   RT81.5.B863 2011
   610.73072—dc22

2010017591

Editor: Maureen Iannuzzi
Associate Developmental Editor: Mary Ann Zimmerman
Publishing Services Manager: Jeff Patterson

Project Manager: Tracey Schriefer
Design Direction: Karen Pauls

Working together to grow
libraries in developing countries

www.elsevier.com | www.bookaid.org | www.sabre.org

ELSEVIER   BOOK AID International   Sabre Foundation

Printed in the United States of America

Last digit is the print number: 9 8 7 6 5 4 3

REVIEWERS

Jennifer Gray, PhD, RN
George W. and Hazel M. Jay Professor, College of
   Nursing
Associate Dean, PhD in Nursing Program
The University of Texas at Arlington
Arlington, Texas

Robyn Nelson, PhD, RN
Dean of Health Services
Touro University
Las Vegas, Nevada

To current and future registered nurses who have dedicated their careers to improving practice with best research evidence.
—Nancy and Susan

To my husband Jay Suggs who is my greatest supporter in all I do.
—Susan

To my brother Richard who is the most courageous person I know.
—Nancy

PREFACE

Research is a major force in nursing, and the evidence generated from research is changing practice, education, and health policy. Our aim in developing this essentials research text, *Understanding Nursing Research: Building an Evidence-Based Practice*, is to create excitement about research in undergraduate students. The text emphasizes the importance of baccalaureate-educated nurses being able to read, critically appraise, and synthesize research so this evidence can be used to make changes in practice. A major goal of professional nursing and health care is the delivery of evidence-based care. By making nursing research an integral part of baccalaureate education, we hope to facilitate the movement of research into the mainstream of nursing. We also hope this text increases student awareness of the knowledge that has been generated through nursing research and that this knowledge is relevant to their practice. Only through research can nursing truly be recognized as a profession with documented effective outcomes for the patient, family, nurse provider, and healthcare system. Because of this expanded focus on evidence-based practice, we have subtitled this edition *Building an Evidence-Based Practice*.

Developing a fifth edition of *Understanding Nursing Research* has provided us with an opportunity to clarify and refine the essential content for an undergraduate research text. The text is designed to assist undergraduate students in overcoming the barriers they frequently encounter in understanding the language used in nursing research. The revisions in this fifth edition are based on our own experiences with the text and input from dedicated reviewers, inquisitive students, and supportive faculty from across the country who provided us with many helpful suggestions.

Chapter 1, Introduction to Nursing Research and Evidence-Based Practice, introduces the reader to nursing research, the history of research, and the significance of research evidence for nursing practice. The discussion of research methodologies and their importance in generating an evidence-based practice for nursing has been expanded.

Chapter 2, Introduction to the Quantitative Research Process, presents the steps of the quantitative research process in a concise, clear manner and introduces students to the focus and findings of quantitative studies. Extensive, recent examples of descriptive, correlational, quasi-experimental, and experimental studies are provided, which reflect the quality of current nursing research.

Chapter 3, Introduction to the Qualitative Research Process, provides details on the common qualitative research methodologies, such as phenomenology, grounded theory, ethnography, and historical research. Suggestions are provided to assist students in reading and critically appraising qualitative studies.

Chapter 4, Examining Ethics in Nursing Research, provides an extensive discussion of the use of ethics in research and the regulations that govern the research process. Detailed content and websites are provided to promote students' understanding of the Health Insurance Portability and Accountability Act (HIPAA), the U.S. Department of Health and Human Services Protection of Human Subjects, and the Federal Drug Administration regulations. Guidelines are provided to assist students in critically appraising the ethics of a study. The ethics chapter is provided much earlier in this edition at the request of reviewers and to provide students with an earlier exposure to the ethics of research.

Chapter 5, Research Problems, Purposes, and Hypotheses, clarifies the difference between a problem and a purpose. Example problem and purpose statements are included from current qualitative, quantitative, and outcome studies. Detailed guidelines are provided with examples to direct students in critically appraising the problems, purposes, hypotheses, and variables in studies.

Chapter 6, Understanding the Literature Review in Published Studies, provides a background for locating, reading, critically appraising, and summarizing research literature to determine the current knowledge in a selected area for use in nursing practice. This chapter details the process for accessing online sources and relevant practice information from the Internet.

Chapter 7, Understanding Theory and Research Frameworks, has been revised to provide a clear and simplified explanation of the importance of frameworks in research. This chapter also includes updated guidelines for critically appraising frameworks in published studies. Frameworks based on middle-range theories, developed for physiological studies, and derived from qualitative studies are described.

Chapter 8, Clarifying Quantitative Research Designs, addresses descriptive, correlational, quasi-experimental, and experimental designs and criteria for critically appraising these designs in studies.

Chapter 9, Examining Populations and Samples in Research, provides a detailed discussion of the concepts of sampling in research. Different types of sampling methods for both qualitative and quantitative research are described. Guidelines are included for critically appraising the sampling criteria, sampling method, and sample size of quantitative and qualitative studies.

Chapter 10, Clarifying Measurement and Data Collection in Quantitative Research, has been updated to reflect current knowledge about measurement methods used in nursing research. New content has been added so students can examine the sensitivity, specificity, and likelihood ratios of diagnostic and screening tests to determine their quality.

Chapter 11, Understanding Statistics in Research, includes the following essential topics: processing data analysis; understanding the reasoning behind statistics; describing, predicting, and testing hypotheses using statistics; examining relationships using statistics; interpreting statistical outcomes; and judging statistical suitability.

Chapter 12, Critical Appraisal of Quantitative and Qualitative Research for Nursing Practice, summarizes and builds on the critical appraisal content provided in previous chapters and offers direction for conducting critical appraisals of quantitative and qualitative studies. The guidelines for critically appraising qualitative studies have been significantly revised and simplified. This chapter also includes a current qualitative and quantitative study, and these two studies are critically appraised using the guidelines provided in the chapter.

Chapter 13, Building an Evidence-Based Nursing Practice, has been significantly updated to reflect the current trends in health care to provide evidence-based nursing care. The types of research synthesis are described (systematic review, meta-analysis, integrative review of research, metasummary, and metasynthesis) and guidelines are provided to assist nurses in determining when research evidence is ready for use in practice. The chapter includes theories to assist nurses and agencies in moving toward evidence-based care. Translational research is introduced as a method for promoting the use of research evidence in practice.

Chapter 14, Introduction to Outcomes Research, is included to provide students an understanding of outcomes research. The content in this chapter will assist students in reading and critically appraising the outcome studies appearing in nursing and other health-care journals.

A variety of changes have been made throughout the fifth edition of this text. Strategies designed to assist the reader in linking research findings to practice are increased; an example of such strategies is selecting study examples with which students as beginning clinicians can easily relate. Research examples have been updated throughout to include recently published quantitative, qualitative, and outcomes nursing studies.

This fifth edition of *Understanding Nursing Research* is appropriate for use in a variety of undergraduate research courses for both RN and general students because it provides an introduction to quantitative, qualitative, and outcomes research methodologies. This text not only will assist students in reading research literature, critically appraising published studies, and summarizing research evidence to make changes in practice, but it also can serve as a valuable resource for practicing nurses in critically appraising studies and implementing research evidence in their clinical settings.

Learning Resources to Accompany *Understanding Nursing Research*, 5th edition

The ancillary package to accompany *Understanding Nursing Research* has been expanded for both the instructor and student to allow a maximum level of flexibility in course design and student review.

Instructor's Electronic Resource

The entire Instructor's Electronic Resource is available online. The Instructor's Electronic Resource consists of an Instructor's Resource Manual, Test Bank, PowerPoint Lecture Slides, Electronic Image Collection, Complimentary Research Article Library, and additional learning activities on the Evolve Resources website.

Instructor's Resource Manual

The Instructor's Resource Manual presents chapter focus, key terms, learning outcomes, learning activities, and higher-level critical appraisal activities for each chapter in the main text. The chapter focus states the concepts to which the reader will be introduced when reading the chapter. Relevant outcomes are developed for undergraduate students. Instructors can select the outcomes that are most appropriate for their particular curricula and courses. The learning activities are a selection of individual and group assignments provided for use in or out of class to facilitate the learning of research content. Higher-level critical appraisal exercises are included for each chapter based on the studies provided in the appendix of the manual. Answer guidelines, with text page references, are provided for each exercise. The Instructor's Resource Manual can be saved, revised, and printed to custom-fit specific classes and individual teaching styles.

Test Bank

The Test Bank is made up of approximately 600 multiple-choice questions, including the topic, learning outcome, cognitive level, correct answer, rationale, and text reference. It is available in ExamView format and can be saved, revised, and printed to custom-fit the needs of the individual instructor.

PowerPoint Lecture Slides

The PowerPoint Lecture Slides contain approximately 800 slides, including important illustrations from the textbook. Slide presentations can be customized by revising or changing the order of existing slides. This teaching aid is provided to facilitate lecture preparation and presentation.

Electronic Image Collection

The electronic image collection consists of all images from the text. This collection can be used in classroom lectures to reinforce student learning.

Research Article Library

A collection of research articles, taken from leading nursing journals, can be found in the appendix of the Instructor's Resource Manual and in the Evolve Learning Resources.

Additional Learning Activities

Two additional learning activities are available on Evolve and may be activated by the instructor for the student's use:

- Critical Appraisal Exercises are a selection of critical-thinking exercises based on supplied research articles and include answer guidelines for the instructor.
- Ideas for Research Projects

Evolve Resources for Students

This edition is web-enhanced, and students are prompted to the Evolve website for further practice. As students log onto the text's website, they will find crossword puzzles, student review questions, WebLinks, and, when activated by the instructor, critical appraisal exercises and ideas for research projects.

- Crossword Puzzles offer a fun review of the material in each chapter.
- Student Review Questions aid the student in reviewing and focusing the chapter material.
- Websites related to and organized by chapter are provided in the WebLinks component.

Study Guide

The Study Guide, available as a companion to the text, includes three recently published nursing studies (two quantitative studies and one qualitative study) that can be used in classroom discussions, as well as to address the study guide questions. The Study Guide provides exercises that target comprehension of the meaning of concepts used in each chapter. Exercises, including fill-in-the-blank, matching, and multiple-choice questions, encourage students to validate their understanding of the chapter content. Critical appraisal activities provide students with opportunities to apply their new research knowledge to evaluate the quantitative and qualitative studies provided in the back of the Study Guide. For students who enjoy a little fun with their learning, crossword puzzles related to chapter content are provided.

Acknowledgments

Developing this essentials research text was a 2-year project, and there are many people we would like to thank. We want to extend a very special thank you to **Dr. Jennifer Gray** who reviewed and assisted with the editing of the chapters in this textbook. We also want to express our appreciation to Dean Elizabeth Poster and Associate Deans Dr. Carolyn Cason, Dr. Mary Schira, and Dr. Beth Mancini of The University of Texas at Arlington College of Nursing who are supportive of this project. We extend our thanks to the faculty of the College of Nursing, for their endless support and encouragement. We also would like to thank other nursing faculty members across the world who are using our book to teach research and have spent valuable time to send us ideas and to identify errors in the text. Special thanks to the students who have read our book and provided honest feedback on its clarity and usefulness to them. We would also like to recognize the excellent reviews of the colleagues, listed on the previous pages, who helped us make important revisions in the text.

In conclusion, we would like to thank the people at Elsevier who helped produce this book. We thank the following individuals who have devoted extensive time to the development of this fifth edition, the instructor's ancillary materials, student study guide, and all of the web-based components. These individuals include, Maureen Iannuzzi, Editor; Mary Ann Zimmerman, Associate Developmental Editor; Tracey Schriefer, Project Manager; and Lisa Godoski, Multimedia Producer.

Nancy Burns
PhD, RN, FCN, FAAN

Susan K. Grove
PhD, RN, ANP-BC, GNP-BC

CONTENTS

1 Introduction to Nursing Research and Evidence-Based Practice, 2

2 Introduction to the Quantitative Research Process, 32

3 Introduction to the Qualitative Research Process, 72

4 Examining Ethics in Nursing Research, 102

5 Research Problems, Purposes, and Hypotheses, 144

6 Understanding the Literature Review in Published Studies, 188

7 Understanding Theory and Research Frameworks, 226

8 Clarifying Quantitative Research Designs, 252

9 Examining Populations and Samples in Research, 288

10 Clarifying Measurement and Data Collection in Quantitative Research, 326

11 Understanding Statistics in Research, 370

12 Critical Appraisal of Quantitative and Qualitative Research for Nursing Practice, 418

13 Building an Evidence-Based Nursing Practice, 464

14 Introduction to Outcomes Research, 506

Glossary, 532

Understanding Nursing Research
BUILDING AN EVIDENCE-BASED PRACTICE

Introduction to Nursing Research and Evidence-Based Practice

Chapter Overview

What Is Nursing Research?   4
What is Evidence-Based Practice?   4
Purposes of Research in Implementing an Evidenced-Based Nursing Practice   6
Description   7
Explanation   8
Prediction   9
Control   9
Nursing's Participation in Research: Past to Present   10
Florence Nightingale   10
Nursing Research: 1900s through 1970s   12
Nursing Research: 1980s and 1990s   13
Nursing Research: Twenty-First Century   14
Acquiring Knowledge in Nursing   15
Traditions   16
Authority   16
Borrowing   16

Trial and Error   17
Personal Experience   17
Role Modeling   18
Intuition   18
Reasoning   18
Acquiring Knowledge through Nursing Research   19
Introduction to Quantitative and Qualitative Research   19
Introduction to Outcomes Research   21
Understanding Best Research Evidence for Practice   22
Strategies Used to Synthesize Research Evidence   22
Levels of Research Evidence   25
Introduction to Evidence-Based Guidelines   26
What Is Your Role in Nursing Research?   26

Learning Outcomes

After completing this chapter, you should be able to:

1. Define research, nursing research, and evidence-based practice.
2. Describe the purposes of research in implementing an evidence-based practice for nursing.
3. Describe the past, present, and future of research in nursing.
4. Describe the ways of acquiring nursing knowledge (tradition, authority, borrowing, trial and error, personal experience, role modeling, intuition, reasoning, and research) that you use in practice.
5. Identify the common types of research—quantitative, qualitative, or outcomes—

conducted to generate essential evidence for nursing practice.
6. Describe the following strategies for synthesizing healthcare research: systematic review, meta-analysis, integrative review, metasummary, and metasynthesis.
7. Identify the levels of research evidence available to nurses for practice.
8. Describe the importance of evidence-based guidelines in implementing evidence-based practice.
9. Identify your role in research as a professional nurse.

Key Terms

Authority, p. 16
Best research evidence,
    p. 4
Borrowing, p. 16
Case study, p. 12
Clinical expertise, p. 5
Control, p. 9
Critical appraisal of research,
    p. 28
Deductive reasoning, p. 19
Description, p. 7
Evidence-based guidelines,
    p. 26

Evidence-based practice,
    p. 4
Explanation, p. 8
Inductive reasoning, p. 18
Integrative review, p. 24
Intuition, p. 18
Knowledge, p. 15
Mentorship, p. 18
Meta-analysis, p. 24
Metasummary, p. 24
Metasynthesis, p. 24
Nursing research, p. 4
Outcomes research, p. 14, 21

Personal experience, p. 17
Prediction, p. 9
Premise, p. 19
Qualitative research, p. 20
Qualitative research
    synthesis, p. 24
Quantitative research, p. 20
Reasoning, p. 18
Research, p. 4
Role modeling, p. 18
Systematic review, p. 23
Traditions, p. 16
Trial and error, p. 17

STUDY TOOLS

Be sure to visit *http://elsevier.com/evolve/Burns/understanding* for additional examples and self-tests. Also, a review of this chapter's concepts and practice exercises can be found in Chapter 1 of the Study Guide for *Understanding Nursing Research: Building an Evidence-Based Practice*, 5th edition.

Welcome to the world of nursing research. You may think it strange to consider research a "world," but it is a truly new way of experiencing reality. Entering a new world means learning a unique language, incorporating new rules, and using new experiences to learn how to interact effectively within that world. As you become a part of this new world, you will modify and expand your perceptions and methods of reasoning. For example, using research to guide your practice involves questioning, and you will be encouraged to ask such questions as these: What is the patient's health care problem? What nursing intervention would effectively manage this problem in your practice? Is this nursing intervention based on sound research evidence? Would another intervention be more effective in improving your patient's outcomes? How can you use research most effectively in promoting an evidence-based practice?

Because research is a new world to many of you, we have developed this textbook to facilitate your entry into and understanding of this world and its contribution to the delivery of quality nursing care. This first chapter clarifies what nursing research is, and its significance in developing an evidence-based practice for nursing. The chapter also explores the past, present, and future of nursing research, including the scientific accomplishments in the profession over the last 160 years. The ways of acquiring knowledge in nursing are discussed and the common research methodologies used in generating research evidence for practice (quantitative, qualitative, and outcomes research) are introduced. The chapter also addresses some of the critical elements of evidence-based practice: strategies for synthesizing research evidence, levels of research evidence, and evidence-based guidelines. This chapter concludes with a description of nurses' roles in research based on their level of education, and their contribution to the development of evidence-based nursing practice.

What Is Nursing Research?

The word **research** means "to search again" or "to examine carefully." More specifically, research is a diligent, systematic inquiry or study that validates and refines existing knowledge and develops new knowledge. Diligent, systematic study indicates planning, organization, and persistence. The ultimate goal of research is the development of an empirical body of knowledge for a discipline or profession, such as nursing.

Defining nursing research requires determining the relevant knowledge needed by nurses. Because nursing is a practice profession, research is essential to develop and refine knowledge that nurses can use to improve clinical practice. Expert researchers have studied many interventions and clinicians have synthesized these studies to provide guidelines and protocols for use in practice. Practicing nurses, like you, need to be able to read research reports and syntheses of research findings to implement evidence-based interventions (protocols and guidelines) in practice to promote positive outcomes for patients and families. For example, extensive research has been conducted to determine the most effective technique for administering medications through an intramuscular (IM) injection. This research was synthesized and used to develop evidence-based guidelines for administering IM injections (Beyea & Nicoll, 1995; Nicoll & Hesby, 2002; Wynaden, Landsborough, McGowan, Baigmohamad, Finn & Pennebaker, 2006).

Nursing research also is needed to generate knowledge about nursing education, nursing administration, healthcare services, characteristics of nurses, and nursing roles. The findings from these studies indirectly influence nursing practice and thus add to nursing's body of knowledge. Research is needed to provide high-quality learning experiences for nursing students. Through research, nurses can develop and refine the best methods for delivering distance nursing education. Nursing administration and health services studies are needed to improve the quality and cost-effectiveness of the healthcare delivery system. Studies of nurses and nursing roles can influence nurses' quality of care, productivity, job satisfaction, and retention. In this era of nursing shortage, additional research is needed to determine effective ways to recruit individuals into and retain them in the profession of nursing. This type of research could have a major impact on the quality and number of nurses providing care to patients and families in the future.

In summary, **nursing research** is a scientific process that validates and refines existing knowledge and generates new knowledge that directly and indirectly influences nursing practice. Nursing research is the key to building an evidence-based practice for nursing.

What Is Evidence-Based Practice?

The ultimate goal of nursing is an evidence-based practice that promotes quality, cost-effective outcomes for patients, families, healthcare providers, and the healthcare system (Brown, 2009; Craig & Smyth, 2007; Cullum, Ciliska, Haynes, & Marks, 2008). **Evidence-based practice** evolves from the integration of the best research evidence with clinical expertise and patient needs and values (Institute of Medicine, 2001; Sackett, Straus, Richardson, Rosenberg, & Haynes, 2000). Figure 1–1 identifies the elements of evidence-based practice and demonstrates the major contribution of the best research evidence to the delivery of this practice. The **best research evidence** is the empirical knowledge generated from

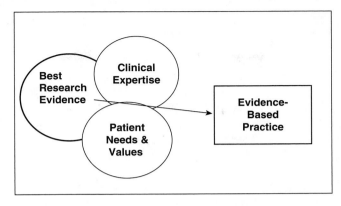

Figure 1–1. Model of evidence-based practice.

the synthesis of quality study findings to address a practice problem. Later, this chapter presents a discussion of the strategies used to synthesize research, the levels of best research evidence, and the sources for this evidence. A team of expert researchers, healthcare professionals, and sometimes policy makers and consumers will synthesize the best research evidence to develop standardized guidelines for clinical practice. For example, a team of experts conducted, critically appraised, and synthesized research related to the chronic health problem of hypertension (HTN) to develop an evidence-based practice guideline. Research evidence from this guideline is presented as an example later in this section.

Clinical expertise is the knowledge and skills of the healthcare professional providing care. The clinical expertise of a nurse depends on his or her years of clinical experience, current knowledge of the research and clinical literature, and educational preparation. The stronger the nurse's clinical expertise, the better his or her clinical judgment is in using the best research evidence in practice (Craig & Smyth, 2007; Sackett et al., 2000). Evidence-based practice also incorporates the needs and values of the patient (see Figure 1–1). The patient's need(s) might focus on health promotion, illness prevention, acute or chronic illness management, or rehabilitation. In addition, patients bring values or unique preferences, expectations, concerns, and cultural beliefs to the clinical encounter. With evidence-based practice, patients and their families are encouraged to take an active role in the management of their health (Pearson, Field, & Jordan, 2007). It is the unique combination of the best research evidence being implemented by an expert nurse clinician in providing quality, cost-effective care to a patient with specific health needs and values that results in evidence-based practice (Brown, 2009; Craig & Smyth, 2007; Sackett et al., 2000).

Extensive research is needed to develop sound empirical knowledge for synthesis into the best research evidence needed for practice. This research evidence might be synthesized to develop guidelines, standards, protocols, or policies to direct the implementation of a variety of nursing interventions. For example, a national guideline was developed for the management of hypertension and is entitled "The Seventh Report of the Joint National Committee on Prevention, Detection, Evaluation, and Treatment of High Blood Pressure: The JNC 7 Report." Experts synthesized the relevant studies and published their findings in the *Journal of the American Medical Association* (Chobanian et al., 2003). The complete guideline for the management of high blood pressure is available online at *www.nhlbi.nih*.

| Table 1–1 | Classification of Blood Pressure with Nursing Interventions for Evidence-Based Practice |

Classification of Blood Pressure (BP)			Nursing Interventions†	
BP Category	Systolic BP, mm Hg*	Diastolic BP, mm Hg*	Life style Modification‡	Cardiovascular (CVD) Disease Risk Factors Education§
Normal	<120	and <80	Encourage	Yes
Prehypertension	120-139	or 80-89	Yes	Yes
Stage 1 hypertension	140-159	or 90-99	Yes	Yes
Stage 2 hypertension	≥160	or ≥100	Yes	Yes

*Treatment is determined by the highest BP category, either systolic or diastolic.
†Treat patients with chronic kidney disease or diabetes to BP goal of less than 130/80 mm Hg.
‡Life Style Modification: Balanced diet, exercise program, normal weight, and nonsmoker.
§CVD risk factors: Hypertension; obesity (body mass index ≥30 kg/m²); dyslipidemia; diabetes mellitus; cigarette smoking; physical inactivity; microalbuminuria, estimated glomerular filtration rate <60 mL/min; age (>55 for men, >65 for women); and family history of premature CVD (men age <55, women age <65).
Table adapted from: National Heart, Lung, and Blood Institute. (2003). *The seventh report of the Joint National Committee on prevention, detection, evaluation, and treatment of high blood pressure: The JNC 7 report.* Bethesda, MD: National Institutes of Health. Retrieved June 6, 2009, from *www.nhlbi.nih.gov/guidelines/hypertension.*

gov/guidelines/hypertension. This guideline provides direction for management of high blood pressure by registered nurses; advanced practice nurses (nurse practitioners, clinical nurse specialists, nurse midwives, and nurse anesthetists); and physicians. For example, the guideline includes the classification of blood pressure (normal, prehypertension, hypertension stage 1, and hypertension stage 2) and the major cardiovascular disease (CVD) risk factors. You need to use this evidence-based guideline in monitoring your patients' blood pressures (BPs) and educating them about life style modifications to improve their BP and CVD risk factors with high BP (Table 1–1).

Figure 1–2 provides an example of the delivery of evidence-based nursing care to women with high BP. In this example, the best research evidence is classification of BP and education on life style modification (LSM) and CVD risk factors based on the JNC 7 National Standardized Guideline for management of high BP (National Heart, Lung, and Blood Institute, 2003). This guideline, based on the best research evidence related to BP, LSM, and CVD risks monitoring and education, is translated by an expert registered nurse and also nursing students to meet the needs and values of elderly African American women with high BP. The outcome of evidenced-based practice is women with a normal blood pressure, less than or equal to 120/80, or referral for medication treatment (see Figure 1–2). A detailed discussion of how to locate, critically appraise, and use national standardized guidelines (such as the JNC 7) in practice is found in Chapter 13.

Purposes of Research in Implementing an Evidence-Based Nursing Practice

Through nursing research, empirical knowledge can be developed to improve nursing care, patient outcomes, and the healthcare delivery system. For example, nurses need a solid research base to implement and document the effectiveness of selected nursing interventions in treating particular patient problems and promoting positive patient and family outcomes.

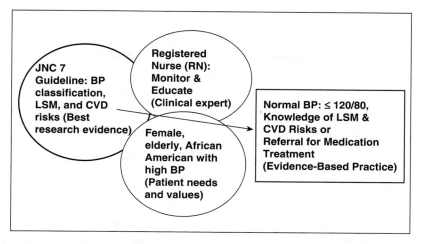

Figure 1–2. Evidence-based practice for elderly African American women with high blood pressure (BP).

In addition, nurses need to use research findings to determine the best way to deliver health-care services to ensure that the greatest number of people receive quality care. Accomplishing these goals will require you to critically appraise, synthesize, and apply research evidence that provides description, explanation, prediction, and control of phenomena in your clinical practice.

Description

Description involves identifying and understanding the nature of nursing phenomena and, sometimes, the relationships among them (Chinn & Kramer, 2008). Through research, nurses are able to (1) describe what exists in nursing practice, (2) discover new information, (3) promote understanding of situations, and (4) classify information for use in the discipline. Some examples of clinically important research evidence that is developed from research focused on description include:

- Identification of the responses of individuals to a variety of health conditions
- Identification of the cluster of symptoms for a particular disease
- Description of the health promotion and illness prevention strategies used by a variety of populations
- Determination of the incidence of a disease locally, nationally, and internationally. (This type of research was a priority in 2009 with the incidence of H1NI [swine] flu.)

For example, Ryan et al. (2007) conducted a study to determine the cluster of symptoms that represent an acute myocardial infarction (AMI). These researchers synthesized their findings as follows:

> Symptoms of AMI occur in clusters, and these clusters vary among persons. None of the clusters identified in this study included all of the symptoms that are included typically as symptoms of AMI (chest discomfort, diaphoresis, shortness of breath, nausea, and light-headedness). These AMI symptom clusters must be communicated clearly to the public in

a way that will assist them in assessing their symptoms more efficiently and will guide their treatment-seeking behavior. Symptom clusters for AMI must also be communicated to the professional community in a way that will facilitate assessment and rapid intervention for AMI. (Ryan et al., 2007, p. 72.)

The findings from this study provide nurses' insights into the varying symptom clusters of patients experiencing an AMI. You can use this research evidence to promote early recognition of the signs and symptoms of AMI in your patients so they might be referred promptly for treatment. This type of research focused on description is essential groundwork for studies that will provide explanation, prediction, and control of nursing phenomena in practice.

Explanation

Explanation clarifies the relationships among phenomena and identifies the reasons why certain events occur. Research focused on explanation provides the following types of evidence essential for practice.

- Determination of the assessment data (both subjective data from the health history and objective data from physical exam) that need to be gathered to address a patient's health need
- The link of assessment data to a diagnosis
- The link of causative risk factors or etiologies to illness, morbidity, and mortality
- Determination of the relationships among health risks, health behaviors, and health status

King, Gerich, Guzick, King, and McDermott (2009) studied women with a history of gestational diabetes mellitus (hGDM) to determine if this condition was related to risk factors for coronary heart disease (CHD) and diabetes mellitus (DM). The CHD risk factors examined included elevated triglycerides and low density lipoprotein cholesterol (LDL-c) and decreased high density lipoprotein cholesterol (HDL-c). These researchers found that the women with hGDM had significantly lower HDL-c ($p = 0.02$) and significantly higher triglycerides ($p = 0.001$) than a control group without hGDM. "The combination of high triglycerides and low HDL-c occurred in 25% of the hGDM cases versus 0% of controls, $p = 0.01$. Two-hour post-load glucose indicated that 45% of hGDM cases were pre-diabetic versus 20% of controls, $p = 0.05$" (King et al., 2009, p. 299). However, the women with hGDM had significantly lower LDL-c versus the controls ($p = 0.01$). The researchers identified the following conclusions, recommendations for future research, and implications for practice.

> In summary, our data suggest that women with a distant hGDM are at risk for developing diabetes and may be at increased risk for CHD. ... Future research focused on long-term follow-up in cohorts of women with hGDM could help to further clarify the relationship between the risk for diabetes and the risk for CHD. Since GDM occurs in relatively young women, long-term risk assessment and follow-up of women with an hGDM may provide an excellent opportunity to enact primary prevention strategies to reduce the risk for diabetes and CHD in the long run (King et al., 2009, p. 304).

Explanatory research such as this promotes an increased understanding of the relationships among the variables hGDM, CHD, and DM. Nurses can use this knowledge in educating their patients with GDM about their potential health risks. In addition, relationships identified through explanatory research provide the basis for conducting research focused on predicting and controlling phenomena in practice.

Prediction

Through prediction, one can estimate the probability of a specific outcome in a given situation (Chinn & Kramer, 2008). However, predicting an outcome does not necessarily enable one to modify or control the outcome. It is through prediction that the risk of illness is identified and linked to possible screening methods to identify the illness. Knowledge generated from research focused on prediction is critical for evidence-based practice and includes the following:

- Prediction of the risk for a disease in different populations
- Prediction of behaviors that promote health and prevent illness
- Prediction of the health care required based on a patient's need and values

For example, Scheetz, Zhang, and Kolassa (2007, p. 399) examined "crash scene variables to predict the need for trauma center care in older persons." The researchers analyzed 26 crash scene variables and developed triage decision rules for managing persons with severe and moderate injuries. Further research is needed to determine whether the triage decision rules improve the health outcomes of the elderly following trauma. Predictive studies isolate independent variables that require additional research to ensure that their manipulation or control results in successful outcomes for patients, healthcare professionals, and healthcare agencies (Creswell, 2009; Kerlinger & Lee, 2000).

Control

If one can predict the outcome of a situation, the next step is to control or manipulate the situation to produce the desired outcome. In health care, control is the ability to write a prescription to produce the desired results. Using the best research evidence, nurses could prescribe specific interventions to meet the needs of patients and their families (Brown, 2009; Craig & Smyth, 2007). Extensive research in the following areas can provide empirical evidence that enables nurses to deliver care that will increase the control over the outcomes desired for practice.

- Testing interventions to improve the health status of individuals, families, and communities
- Testing interventions to improve healthcare delivery

Extensive research has been conducted in the area of safe administration of IM injections. This research has been critically appraised, synthesized, and developed into an evidence-based guideline to direct the administration of medications by an IM route to infants, children, and adults in a variety of practice settings (Beyea & Nicoll, 1995; Nicoll & Hesby, 2002; Wynaden et al., 2006). The guideline for IM injections is based on the best research evidence and identifies the appropriate needle size and length to use for administering different types of medications; the safest injection site (ventrogluteal site) for many medications;

and the best injection technique to deliver a medication, minimize patient discomfort, and prevent physical damage (Beyea & Nicoll, 1995; Greenway, 2004; Nicoll & Hesby, 2002; Rodger & King, 2000). The outcomes from using this evidence-based guideline in practice include (1) adequate administration of medication to promote patient health, (2) minimal patient discomfort, and (3) no physical damage to the patient, all of which promote high-quality, cost-effective care. Using this guideline in your practice promotes the delivery of evidence-based nursing care. More details on the evidenced-based guideline for the administrations of IM injections are in Chapter 13.

Broadly, the nursing profession is accountable to society for providing high-quality, cost-effective care for patients and families. Thus, the care provided by nurses must be constantly evaluated and improved on the basis of new and refined research knowledge. Studies that document the effectiveness of specific nursing interventions make it possible to implement evidence-based care that will produce the best outcomes for patients and their families. The quality of research conducted in nursing affects not only the quality of care delivered but also the power of nurses in making decisions about the healthcare delivery system. The extensive number of nursing studies conducted in the last 30 years has greatly expanded the scientific knowledge available to you for describing, explaining, predicting, and controlling phenomena within your nursing practice.

Nursing's Participation in Research: Past to Present

Nursing's participation in research has changed drastically over the last 160 years and holds great promise for the twenty-first century. Initially, nursing research evolved slowly, from the investigations of Nightingale in the nineteenth century to the studies of nursing education in the 1930s and 1940s and the research of nurses and nursing roles in the 1950s and 1960s. In the 1970s through the 1990s, an increasing number of nursing studies focused on clinical problems and produced findings that had a direct impact on practice. Clinical research continues to be a major focus for the twenty-first century, with the goal of developing an evidence-based practice for nursing. Reviewing the history of nursing research enables you to identify the accomplishments and understand the need for further research to determine the best research evidence for use in practice. Table 1–2 outlines the key historical events that have influenced the development of research in nursing.

Florence Nightingale

Nightingale's (1859) initial research focused on the importance of a healthy environment in promoting patients' physical and mental well-being. She studied aspects of the environment such as ventilation, cleanliness, purity of water, and diet to determine the influence on patients' health, which continue to be important areas of study today (Herbert, 1981). However, Nightingale is most noted for her collection and analysis of soldier morbidity and mortality data during the Crimean War. This research enabled her to change the attitudes of the military and society toward the care of the sick. The military began to view the sick as having the right to adequate food, suitable quarters, and appropriate medical treatment. These interventions drastically reduced the mortality rate from 43% to 2% in the Crimean War (Cook, 1913). Nightingale also used research knowledge to make significant changes in

Table 1-2	Historical Events Influencing Research in Nursing
Year	**Event**
1850	Florence Nightingale is the first nurse researcher.
1900	*American Journal of Nursing* is first published.
1923	Teachers College at Columbia University offers the first educational doctoral program for nurses.
1929	First Master's in Nursing Degree is offered at Yale University.
1932	The Association of Collegiate Schools of Nursing is organized.
1950	American Nurses Association (ANA) publishes study of nursing functions and activities.
1952	*Nursing Research* is first published.
1953	Institute of Research and Service in Nursing Education is established.
1955	American Nurses Foundation is established to fund nursing research.
1963	*International Journal of Nursing Studies* is first published.
1965	ANA sponsors of the first nursing research conferences.
1967	*Image* (Sigma Theta Tau Journal) is first published, now entitled *Journal of Nursing Scholarship*. Stetler/Marram Model for Application of Research Findings to Practice is first published.
1970	ANA Commission on Nursing Research is established.
1972	Professor Archie Cochrane, a Scottish epidemiologist, publishes his book *Effectiveness and Efficiency: Random Reflections on Health Services*, which promoted the acceptance of the concepts behind evidence-based practice. ANA Council of Nurse Researchers is established.
1973	First Nursing Diagnosis Conference is held.
1978	*Research in Nursing & Health* is first published. *Advances in Nursing Science* is first published.
1979	*Western Journal of Nursing Research* is first published.
1980s-1990s	David Sackett and his research team developed methodologies to determine "best evidence" for practice.
1982-1983	Conduct and Utilization of Research in Nursing (CURN) Project is published.
1983	*Annual Review of Nursing Research* is first published.
1985	National Center for Nursing Research (NCNR) was established within the National Institutes of Health.
1987	*Scholarly Inquiry for Nursing Practice* first published
1988	*Applied Nursing Research* is first published. *Nursing Science Quarterly* is first published.
1989	Agency for Health Care Policy and Research (AHCPR) is established. Clinical practice guidelines are first published by the AHCPR.
1992	*Healthy People 2000* is published by U.S. Department of Health and Human Services. *Clinical Nursing Research* is first published.
1993	NCNR is renamed the National Institute of Nursing Research (NINR). *Journal of Nursing Measurement* is first published. Cochrane Collaboration is initiated providing systematic reviews and evidence-based guidelines for practice (*http://www.cochrane.org*).
1994	*Qualitative Health Research* is first published.
1999	AHCPR is renamed the Agency for Healthcare Research and Quality (AHRQ).
2000	*Healthy People 2010* is published by the U.S. Department of Health and Human Services. *Biological Research for Nursing* is first published.
2001	Stetler publishes her model, "Steps of Research Utilization to Facilitate Evidence-Based Practice."
2002	The Joint Commission revises the accreditation policies for hospitals to support the implementation of evidence-based health care.
2004	*Worldviews on Evidence-Based Nursing* is first published.
2006	The American Association of Colleges of Nursing releases its current Position Statement on Nursing Research.
2009	NINR identifies mission and funding priorities (*http://www.ninr.nih.gov*).
2009	AHRQ identifies mission and funding priorities (*http://www.ahrq.gov*).

society, such as testing public water, improving sanitation, preventing starvation, and decreasing morbidity and mortality (Palmer, 1977).

Nursing Research: 1900s through 1970s

The *American Journal of Nursing* was first published in 1900, and late in the 1920s and 1930s, case studies began appearing in this journal. A **case study** involves an in-depth analysis and a systematic description of one patient or a group of similar patients to promote understanding of healthcare interventions. Case studies are one example of the practice-related research that has been conducted in nursing over the last century.

Nursing educational opportunities expanded with Teachers College at Columbia University offering the first educational doctoral program for nurses in 1923, and Yale University offering the first master's degree in nursing in 1929. In 1950 the ANA initiated a 5-year study on nursing functions and activities. In 1959 the findings from this study were used to develop statements on functions, standards, and qualifications for professional nurses. During that time, clinical research began expanding as nursing specialty groups, such as community health, psychiatric-mental health, medical-surgical, pediatrics, and obstetrics, developed standards of care. The research conducted by the ANA and specialty groups provided the basis for the nursing practice standards that currently guide professional practice (Gortner & Nahm, 1977). The increase in research activity during the 1940s prompted the publication of the first research journal, *Nursing Research*, in 1952.

In the 1950s and 1960s, nursing schools began introducing research and the steps of the research process at the baccalaureate level, and MSN-level nurses were provided a background for conducting small, replication studies. In 1953 the Institute for Research and Service in Nursing Education established at Teachers College of Columbia University began providing research experiences for doctoral students (Gortner & Nahm, 1977).

In the 1960s an increasing number of clinical studies focused on quality care and the development of criteria to measure patient outcomes. Intensive care units were developed, which promoted the investigation of nursing interventions, staffing patterns, and cost-effectiveness of care (Gortner & Nahm, 1977). An additional research journal, the *International Journal of Nursing Studies*, was published in 1963. In 1965 the ANA sponsored the first of a series of nursing research conferences to promote the communication of research findings and the use of these findings in clinical practice.

In the late 1960s and 1970s, nurses were involved in the development of models, conceptual frameworks, and theories to guide nursing practice. The nursing theorists' work provided direction for future nursing research. In 1978 Chinn became the editor of a new journal *Advances in Nursing Science*, which included nursing theorists' work and related research. Another event influencing research during the 1970s was the establishment of the ANA Commission on Nursing Research in 1970. In 1972 the commission established the Council of Nurse Researchers to advance research activities, provide an exchange of ideas, and recognize excellence in research. The commission also influenced the development of federal guidelines concerning research with human subjects and sponsored research programs nationally and internationally (See, 1977).

The communication of research findings was a major issue in the 1970s (Barnard, 1980). Sigma Theta Tau, the International Honor Society for Nursing, sponsored national and international research conferences; the chapters of this organization sponsored many local conferences to communicate research findings. Sigma Theta Tau first published *Image*, now entitled *Journal of Nursing Scholarship*, in 1967 and it includes research articles and summaries of research conducted on selected topics. Stetler and Marram developed the first model in nursing to promote the application of research findings to practice in 1967. Two additional research journals were first published in the 1970s: *Research in Nursing & Health* in 1978 and *Western Journal of Nursing Research* in 1979.

In the 1970s, Professor Archie Cochrane originated the concept of evidence-based practice with a book he published in 1972 entitled *Effectiveness and Efficiency: Random Reflections on Health Services*. Cochrane advocated the provision of health care based on research to improve the quality. To facilitate the use of research evidence in practice, the Cochrane Center was established in 1992 and the Cochrane Collaboration in 1993. The Cochrane Collaboration and Library house numerous resources to promote evidence-based practice, such as systematic reviews of research and evidence-based guidelines for practice (discussed later in this chapter) (see the Cochrane Collaboration at *http://www.cochrane.org*).

Nursing Research: 1980s and 1990s

The conduct of clinical research was the focus of the 1980s, and clinical journals began publishing more studies. One new research journal was published in 1987, *Scholarly Inquiry for Nursing Practice*, and two in 1988, *Applied Nursing Research* and *Nursing Science Quarterly*. Although the body of empirical knowledge generated through clinical research increased rapidly in the 1980s, little of this knowledge was used in practice. During 1982 and 1983 the materials from a federally funded project, Conduct and Utilization of Research in Nursing (CURN), were published to facilitate the use of research to improve nursing practice (Horsley, Crane, Crabtree, & Wood, 1983).

In 1983 the first volume of the *Annual Review of Nursing Research* was published (Werley & Fitzpatrick, 1983). These volumes include experts' reviews of research organized into four areas: nursing practice, nursing care delivery, nursing education, and the nursing profession. These summaries of current research knowledge encourage the use of research findings in practice and provide direction for future research. Publication of the *Annual Review of Nursing Research* continues today, with leading expert nurse scientists providing summaries of research in their areas of expertise.

Qualitative research was introduced in the late 1970s, with the first studies appearing in nursing journals in the 1980s. The focus of qualitative research was holistic, with the intent to discover meaning and gain new insight and understanding of phenomena relevant to nursing. The number of qualitative researchers and studies expanded greatly in the 1990s, with qualitative studies appearing in most of the nursing research and clinical journals. In 1994 a journal focused on disseminating qualitative research, *Qualitative Health Research*, was first published. However, quantitative research has been and continues to be the most frequently used research methodology in conducting nursing research. In the 1990s, more new research journals were added, with *Clinical Nursing Research* first published in 1992 and the *Journal of Nursing Measurement* in 1993.

Another priority of the 1980s was to obtain increased funding for nursing research. Most of the federal funds in the 1980s were designated for medical studies involving the diagnosis and treatment of diseases. However, the ANA achieved a major political victory for nursing research with the creation of the National Center for Nursing Research (NCNR) in 1985.

The purpose of this center is to support the conduct and dissemination of knowledge developed through basic and clinical nursing research, training, and other programs in patient care research (Bauknecht, 1985). Under the direction of Dr. Ada Sue Hinshaw, the NCNR became the National Institute of Nursing Research (NINR) in 1993. During the rest of the decade, the NINR (1993) focused its support on five research priorities: community-based nursing models, effectiveness of nursing interventions in human immunodeficiency virus and acquired immunodeficiency syndrome (HIV/AIDS), cognitive impairment, living with chronic illness, and biobehavioral factors related to immunocompetence.

Outcomes research emerged as an important methodology for documenting the effectiveness of healthcare services in the 1980s and 1990s. This effectiveness research evolved from the quality assessment and quality assurance functions that originated with the professional standards review organizations (the PSROs) in 1972. William Roper, director of the Health Care Finance Administration (HCFA), promoted outcomes research during the 1980s to determine quality and cost-effectiveness of patient care. In 1989 the Agency for Health Care Policy and Research (AHCPR) was established to facilitate the conduct of outcomes research (Rettig, 1991). AHCPR also had an active role in communicating research findings to healthcare practitioners and was responsible for publishing the first clinical practice guidelines in 1989. These guidelines included a synthesis of the best research evidence with directives for practice developed by healthcare experts in a variety of areas. Several of these evidence-based guidelines were published in the 1990s and provided standards for practice in nursing and medicine. The Healthcare Research and Quality Act of 1999 reauthorized the AHCPR, changing its name to the Agency for Healthcare Research and Quality (AHRQ). This significant change positioned the AHRQ as a scientific partner with the public and private sectors to improve the quality and safety of patient care.

Building on the process of research utilization, physicians, nurses, and other healthcare professions focused on the development of evidence-based practice for health care during the 1990s. A research group lead by Dr. David Sackett at McMaster University in Canada developed explicit research methodologies to determine the "best evidence" for practice. David Eddy first used the term "evidence-based" in 1990 with the focus on providing evidence-based practice for medicine (Craig & Smyth, 2007; Sackett et al., 2000). In 2002, the Joint Commission revised the accreditation policies for hospitals to support the implementation of evidence-based health care. To facilitate the movement of nursing toward evidence-based practice, Stetler (2001) developed a model entitled "Research Utilization to Facilitate EBP" (see Chapter 13 for a description of this model).

Nursing Research: Twenty-First Century

The vision for nursing in the twenty-first century is the development of a scientific knowledge base that enables nurses to implement an evidence-based practice (Brown, 2009; Melnyk & Fineout-Overholt, 2005). This vision is consistent with the mission of NINR, which is to

> support clinical and basic research to establish a scientific basis for the care of individuals across the lifespan—from management of patients during illness and recovery to the reduction of risks for disease and disability, the promotion of healthy lifestyles, promoting quality of life in those with chronic illness, and care for the individuals at the end of life (NINR, 2009).

NINR is seeking expanded funding for nursing research and is encouraging a variety of methodologies (quantitative, qualitative, and outcomes research) to be used to generate essential knowledge for nursing practice. The NINR (2009) website *(http://ninr.nih.gov/)* provides the most current information on the institute's research priorities and activities (see Chapter 5).

The AHRQ is the lead agency supporting research designed to improve the quality of health care, reduce its cost, improve patient safety, decrease medical errors, and broaden access to essential services. AHRQ (2009) conducts and sponsors research that provides evidence-based information on healthcare outcomes, quality, cost, use, and access. This research information is needed to promote effective healthcare decision making by patients, clinicians, health system executives, and policy makers. The AHRQ (2009) website *(http://www.ahrq.gov)* provides the most current information on this agency and includes current guidelines for clinical practice.

The expansion of biological research and the movement toward evidence-based practice in nursing has resulted in the publication of two new research journals, *Biological Research for Nursing* in 2000 and *Worldviews on Evidence-Based Nursing* in 2004. However, the focus of healthcare research and funding is expanding from the treatment of illness to include health promotion and illness prevention interventions. *Healthy People 2010*, published by the U.S. Department of Health and Human Services (DHHS, 2000), increased the visibility of and identified priorities for health promotion research. In the twenty-first century, nurses could play a major role in the development of interventions to promote health and prevent illness in individuals, families, and communities (ANA, 2004). *Healthy People 2020* will be published in 2010 and will identify updated priorities for health promotion research *(http://www.healthypeople.gov/hp2020/default.asp)*.

The American Association of Colleges of Nursing (AACN), developed in 1932 to promote the quality of nursing education, revised their position statement of nursing research in 2006 and provided future direction for the discipline in moving toward evidence-based practice. To ensure an effective research enterprise in nursing, the discipline must (1) create a research culture; (2) provide high-quality educational programs (baccalaureate, master's, practice-focused doctorate, research-focused doctorate, and postdoctorate) to prepare a workforce of nurse scientists; (3) develop a sound research infrastructure; and (4) obtain sufficient funding for essential research (AACN, 2006). The complete AACN position statement on nursing research is online at *http://www.aacn.nche.edu/Publications/pdf/NsgResearch.pdf*.

Acquiring Knowledge in Nursing

Acquiring knowledge in nursing is essential for the delivery of quality patient and family nursing care. Some key questions about knowledge include the following: What is knowledge? How is knowledge acquired in nursing? Is most of nursing's knowledge based on research? Knowledge is essential information acquired in a variety of ways, expected to be an accurate reflection of reality, and incorporated and used to direct a person's actions (Kaplan, 1964). During your nursing education, you acquired an extensive amount of knowledge from your classroom and clinical experiences. You had to learn, synthesize, incorporate, and apply this knowledge so that you could practice as a nurse.

The quality of your nursing practice depends on the quality of the knowledge that you acquired. Thus, you need to question the quality and credibility of new information that you hear or read. For example, what were the sources of the knowledge that you acquired during your nursing education? Were the nursing interventions taught based more on research or tradition? Which interventions were based on research, and which need further study to determine their effectiveness? Nursing has historically acquired knowledge through traditions, authority, borrowing, trial and error, personal experience, role modeling, intuition, and reasoning. However, in the last 20 years, most nursing textbooks include content that is based on research evidence and most faculty members support their lectures and educational strategies with research evidence. This section introduces different ways of acquiring knowledge in nursing.

Traditions

Traditions include "truths" or beliefs that are based on customs and trends. Nursing traditions from the past have been transferred to the present by written and oral communication and role modeling, and they continue to influence the practice of nursing. For example, some of the policy and procedure manuals in hospitals contain traditional ideas. Traditions can positively influence nursing practice because they were developed from effective past experiences. However, traditions also can narrow and limit the knowledge sought for nursing practice. For example, nursing units are frequently organized and run according to set rules or traditions that may not be efficient or effective. Often these traditions are neither questioned nor changed because they have existed for years and are frequently supported by people with power and authority. Nursing's body of knowledge needs to be more evidence-based than traditional if nurses are to have a powerful impact on patient outcomes.

Authority

An **authority** is a person with expertise and power who is able to influence opinion and behavior. A person is given authority because it is thought that she or he knows more in a given area than others do. Knowledge acquired from an authority is illustrated when one person credits another as the source of information. Nurses who publish articles and books or develop theories are frequently considered authorities. Students usually view their instructors as authorities, and clinical nursing experts are considered authorities within the clinical practice setting. It is important that nurses with authority act based on research evidence versus customs and traditions.

Borrowing

Some nursing leaders have described part of nursing's knowledge as information borrowed from disciplines such as medicine, sociology, psychology, physiology, and education (McMurrey, 1982). **Borrowing** in nursing involves the appropriation and use of knowledge from other fields or disciplines to guide nursing practice. Nursing has borrowed in two ways. For years, some nurses have taken information from other disciplines and applied it directly to nursing practice. This information was not integrated within the unique focus of nursing. For example, some nurses have used the medical model to guide their nursing practice, thus focusing on the diagnosis and treatment of disease. This type of borrowing continues today as nurses use advances in technology to become highly specialized and focused on the detection and treatment of disease. The second way of borrowing, which is more useful in nursing, involves integrating information from other disciplines within the focus of nursing. For example, nurses borrow knowledge from other disciplines like medicine but integrate this knowledge in their holistic care of patients and families experiencing acute and chronic illnesses.

Trial and Error

Trial and error is an approach with unknown outcomes that is used in a situation of uncertainty in which other sources of knowledge are unavailable. Because each patient responds uniquely to a situation, there is uncertainty in nursing practice. Hence, nurses must use trial and error in providing nursing care. However, trial and error frequently involves no formal documentation of effective and ineffective nursing actions. With this strategy, knowledge is gained from experience, but often it is not shared with others. The trial-and-error approach to acquiring knowledge also can be time consuming because you may implement multiple interventions before finding one that is effective. There also is a risk of implementing nursing actions that are detrimental to patients' health. If studies are conducted on nursing interventions, selection and implementation of interventions need to be based on scientific knowledge rather than trial and error.

Personal Experience

Personal experience involves gaining knowledge by being personally involved in an event, situation, or circumstance. Personal experience enables the nurse to gain skills and expertise by providing care to patients and families in clinical settings. Learning that occurs from personal experience enables the nurse to cluster ideas into a meaningful whole. For example, you may read about giving an IM injection or be told how to give an injection in a classroom setting, but you do not "know" how to give an injection until you observe other nurses giving injections to patients and actually give several injections yourself.

The amount of personal experience affects the complexity of a nurse's knowledge base. Benner (1984) conducted a phenomenological qualitative study to identify the levels of experience in the development of clinical knowledge and expertise, and these include: (1) novice, (2) advanced beginner, (3) competent, (4) proficient, and (5) expert. Novice nurses have no personal experience in the work they are to perform, but they have some preconceptions and expectations about clinical practice that they obtained during their education. These preconceptions and expectations are challenged, refined, confirmed, or refuted by personal experience in a clinical setting. The advanced beginner nurse has just enough experience to recognize and intervene in recurrent situations. For example, the advanced beginner is able to recognize and intervene in managing patients' pain. Competent nurses are able to generate and achieve long-range goals and plans because of years of personal experience. The competent nurse also is able to use personal knowledge to take conscious, deliberate actions that are efficient and organized. From a more complex knowledge base, the proficient nurse views the patient as a whole and as a member of a family and community. The proficient nurse recognizes that each patient and family responds differently to illness and health. The expert nurse has an extensive background of experience and is able to identify accurately and intervene skillfully in a situation. Personal experience increases the ability of the expert nurse to grasp a situation intuitively with accuracy and speed. Benner's (1984) qualitative research provided an increased understanding of how knowledge is acquired through personal experience. As you gain clinical experience during your educational program and after you graduate, you will note your movement through these different levels of knowledge.

Role Modeling

Role modeling is learning by imitating the behaviors of an expert. In nursing, role modeling enables the novice nurse to learn through interactions with or examples set by highly competent, expert nurses. Role models include admired teachers, expert clinicians, researchers, or persons who inspire others through their examples. An intense form of role modeling is **mentorship**, in which the expert nurse serves as a teacher, sponsor, guide, and counselor for the novice nurse. The knowledge gained through personal experience is greatly enhanced by a high-quality relationship with a role model or mentor. Many new graduates enter internship programs provided by clinical agencies so that expert nurses can mentor them during the novices' first few months of employment.

Intuition

Intuition is an insight into or understanding of a situation or event as a whole that usually cannot be explained logically (Rew & Barrow, 1987). Because intuition is a type of knowing that seems to come unbidden, it may also be described as a "gut feeling" or a "hunch." Because intuition cannot be explained scientifically with ease, many people are uncomfortable with it. Some even believe that it does not exist. However, intuition is not the lack of knowing; rather, it is a result of "deep" knowledge (Benner, 1984). The knowledge is so deeply incorporated that it is difficult to bring it to the surface consciously and express it in a logical manner. Some nurses can intuitively recognize when a patient is experiencing a health crisis. Using this intuitive knowledge, they can assess the patient's condition and contact the physician for medical intervention.

Reasoning

Reasoning is the processing and organizing of ideas in order to reach conclusions. Through reasoning, people are able to make sense of their thoughts, experiences, and research evidence. This type of logical thinking is often evident in the oral presentation of an argument in which each part is linked to reach a logical conclusion. The science of logic includes inductive and deductive reasoning. **Inductive reasoning** moves from the specific to the general; particular instances are observed and then combined into a larger whole or a general statement (Chinn & Kramer, 2008). An example of inductive reasoning follows:

PARTICULAR INSTANCES
    A headache is an altered level of health that is stressful.
    A terminal illness is an altered level of health that is stressful.

GENERAL STATEMENT

Therefore it can be induced that all altered levels of health are stressful.

Deductive reasoning moves from the general to the specific or from a general premise to a particular situation or conclusion (Chinn & Kramer, 2008). A premise or proposition is a statement of the proposed relationship between two or more concepts. An example of deductive reasoning follows:

PREMISES

All human beings experience loss.

All adolescents are human beings.

CONCLUSION

Therefore it can be deduced that all adolescents experience loss.

In this example, deductive reasoning is used to move from the two general premises about human beings and adolescents to the conclusion that "All adolescents experience loss." However, the conclusions generated from deductive reasoning are valid only if they are based on valid premises. Research is a means to test and confirm or refute a premise or proposition so that valid premises can be used as a basis for reasoning in nursing practice.

Acquiring Knowledge through Nursing Research

Acquiring knowledge through traditions, authority, borrowing, trial and error, personal experience, role modeling, intuition, and reasoning is important in nursing. However, these ways of acquiring knowledge are inadequate in providing evidence-based practice (Brown, 2009; Craig & Smyth, 2007). The knowledge needed for practice is specific and holistic, as well as process-oriented and outcomes-focused (ANA, 2003). Thus, a variety of research methods are needed to generate this knowledge. This section introduces quantitative, qualitative, and outcomes research methods that are used to generate empirical knowledge for nursing practice. These research methods are essential to generate research evidence for specific goals of the nursing profession:

- Promoting an understanding of patients' and families' experiences with health and illness (a common focus of qualitative research)
- Implementing effective nursing interventions to promote patient health (a common focus of quantitative research)
- Providing high-quality, cost-effective care within the health care system (a common focus of outcomes research)

Introduction to Quantitative and Qualitative Research

Quantitative and qualitative research methods complement each other because they generate different kinds of knowledge that are useful in nursing practice. Familiarity with these two types of research will help you identify, understand, and critically appraise these studies in journals and books. Quantitative and qualitative research methodologies have some

Table 1-3	Quantitative and Qualitative Research Characteristics	
Characteristic	Quantitative Research	Qualitative Research
Philosophical origin	Logical positivism	Naturalistic, interpretive, humanistic
Focus	Concise, objective, reductionistic	Broad, subjective, holistic
Reasoning	Logistic, deductive	Dialectic, inductive
Basis of knowing	Cause-and-effect relationships	Meaning, discovery, understanding
Theoretical focus	Theory testing	Theory development

similarities; both require researcher expertise, involve rigor in implementation, and generate scientific knowledge for nursing practice. Some of the differences between the two methodologies are presented in Table 1–3.

A majority of the studies conducted in nursing have used quantitative research methods. **Quantitative research** is a formal, objective, systematic process in which numerical data are used to obtain information about the world. The quantitative approach toward scientific inquiry emerged from a branch of philosophy called *logical positivism*, which operates on strict rules of logic, truth, laws, and predictions. Quantitative researchers hold the position that "truth" is absolute and that a single reality can be defined by careful measurement. To find truth, the researcher must be objective, which means that values, feelings, and personal perceptions cannot enter into the measurement of reality. Quantitative research is conducted to test theory by describing variables (descriptive research), examining relationships among variables (correlational research), and determining cause-and-effect interactions between variables (quasi-experimental and experimental research) (Burns & Grove, 2009; Creswell, 2009). Chapter 2 describes the different types of quantitative research and the quantitative research process.

Qualitative research is a systematic, subjective approach used to describe life experiences and situations and give them meaning (Munhall, 2007). This research methodology evolved from the behavioral and social sciences as a method of understanding the unique, dynamic, holistic nature of human beings. The philosophical base of qualitative research is interpretive, humanistic, and naturalistic and is concerned with understanding the meaning of social interactions by those involved (Standing, 2009). Qualitative researchers believe that "truth" is both complex and dynamic and can be found only by studying people as they interact with and in their sociohistorical settings (Creswell, 2009; Munhall, 2007; Patton, 2002). Nurses' interest in conducting qualitative research began in the late 1970s. Currently, an extensive number of qualitative studies are conducted using a variety of qualitative research methods. Qualitative research is conducted to promote understanding of human experiences and situations and develop theories that describe these experiences and situations. Because human emotions are difficult to quantify (i.e., assign a numerical value to), qualitative research seems to be a more effective method of investigating emotional responses than quantitative research (see Table 1–3). Chapter 3 introduces the different types of qualitative research.

Several types of quantitative and qualitative research have been conducted to generate nursing knowledge for practice. These types of research can be classified in a variety of ways. The classification system for this book (Table 1–4) includes the most common types of quantitative and qualitative research conducted in nursing. The quantitative research methods

Table 1–4	Classification System for Nursing Research Methods

I. Types of Quantitative Research
Descriptive research
Correlational research
Quasi-experimental research
Experimental research

II. Types of Qualitative Research
Phenomenological research
Grounded theory research
Ethnographical research
Historical research

III. Outcomes Research

are classified into four categories: descriptive, correlational, quasi-experimental, and experimental. Descriptive research explores new areas of research and describes situations as they exist in the world. Correlational research examines relationships and is conducted to develop and refine explanatory knowledge for nursing practice. Quasi-experimental and experimental studies determine the effectiveness of nursing interventions in predicting and controlling the outcomes desired for patients and families (Burns & Grove, 2009; Kerlinger & Lee, 2000). (These types of research are discussed in detail in Chapter 2.)

The qualitative research methods included in this text are phenomenological, grounded theory, ethnographic, and historical research (see Table 1–4). Phenomenological research is an inductive descriptive approach used to describe an experience as it is lived by an individual, such as the lived experience of chronic pain (Thomas, 2000). Grounded theory research is an inductive research technique that is used to formulate, test, and refine a theory about a particular phenomenon. Grounded theory research initially was developed by Glaser and Strauss (1967) and was used to formulate a theory about the grieving process. Ethnographic research was developed by the discipline of anthropology for investigating cultures through an in-depth study of the members of the culture. Health practices vary among cultures, and these practices need to be recognized in delivering care to patients, families, and communities. Nurse researchers have also used ethnography to better understand work cultures (Hunter, Spence, McKenna, & Iedema, 2008). Historical research is a narrative description or analysis of events that occurred in the remote or recent past. Through historical research, past mistakes are examined to facilitate an understanding of and an effective response to present situations (Munhall, 2007). (Qualitative research methods are the focus of Chapter 3.)

Introduction to Outcomes Research

The spiraling cost of health care has generated many questions about the quality and effectiveness of healthcare services and the patient's outcomes related to these services. Consumers want to know what services they are purchasing and if these services will improve their health. Healthcare policy makers want to know whether the care is cost effective and high in quality. These concerns have promoted the conduct of **outcomes research**, which focuses on examining the result of care or determining the changes in health status for the patient (Doran, 2003; Rettig, 1991). Four essential areas that require examination through outcomes research are the following: (1) patient responses to medical and nursing interventions; (2) functional maintenance or improvement of physical functioning for the patient; (3) financial outcomes achieved with the provision of healthcare services; and (4) patient satisfaction with the health outcomes, care received, and healthcare providers (Jones & Burney, 2002). Nurses are playing an active role in conducting outcomes research by participating in multidisciplinary research teams that examine the outcomes of healthcare services. This knowledge provides a basis for improving the quality of care nurses deliver in practice. Chapter 14 provides a detailed discussion of outcomes research. Quantitative, qualitative, and outcomes research are essential for the development of the best research evidence for practice.

Understanding Best Research Evidence for Practice

Evidence-based practice involves the use of best research evidence to support clinical decisions in practice. Best research evidence was previously defined as a summary of the highest quality, current empirical knowledge in a specific area of health care that is developed from a synthesis of quality studies (quantitative, qualitative, and outcomes) in that area. As a nurse, you make numerous clinical decisions each day that affect the health outcomes of your patients. By using the best research evidence available, you can make quality clinical decisions that will improve patients' and families' health outcomes. This section was developed to expand your understanding of the concept of best research evidence for practice by providing the following: (1) a description of the strategies used to synthesize research evidence, (2) a model of the levels of research evidence available, and (3) a link of the best research evidence to evidence-based guidelines for practice.

Strategies Used to Synthesize Research Evidence

The synthesis of study findings is a complex, highly structured process that is best conducted by at least two or even a team of expert researchers and healthcare providers. There are various types of research synthesis and the type of synthesis conducted varies based on the quality and types of research evidence available.

The quality of the research evidence available in an area is dependent on the number and strength of studies that have been conducted in an area. The types of research commonly conducted in nursing were identified earlier in this chapter as quantitative, qualitative, and outcomes. The research synthesis process used to summarize knowledge varies for quantitative and qualitative research. In building best research evidence for practice, the quantitative experimental study, such as a randomized clinical trial (RCT), is identified as producing the strongest research evidence for practice (Brown, 2009; Craig & Smyth, 2007; Cullum et al., 2008; Institute of Medicine, 2001; Melnyk & Fineout-Overholt, 2005; Pearson et al., 2007; Sackett et al., 2000). The number and strengths of the studies conducted in an area are determined by the critical appraisal of the studies and the validity or credibility of the study outcomes (see Chapter 12).

Research evidence in nursing and health care is synthesized using the following processes: (1) systematic review, (2) meta-analysis, (3) integrative review, (4) metasummary, and (5) metasynthesis. Table 1–5 identifies the processes used in research evidence synthesis, the purpose of each synthesis process, the types of research included in the synthesis (sampling frame), and the analysis techniques used to achieve the synthesis of research evidence (Whittemore, 2005). A systematic review is a structured, comprehensive synthesis of quantitative and outcomes studies in a particular healthcare area to determine the best research evidence available for expert clinicians to use to promote an evidence-based practice. Sys-

Table 1–5	Processes Used to Synthesize Research Evidence		
Synthesis Process	Purpose of Synthesis	Types of Research Included in the Synthesis (Sampling Frame)	Analysis Achieving Synthesis
Systematic Review	Summary of research evidence from highly controlled studies about a particular problem in practice.	Quantitative and outcomes studies with similar methodology usually randomized clinical trials (RCT). Also includes meta-analyses and integrative reviews focused on the practice problem.	Narrative and Statistical
Meta-analysis	Synthesis or pooling of the results from several previous studies using statistical analysis to determine the effect of an intervention or the strengths or types of relationships among variables.	Quantitative studies with similar methodology, such as quasi-experimental and experimental studies focused on the effect of an intervention or correlational studies focused on a relationship. Also includes outcomes studies.	Statistical
Integrative Review	Synthesis of the findings from a variety of independent studies to determine the current knowledge in an area.	Quantitative, outcomes, and qualitative studies. Quantitative studies test theory and qualitative studies generate theory so the synthesis also includes the theoretical literature.	Narrative
Metasummary	Quantitative oriented aggregation or synthesis of qualitative research findings to sum the findings across reports in a target area (Sandelowski & Barroso, 2007).	Summarizes existing qualitative studies and provides basis for metasynthesis.	Narrative
Metasynthesis	Integration of qualitative study findings that offers a "novel interpretation of findings that is the result of interpretive transformations far removed from these findings as given in the research reports" (Sandelowski & Barroso, 2007, p. 18).	Use of original qualitative studies and metasummaries to produce synthesis.	Narrative

Table adapted from: Whittemore, R. (2005). Combining evidence in nursing research: Methods and implications. *Nursing Research*, 54(1), 57.

tematic reviews are conducted to synthesis research evidence from numerous, high-quality studies with similar methodologies (Craig & Smyth, 2007). These reviews are often conducted by teams or panels of expert researchers and clinicians using rigorous synthesis processes. The results of these reviews are used to produce the national and international standardized guidelines. These guidelines are used by nurses and other healthcare providers to manage healthcare problems such as high blood pressure (Chobanian et al., 2003). These standardized guidelines are made available online, published in articles and books, and presented at conferences and professional meetings. Some of the common sources for these standardized guidelines are presented toward the end of this chapter.

Meta-analysis is a type of study that statistically pools the results from previous studies into a single quantitative analysis that provides one of the highest levels of evidence for an intervention's efficacy (Conn & Rantz, 2003). In addition, a meta-analysis can be preformed on correlational studies to determine the type (positive or negative) or strength of relationships among selected variables (see Table 1–5). Because meta-analyses require statistical analysis to combine study findings, it is possible to be objective rather than subjective in synthesizing research evidence. Some of the strongest evidence for using an intervention in practice is generated from a meta-analysis of multiple, controlled studies such as RCT. Thus, many systematic reviews conducted to generate evidence-based guidelines include meta-analyses. Chapter 13 provides details on how to locate meta-analyses and critically appraise their quality.

An **integrative review** of research includes the identification, analysis, and synthesis of research findings from independent quantitative, outcomes, and qualitative studies to determine the current knowledge (what is known and not known) in a particular area. Most of the studies synthesized in an integrative review are quantitative (descriptive, correlational, quasi-experimental, and experimental) and outcomes but some reviews also include important findings from qualitative studies (see Table 1–5). Integrative reviews of research provide direction for future studies and are sometimes included in systematic reviews. The value of an integrative review depends on the standards used to the conduct the review, which are similar to the standards of clarity, rigor, and replication required for conducting primary research. Chapter 13 presents the process for critically appraising an integrative review of research.

Qualitative research synthesis is the process and product of systematically reviewing and formally integrating the findings from qualitative studies (Sandelowski & Barroso, 2007). Qualitative research synthesis includes two categories: qualitative metasummary and qualitative metasynthesis (see Table 1–5). Qualitative **metasummary** is the synthesis or summing of the findings across qualitative reports to develop a description of current knowledge in an area. Metasummary can be an end in itself to identify current knowledge or can provide a foundation for conducting qualitative metasynthesis. Qualitative **metasynthesis** provides a fully integrated, novel description or explanation of a target event or experience versus a summary view of that event or experience. Metasynthesis requires more complex, integrative thought in developing a new perspective or theory based on the findings of previous qualitative studies. These qualitative research synthesis processes have been used to generate research evidence that contributes to the knowledge needed for evidence-based practice. Sandelowski and Barroso (2007) have developed a book focused on synthesis of qualitative research and Chapter 13 addresses their processes for critically appraising qualitative metasummary and metasynthesis.

Levels of Research Evidence

The strength or validity of the best research evidence in an area depends on the quality and quantity of the studies that have been conducted in the area. Quantitative studies, especially experimental studies like the RCT, provide the strongest research evidence (see Chapter 8). Also the replication or repeating of studies with similar methodology increases the strength of the research evidence generated. The levels of the research evidence are a continuum, with the highest quality of research evidence at one end and weakest research evidence at the other (see Figure 1–3) (Brown, 2009; Craig & Smyth, 2007; Melnyk & Fineout-Overholt, 2005; Pearson et al., 2007). The systematic research reviews and meta-analyses of high quality experimental studies provide the strongest or best research evidence for use by expert clinicians in practice. Meta-analyses and integrative reviews of quasi-experimental, experimental, and outcomes studies also provide very strong research evidence for managing practice problems. Correlational, descriptive, and qualitative studies often provide initial knowledge, which serves as a basis for generating quasi-experimental and outcomes studies (see Figure 1–3). The weakest evidence comes from expert opinions, which can include expert clinicians' opinions or the opinions expressed in committee reports. When making a

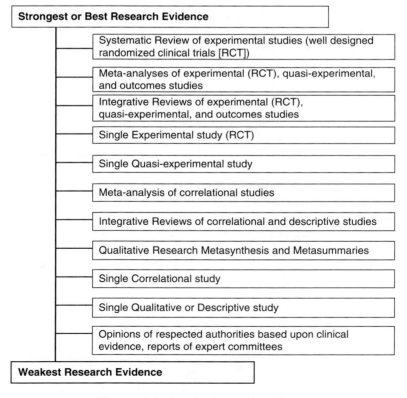

Figure 1–3. Levels of research evidence.

decision in your clinical practice, be sure to base that decision on the best research evidence available.

The levels of research evidence identified in Figure 1–3 will help you to determine the quality and validity of the evidence that is available for practice. The best research evidence generated from systematic reviews, meta-analyses, and integrative reviews is used to develop standardized evidence-based guidelines for practice.

Introduction to Evidence-Based Guidelines

Evidence-based guidelines are rigorous, explicit clinical guidelines developed based on the best research evidence available in that area. These guidelines are usually developed by a team or panel of expert clinicians (physicians, nurses, pharmacists, and other health professionals); researchers; and sometimes consumers, policy makers, and economists. The expert panel works to achieve consensus on the content of the guideline to provide clinicians with the best information for making clinical decisions in practice. There has been a dramatic growth in the production of evidence-based guidelines to assist healthcare providers in building an evidence-based practice and improving healthcare outcomes for patients, families, providers, and healthcare agencies.

Every year, new guidelines are developed and some of the existing guidelines are revised based on new research evidence. These guidelines have become the gold standard (or standard of excellence) for patient care, and nurses and other healthcare providers are encouraged to incorporate these standardized guidelines into their practice. Many of these evidence-based guidelines have been made available online by national and international government agencies, professional organizations, and centers of excellence. When selecting a guideline for practice, be sure the guideline was developed by a credible agency or organization and that the reference list reflects the synthesis of extensive research evidence.

An extremely important source for evidence-based guidelines in the United States is the National Guideline Clearinghouse (NGC), initiated in 1998 by the Agency for Healthcare Research and Quality (AHRQ). The NGC started with 200 guidelines and has expanded to more than 1000 evidence-based guidelines (see *http://www.guideline.gov/*). Another excellent source of systematic reviews and evidence-based guidelines is the Cochrane Collaboration and Library in the United Kingdom that can be accessed at *http://cochrane.org*. Professional nursing organizations, such as Oncology Nursing Society *(http://www.ons.org)* and National Association of Neonatal Nurses *(http://www.nann.org)*, have also developed evidence-based guidelines for nursing practice. These websites will introduce you to some of evidence-based guidelines that exist nationally and internationally. Chapter 13 provides you direction in critically appraising the quality of an evidence-based guideline and implementing that guideline in your practice.

What Is Your Role in Nursing Research?

Now that you have been introduced to the world of nursing research and evidence-based practice, what do you think will be your research role? You may believe that you have no role in research, that research is the responsibility of other nurses. However, generating a scientific knowledge base and using this research evidence in practice requires the participation of all nurses in a variety of research activities. Some nurses are developers of research and conduct studies to generate and refine the knowledge needed for nursing practice. Others are consumers of research and use research evidence to improve their nursing practice.

Professional nursing organizations, such as American Association of Colleges of Nursing (AACN) (2006) and American Nurses Association (ANA) (1989), have published position statements that identify the participation of nurses in research based on their educational preparation. Nurses with a Bachelor of Science in Nursing (BSN), a Master of Science in Nursing (MSN), a doctorate degree, or postdoctorate education have clearly designated roles in research (AACN, 2006; ANA, 1989). Figure 1–4 identifies nurses' participation in research activities based on their level of education. The research role a nurse assumes expands with his or her advanced education and expertise. Thus, nurses with a BSN degree have a significant role in identifying the best research evidence for use in practice by searching databases and Internet sites for evidence-based guidelines, protocols, and policies. They also have a role in planning and implementing research-based changes in nursing care and in the health-

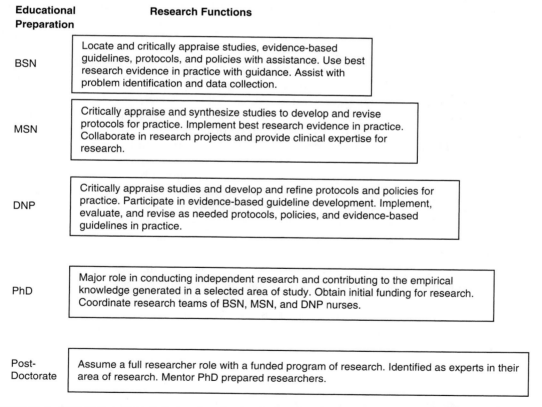

Educational Preparation | **Research Functions**

BSN — Locate and critically appraise studies, evidence-based guidelines, protocols, and policies with assistance. Use best research evidence in practice with guidance. Assist with problem identification and data collection.

MSN — Critically appraise and synthesize studies to develop and revise protocols for practice. Implement best research evidence in practice. Collaborate in research projects and provide clinical expertise for research.

DNP — Critically appraise studies and develop and refine protocols and policies for practice. Participate in evidence-based guideline development. Implement, evaluate, and revise as needed protocols, policies, and evidence-based guidelines in practice.

PhD — Major role in conducting independent research and contributing to the empirical knowledge generated in a selected area of study. Obtain initial funding for research. Coordinate research teams of BSN, MSN, and DNP nurses.

Post-Doctorate — Assume a full researcher role with a funded program of research. Identified as experts in their area of research. Mentor PhD prepared researchers.

Figure 1–4. Research participation at various levels of education preparation. Table adapted from American Nurses Association. (1989). *Education for participation in nursing research*. Kansas City, MO: Author. And American Association of Colleges of Nursing (AACN). (2006). AACN Position Statement on Nursing Research. Washington, DC: AACN. Retrieved June 1, 2009, from *http://www.aacn.nche.edu/Publications/positions/NsgRes.htm*.

care system (AACN, 2006). The educational preparation of BSN nurses includes a background in reading and critically appraising research reports. In addition, these nurses provide valuable assistance in identifying research problems and collecting data for studies.

Nurses with an MSN are provided the educational preparation to critically appraise and synthesize findings from studies to revise or develop protocols for use in practice. They also have the ability to identify and critically appraise the quality of evidence-based guidelines developed by national organizations. In addition, they have the ability to lead healthcare teams in making essential changes in nursing practice and the healthcare system that are based on evidence-based guidelines, protocols, and policies. MSN-prepared nurses also conduct narrowly focused quantitative studies and replication studies in collaboration with other nurse scientists (AACN, 2006; ANA, 1989).

The doctorate in nursing can be practice focused (doctorate of nursing practice [DNP]) or research focused (doctorate of philosophy [PhD]). DNPs are educated to have the highest level of practice expertise with the ability to translate scientific knowledge into complex guidelines and protocols for practice. These nurses have the ability to individualize guidelines and protocols to meet the specific needs of patients, families, and communities. DNPs also have advanced leadership knowledge and skills to evaluate the effectiveness of evidence-based guidelines used in practice and revise them as needed. In addition, DNP prepared nurses have the expertise to assume all the research activities performed by BSN- and MSN-prepared nurses (Webber, 2008).

PhD-prepared nurses assume a major role in the conduct of research and the generation of nursing knowledge in a selected area of interest. These nurse scientists often coordinate research teams that include DNP-, MSN-, and BSN-prepared nurses to facilitate the conduct of high-quality studies in a variety of healthcare agencies. PhD-prepared nurses sometimes want additional educational preparation and mentoring in research and seek a postdoctorate program. The postdoctorally-prepared nurse usually assumes a full-time researcher role and has a funded program of research. These scientists are often experts in selected areas and provide mentoring of new PhD-prepared nurse researchers. The maximum preparation of postdoctorate education provides a background for doing all the research activities identified for the other levels of educational preparation (see Figure 1–4).

The following chapters in this textbook were developed to expand your understanding of quantitative, qualitative, and outcomes research processes and increase your ability to critically appraise studies. A **critical appraisal of research** involves careful examination of all aspects of a study to judge its strengths, limitations, meaning, and significance. You will also be provided assistance in identifying and implementing the best research evidence in practice. We think you will find that nursing research is an exciting adventure that holds much promise for the future practice of nursing. We hope that this book will increase your understanding of research and facilitate your implementation of an evidence-based practice as a nurse.

KEY CONCEPTS

- Research is defined as diligent, systematic inquiry to validate and refine existing knowledge and generate new knowledge.

- Nursing research is defined as a scientific process that validates and refines existing knowledge and generates new knowledge that directly and indirectly influences nursing practice.
- Evidence-based practice is the conscientious integration of best research evidence with clinical expertise and patient values and needs in the delivery of high-quality, cost-effective health care.
- The purposes of research in nursing include description, explanation, prediction, and control of phenomenon in practice.
- Nightingale was the first nurse researcher who developed empirical knowledge to improve practice in the nineteenth century.
- The conduct of clinical research continues to be a major focus in the twenty-first century, with the goal of developing an evidence-based practice for nursing.
- Knowledge is acquired in nursing in a variety of ways, including tradition, authority, borrowing, trial and error, personal experience, role modeling, intuition, reasoning, and most importantly, research.
- Quantitative research is a formal, objective, systematic process using numerical data to obtain information about the world. This research method is used to describe, examine relationships, and determine cause and effect.
- Qualitative research is a systematic, subjective approach used to describe life experiences and give them meaning. Knowledge generated from qualitative research will provide meaning and understanding of specific emotions, values, and life experiences.
- A third research method is outcomes research, which focuses on examining the results of care or determining the changes in health status for the patient.
- Research evidence in nursing and health care is synthesized using the following processes: (1) systematic review, (2) meta-analysis, (3) integrative review, (4) metasummary, and (5) metasynthesis.
- A systematic review is a structured, comprehensive synthesis of quantitative studies in a particular healthcare area to determine the best research evidence available for expert clinicians to use to promote an evidence-based practice.
- Meta-analysis is a type of study that statistically pools the results from previous studies into a single quantitative analysis that provides one of the highest levels of evidence for an intervention's efficacy.
- An integrative review of research includes the identification, analysis, and synthesis of research findings from independent quantitative, outcomes, and qualitative studies to determine the current knowledge (what is known and not known) in a particular area.
- Qualitative research synthesis includes two categories: qualitative metasummary and qualitative metasynthesis.
- Qualitative metasummary is the synthesis or summing of the findings across qualitative reports to describe the current knowledge in an area.
- Qualitative metasynthesis provides a fully integrated, novel description or explanation of a target event or experience verses a summary view of that event or experience.
- The levels of the research evidence are a continuum with the highest quality of research evidence at one end and weakest research evidence at the other. The systematic research reviews and meta-analyses of high-quality experimental studies provide the strongest or best research evidence for practice.

- Evidence-based guidelines are rigorous, explicit clinical guidelines developed based on the best research evidence available in that area.
- Nurses with a BSN, MSN, a doctorate degree (both DNP and PhD), and postdoctorate education have clearly designated roles in research based on the breadth and depth of the research knowledge gained during their educational programs.

REFERENCES

Agency for Healthcare Research and Quality (AHRQ). (2009). Research priorities. Rockville, Maryland: Author. Retrieved June 1, 2009, from *http://www.ahrq.gov/about/nursing/*.

American Association of Colleges of Nursing (AACN). (2006). AACN Position Statement on Nursing Research. Washington, DC: AACN. Retrieved June 1, 2009, from *http://www.aacn.nche.edu/Publications/positions/NsgRes.htm*.

American Nurses Association (1989). *Education for participation in nursing research*. Kansas City, MO: Author.

American Nurses Association (2003). *Nursing's social policy statement* (2nd ed.). Washington, DC: Author.

American Nurses Association (2004). *Nursing: Scope and standards of practice*. Washington, DC: Author.

Barnard, K. E. (1980). Knowledge for practice: Directions for the future. *Nursing Research, 29*(4), 208-212.

Bauknecht, V. L. (1985). Capital commentary: NIH bill passes, includes nursing research center. *American Nurse, 17*(10), 2.

Benner, P. (1984). *From novice to expert: Excellence and power in clinical nursing practice*. Menlo Park, CA: Addison-Wesley.

Beyea, S. C., & Nicoll, L. H. (1995). Administration of medications via the intramuscular route: An integrative review of the literature and research-based protocol for the procedure. *Applied Nursing Research, 8*(1), 23-33.

Brown, S. J. (2009). *Evidence-based nursing: The research-practice connection*. Sudbury, MA: Jones & Bartlett.

Burns, N., & Grove, S. K. (2009). *The practice of nursing research: Appraisal, synthesis, and generation of evidence* (6th ed.). Philadelphia: Saunders.

Chinn, P. L., & Kramer, M. K. (2008). *Integrated theory and knowledge development in nursing* (7th ed.). St. Louis: Mosby Elsevier.

Chobanian, A. V., Bakris, G. L., Black, H. R., Cushman, W. C., Green, L. A., Izzo, J. L., et al. (2003). The seventh report of the Joint National Committee on prevention, detection, evaluation, and treatment of high blood pressure: The JNC 7 report. *Journal of the American Medical Association, 289*(19), 2560-2572.

Cook, E. (1913). *The life of Florence Nightingale* (Vol. 1). London: Macmillan.

Conn, V. S., & Rantz, M. J. (2003). Research methods: Managing primary study quality in meta-analyses. *Research in Nursing & Health, 26*(4), 322-333.

Craig, J., & Smyth, R. (2007). *The evidence-based practice manual for nurses* (2nd ed.). Edinburgh: Churchill Livingstone Elsevier.

Creswell, J. W. (2009). *Research design: Qualitative, quantitative and mixed methods approaches* (3rd ed.). Thousand Oaks: CA: Sage Publications.

Cullum, N., Ciliska, D., Haynes, R. B., & Marks, S. (2008). *Evidence-based nursing: An introduction*. Oxford, UK: Blackwell.

Doran, D. M. (2003). *Nursing sensitive outcomes: The state of the science*. Sudbury, MA: Jones & Bartlett.

Glaser, B. G., & Strauss, A. L. (1967). *The discovery of grounded theory: Strategies for qualitative research*. Chicago: Aldine.

Gortner, S. R., & Nahm, H. (1977). An overview of nursing research in the United States. *Nursing Research, 26*(1), 10-33.

Greenway, K. (2004). Using the ventrogluteal site for intramuscular injection. *Nursing Standard, 18*(25), 39-42.

Herbert, R. G. (1981). *Florence Nightingale: Saint, reformer or rebel?* Malabar, FL: Robert E. Krieger.

Horsley, J. A., Crane, J., Crabtree, M. K., & Wood, D. J. (1983). *Using research to improve nursing practice: A guide, CURN Project*. New York: Grune & Stratton.

Hunter, C. L., Spence, K., McKenna, K., & Iedema, R. (2008). Learning how we learn: An ethnographic study in a neonatal intensive care unit. *Journal of Advanced Nursing, 62*(6), 657-664.

Institute of Medicine. (2001). *Crossing the quality chasm: A new health system for the 21st century*. Washington, DC: National Academy Press.

Jones, K. R., & Burney, R. E. (2002). Outcomes research: An interdisciplinary perspective. *Outcomes Management, 6*(3), 103-109.

Kaplan, A. (1964). *The conduct of inquiry; Methodology for behavioral science*. San Francisco: Chandler.

Kerlinger, F. N., & Lee, H. B. (2000). *Foundations of behavioral research* (4th ed.). Fort Worth, TX: Harcourt College Publishers.

King, K. B., Gerich, J. E., Guzick, D. S., King, K. U., & McDermott, M. P. (2009). Is a history of gestational diabetes related to risk factors for coronary heart disease? *Research in Nursing & Health, 32*(3), 298-306.

McMurrey, P. H. (1982). Toward a unique knowledge base in nursing. *Image, 14*(1), 12-15.

Melnyk, B. M., & Fineout-Overholt, E. (2005). *Evidence-based practice in nursing & healthcare: A guide to best practice*. Philadelphia: Lippincott Williams & Wilkins.

Munhall, P. L. (2007). *Nursing research: A qualitative perspective* (4th ed.). Sudbury, MA: Jones & Bartlett.

National Heart, Lung, and Blood Institute. (2003). *The seventh report of the Joint National Committee on prevention,* detection, evaluation, and treatment of high blood pressure: The JNC 7 report. Bethesda, MD: National Institutes of Health. Retrieved June 6, 2009 from *www.nhlbi.nih.gov/guidelines/hypertension*.

National Institute of Nursing Research (NINR) (September 23, 1993). *National nursing research agenda: Setting nursing research priorities*. Bethesda, MD: National Institutes of Health.

National Institute of Nursing Research (2009). About the NINR. Retrieved June 1, 2009 from *http://ninr.nih.gov/*.

Nicoll, L. H., & Hesby, A. (2002). Intramuscular injections: An integrative research review and guideline for evidence-based practice. *Applied Nursing Research, 16*(2), 149-162.

Nightingale, F. (1859). *Notes on nursing: What it is, and what it is not*. Philadelphia: Lippincott.

Palmer, I. S. (1977). Florence Nightingale: Reformer, reactionary, researcher. *Nursing Research, 26*(2), 84-89.

Patton, M. Q. (2002). *Qualitative research & evaluation methods* (3rd ed.). Thousand Oaks, CA: Sage Publications.

Pearson, A., Field, J., & Jordan, Z. (2007). *Evidence-based clinical practice in nursing and health care: Assimilating research, experience, and expertise*. Oxford, UK: Blackwell.

Rettig, R. (1991). History, development, and importance to nursing of outcomes research. *Journal of Nursing Quality Assurance, 5*(2), 13-17.

Rew, L., & Barrow, E. M. (1987). Intuition: A neglected hallmark of nursing knowledge. *Advances in Nursing Science, 10*(1), 49-62.

Rodger, M. A., & King, L. (2000). Drawing up and administering intramuscular injections: A review of the literature. *Journal of Advanced Nursing, 31*(3), 574-582.

Ryan, C. J., DeVon, H. A., Horne, R., King, K. B., Milner, K., Moser, D. K., et al. (2007). Symptom clusters in acute myocardial infarction: A secondary data analysis. *Nursing Research, 56*(2), 72-81.

Sackett, D. L., Straus, S. E., Richardson, W. S., Rosenberg, W., & Haynes, R. B. (2000). *Evidence-based medicine: How to practice and teach EBM* (2nd ed.). London: Churchill Livingstone.

Sandelowski, M., & Barroso, J. (2007). *Handbook for synthesizing qualitative research*. New York: Springer.

Scheetz, L. J., Zhang, J., & Kolassa, J. E. (2007). Using crash scene variables to predict the need for trauma center care in older persons. *Research in Nursing & Health, 30*(4), 399-412.

See, E. M. (1977). The ANA and research in nursing. *Nursing Research, 26*(3), 165-171.

Standing, M. (2009). A new critical framework for applying hermeneutic phenomenology. (2009). *Nurse Researcher, 16*(4), 20-30.

Stetler, C. B. (2001). Updating the Stetler model of research utilization to facilitate evidence-based practice. *Nursing Outlook, 49*(6), 272-279.

Thomas, S. P. (2000). A phenomenologic study of chronic pain. *Western Journal of Nursing Research, 22*(6), 683-706.

U.S. Department of Health and Human Services. (2000). *Healthy people 2010: Understanding and improving health*. Washington, DC: U.S. Department of Health and Human Services.

Webber, P. B. (2008). The doctor of nursing practice degree and research: Are we making an epistemological mistake? *Journal of Nursing Education, 47*(10), 466-472.

Werley, H. H., & Fitzpatrick, J. J. (1983). *Annual review of nursing research* (Vol. 1). New York: Springer.

Whittemore, R. (2005). Combining evidence in nursing research: Methods and implications. *Nursing Research, 54*(1), 56-62.

Wynaden, D., Landsborough, I., McGowan, S., Baigmohamad, Z. Finn, M., and Pennebaker, D. (2006). Best practice guidelines for the administration of intramuscular injections in the mental health setting. *International Journal of Mental Health Nursing, 15*(3), 195-200.

2

Introduction to the Quantitative Research Process

Chapter Overview

What Is Quantitative Research? 34
  Types of Quantitative Research 34
  Defining Terms Relevant to Quantitative
    Research 36
**Problem-Solving and Nursing Processes:
  Basis for Understanding the Quantitative
  Research Process** 41
  Comparing Problem Solving with the Nursing
    Process 42
  Comparing the Nursing Process with the
    Research Process 42
**Identifying the Steps of the Quantitative
  Research Process** 43
  Research Problem and Purpose 44
  Literature Review 44
  Study Framework 45
  Research Objectives, Questions, and
    Hypotheses 46

Study Variables 47
Assumptions 48
Limitations 48
Research Design 49
Population and Sample 51
Methods of Measurement 51
Data Collection 52
Data Analysis 52
Research Outcomes 53
Reading Research Reports 54
  Sources of Research Reports 54
  Content of Research Reports 55
  Tips for Reading Research Reports 59
**Practice Reading Quasi-experimental and
  Experimental Studies** 61
  Quasi-experimental Study 61
  Experimental Study 66

Learning Outcomes

After completing this chapter, you should be able to:

1. Define terms relevant to the quantitative research process: basic research, applied research, rigor, and control.
2. Compare and contrast the problem-solving process, nursing process, and research process.
3. Identify the steps of the quantitative research process in descriptive, correlational, quasi-

experimental, and experimental published studies.
4. Read research reports.
5. Conduct an initial critical appraisal of a research report.

Key Terms

Abstract, p. 55
Analyzing a research report,
  p. 60

Applied (practical) research,
  p. 37
Assumptions, p. 48

Basic (pure) research, p. 36
Comprehending a research
  report, p. 60

Conceptual definition, p. 47
Control, p. 39
Correlational research, p. 35
Data analysis, p. 52
Data collection, p. 52
Descriptive research, p. 34
Design, p. 49
Experiment, p. 33
Experimental research,
    p. 35
Extraneous variables, p. 40
Framework, p. 45
Generalization, p. 48
Highly controlled setting,
    p. 41
Interpretation of research
    outcomes, p. 53
Limitations, p. 48

Literature review, p. 44
Measurement, p. 51
Methodological limitations,
    p. 48
Natural (field) setting, p. 40
Nursing process, p. 42
Operational definition, p. 47
Partially controlled setting,
    p. 40
Pilot study, p. 49
Population, p. 51
Precision, p. 39
Problem-solving process,
    p. 42
Process, p. 41
Quantitative research, p. 34
Quantitative research
    process, p. 43

Quasi-experimental research,
    p. 35
Reading a research report,
    p. 60
Research problem, p. 44
Research process, p. 42
Research purpose, p. 44
Research report, p. 54
Rigor, p. 39
Sample, p. 51
Sampling, p. 40, 51
Setting, p. 40
Skimming a research report,
    p. 60
Theoretical limitations, p. 48
Theory, p. 45
Variables, p. 47

STUDY TOOLS

Be sure to visit *http:/elsevier.com/evolve/Burns/understanding* for additional examples and self-tests. Also, a review of this chapter's concepts and practice exercises can be found in Chapter 2 of the Study Guide for *Understanding Nursing Research: Building an Evidence-Based Practice*, 5th edition.

What do you think of when you hear the word *research?* Frequently, the idea of experimentation comes to mind. Typical features of an **experiment** include randomizing subjects into groups, collecting data, and conducting statistical analyses. You may think of researchers conducting an experiment to determine the effectiveness of an intervention, such as determining the effectiveness of a walking exercise program on body mass index (BMI) of patients with type 2 diabetes. These ideas are associated with quantitative research. Quantitative research includes specific steps that are detailed in research reports. Reading and critically appraising quantitative studies require learning new terms, understanding the steps of the quantitative research process, and applying a variety of analytical skills.

This chapter provides an introduction to quantitative research to promote the development of expertise in reading quantitative research reports. Relevant terms are defined, and the problem-solving and nursing processes are presented to provide a background for understanding the quantitative research process. The steps of the quantitative research process are introduced, and a descriptive correlational study is presented as an example to promote understanding of the process. Also included are a discussion of the critical thinking skills needed for reading research reports and guidelines for conducting an initial critical appraisal of these reports. The chapter concludes with the identification of the steps of the research process from published quasi-experimental and experimental studies with an initial critical appraisal of these studies.

What Is Quantitative Research?

Quantitative research is a formal, objective, rigorous, systematic process for generating numerical information about the world. Quantitative research is conducted to describe new situations, events, or concepts; examine relationships among variables; and determine the effectiveness of treatments in the world. Some examples are:

1. Describing the spread of swine flu and its potential influence on global health (descriptive study)
2. Examining the relationships among the variables—minutes watching television per week, minutes playing video games per week, and BMI of a school age child (correlational study)
3. Determining the effectiveness of calcium with vitamin D_3 on the bone density of patients (quasi-experimental study)

The classic experimental designs to test the effectiveness of treatments were originated by Sir Ronald Fisher (1935). He is noted for adding structure to the steps of the quantitative research process with such ideas as the hypothesis, research design, and statistical analysis. Fisher's studies provided the groundwork for what is now known as experimental research.

Throughout the years, a number of other quantitative approaches have been developed. Campbell and Stanley (1963) developed quasi-experimental approaches to study the effects of treatments under less controlled conditions. Karl Pearson (Porter, 2004) developed statistical approaches for examining relationships between variables, which increased the conduct of correlational research. The fields of sociology, education, and psychology are noted for their development and expansion of strategies for conducting descriptive research. A broad range of quantitative research approaches is needed to develop the empirical knowledge essential for evidence-based nursing practice (Brown, 2009; Craig & Smyth, 2007). This section introduces you to the different types of quantitative research and provides definitions of terms relevant to the quantitative research process.

Types of Quantitative Research

Four types of quantitative research are included in this textbook:

- Descriptive
- Correlational
- Quasi-experimental
- Experimental

The type of quantitative research conducted is influenced by the current knowledge of a research problem. When little knowledge is available, descriptive studies often are conducted. As the knowledge level increases, correlational, quasi-experimental, and experimental studies are conducted.

Descriptive Research

Descriptive research is the exploration and description of phenomena in real-life situations. It provides an accurate account of characteristics of particular individuals, situations, or groups (Kerlinger & Lee, 2000). Descriptive studies are usually conducted with large numbers of subjects, in natural settings, with no manipulation of the situation in anyway. Through descriptive studies, researchers discover new meaning, describe what exists, determine the frequency with which something occurs, and categorize information. The outcomes of descriptive research include the description of concepts, identification of possible relationships between concepts, and development of hypotheses that provide a basis for future quantitative research.

Correlational Research

Correlational research involves the systematic investigation of relationships between or among variables. To do this, the researcher measures the selected variables in a sample and then uses correlational statistics to determine the relationships among the variables. Using correlational analysis, the researcher is able to determine the degree or strength and type (positive or negative) of a relationship between two variables. The strength of a relationship varies, ranging from -1 (perfect negative correlation) to $+1$ (perfect positive correlation), with 0 indicating no relationship (Grove, 2007).

The positive relationship indicates that the variables vary together; that is, both variables either increase or decrease together. For example, research has shown that the more people smoke, the more lung damage they experience. The negative relationship indicates that the variables vary in opposite directions; thus, as one variable increases, the other will decrease (Grove, 2007). As an example, research has shown that an increase in the number of smoking pack-years (number of years smoked times the number of packs smoked per day) is correlated with a decrease in life span. The primary intent of correlational studies is to explain the nature of relationships in the real world, not to determine cause and effect (Porter, 2004). However, the relationships identified with correlational studies are the means for generating hypotheses to guide quasi-experimental and experimental studies that do focus on examining cause-and-effect relationships.

Quasi-experimental Research

The purpose of quasi-experimental research is to examine causal relationships or determine the effect of one variable on another. Thus, these studies involve implementing a treatment and examining the effects of this treatment using selected methods of measurement (Cook & Campbell, 1979). In nursing research, a treatment is an intervention implemented by researchers to improve the outcomes of clinical practice. For example, a treatment of a swimming exercise program might be implemented to improve the balance and muscle strength of elderly women. Quasi-experimental studies differ from experimental studies by the level of control achieved by the researcher. Quasi-experimental studies usually lack a certain amount of control over the manipulation of the treatment, management of the setting, and/or selection of the subjects. When studying human behavior, especially in clinical settings, researchers frequently are unable to randomly select the subjects or manipulate or control certain variables related to the subjects or the setting. Thus, nurse researchers conduct more quasi-experimental studies than experimental studies.

Experimental Research

Experimental research is an objective, systematic, highly controlled investigation for the purpose of predicting and controlling phenomena in nursing practice. In an experimental study, causality between the independent and the dependent variables is examined under highly controlled conditions (Kerlinger & Lee, 2000). Experimental research is the most powerful quantitative method because of the rigorous control of variables. The three main characteristics of experimental studies are: (1) controlled manipulation of at least one treatment variable (independent variable); (2) exposure of some of the subjects to the treatment (experimental group), and no exposure of the remaining subjects (control group); and (3) random assignment of subjects to either the control or experimental group. Random selection of subjects and the conduct of the study in a laboratory or research facility strengthen control in an experimental study. The degree of control achieved in experimental studies varies according to the population studied, the variables examined, and the environment of the study.

Defining Terms Relevant to Quantitative Research

Understanding quantitative research requires comprehension of the following important terms: basic research, applied research, rigor, and control. These terms are defined in the following sections with examples provided from published studies.

Basic Research

Basic research (or pure research) is scientific investigation that involves the pursuit of "knowledge for knowledge's sake" or for the pleasure of learning and finding truth (Miller & Salkind, 2002). Basic scientific investigation seeks new knowledge about health phenomena with the hope of establishing general principles. The purpose of basic research is to generate and refine theory; thus, the findings frequently are not directly useful in practice (Wysocki, 1983). Basic nursing research focused on physiological or pathological variables might include laboratory investigations in animals or humans to develop principles regarding physiological functioning or pathologic processes or the effects of treatments on physiological and pathological functioning. These studies might focus on increasing understanding of oxygenation, perfusion, fluid and electrolyte balance, acid-base status, eating and sleeping patterns, and comfort status, as well as pathophysiology of the immune system (Bond & Heitkemper, 1987).

You might conduct an initial critical appraisal of quantitative studies and identify if basic or applied research was conducted. Yamakage, Iwasaki, Jeong, Satoh, and Namiki (2009) conducted basic research to examine the safe use of selective drugs in animals with airway hyperreactivity. This study is introduced and then critically appraised using the following questions.

CRITICAL APPRAISAL GUIDELINES

Basic versus Applied Research

1. What type of quantitative study was conducted: descriptive, correlational, quasi-experimental, or experimental?
2. Was the study basic or applied research?
3. Were animals or humans used as subjects in the study?

RESEARCH EXAMPLE Basic Research

Yamakage and colleagues (2009) examined the effect of propranolol (Inderal) versus esmolol (Brevibloc) and Landiolol on guinea pigs with asthma induced by ovalbumin (primary protein in chicken eggs). Beta-blockers, such as Inderal, have established benefits to control tachycardia, tachyarrhythmia, and hypertension in patients perioperatively and in intensive care units (ICUs). "However, beta-blockers are contraindicated in patients with airway hyperreactivity, such as patients with asthma and/or chronic obstructive pulmonary disease (COPD), because of its concomitant beta-2 blocking effect, which causes bronchoconstriction" (Yamakage et al., 2009, p. 48). However, the two ultra-short-acting beta-1 selective adrenergic antagonist esmolol (Brevibloc) and Landiolol (a new drug used mainly in Japan) are hypothesized to be better pharmacological agents to use to control tachycardia and tachyarrhythmia in patients who have asthma and/or COPD in perioperative and ICU settings.

CRITICAL APPRAISAL

Yamakage et al. (2009) conducted an experimental study of the effects of Inderal, Brevibloc, and Landiolol on guinea pigs with induced asthma. This is an experimental study since treatments were implemented in a highly controlled laboratory setting with animals. This is basic research since the focus was on understanding the effects of drug treatments on physiological responses of pulmonary resistance and dynamic lung compliance in animals (guinea pigs). Thus, the focus was on the generation of knowledge for knowledge sake without direct application to clinical practice.

IMPLICATIONS FOR PRACTICE

Yamakage and colleagues (2009) found that both Brevibloc and the new drug Landiolol were safer drugs than Inderal to use in the guinea pigs with induced asthma. Basic research such as this usually precedes or is the basis for applied research with patients. Thus, applied research is needed to determine the effectiveness and safety of both Brevibloc and Landiolol in the management of tachycardia and tachyarrhythmia of patients with asthma and/or COPD in perioperative and ICU settings.

Applied Research

Applied research (or practical research) is scientific investigation conducted to generate knowledge that will directly influence or improve clinical practice. The purpose of applied research is to solve problems, make decisions, or predict or control outcomes in real-life practice situations. The findings from applied studies also can be invaluable to policy makers as a basis for making changes to address health and social problems (Miller & Salkind, 2002). Many of the studies conducted in nursing are applied because researchers have chosen to focus on clinical problems and the testing of nursing interventions to improve patient outcomes. Applied research also is used to test theory and validate its usefulness in clinical practice. Researchers often examine the new knowledge discovered through basic research for usefulness in practice by applied research, making these approaches complementary (Wysocki, 1983). An example of applied research is on the next page.

RESEARCH EXAMPLE Applied Research

Lacey, Finkelstein, and Thygeson (2008) conducted an applied study to determine the effect of positioning, supine versus sitting, on the fear children experience during immunizations. The researchers noted from their review of the literature that "low rates of immunizations have been attributed to the parental fear of not wanting to see their child cry. ... We hypothesized that a child sitting up when receiving an injection would feel more in control and be less fearful than when lying down. ... They [child subjects] were randomly assigned to one of two groups, where Group 1 was placed in the supine position and Group 2 in the sitting position prior to immunizations" (Lacey et al., 2008, pp. 195-196). Thus, the position (supine or sitting) was the treatment or independent variable and fear (as measured by crying time, Child Medical Fear Scale [CMFS], and Fearmometer) and pain (as measured by the FACES scale) were the outcome or dependent variables.

CRITICAL APPRAISAL

Lacey and colleagues (2008) conducted a quasi-experimental study that examined the effects of the treatment positioning (supine versus sitting up) on the outcomes fear and pain children experienced during immunizations. This is a quasi-experimental study since it was conducted with a convenience sample of children in a clinic setting. Thus, this study lacked the control of setting and subject selection that is usually present in an experimental study. Lacey et al. (2008) chose to conduct an applied study to generate knowledge that could directly influence or improve practice. These researchers noted the problem of low immunization rates related to children's fear of injections and tested the effectiveness of an intervention to reduce that fear.

IMPLICATIONS FOR PRACTICE

Lacey and colleagues' (2008, p. 198) "study provides evidence that children are significantly less fearful of an immunization injection when they are sitting up as compared to when they are lying down [supine]. A smaller percentage of the children cried prior to the injection, and crying time postinjection was significantly less for children who were sitting up." However, the researchers did not find significant differences between the sitting and supine positions for immunization injections with the CMFS, Fearmometer, or FACES scales. In addition, the nurses expressed safety concerns about giving immunizations to children in the sitting position due to the possibility of the parent, child, or nurse being accidently stuck by a needle during the injections. Based on the study findings related to crying time, the researchers recommended that health professionals consider giving immunization injections to children in the sitting position. Parents and health professionals were encouraged to be supportive of children during immunizations by providing them more control and comfort to decrease their fears. We recommend that this study be repeated with a larger sample and different measurement methods other than scales before the findings are used in practice. These applied study findings, combined with the findings of additional studies in this area, have the potential to generate important knowledge for the delivery of evidence-based care to children during their immunization injections.

Rigor in Quantitative Research

Rigor is the striving for excellence in research, and it requires discipline, adherence to detail, and strict accuracy. A rigorously conducted quantitative study has precise measuring tools, a representative sample, and a tightly controlled study design. Critically appraising the rigor of a study involves examining the reasoning and precision used in conducting the study. Logical reasoning, including deductive and inductive reasoning, is essential to the development of quantitative studies. The research process includes specific steps that are developed with meticulous detail and are logically linked. These steps, such as design, measurement, sample, data collection, and statistical analysis, need to be examined for weaknesses and errors.

Another aspect of rigor is precision, which encompasses accuracy, detail, and order. Precision is evident in the concise statement of the research purpose and detailed development of the study design. But the most explicit example of precision is the measurement or quantification of the study variables. For example, a researcher might use a cardiac monitor to measure and record the heart rate of subjects during an exercise program, rather than palpating a radial pulse for 30 seconds and recording it on a data collection sheet. In the Lacey et al. (2008) study, the child's crying time might be a more objective and precise measure of fear than paper and pencil scales like the CMFS and Fearmometer completed by the children.

Control in Quantitative Research

Control involves the imposing of rules by the researcher to decrease the possibility of error, thereby increasing the probability that the study's findings are an accurate reflection of reality. The rules used to achieve control in research are referred to as design. Thus, quantitative research includes various degrees of control, ranging from uncontrolled to highly controlled, depending on the type of study (Table 2–1). Descriptive and correlational studies often are designed with little or no researcher control because subjects are examined as they exist in their natural setting, such as home, work, school, or a health clinic. Quasi-experimental studies focus on determining the effectiveness of a treatment (independent variable) in producing a desired outcome (dependent variable) in a partially controlled setting. Thus, these studies are conducted with more control in the selection of subjects, implementation of the treatment, and measurement of the dependent variables. However, experimental studies are the most highly controlled type of quantitative research conducted to examine the effect of treatments on dependent variables. Experimental studies often are

Table 2–1	Control in Quantitative Research	
Type of Quantitative Research	Researcher Control Treatment and Extraneous Variables	Research Setting
Descriptive	No treatment	Natural or partially controlled setting
Correlational	No treatment	Natural or partially controlled setting
Quasi-experimental	Controlled treatment and extraneous variables	Partially controlled setting
Experimental	Highly controlled treatment and extraneous variables	Laboratory or research unit

conducted on subjects in experimental units in healthcare agencies or on animals in laboratory settings (see Table 2–1).

Extraneous Variables

Through control, the researcher can reduce the influence of extraneous variables. **Extraneous variables** exist in all studies and can interfere with obtaining a clear understanding of the relationships among the study variables. For example, if a study focused on the effect of relaxation therapy on perception of incisional pain, the researchers would have to control the extraneous variables (such as type of surgical incision and time, amount, and type of pain medication administered following surgery) to prevent their influence on the patient's perception of pain. Selecting only patients with abdominal incisions who are hospitalized and intravenously receiving only one type of pain medication after surgery would control some of these extraneous variables. In critically appraising quantitative studies, try to determine if the study was designed to decrease the influence of extraneous variables through the selection of subjects (sampling) and the research setting. Controlling extraneous variables enables the researcher to more accurately determine the effect of an independent or treatment variable on a dependent or outcome variable.

Sampling

Sampling is a process of selecting subjects who are representative of the population being studied. Random sampling usually provides a sample that is representative of a population because each member of the population is selected independently and has an equal chance or probability of being included in the study. In quantitative research, both random and nonrandom samples are used. Descriptive studies often are conducted with nonrandom or nonprobability samples, in which the subjects are selected on the basis of convenience. Correlation and quasi-experimental studies include either nonrandom or random sampling methods, but having a randomly selected sample strengthens highly controlled experimental studies. A randomly selected sample is very difficult to obtain in nursing research, so quantitative studies often are conducted with convenience samples. To increase the control and rigor of a study and decrease the potential for bias (slanting of findings away from what is true or accurate), the subjects who are part of a convenience sample often are randomly assigned to the treatment group or the control (no treatment) group in quasi-experimental and experimental studies. Lacey and colleagues' (2008) study was strengthen by the random assignment of the children to either the sitting or supine position for their immunization injections.

Research Settings

The **setting** is the location in which a study is conducted. There are three common settings for conducting research: Natural, partially controlled, and highly controlled (see Table 2–1). A **natural setting**, or **field setting**, is an uncontrolled, real-life situation or environment (Miller & Salkind, 2002). Conducting a study in a natural setting means that the researcher does not manipulate or change the environment for the study. Descriptive and correlational studies often are conducted in natural settings. A **partially controlled setting** is an environment that the researcher has manipulated or modified in some way. An increasing number of nursing studies are occurring in partially controlled settings. Lacey and colleagues (2008) conducted their study in a general pediatric clinic within a Midwest hospital. This partially controlled setting was selected to limit the effects of extraneous variables on the study outcomes. Children in one group were sitting for their immunization injections and children in the other group were supine. The exam rooms were similar for both groups and included the parent and a health professional to limit the impact of the environment on the child's fear.

A highly controlled setting is an artificially constructed environment developed for the sole purpose of conducting research. Laboratories, research or experimental centers, and test units in hospitals or other healthcare agencies are highly controlled settings in which experimental studies often are conducted. This type of setting reduces the influence of extraneous variables, which enables the researcher to examine accurately the effect of one variable on another. Yamakage et al. (2009) conducted their study with guinea pigs in a laboratory setting. This setting is highly controlled by the researchers, which results in limited effects by extraneous variables in the environment. Using animals in a study ensures that the subjects are similar for the treatment and control groups, which limits the effects of extraneous variables in the sampling process.

Problem-Solving and Nursing Processes: Basis for Understanding the Quantitative Research Process

Research is a process, and it is similar in some ways to other processes. Therefore, the background acquired early in nursing education in problem solving and the nursing process also is useful in research. A process includes a purpose, a series of actions, and a goal. The purpose provides direction for the implementation of a series of actions to achieve an identified goal. The specific steps of the process can be revised and reimplemented in order to reach the endpoint or goal. Table 2–2 presents the problem-solving process, nursing process,

Table 2-2	Comparison of the Problem-Solving Process, Nursing Process, and Research Process

Problem-Solving Process	Nursing Process	Research Process
Data Collection	**Assessment**	**Knowledge of Nursing World**
	Data collection	Clinical experiences
	Data interpretation	Literature review
Problem Definition	**Nursing Diagnosis**	**Problem and Purpose Identification**
Plan	**Plan**	**Methodology**
Setting goals	Setting goals	Design
Identifying solutions	Planning interventions	Sample
		Measurement methods
		Data collection
		Data analysis
Implementation	**Implementation**	**Implementation**
Evaluation and Revision	**Evaluation and Modification**	**Outcomes, Communication, and Synthesis of Study Findings to Promote Evidence-Based Nursing Practice**

and research process. Relating the research process to problem solving and the nursing process may be helpful in understanding the steps of the quantitative research process.

Comparing Problem Solving with the Nursing Process

The problem-solving process involves the systematic identification of a problem, determination of goals related to the problem, identification of possible approaches to achieve those goals (planning), implementation of selected approaches, and evaluation of goal achievement. Problem solving frequently is used in daily activities and nursing practice. For example, you use problem solving when you select your clothing, decide where to live, or turn a patient with a fractured hip.

The nursing process is a subset of the problem-solving process. The steps of the nursing process are assessment, diagnosis, planning, implementation, evaluation, and modification (see Table 2–2). Assessment involves the collection and interpretation of data for the development of nursing diagnoses. These diagnoses guide the remaining steps of the nursing process, just as the step of identifying the problem, directs the remaining steps of the problem-solving process. The planning step in the nursing process is the same as in the problem-solving process. Both processes involve implementation (putting the plan into action) and evaluation (determining the effectiveness of the process). If the process is ineffective, the nurse reviews all steps and revises (modifies) as necessary. The nurse implements the process until the problems/diagnoses are resolved and the identified goals are achieved.

Comparing the Nursing Process with the Research Process

The nursing process and research process have important similarities and differences. The two processes are similar because they both involve abstract, critical thinking and complex reasoning (Wilkinson, 2006). These processes help to identify new information, discover relationships, and make predictions about phenomena. In both processes, information is gathered, observations are made, problems are identified, plans are developed (methodology), and actions are taken (data collection and analysis). Both processes are reviewed for effectiveness and efficiency; the nursing process is evaluated, and outcomes are determined in the research process (see Table 2–2). Implementing the two processes expands and refines the user's knowledge. With this growth in knowledge and critical thinking, the user is able to implement increasingly complex nursing processes and studies.

The research and nursing processes also have definite differences. Knowledge of the nursing process will assist you in understanding the research process. However, the research process is more complex than the nursing process. It requires an understanding of a unique language and involves the rigorous application of a variety of research methods (Burns, 1989; Burns & Grove, 2009). The research process also has a broader focus than that of the nursing process, in which the nurse focuses on a specific patient and family. During the research process, the researcher focuses on large groups of individuals, such as a population of patients with hypertension. In addition, researchers must be knowledgeable about the world of nursing to identify problems that require study. This knowledge comes from clinical and other personal experiences and by conducting a review of the literature.

The theoretical underpinnings of the research process are much stronger than those of the nursing process. All steps of the research process are logically linked to each other, as well as to the theoretical foundations of the study. The conduct of research requires greater precision, rigor, and control than are needed in implementation of the nursing process. The outcomes from research frequently are shared with a large number of nurses and other healthcare professionals through presentations and publications. In addition, the outcomes from several studies can be synthesized to provide sound evidence for nursing practice (Brown, 2009; Melnyk & Fineout-Overholt, 2005; Whittemore, 2005).

Identifying the Steps of the Quantitative Research Process

The quantitative research process involves conceptualizing a research project, planning and implementing that project, and communicating the findings. Figure 2–1 identifies the steps of the quantitative research process that usually are included in a research report. This figure indicates the logical flow of the process as one step builds progressively on another. The steps of the quantitative research process are briefly reviewed here; Chapters 4 to 11 discuss them in detail. The descriptive correlational study conducted by Hulme and Grove (1994) on the symptoms of female survivors of child sexual abuse is used as an example to introduce the steps of the quantitative research process.

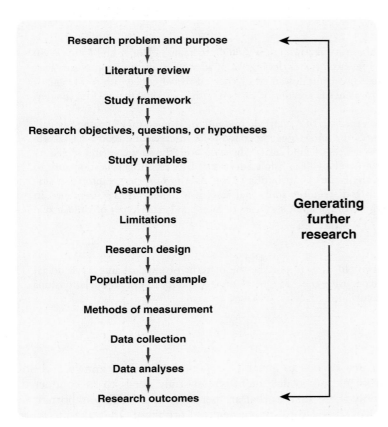

Research problem and purpose
↓
Literature review
↓
Study framework
↓
Research objectives, questions, or hypotheses
↓
Study variables
↓
Assumptions
↓
Limitations
↓
Research design
↓
Population and sample
↓
Methods of measurement
↓
Data collection
↓
Data analyses
↓
Research outcomes

Generating further research

Figure 2–1. Steps of the quantitative research process.

Research Problem and Purpose

A **research problem** is an area of concern in which there is a gap in the knowledge base needed for nursing practice. The problem statement in a study usually identifies an area of concern for a particular population that requires investigation. Research is then conducted to generate essential knowledge that addresses the practice concern, with the ultimate goal of providing an evidence-based practice in nursing (Brown, 2009; Craig & Smyth, 2007). The research problem is usually broad and could provide the basis for several studies. The **research purpose** is generated from the problem and identifies the specific goal of the study. The goal of a study might be to identify, describe, or explain a situation; predict a solution to a situation; or control a situation to produce positive outcomes in practice. The purpose includes the variables, population, and often the setting for the study. Chapter 5 presents a detailed discussion of the research problem and purpose.

 RESEARCH EXAMPLE Problem and Purpose

Hulme and Grove (1994) conducted an initial study of female adult survivors of child sexual abuse and identified the following problem and purpose for their study. Hulme (2000; Hulme & Agrawal, 2004) continues to conduct studies in this significant problem area of adult survivors of child abuse.

Research Problem

"The actual prevalence of child sexual abuse is unknown but is thought to be high. Bagley and King (1990) were able to generalize from compiled research that at least 20% of all women in the samples surveyed had been victims of serious sexual abuse involving unwanted or coerced sexual contact up to the age of 17 years. Evidence indicates that the prevalence is greater for women born after 1960 than before (Bagley, 1990).

The impact of child sexual abuse on the lives of the girl victims and the women they become has only lately received the attention it deserves … the knowledge generated from research and theory has slowly forced the recognition of the long-term effects of child sexual abuse on both the survivors and society as a whole … Brown and Garrison (1990) developed the Adult Survivors of Incest (ASI) Questionnaire to identify the patterns of symptoms and the factors contributing to the severity of these symptoms in survivors of childhood sexual abuse. This tool requires additional testing to determine its usefulness in identifying symptoms and contributing factors of adult survivors of incest and other types of child sexual abuse." (Hulme & Grove, 1994, pp. 519-520)

Research Purpose

Thus, the purpose of this study was twofold: "(a) to describe the patterns of physical and psychosocial symptoms in female sexual abuse survivors using the ASI Questionnaire, and (b) to examine relationships among the symptoms and identified contributing factors." (Hulme & Grove, 1994, p. 520)

Literature Review

Researchers conduct a literature review to generate a picture of what is known and not known about a particular problem and to document why a study needs to be conducted. Relevant literature includes only those sources that are pertinent to or highly important in providing the in-depth knowledge needed to study a selected problem. Often the literature review section concludes with a summary paragraph that indicates the current knowledge of a problem area and identifies the additional research that is needed to generate essential evidence for practice (research problem). Chapter 6 describes the process for reviewing the literature.

Hulme and Grove's (1994) review of the literature covered relevant theories and studies related to child sexual abuse and its contributing factors and long-term effects.

Theorists indicated that … the act of child sexual abuse can be explained as an abuse of power by a trusted parent figure, usually male, on a dependent child, violating the child's body, mind, and spirit. The family, which normally functions to nurture and protect the child from harm, is viewed as not fulfilling this function, leaving the child to feel further betrayed and powerless. Acceptance of the immediate psychological trauma of child sexual abuse has given impetus for acknowledging the long-term effects.

Studies of both nonclinical and clinical populations have lent support to these theoretical developments. When compared with control groups consisting of women who had not been sexually abused as children, survivors of child sexual abuse consistently have higher incidence of depression and lower self-esteem. Other psychosocial long-term effects encountered include suicidal plans, anxiety, distorted body image, decreased sexual satisfaction, poor general social adjustment, lower positive affect, negative personality characteristics, and feeling different from significant others. … The physical long-term effects suggested by research include gastrointestinal problems such as ulcers, spastic colitis, irritable bowel syndrome, and chronic abdominal pain; gynecological disorders; chronic headache; obesity; and increased lifetime surgeries.

Studies of contributing factors that may affect the traumatic impact of child sexual abuse are less in number and less conclusive than those identifying long-term effects. However, poor family functioning, increased age difference between the victim and perpetrator, threat or use of force or violence, multiple abusers, parent or primary caretaker as perpetrator, prolonged or intrusive abuse, and strong emotional bond to the perpetrator with betrayal of trust may all contribute to the increased severity of the long-term effects. (pp. 521-522)

Study Framework

A **framework** is the abstract, theoretical basis for a study that enables the researcher to link the findings to nursing's body of knowledge. In quantitative research, the framework is a testable theory that has been developed in nursing or another discipline, such as psychology, physiology, pathology, or sociology. A **theory** consists of an integrated set of defined concepts and relational statements that present a view of a phenomenon and can be used to describe, explain, predict, or control the phenomenon. Researchers test the relational statements of the theory, not the theory itself, through research. A study framework can be expressed as a map or a diagram of the relationships that provide the basis for a study, or the framework can be presented in narrative format. Chapter 7 provides you with a background for understanding and critically appraising study frameworks.

The framework for Hulme and Grove's (1994) study is Browne and Finkelhor's (1986) theory of Traumagenic Dynamics in the Impact of Child Sexual Abuse. Over the years, Finkelhor (2008) continued to expand his theory of the impact of child victimization. Hulme and Grove (1994) developed a map of Browne and Finkelhor's (1986) concepts and relationships and it is presented as follows.

Continued

As shown in the illustration below child sexual abuse is at the center of the adult survivor's existence. Arising from the abuse are four trauma-causing dynamics: traumatic sexualization, betrayal, powerlessness, and stigmatization. These traumagenic dynamics lead to behavioral manifestations and collectively indicate a history of child sexual abuse. The behavioral manifestations were operationalized as physical and psychosocial symptoms for the purposes of this study. Penetrating the core of the adult survivors are the contributing factors, including the characteristics of the child sexual abuse and other factors occurring later in the survivor's life, that affect the severity of behavioral manifestations (Follette, Alexander, & Follette, 1991). The contributing factors examined in this study were age when the abuse began, duration of the abuse, and other victimizations. Other victimizations included past or present physical and emotional abuse, rape, control by others, and prostitution. (Hulme & Grove, 1994, pp. 522-523)

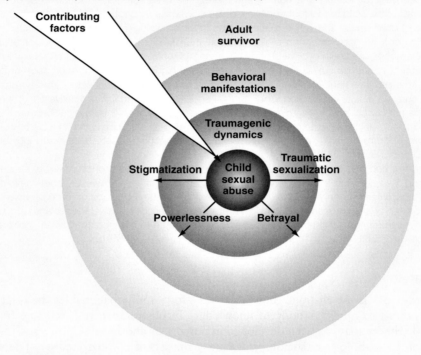

Long-term effects of child sexual abuse.
(Adapted from Hulme, P. A., & Grove, S. K. [1994]. Symptoms of female survivors of sexual abuse. *Issues in Mental Health Nursing*, 15[5], p. 123. Washington, DC: Taylor & Francis. Reproduced with permission. All rights reserved.)

Research Objectives, Questions, and Hypotheses

Investigators formulate research objectives, questions, or hypotheses to bridge the gap between the more abstractly stated research problem and purpose and the study design and plan for data collection and analysis. Objectives, questions, and hypotheses are narrower in focus than the purpose and often specify only one or two research variables. They also identify the relationship between the variables, and indicate the population to be studied. Some descriptive studies include only a research purpose, whereas others include a purpose and either objectives or questions to direct the study. Some correlational studies include a purpose and specific questions or hypotheses. Quasi-experimental and experimental studies need to include hypotheses to direct the conduct of the studies and the interpretation of findings. Chapter 5 provides guidelines for critically appraising the objectives, questions, and hypotheses in research reports.

Hulme and Grove (1994) developed the following research questions to direct their study:

1. What patterns of physical and psychosocial symptoms are present in women 18 to 40 years of age who have experienced child sexual abuse?
2. Are there relationships among the number of physical and psychosocial symptoms, the age when the abuse began, the duration of abuse, and [the] number of other victimizations? (p. 523)

Study Variables

The research purpose and the objectives, questions, or hypotheses identify the variables to be examined in a study. **Variables** are concepts at various levels of abstraction that are measured, manipulated, or controlled in a study. More concrete concepts, such as temperature, weight, or blood pressure are referred to as variables in a study. The more abstract concepts such as creativity, empathy, or social support sometimes are referred to as research concepts.

Researchers operationalize the variables or concepts in a study by identifying conceptual and operational definitions. A **conceptual definition** provides a variable or concept with theoretical meaning (Burns & Grove, 2009), and it either comes from a theorist's definition of the concept or is developed through concept analysis. The conceptual definitions of variables provide a link from selected concepts in the study framework to the study variables. Researchers develop an **operational definition** so that the variable can be measured or manipulated in a study. The knowledge gained from studying the variable will increase understanding of the theoretical concept from the study framework that the variable represents. Chapter 5 provides a more extensive discussion of variables.

Hulme and Grove (1994) provided conceptual and operational definitions of the study variables— physical and psychosocial symptoms, age when the abuse began, duration of abuse, and victimizations—identified in their purpose and/or research questions. Only the definitions for physical symptoms and victimizations are presented as examples.

Physical Symptoms

Conceptual definition

Physical symptoms are behavioral manifestations that result directly from the traumagenic dynamics of child sexual abuse (Browne & Finkelhor, 1986).

Operational definition

ASI Questionnaire was used to measure physical symptoms.

Victimizations

Conceptual definition

Experiences of any of multiple forms of abuse and betrayal, including past and present physical and emotional abuse, rape, control by others, and prostitution in an adult survivor of child abuse (Browne & Finkelhor, 1986).

Operational definition

ASI Questionnaire was used to measure victimizations.

Assumptions

Assumptions are statements that are taken for granted or are considered true, even though they have not been scientifically tested. Assumptions often are embedded (unrecognized) in thinking and behavior, and uncovering these assumptions requires introspection and a strong knowledge base in a research area. Sources of assumptions are universally accepted truths (e.g., "all humans are rational beings"), theories, previous research, and nursing practice. Two common assumptions in nursing research are: "People want to assume control of their health" and Health is a priority for most people" (Williams, 1980, p. 48).

In studies, assumptions are embedded in the philosophical base of the framework, study design, and interpretation of findings. Theories and research instruments are developed on the basis of assumptions that may or may not be recognized by the researcher. These assumptions influence the development and implementation of the research process. Thus, the recognition of assumptions by the researcher is a strength, not a weakness. Assumptions influence the logic of the study, and their recognition leads to more rigorous study development (Burns & Grove, 2009).

Hulme and Grove (1994) did not identify assumptions for their study, but the following assumptions seem to provide a basis for this study: (1) the child victim bears no responsibility for the sexual contact; (2) survivors can remember and are willing to report their past child sexual abuse; and (3) behavioral manifestations (physical and psychological symptoms) indicate altered health and functioning.

Limitations

Limitations are restrictions in a study that may decrease the credibility and generalizability of the findings. **Generalization** is the extension of the implications of the research findings from the sample studied to a larger population. For example, the findings from studying a sample of adult female survivors of child sexual abuse might be extended to a population of women who have survived child sexual abuse. The two types of limitations are theoretical and methodological. **Theoretical limitations** restrict the abstract generalization of the findings and are reflected in the study framework and the conceptual and operational definitions of the variables. Theoretical limitations might include (1) a concept that lacks clarity of definition in the theory used to develop the study framework; (2) the unclear relationships among some concepts in the theorist's work; (3) a study variable that lacks a clear link to a concept in the framework; and (4) an objective, question, or hypothesis that lacks a clear link to a relationship (or proposition) expressed in the study framework.

Methodological limitations can limit the credibility of the findings and restrict the population to which the findings can be generalized. Methodological limitations result from such factors as unrepresentative sample, weak design, single setting, limited control over treatment implementation, measurement instruments with limited reliability and validity, limited control over data collection, and improper use of statistical analyses.

Hulme and Grove (1994) identified the following methodological limitation.

... [T]his study has limited generalizability due to the relatively small nonprobability sample ... (p. 528). Additional replications drawing from various social classes and age groups are needed to improve the generalizability of Brown and Garrison's (1990) findings and establish reliability and validity of their tool. (p. 529)

Research Design

Research **design** is a blueprint for the conduct of a study that maximizes control over factors that could interfere with the study's desired outcome. The type of design directs the selection of a population, procedures for sampling, methods of measurement, and plans for data collection and analysis. The choice of research design depends on what is known and not known about the research problem, the researcher's expertise, the purpose of the study, and the intent to generalize the findings.

Sometimes the design of a study indicates that a pilot study was conducted. A **pilot study** is a smaller version of a proposed study, and researchers frequently conduct these to refine the methodology. Researchers might conduct pilot studies in a manner similar to that for the proposed study, using similar subjects, the same setting, the same treatment, and the same data collection and analysis techniques. Prescott and Soeken (1989), however, believe a pilot study can be conducted to develop and refine any of the steps in the research process. The reasons for conducting pilot studies are to:

1. Determine whether the proposed study is feasible. (For example, are the subjects available? Does the researcher have the time and money to do the study?)
2. Develop or refine a research treatment.
3. Develop a protocol for the implementation of a treatment.
4. Identify problems with the design.
5. Determine whether the sample is representative of the population or whether the sampling technique is effective. Hertzog (2008) provided sample size guidelines for pilot studies.
6. Examine the reliability and validity of the research instruments.
7. Develop or refine data collection instruments.
8. Refine the data collection and analysis plans.
9. Collect preliminary data.
10. Give the researcher experience with the subjects, setting, methodology, and methods of measurement.
11. Implement data analysis techniques.
12. Convince funding organizations that the research team is knowledgeable and competent to implement the study (Prescott & Soeken, 1989; van Teijlingen & Hundley, 2001).

Thus, conducting a pilot study is usually beneficial to strengthen the major study design. When critically appraising a study, note if a pilot study was conducted and how did the pilot study contribute to the conduct of the current study.

Designs have been developed to meet unique research needs as they emerge; thus, a variety of descriptive, correlational, quasi-experimental, and experimental designs have been generated over time. In descriptive and correlational studies, no treatment is administered, so the purposes of these study designs include improving the precision of measurement, describing what exists, and clarifying relationships that provide a basis for quasi-experimental and experimental studies. Quasi-experimental and experimental study designs usually involve treatment and control groups, and focus on achieving high levels of control as well as precision in measurement. A study's design usually is in the methodology section of a research report.

Hulme and Grove (1994) used a descriptive correlational design to direct their study. The diagram of the design, presented in the illustration below, indicates the variables described and the relationships examined. The findings generated from correlational research provide a basis for generating hypotheses for testing in future research.

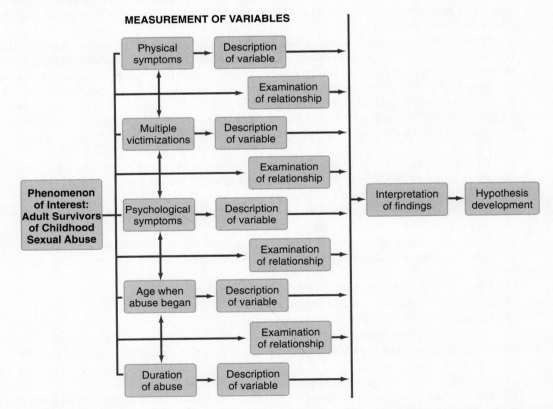

Proposed descriptive correlational design for Hulme and Grove's study of symptoms of female survivors of child sexual abuse.
(From Hulme, P. A., & Grove, S. K. [1994]. Symptoms of female survivors of sexual abuse. *Issues in Mental Health Nursing,* 15[5], p. 55. Reproduced with permission.)

Population and Sample

The **population** is all elements (individuals, objects, or substances) that meet certain criteria for inclusion in a study (Kerlinger & Lee, 2000). A **sample** is a subset of the population that is selected for a particular study, and the members of a sample are the subjects or participants. In many quantitative studies, the members of the study are referred to as subjects but the term participants is used to describe the individuals studied in qualitative research. **Sampling** defines the process of selecting a group of people, events, behaviors, or other elements with which to conduct a study. Chapter 9 provides you a background for critically appraising populations and samples in research reports.

The following excerpt identifies the sampling method, setting, sample size, population, sample criteria, and sample characteristics for the study conducted by Hulme and Grove (1994).

The convenience sample [sampling method] was obtained by advertising for subjects at three state universities in the southwest [setting]. Despite the sensitive nature of the study, 22 [sample size] usable interviews were obtained. The sample included women between the ages of 18 and 39 years ($\bar{X}$ = 28 years, SD = 6.5 years) [sample characteristics] who were identified as survivors of child sexual abuse [population] [sample criteria]. The majority of these women were white (91%) and students (82%). A little more than half (54%) were single, seven (32%) were divorced, and three (14%) were married. Most (64%) had no children. A small percentage (14%) was on some form of public assistance and only 14% had been arrested. Although 27% of the subjects had step family members, the parents of 14 subjects (64%) were still married. Half the fathers were working class or self-employed; the rest were professionals. Mothers were either working class or self-employed (50%), homemakers (27%), or professionals (11%). Most subjects (95%) had siblings, and 36% knew or suspected their siblings also had been abused [sample characteristics]. (pp. 523-524)

Methods of Measurement

Measurement is the process of assigning "numbers to objects (or events or situations) in accord with some rule" (Kaplan, 1964, p. 177). A component of measurement is instrumentation, which is the application of specific rules to the development of a measurement device or instrument. An instrument is selected to measure a specific variable in a study. The numerical data generated with an instrument may be at the nominal, ordinal, interval, or ratio level of measurement. The level of measurement, with nominal being the lowest form of measurement and ratio being the highest, determines the type of statistical analysis that can be performed on the data (Grove, 2007). Chapter 10 introduces you to the concept of measurement, describes different types of measurement methods, and provides you direction to critically appraise measurement techniques in studies.

Hulme and Grove (1994) used the ASI Questionnaire to measure their study variables.

The ASI Questionnaire contains 10 sections: demographics; family origin; educational history, occupational history and public assistance; legal history; characteristics of the child sexual abuse (duration, perpetrator, pregnancy, type, and threats); past and present other victimizations; past and present physical symptoms; past and present psychosocial symptoms; and relationship with own children. Each section is followed by a response set that includes space for 'other'. Content validity was established by Brown and Garrison (1990) using an in-depth review of 132 clinical records. ... For this descriptive correlational study ... content validity of the tool was examined by asking an open-ended question: "Is there additional information you would like to share?" (p. 524)

Data Collection

Data collection is the precise, systematic gathering of information relevant to the research purpose or the specific objectives, questions, or hypotheses of a study. To collect data, the researcher must obtain permission from the setting or agency where the study will be conducted. Researchers must also obtain consent from all research subjects to indicate their willingness to participate in the study. Frequently, the researcher asks the subject to sign a consent form, which describes the study, promises the subject confidentiality, and indicates that the subject can withdraw from the study at any time. The research report should document permission from an agency to conduct a study and consent from the subject to participate in the study (see Chapter 4).

During data collection, investigators will use a variety of techniques for measuring study variables, such as observation, interview, questionnaires, or scales. In an increasing number of studies, nurses are measuring physiological variables with high-technology equipment. Researchers collect and systematically record data on each subject, organizing the data in a way that facilitates computer entry. Data collection is usually described in the "Methodology" section of a research report under the subheading of "Procedures."

Hulme and Grove (1994) identified the following procedure for data collection.

Although the tool can be self-reporting, it was administered by personal interview to allow for elaboration of 'other' responses. The interviews lasted about one hour and were conducted in a private room provided by The University of Texas at Arlington. Each interview started with a discussion of the study benefits and risks and included signing a consent form. Risks included possible painful memories, anger, and sadness during the interview as well as emotional and physical discomfort after the interview. Sources of public and private counseling were provided to assist subjects with any difficulties experienced related to the study. (pp. 524-525)

Data Analysis

Data analysis reduces, organizes, and gives meaning to the data. Analysis techniques conducted in quantitative research include descriptive and inferential analyses (see Chapter 11) and some sophisticated, advanced analyses. Investigators base their choice of analysis techniques primarily on the research objectives, questions, or hypotheses, and the level of measurement achieved by the research instruments. You can find the data analysis process in the "Results" section of the research report; this section usually is organized by the research objectives, questions, or hypotheses.

Hulme and Grove (1994) used frequencies, percents, means, standard deviations, and Pearson correlations to address their research questions.

RESULTS

The first research question focused on patterns of physical and psychosocial symptoms. Six physical symptoms occurred in 50% or more of the subjects: insomnia, sexual dysfunction, overeating, drug abuse, severe headache, and two or more major surgeries. ... Eleven psychosocial symptoms occurred in 75% or more of the subjects: depression, guilt, low self-esteem, inability to trust others, mood swings, suicidal thoughts, difficulty in relationships, confusion, flashbacks of the abuse, extreme anger, and memory lapse. ... Self-injurious behavior was reported by eight subjects (33%). (pp. 527-528)

The second research question focused on the relationships among the number of physical and psychosocial symptoms and three contributing factors (age abuse began, duration of abuse, and other victimizations). There were five significant correlations among study variables: physical symptoms with other victimizations ($r = 0.59$, $p = 0.002$), physical symptoms with psychosocial symptoms ($r = 0.56$, $p = 0.003$), age abuse began with duration of abuse ($r = -0.50$, $p = 0.009$), psychosocial symptoms with other victimizations ($r = 0.40$, $p = 0.033$), and duration of abuse with psychosocial symptoms ($r = 0.40$, $p = 0.034$). (p. 528)

Research Outcomes

The results obtained from data analyses require interpretation to be meaningful. **Interpretation of research outcomes** involves examining the results from data analysis, exploring the significance of the findings, forming conclusions, generalizing the findings, considering the implications for nursing, and suggesting further studies. You can find the research outcomes in the "Discussion" section of a research report.

Hulme and Grove (1994) provided the following discussion of their findings, with implications for nursing and suggestions for further study.

DISCUSSION

While this study may have limited generalizability due to the relatively small nonprobability sample, the findings do support previous research. ... In addition, the findings support Browne and Finkelhor's (1986) framework that a wide range of behavioral manifestations (physical and psychosocial symptoms) comprise the long-term effects of child sexual abuse. (p. 528)

Brown and Garrison's (1990) ASI Questionnaire was effective in identifying patterns of physical and psychosocial symptoms in women with a history of child sexual abuse. ... As data on the behavioral manifestations (physical and psychosocial symptoms) and the effect of each of the contributing factors accumulate, hypotheses need to be formulated to further test Browne and Finkelhor's (1986) framework explaining the long-term effects of child sexual abuse. ... With additional research, the ASI Questionnaire might be adapted for use in clinical situations. This questionnaire might facilitate identification and delivery of appropriate treatment to female survivors of child sexual abuse in clinical settings. (pp. 529-530)

Reading Research Reports

Understanding the steps of the research process and learning new terms related to those steps will assist you in reading research reports. A **research report** summarizes the major elements of a study and identifies the contributions of that study to nursing knowledge. Research reports are presented at professional meetings and conferences and are published in journals and books. These reports often are overwhelming to nursing students and new graduates. Maybe you have had difficulty locating research articles or understanding the content of these articles. Research reports usually are written to communicate with other researchers, not with clinicians. Thus, the style of the report often is technical, and the report sometimes is filled with jargon, which is very confusing to students and practicing nurses. We would like to help you overcome some of these barriers and assist you in understanding the research literature by (1) identifying sources that publish research reports, (2) describing the content of a research report, and (3) providing tips for reading the research literature.

Sources of Research Reports

The most common sources for nursing research reports are professional journals. Research reports are the major focus of several nursing research journals: *Advances in Nursing Science, Applied Nursing Research, Biological Research for Nursing, Clinical Nursing Research: An International Journal, Journal of Nursing Scholarship, International Journal of Nursing Studies, Nursing Research, Nursing Science Quarterly, Qualitative Health Research, Qualitative Nursing Research, Research in Nursing & Health, Scholarly Inquiry for Nursing Practice: An International Journal,* and *Western Journal of Nursing Research.* Two journals in particular, *Applied Nursing Research* and *Clinical Nursing Research,* focus on communicating research findings to practicing nurses. Thus, these journals usually include less detail on the framework, methodology, and the statistical results of a study and more on discussion of the findings and the implications for practice. *Worldviews on Evidence-Based Nursing* is a journal published in 2004 that focuses on innovative ideas for using evidence to improve patient care globally.

Many of the nursing clinical specialty journals also place a high priority on publishing research findings. Table 2–3 identifies the clinical journals in which research reports constitute a major portion of the journal content. More than 100 nursing journals are published in the United States, and most of them include research articles.

Some research reports, such as those for complex qualitative studies, are lengthy and might be published as books or as chapters in books. Research reports of master's degree candidates are presented as theses. Doctoral candidates produce dissertations summarizing their research projects. Before publication, many research reports are presented at local, national, and international nursing and healthcare conferences. Often, brochures for conferences will indicate whether research reports are part of the program. The findings from many studies are now communicated through the Internet as journals are placed online, and selected websites include the most current healthcare research.

Table 2-3	Clinical Journals That Focus on Research Articles

Clinical Journals

American Journal of Alzheimer's Care & Related Disorders and Research
Birth
Cardiovascular Nursing
Computers in Nursing
Heart & Lung: The Journal of Acute and Critical Care
Issues in Comprehensive Pediatric Nursing
Issues in Mental Health Nursing
Journal of Child and Adolescent Psychiatric and Mental Health Nursing
Journal of Continuing Education in Nursing
Journal of Holistic Nursing
Journal of National Black Nurses' Association
Journal of Nursing Education
Journal of Pediatric Nursing: Nursing Care of Children and Families
Journal of Transcultural Nursing
Maternal-Child Nursing Journal
Nursing Diagnosis
Public Health Nursing
Rehabilitation Nursing
The Diabetes Educator

Content of Research Reports

At this point, you may be overwhelmed by the seeming complexity of a research report. You will find it easier to read and comprehend these reports if you understand each of the component parts. A research report often includes six parts: (1) "Abstract," (2) "Introduction," (3) "Methods," (4) "Results," (5) "Discussion," and (6) "References." These parts are described in this section, and the study by Twiss, Waltman, Berg, Ott, Gross, and Lindsey (2009) that examined the effects of an exercise intervention on the muscle strength and balance of breast cancer survivors with bone loss is presented as an example.

Abstract

The report usually begins with an **abstract**, which is a clear, concise summary of a study (Burns & Grove, 2009; Crosby, 1990). Abstracts range from 100 to 250 words and usually include the study purpose, design, setting, sample size, major results, and conclusions. Researchers hope their abstracts will concisely convey the findings from their study and capture your attention so that you will read the entire report.

Usually, four major content sections of a research report follow the abstract: "Introduction," "Methods," "Results," and "Discussion." Table 2–4 outlines the content covered in each of these sections. It is also briefly discussed in the following sections.

Table 2–4	Major Sections of a Research Report

Introduction
Statement of the problem, with background and significance
Statement of the purpose
Brief literature review
Identification of the framework
Identification of the research objectives, questions, or hypotheses (if applicable)

Methods
Identification of the research design
Description of the treatment or intervention (if applicable)
Description of the sample and setting
Description of the methods of measurement (including reliability and validity)
Discussion of the data collection process

Results
Description of the data analysis procedures
Presentation of results in tables, figures, or narrative organized by the purpose(s) and/or objectives,
  questions, or hypotheses

Discussion
Discussion of major findings
Identification of the limitations
Presentation of conclusions
Implications of the findings for nursing practice
Recommendations for further research

RESEARCH EXAMPLE Abstract

Twiss and colleagues (2009) developed the following clear, comprehensive abstract, which conveys the critical information about their quasi-experimental study and also includes the study's clinical relevance. However, the abstract might be considered a little long at 325 words.

PURPOSE

(a) to determine if 110 postmenopausal breast cancer survivors (BCS) with bone loss who participated in 24 months of strength and weight training (ST) exercises had improved muscle strength and balance and had fewer falls compared to BCS who did not exercise; and (b) to describe type and frequency of ST exercises; adverse effects of exercises; and participants' adherence to exercise at home, at fitness centers, and at 36-month follow-up.

DESIGN

Findings reported are from a federally funded multi-component intervention study of 223 postmenopausal BCS with either osteopenia or osteoporosis who were randomly assigned to an exercise ($n = 110$) or comparison ($n = 113$) groups.

METHODS

Time points for testing outcomes were baseline, 6, 12, and 24 months into intervention. Muscle strength was tested using Biodex Velocity Spectrum Evaluation, and dynamic balance using Timed Backward

Tandem Walk. Adherence to exercises was measured using self-report of number of prescribed sessions attended and participants' reports of falls.

FINDINGS

Mean adherence over 24 months was 69.4%. Using generalized estimating equation (GEE) analyses, compared to participants not exercising, participants who exercised for 24 months had significantly improve hip flexion ($p = 0.011$), hip extension ($p = 0.0006$), knee flexion ($p < 0.0001$), knee extension ($p = 0.0018$), wrist flexion ($p = 0.031$), and balance ($p = 0.010$). Gains in muscle strength were 9.5% and 28.5% for hip flexion and extension, 50.0% and 19.4% for wrist flexion and extension, and 21.1% and 11.6% for knee flexion and extension. Balance improved by 39.4%. Women who exercised had fewer falls, but difference in number of falls between the two groups was not significant.

CONCLUSIONS

Many postmenopausal BCS with bone loss can adhere to a 24 month ST exercise intervention, and exercises can result in meaningful gains in muscle strength and balance.

CLINICAL RELEVANCE

More studies are needed for examining relationships between muscle strength and balance in postmenopausal BCS with bone loss and their incidence of falls and fractures (Twiss et al., 2009, p. 20).

Introduction

The Introduction section of a research report identifies the nature and scope of the problem being investigated and provides a case for the conduct of the study. You should be able to clearly identify the significance of conducting the study to generate knowledge for nursing practice. Twiss and colleagues' (2009) study was significant because an estimated 182,460 women in the United States are diagnosed with breast cancer each year and these women are at risk for osteoporosis because of their cancer therapies. An exercise intervention could be an effective way to increase these women's muscle strength and balance and decrease their falls. The purpose of this study was clearly stated in the abstract.

Depending on the type of research report, the literature review and the framework may be separate sections or part of the introduction. The literature review documents the current knowledge of the problem investigated and includes the sources that were used to develop the study and interpret the findings. For example, Twiss et al. (2009) summarized the literature in a Background section that included research in the areas of ST exercises, adherence to exercise, adverse effects of exercise, muscle strength, balance, and falls. A research report also needs to include a framework, but only about half of the published studies identify one. Twiss et al. (2009) did not identify a framework for their study. The inclusion of a physiological framework that focused on the impact of exercise on the physiological function of the musculoskeletal system would have strengthened this study. The relationships in the framework provide a basis for the formulation of hypotheses to be tested in quasi-experimental and experimental studies.

Investigators often end the introduction by identifying the objectives, questions, or hypotheses that they used to direct the study. However, the Twiss et al. (2009) study lacked a framework and no hypotheses were developed to direct this quasi-experimental study.

Methods

The Methods section of a research report describes how the study was conducted and usually includes the study design, treatment (if appropriate), sample, setting, methods of measurement, and data collection process. This section of the report needs to be presented in enough detail so that the reader can critically appraise the adequacy of the study methods to produce reliable findings (Tornquist, Funk, Champagne, & Wiese, 1993).

Twiss et al. (2009) provided extensive coverage of their study methodology. The design was clearly identified as a multisite, randomized controlled trial. They also included the subsection Sample, which described the population, sampling method, sample criteria, sample size, and attrition and reasons for withdrawing from the study. Institutional approval for the conduct of this study and consent of the participants and their physicians were also discussed in this subsection. A subsection Setting was included that clearly indicated the sites where the study was conducted.

ST Exercises was another subsection and provided a detailed description of the exercise intervention and how it was implemented in this study. A protocol for the intervention was also included in a table in the article. Measures was another subsection of the study methodology that detailed the quality of the measurement methods used to measure the dependent variables of muscle strength, balance, falls, adherence to the exercise sessions, and any adverse effects from the exercise. The measurements used in this study were identified previously in the study abstract. The Methods section concluded with a subsection Statistical Analysis that detailed the analysis techniques used to analyze the study data.

Results

The Results section presents the outcomes of the statistical tests used to analyze the study data and the significance of these outcomes. The research purpose or objectives, questions, and hypotheses formulated for the study are used to organize this section. Researchers identify the statistical analyses conducted to address the purpose or each objective, question, or hypothesis, and present the specific results obtained from the analyses in tables, figures, or narrative of the report (Burns & Grove, 2009). Focusing more on the summary of the study results and their significance than on the statistical results can help to reduce the confusion that may be caused by the numbers.

Twiss and colleagues' (2009) had a Findings section that might have been more clearly identified as "Results." This section began with a description of the sample and the sample characteristics were presented in a table. The study results were organized by the study variables of adverse effects of exercises, adherence to exercises, muscle strength and balance, and falls. As indicated in the abstract, the study results were significant for all study variables except falls.

Discussion

The Discussion section ties together the other sections of the research report and gives them meaning. This section includes the major findings, limitations of the study, conclusions drawn from the findings, implications of the findings for nursing, and recommendations for further research.

Twiss et al. (2009) discussed their findings in detail, and compared and contrasted them with the findings of previous research. They also included a separate section in the study, Limitations, which included the following: participants were not obtaining sufficient vitamin D, stronger intervention fidelity was needed, self-report of adherence often results in an overestimation of true levels of adherence, a lack of test-retest reliability for the investigator-developed instruments used in the study, and the small number of minority women who completed the study were not representative of this Midwestern state.

The Discussion section also included a subsection Conclusions that presented the implications for practice and identified the future studies needed. The conclusions drawn from a research project can be useful in at least three different ways. First, you can use the intervention or treatment tested in a study with patients to improve their care and promote a positive health outcome. Second, reading research reports might change your view of a patient's situation or give you greater insight into the situation. Last, studies heighten your awareness of the problems experienced by patients and assist you in assessing and working toward solutions for these problems. Twiss and colleagues (2009) also provided a Clinical Resources section that included websites with research evidence about osteoporosis, breast cancer, and BCS support that would be useful for your practice.

References

A References section that includes all sources cited in the research report follows the Discussion section. The reference list includes the studies, theories, and methodology resources that provide a basis for the conduct of the study. These sources provide an opportunity to read about the research problem in greater depth. We strongly encourage you to read the Twiss et al. (2009) article to identify the sections of a research report and to examine the content in each of these sections. These researchers detailed a rigorously conducted quasi-experimental study, provided findings that are supportive of previous research, and identified conclusions that provide sound evidence to direct the care of patients who are breast cancer survivors with bone loss.

Tips for Reading Research Reports

When you start reading research reports, you may be overwhelmed by the new terms and complex information presented. We hope that you will not be discouraged but will see the challenge of examining new knowledge generated through research. You probably will need to read the report slowly two or three times. You can also use the glossary at the end of this book to review the definitions of unfamiliar terms. We recommend that you read the abstract first and then the Discussion section of the report. This approach will enable you to determine the relevance of the findings to you personally and to your practice. Initially, your focus should be on research reports you believe can provide relevant knowledge for your practice.

Reading a research report requires the use of a variety of critical thinking skills, such as skimming, comprehending, and analyzing, to facilitate an understanding of the study (Wilkinson, 2006). **Skimming a research report** involves quickly reviewing the source to gain a broad overview of the content. Try this approach: First, familiarize yourself with the title and check the author's name. Next, scan the Abstract or Introduction and the Discussion section. Knowing the findings of the study will provide you with a standard for evaluating the rest of the article (Tornquist et al., 1993). Then read the major headings and perhaps one or two sentences under each heading. Finally, reexamine the conclusions and implications for practice from the study. Skimming enables you to make a preliminary judgment about the value of a source and a determination about reading the report in depth.

Comprehending a research report requires that the entire study be read carefully. During this reading, focus on understanding major concepts and the logical flow of ideas within the study. You may wish to highlight information about the researchers, such as their education, their current positions, and any funding they received for the study. As you read the study, steps of the research process also might be highlighted. Record any notes in the margin so that you can easily identify the problem, purpose, framework, major variables, study design, treatment, sample, measurement methods, data collection process, analysis techniques, results, and study outcomes. Also record any creative ideas or questions you have in the margin of the report.

We encourage you to highlight the parts of the article that you do not understand and ask your instructor or other nurse researchers for clarification. Your greatest difficulty in reading the research report probably will be in understanding the statistical analyses. Information in Chapter 11 should help you comprehend the analyses. Basically, you must identify the particular statistics used, the results from each statistical analysis, and the meaning of the results. Statistical analyses describe variables, examine relationships among variables, or determine differences among groups. The study purpose or specific objectives, questions, or hypotheses indicate whether the focus is on description, relationships, or differences. Therefore, you need to link each analysis technique to its results and then to the study purpose or objectives, questions, or hypotheses presented in the study.

The final reading skill, **analyzing a research report**, involves determining the value of the report's content. Break the content of the report into parts, and examine the parts in depth for accuracy, completeness, uniqueness of information, and organization. Note whether the steps of the research process build logically on each other or whether steps are missing or incomplete. Examine the discussion section of the report to determine whether the researchers have provided a critical argument for using the study findings in practice. Using the skills of skimming, comprehending, and analyzing while reading research reports will increase your comfort with studies, allow you to become an informed consumer of research, and expand your knowledge for making changes in practice. These skills for reading research reports are essential for conducting a comprehensive critical appraisal of a study. Chapter 12 focuses on the guidelines for critically appraising quantitative and qualitative studies.

Practice Reading Quasi-experimental and Experimental Studies

Knowing the parts of the research report—introduction, methods, results, and discussion—provides a basis for reading research reports of quantitative studies. You can apply the critical thinking skills of skimming, comprehending, and analyzing to your reading of the example quasi-experimental and experimental studies provided here. Being able to read research reports and identify the steps of the research process should enable you to conduct an initial critical appraisal of a report. Throughout this book you'll find boxes, entitled Critical Appraisal Guidelines, which provide questions you will want to consider in your critical appraisal of various research elements. This chapter concludes with critical appraisals of both a quasi-experimental study and an experimental study.

INITIAL CRITICAL APPRAISAL GUIDELINES

Quantitative Research

The following questions are important in conducting an initial critical appraisal of a quantitative research report.

1. What type of quantitative study was conducted: descriptive, correlational, quasi-experimental, or experimental?
2. Can you identify the following sections in the research report: Introduction, Methods, Results, and Discussion as identified in Table 2–4?
3. Were the steps of the study clearly identified? Figure 2–1 identifies the steps of the quantitative research process.
4. Were any of the steps of the research process missing?

Quasi-experimental Study

The purpose of *quasi-experimental research* is to examine cause-and-effect relationships among selected independent and dependent variables. Researchers conduct quasi-experimental studies in nursing to determine the effects of nursing interventions or treatments (independent variables) on patient outcomes (dependent variables) (Cook & Campbell, 1979). Artinian et al. (2007) conducted a quasi-experimental study to determine the effects of nurse-managed telemonitoring (TM) on the blood pressure (BP) of African Americans. The steps for this study are described here and illustrated with extracts from the study.

RESEARCH EXAMPLE Quasi-experimental Study

Steps of the Research Process in a Quasi-experimental Study

1. Introduction

Research Problem

Nearly one in three, or approximately 65 million adults in the United States have hypertension, defined as (a) having systolic blood pressure (SBP) of 140 mm Hg or higher or diastolic blood pressure (DBP) of at least 90 mm Hg or higher, (b) taking antihypertensive medication, or (c) being told at least twice by a physician or other health professional about having high blood pressure (BP) (American Heart Association [AHA], 2004; AHA Statistics Committee & Stroke Statistics Subcommittee [AHASC], 2006; Fields et al., 2004). … Estimated direct and indirect costs associated with hypertension total $63.5 billion (AHA, 2004). … The crisis of high BP (HBP) is particularly apparent among African Americans; their prevalence of HBP is among the highest in the world … Unless healthcare professionals can improve care for individuals with hypertension, approximately two thirds of the population will continue to have uncontrolled BP and face other major health risks (Chobanian et al., 2003). … There is a need to test alternative treatment strategies. (Artinian et al., 2007, pp. 312-313)

Research Purpose

The purpose of this randomized controlled trial with urban African Americans was to compare usual care (UC) only with BP telemonitoring (TM) plus UC to determine which leads to greater reduction in BP from baseline over 12 months of follow-up, with assessments at 3, 6, and 12 months postbaseline. (Artinian et al., 2007, p. 313)

Literature Review

The literature review for this study included relevant, current studies that summarized what is known about the impact of TM on BP. The sources were current and ranged in publication dates from 1998 to 2005, with the majority of the studies published in the last 5 years. The study was accepted for publication on May 31, 2007 and published in the September/October 2007 issue of *Nursing Research*. Artinian et al. (2007, p. 314) summarized the current knowledge about the effect of TM on BP by stating, "Although promising, the effects of TM on BP have been tested in small, sometimes nonrandomized, samples, with one study suggesting that patients may not always adhere to measuring their BP at home. The influence of TM on BP control warrants further study."

Framework

Artinian et al. (2007) developed a model that identified the theoretical basis for their study. The model is presented in Figure 2–2 and indicates that "Nurse-managed TM is an innovative strategy that may offer hope to hypertensive African Americans who have difficulty accessing care for frequent BP checks … In other words, TM may lead to a reduction in opportunity costs or barriers for obtaining follow-up care by minimizing the contextual risk factors that interfere with frequent healthcare visits. … Combined with information about how to control hypertension, TM may both help individuals gain conscious control over their HBP and contribute to feelings of confidence for carrying out hypertension self-care actions. … Home TM appeared to contribute to individuals' increased personal control and self-responsibility for managing their BP, which ultimately led to improved BP control (Artinian et al., 2004; Artinian, Washington, & Templin, 2001)." (Artinian et al., 2007, pp. 313-314). The framework for this study was

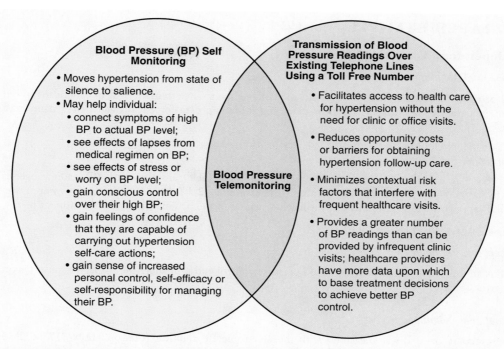

Figure 2–2. Theoretical basis for the effects of telemonitoring on blood pressure. From Artinian, N. T., Flack, J. M., Nordstrom, C. K., Hockman, E. M., Washington, O. G. M., Jen, K. C., & Fathy, M. (2007). Effects of nurse-managed telemonitoring on blood pressure at 12-month follow-up among urban African Americans. *Nursing Research, 56*(5), p. 313, Figure 2 in this publication.

based on tentative theory that was develop from the findings of previous research by Artinian et al. (2001; 2004) and other investigators. This framework provides a basis for interpreting the study findings and giving them meaning.

Hypothesis Testing

H1: Individuals who participate in UC plus nurse-managed TM will have a greater reduction in BP from baseline at 3-, 6-, and 12-month follow-up than would individuals who receive UC only. (Artinian et al., 2007, p. 317)

Variables

The independent variable was TM Program and the dependent variables were SBP and DBP. Only the TM Program and SBP are defined with conceptual and operational definitions. The conceptual definitions are derived from the study framework and the operational definitions are often found in the methods section under measurement methods and intervention headings.

Continued

RESEARCH EXAMPLE—cont'd

Independent Variable: TM Program

Conceptual Definition

TM program is an innovative strategy that may offer hope to hypertensive African Americans to reduce their opportunity costs and barriers for obtaining follow-up care for BP management (Artinian et al., 2007).

Operational Definition

TM "refers to individuals self-monitoring their BP at home, then transmitting the BP readings over existing telephone lines using a toll-free number" (Artinian et al., 2007, p. 313). The readings were reviewed by the care providers with immediate feedback provided to the patients about their treatment plan.

Dependent Variable: SBP

Conceptual Definition

SBP is an indication of the patient's blood pressure control and ultimately the management of his or her hypertension.

Operational Definition

The outcome of SBP was measured with the electronic BP monitor (Omron HEM-737 Intellisense, Omron Health Care, Inc., Bannockburn, IL) (Artinian et al., 2007).

2. Methods

Design

"A randomized, two-group, experimental, longitudinal design was used. The treatment group received nurse-managed TM and the control group received enhanced UC. Data were collected at baseline and 3-, 6-, and 12-month follow-ups" (Artinian et al., 2007, p. 314).

Sample

"African Americans with hypertension [population] were recruited through free BP screenings offered at community centers, thrift stores, drug stores, and grocery stores located on the east side of Detroit" [natural settings] (Artinian et al., 2007, p. 315). The sample criteria for including and excluding subjects from the study were detailed and provided a means of identifying patients with hypertension. The sample size was 387 (194 in the TM group and 193 in the UC group) with a 13% attrition or loss of subjects over the 12-month study. The subjects' recruitment and participation in the study are detailed in a figure in the article (see Artinian et al., 2007, p. 316).

Intervention

Artinian et al. (2007) detailed the nurse-managed TM intervention on pages 315-316 of their research article. LifeLink Monitoring, Inc. (Bearsville, NY) was used to provide the TM services for this study. The researchers also describe the enhanced UC (usual care) that was received by both the experimental and control groups.

Outcome Measurement

The BP was measured with the electronic Omron BP monitor "after a 5-minute rest period; at least two BPs were measured, and the average of all was used for analyses. Participants wore unrestrictive clothing and sat next to the interviewer's table, their feet on the floor; their back supported; and their arm abducted, slightly flexed, and supported at heart level by the smooth, firm surface of a table" (Artinian et al., 2007, pp. 316-317).

Data Collection

"Most of the data were collected during 2-hour structured face-to-face interviews and brief physical exams, which were conducted by trained interviewers in a private room at one of the project-affiliated neighborhood community centers. Mailed postcards provided interview appointment reminders 1 week before the scheduled interview; telephone call reminders were made the evening before the interview. ... Participants were compensated $25.00 after the completion of each interview" (Artinian et al., 2007, p. 316). The study was approved by the Wayne State University Human Investigation Committee and all participants signed consent forms indicating their willingness to be subjects in the study.

3. Results

"The hypothesis was supported partially by the data. Overall, the TM intervention group had a greater reduction in SBP (13.0 mm Hg) than the UC group did (7.5 mm Hg; $t = -2.09$, $p = .04$) from baseline to the 12-month follow-up. Although the TM intervention group had a greater reduction in the DBP (6.3 mm Hg) compared with the UC group (4.1 mm Hg), the differences were not statistically significant ($t = -1.56$, $p = .12$)" (Artinian et al., 2007, pp. 317-318).

4. Discussion

"The nurse-managed TM group experienced both clinically and statistically significant reductions in SBP (13.0 mm Hg) and clinically significant reductions in DBP (6.3 mm Hg) over a 12-month monitoring period [study conclusions]. ... The BP reductions achieved here are important results, which, if maintained over time, could improve care and outcomes significantly for urban African Americans with hypertension. ... This may mean that an individual could avoid starting a drug regimen or may achieve BP control using a one-drug regimen rather than a two-drug regimen and thus be at risk for fewer medication side effects [implications of the findings for nursing practice]. ... Future research needs to determine if this intervention effect maintained over time leads to reducing the number of complications associated with uncontrolled BP and if it leads to reducing the number of drugs necessary to achieve BP control" (Artinian et al., 2007, pp. 320-321).

INITIAL CRITICAL APPRAISAL

Quasi-experimental Study

Artinian and colleagues (2007) presented a clear, concise, and comprehensive report of their quasi-experimental study of the effect of TM on BP in urban African Americans. Artinian et al. also clearly organized their research article using the four major sections: introduction, methods, results, and discussion. Each section clearly detailed the steps of the quantitative research process and no steps of the research process were omitted.

Experimental Study

The purpose of experimental research is to examine cause-and-effect relationships between independent and dependent variables under highly controlled conditions. The planning and implementation of experimental studies are highly controlled by the researcher, and often these studies are conducted in a laboratory setting on animals or objects. Few nursing studies are "purely" experimental. Lee, Lin, Chao, Lin, Harn, and Chen (2007) conducted an experimental study of the effects of high-density lipoprotein (HDL) on organ damage in rats with sepsis. We encourage you to read this study, identify the sections of the research report, determine the steps of the quantitative research process, and then compare your findings with those presented in this section.

RESEARCH EXAMPLE Experimental Study

Steps of the Research Process in an Experimental Study

1. Introduction

Research Problem

Sepsis from gram-negative bacteria produces a systemic inflammatory reaction that is overwhelming and life threatening, in part, due to the bacterial release of endotoxins. Endotoxemia is associated with the progressive release of proinflammatory mediators that aggravate multiple organ dysfunctions. Despite enormous investments in intensive care, septic shock has been associated with mortality rates ranging from 20% to 46%). ... HDL and low-density lipoprotein cholesterol (LDL) are two major components in the lipoprotein family. There is evidence that plasma cholesterol levels, especially HDL, are lower in patients with sepsis, particularly in non-survivors (Giovannini, Chiarla, & Greco, 2003). ... No evidence was available indicating whether an increase in HDL or LDL before endotoxemia can prevent organ damage in gram-negative sepsis. (Lee et al., 2007, pp. 250-251)

Research Purpose

This laboratory study "was designed using an animal model to mimic people who had a high HDL level and to test HDL effects on preventing organ damage in endotoxemia" (Lee et al., 2007, p. 250).

Review of Literature

The literature review included current sources, based on the publication of the study in 2007, with publication dates that ranged from 1999 to 2005. This article was accepted for publication in November 2006 and published in June of 2007. The literature review included mainly studies focused on therapeutic interventions to reduce sepsis and prevent organ damage in endotoxemia. The researchers also covered studies that described the anti-inflammatory effects of HDL in sepsis and the link of HDL levels in patients with sepsis, particularly the non-survivors.

Lee et al. (2007) did not identify a framework for their study but the study seemed to be based on the physiology of HDL and the pathology of sepsis and organ damage in endotoxemia, which were presented in the literature review. The framework provides relationships that guide the development of study hypotheses for experimental studies (Burns & Grove, 2009). No hypotheses were identified to direct the conduct of this experimental study.

Variables

Endotoxemia was induced by an infusion of lipopolysaccharide (LPS) of *Klebsiella pneumoniae*. The two independent (treatment) variables were infusion of HDL and LDL into the rats' femoral arteries. The dependent (outcome) variables were plasma levels of tumor necrosis factor alpha (TNF-α), white blood cells (WBCs), and platelets. Other dependent variables include parameters "typically used to evaluate the clinical status of multiple organ functions, such as AST [aspartate aminotransferase] and ALT [alanine aminotransferase] for hepatic function, BUN [blood urea nitrogen] and Cr [creatine] for renal, LDL [lactate dehydrogenase] and CPK [creatine phosphokinase] for cardiac function and possibly other organ functions, and amylase for pancreatic function" (Lee et al., 2007, p. 252). Conceptual and operational definitions are provided for HDL and BUN only as examples.

Conceptual Definition of HDL is a lipoprotein cholesterol with an anti-inflammatory effect in sepsis.
Operational Definition of HDL is intravenous (IV) infusion of 1 mg of HDL in 1 mL of sterile physiological
  saline solution (PSS) into the femoral arteries of rats.
Conceptual Definition of BUN is the blood urea nitrogen plasma level that is reflective of organ damage to
  the kidney.
Operational Definition of BUN plasma level was "measured with an autoanalyzer (Vitros 750, Johnson-
  Johnson Co., New Brunswick, NJ)" (Lee et al., 2007, p. 252).

2. Materials and Methods

Sample and Setting

Lee and colleagues (2007) clearly described the approval of their study by the University Committee for Animal Use and Care. The sample included 32 rats that were purchased from the National Laboratory Animal Center. The animals were housed in the University Animal Center where the environment was highly controlled. "Room temperature was kept at 22 ± 1° C with a 12-hour light/dark cycle. Food and water were provided" (setting) (Lee et al., p. 251). The rats' preparation for the study and their IV exposure to LPS to induce endotoxemia were described in detail.

Experimental Design

Lee et al. (2007) described in depth the experimental design used to conduct their study. The design included four groups of eight rats each: (1) the PSS or control group that received PSS only, (2) the LPS grouped received LPS only, (3) the HDL group received 1 mg of HDL in 1 mL PSS before the LPS administration, and (4) the LDL group received 1 mg of LDL in 1 mL PSS before the LPS administration.

Measurements

Lee et al. (2007) provided detailed descriptions of the measurement of the dependent variables. "The amount of TNF-α in the plasma (100L) was diluted (1:2) and measured using Quantikine M ELISA kits (R & D Systems, Minneapolis, MN)" (p. 251). The "WBCs and platelets (Sysmex K-1000, NY) were measured by immediate centrifugation of the blood at 12,000 rpm for 5 minutes" (p. 252). The plasma levels of "AST, ALT, BUN, Cr, LDH, CPK, and amylase were measured with autoanalyzer (Vitros 750, Johnson-Johnson Co., New Brunswick, NJ)" (p. 252). In addition, "animals were sacrificed by decapitation at the end of the experiment. The liver, the heart, and the lung were excised and stored immediately in 10% formaldehyde. The tissues were subsequently embedded in paraffin, sectioned using microtome (5 m), stained with hematoxylin and eosin (H&E) and microscopically examined" (Lee et al., 2007, p. 252).

Continued

RESEARCH EXAMPLE—cont'd

3. Results

Detailed results are presented for the four groups of rats for all dependent variables (TNF-α, WBCs, platelets, AST, ALT, BUN, Cr, LDH, CPK, and amylase). The results were presented in complex line figures, tables, and narrative. The results indicated that HDL had a significant effect in preventing organ damage in endotoxemia. The researchers also presented pictures of the liver, heart, and lung tissues for the four groups (LPS, LDL, HDL, and PSS). "In the heart and lung, inflammatory changes were found in the LPS group. ... LDL worsened these pathological changes but HDL improved them" (Lee et al., p. 258).

4. Discussion

Lee et al. (2007) discussed their research findings and linked them to previous research. They concluded "HDL pretreatment alleviated organ dysfunction and injury due to endotoxemia. ... In contrast, LDL induced cardiovascular impairment and organ deterioration. Our study provides evidence of HDL alleviation of endotoxemia and a potential effect of HDL for the prevention and treatment of endotoxemia" (Lee et al., 2007, p. 259). This basic research provides a basis for conducting applied research to determine the impact of HDL levels on patients' organ damage with endotoxemia.

INITIAL CRITICAL APPRAISAL

Experimental Study

Lee and colleagues (2007) presented a complex, comprehensive report of their experimental study of the effects of HDL on organ damage in endotoxemia. These researchers also clearly organized their article using the four major sections: introduction, methods, results, and discussion. Each section clearly detailed many of the steps of the quantitative research process. However, the study does lack a framework and hypotheses to direct its implementation. In addition, the study would have been strengthened by a discussion of the study limitations, an expansion of the implications for practice, and the need for future research.

KEY CONCEPTS

- Quantitative research is the traditional research approach in nursing and includes descriptive, correlational, quasi-experimental, and experimental types of research.
- Basic, or pure, research is a scientific investigation that involves the pursuit of "knowledge for knowledge's sake," or for the pleasure of learning and finding truth.
- Applied, or practical, research is a scientific investigation conducted to generate knowledge that will directly influence or improve clinical practice.
- Conducting quantitative research requires rigor and control.
- A comparison of the problem-solving process, the nursing process, and the research process shows the similarities and differences in these processes and provides a basis for understanding the research process.
- The quantitative research process involves conceptualizing a research project, planning and implementing that project, and communicating the findings. The following steps of the quantitative research process are briefly introduced in this chapter.

- The research problem is an area of concern in which there is a gap in the knowledge needed for nursing practice. The research purpose is generated from the problem and identifies the specific goal or aim of the study.
- The review of relevant literature is conducted to generate a picture of what is known and unknown about a particular topic and provides a rationale for why the study needs to be conducted.
- The study framework is the theoretical basis for a study that guides the development of the study and enables the researcher to link the findings to nursing's body of knowledge.
- Research objectives, questions, or hypotheses are formulated to bridge the gap between the more abstractly stated research problem and purpose and the study design and plan for data collection and analysis.
- Study variables are concepts, at various levels of abstraction that are measured, manipulated, or controlled in a study.
- Assumptions are statements that are taken for granted or are considered true even though they have not been scientifically tested.
- Limitations are theoretical or methodological restrictions in a study that may decrease the generalizability of the findings.
- Research design is a blueprint for conducting a study that maximizes control over factors that could interfere with the study's desired outcomes.
- The population is all of the elements that meet certain criteria for inclusion in a study. A sample is a subset of the population that is selected for a particular study; the members of a sample are the subjects.
- Measurement is the process of assigning numerical values to objects, events, or situations in accord with some rule. Methods of measurement are identified to measure each of the variables in a study.
- The data collection process involves the precise, systematic gathering of information relevant to the research purpose or the objectives, questions, or hypotheses of a study.
- Data analyses are conducted to reduce, organize, and give meaning to the data and to address the research purpose and/or objectives, questions, and hypotheses.
- Research outcomes include the conclusions or findings, generalization of findings, implications for nursing, and suggestions for further research.
- The content of a research report includes six parts: abstract, introduction, methods, results, discussion, and references.
- Reading research reports involves skimming, comprehending, and analyzing the report.
- The guidelines for conducting an initial critical appraisal of a quantitative study are provided.

REFERENCES

American Heart Association. (2004). *Heart disease and stroke statistics-2005 update*. Dallas, TX: Author.

American Health Association Statistics Committee and Stroke Statistics Subcommittee. (2006). Heart disease and stroke statistics—2006 update. *Circulation*, *113*(6), e85-e152.

Artinian, N. T., Flack, J. M., Nordstrom, C. K., Hockman, E. M., Washington, O. G. M., Jen, K. C., & Fathy, M. (2007). Effects of nurse-managed telemonitoring on blood pressure at 12-month follow-up among urban African Americans. *Nursing Research*, *56*(5), 312-322.

Artinian, N., Washington, O., Klymko, K., Marbury, C., Miller, W., & Powell, J. (2004). What you need to know about home blood pressure telemonitoring, but may not know to ask. *Home Healthcare Nurse*, *22*(10), 680-686.

Artinian, N., Washington, O., & Templin, T. (2001). Effects of home telemonitoring and community-based monitoring on blood pressure control in urban African Americans: A pilot study. *Heart & Lung, 30*(3), 191-199.

Bagley, C. (1990). Development of a measure of unwanted sexual contact in childhood, for use in community mental health surveys. *Psychology Reports, 66*(2), 401-402.

Bagley, C., & King, K. K. (1990). *Child sexual abuse: The search for healing*. New York: Travistock/Routledge.

Bond, E. F., & Heitkemper, M. M. (1987). Importance of basic physiologic research in nursing science. *Heart & Lung: The Journal of Acute and Critical Care, 16*(4), 347-349.

Brown, B. E., & Garrison, C. J. (1990). Patterns of symptomatology of adult women incest survivors. *Western Journal of Nursing Research, 12*(5), 587-600.

Brown, S. J. (2009). *Evidence-based nursing: The research-practice connection*. Sudbury, MA: Jones & Bartlett.

Browne, A., & Finkelhor, D. (1986). Initial and long-term effects: A review of the research. In D. Finkelhor (Ed.), *A sourcebook on child sexual abuse* (pp. 143-179). Beverly Hills: Sage.

Burns, N. (1989). The research process and the nursing process: Distinctly different. *Nursing Science Quarterly, 2*(4), 157-158.

Burns, N., & Grove, S. K. (2009). *The practice of nursing research: Appraisal, synthesis, and generation of evidence* (6th ed.). Philadelphia: Saunders.

Campbell, D. T., & Stanley, J. C. (1963). *Experimental and quasi-experimental designs for research*. Chicago: Rand McNally.

Chobanian, A., Bakris, G., Black, H., Cushman, W., Green, L., Izzo, J., Jr., et al. (2003). Seventh report of the Joint National Committee on Prevention, Detection, Evaluation, and Treatment of High Blood Pressure. *Hypertension, 42*(6), 1206-1252.

Cook, T. D., & Campbell, D. T. (1979). *Quasi-experimentation: Design and analysis issues for field settings*. Chicago: Rand McNally.

Craig, J., & Smyth, R. (2007). *The evidence-based practice manual for nurses* (2nd ed.). Edinburgh: Churchill Livingstone Elsevier.

Crosby, L. J. (1990). The abstract: An important first impression. *Journal of Neuroscience Nursing, 22*(3), 192-194.

Fields, L., Burt, V., Cutler, J., Hughers, J., Roccella, E., & Sorlie, P. (2004). The burden of adult hypertension in the United States 1999-2000: A rising tide. *Hypertension, 44*(4), 398-404.

Finkelhor, D. (2008). *Child victimization*. Oxford, UK: Oxford University Press.

Fisher, Sir R. A. (1935). *The designs of experiments*. New York: Hafner.

Follette, N. M., Alexander, P. C., & Follette, W. C. (1991). Individual predictors of outcome in group treatment for incest survivors. *Journal of Consulting and Clinical Psychology, 59*(1), 150-155.

Giovannini, I., Chiarla, C., & Greco, F. (2003). Characterization of biochemical and clinical correlates of hypocholesterolemia after hepatectomy. *Clinical Chemistry, 49*(2), 317-319.

Grove, S. K. (2007). *Statistics for health care research: A practical workbook*. St. Louis: Saunders Elsevier.

Hertzog, M. A. (2008). Considerations in determining sample size for pilot studies. *Research in Nursing & Health, 31*(2), 180-191.

Hulme, P. A. (2000). Symptomatology and health care utilization of women primary care patients who experienced childhood sexual abuse. *Child Abuse & Neglect, 24*(11), 1471-1484.

Hulme, P. A., & Agrawal, S. (2004). Patterns of childhood sexual abuse characteristics and their relationships to other childhood abuse and adult health. *Journal of Interpersonal Violence, 19*(4), 389-405.

Hulme, P. A., & Grove, S. K. (1994). Symptoms of female survivors of child sexual abuse. *Issues in Mental Health Nursing, 15*(5), 519-532.

Kaplan, A. (1964). *The conduct of inquiry: Methodology for behavioral science*. San Francisco: Chandler.

Kerlinger, F. N., & Lee, H. B. (2000). *Foundations of behavioral research* (4th ed.). Fort Worth, TX: Harcourt.

Lacey, C. M., Finkelstein, M., & Thygeson, M. V. (2008). The impact of positioning on fear during immunizations: Supine versus sitting up. *Journal of Pediatric Nursing, 23*(3) 195-200.

Lee, R., Lin, N., Chao, Y. C., Lin, C., Harn, H., & Chen, H. (2007). High density lipoprotein prevents organ damage in endotoxemia. *Research in Nursing & Health, 30*(3), 250-260.

Melnyk, B. M., & Fineout-Overholt, E. (2005). *Evidence-based practice in nursing & healthcare: A guide to best practice*. Philadelphia: Lippincott.

Miller, D. C., & Salkind, N. J. (2002). *Handbook of research design & social measurement* (5th ed.). Newbury Park, CA: Sage.

Porter, T. M. (2004). *Karl Pearson: The scientific life in a statistical age*. United Kingdom: Princeton University Press.

Prescott, P. A., & Soeken, K. L. (1989). The potential uses of pilot work. *Nursing Research, 38*(1), 60-62.

Tornquist, E. M., Funk, S. G., Champagne, M. T., & Wiese, R. A. (1993). Advice on reading research: Overcoming the barriers. *Applied Nursing Research, 6*(4), 177-183.

Twiss, J. J., Waltman, N. L., Berg, K., Ott, C. D., Gross, G. J., & Lindsey, A. M. (2009). An exercise intervention for breast cancer survivors with bone loss. *Journal of Nursing Scholarship, 41*(1), 20-27.

van Teijlingen, E. R., & Hundley, V. (2001). The importance of pilot studies. *Social Research Update, 35*(4). Retrieved April 22, 2009 from *http://sru.soc.surrey.ac.uk/SRU35.html*.

Whittemore, R. (2005). Combining evidence in nursing research: Methods and implications. *Nursing Research, 54*(1), 56-62.

Wilkinson, J. M. (2006). *Nursing process and critical thinking* (4th ed.). Englewood Cliffs, NJ: Prentice Hall.

Williams, M. A. (1980). Editorial: Assumptions in research. *Research in Nursing & Health, 3*(2), 47-48.

Wysocki, A. B. (1983). Basic versus applied research: Intrinsic and extrinsic considerations. *Western Journal of Nursing Research, 5*(3), 217-224.

Yamakage, M., Iwasaki, S., Jeong, S., Satoh, J., & Namiki, A. (2009). Beta-1 selective adrenergic antagonist landiolol and esmolol can be safely used in patients with airway hyperreactivity. *Heart & Lung, 38*(1), 48-55.

3

Introduction to the Qualitative Research Process

Chapter Overview

Values of Qualitative Research   73
Gestalt   74
Rigor in Qualitative Research   75
Qualitative Research Approaches   75
Phenomenological Research   75
Grounded Theory Research   77
Ethnographic Research   79
Historical Research   81
Qualitative Research Methods   83
Selection of Participants   84
Researcher-Participant Relationships   84
Data Collection Methods   85
Interviews   85
Focus Groups   87
Observation   88
Text as a Source of Qualitative Data   90

**Other Qualitative Methods of Data
Collection**   90
Collecting Stories   90
Constructing Life Stories   91
Case Studies   92
Data Management   93
Transcribing Interviews   93
Immersion in the Data   94
Data Reduction   94
Data Analysis   94
Codes and Coding   94
Reflection   96
Identifying Themes   96
Analysis of Focus Group Data   96
Interpretation   97

Learning Outcomes

After completing this chapter, you should be able to:

1. Describe differences between quantitative and qualitative research.
2. Describe four qualitative research approaches: phenomenological research, grounded theory research, ethnography, and historical research.
3. Describe the intended outcome of each qualitative approach.
4. Describe three ways that data may be collected in a qualitative study.

5. Describe strategies used by qualitative researchers to set aside their own values and allow the findings to emerge from the data.
6. Compare how data collected in an interview might be different than data collected in a focus group.
7. Critically appraise the data collection, analysis, and interpretation of qualitative studies.

Key Terms

Bracketing, p. 96
Case study, p. 92
Coding, p. 94

Data reduction, p. 94
Dwelling with the data, p. 94
Emic approach, p. 80

Ethnographic research, p. 79
Ethnonursing research, p. 80
Etic approach, p. 80

Field notes, p. 89
Focus groups, p. 87
Gestalt, p. 74
Going native, p. 85
Grounded theory research,
   p. 77
Historical research, p. 81
Immersed, p. 85
Interpretation, p. 97
Life story, p. 91

Moderator or facilitator, p. 87
Observation, p. 88
Open-ended interview, p. 85
Participants, p. 84
Phenomenology, p. 75
Primary source, p. 82
Probes, p. 85
Qualitative research, p. 73
Reflexive thought, p. 95

Researcher-participant
   relationship, p. 84
Rigor, p. 75
Secondary source, p. 82
Semi-structured interview,
   p. 85
Text analysis, p. 90
Transcription, p. 90

STUDY TOOLS

Be sure to visit *http://evolve.elsevier.com/Burns/understanding* for additional examples and self-tests. Also, a review of this chapter's concepts and practice exercises can be found in Chapter 3 of the Study Guide for *Understanding Nursing Research: Building an Evidence-Based Practice,* 5th edition.

Qualitative research is a systematic, subjective approach used to describe life experiences and give them meaning. Qualitative research is not a new idea in the social or behavioral sciences. The nursing profession's interest in qualitative research began in the late 1970s and has continued to grow since that time.

This chapter introduces the values upon which qualitative research is based and presents an overview of four specific qualitative perspectives: phenomenological research, grounded theory research, ethnographic research, and historical research. An example of each type of study will be described. You will be introduced to some of the more common methods used to collect, analyze, and interpret qualitative data. This content provides a background for you to use in reading and comprehending published qualitative studies, critically appraising qualitative studies, and applying study findings to your practice.

Values of Qualitative Research

The values underlying qualitative research differ from those of quantitative research. Qualitative research approaches are based on a worldview that is holistic, and may draw upon the following beliefs:

1. There are multiple, constructed realities (Nicholls, 2009).
2. The knower and the known are inseparable and knowledge is co-constructed (Haverkamp & Young, 2007).
3. Inquiry is value bound (Haverkamp & Young, 2007).
4. All generalizations are bounded by time and context (Grace & Powers, 2009; Lincoln & Guba, 1985).

The reasoning process used in qualitative research involves perceptually putting pieces together to make wholes. From this process, meaning is produced. Because perception varies with the individual, many different meanings are possible (Munhall, 2007). Still, it is possible for the identified meanings to be considered "wrong" because the researcher failed to accurately reflect the perspectives of the participants. Qualitative researchers believe that there are better and worse interpretations of data (Ayres & Poirier, 1996).

Frameworks are used in a different sense in qualitative research. Instead of identifying hypotheses based on theorized relationships and testing the hypotheses in a quantitative study, qualitative researchers use theories during data analysis to further expand their understanding of the data. From qualitative data, researchers using grounded theory methods may develop a new theory as a result of the study.

The findings from a qualitative study lead to an understanding of a phenomenon in a particular situation and are not generalized in the same way as quantitative studies. However, denoting the meanings of a phenomenon in a particular situation offers insights that can be applied more broadly. The insights from qualitative studies can guide nursing practice and aid in the important process of theory development for building nursing knowledge (Sandelowski & Barroso, 2007; Schwartz-Barcott & Kim, 1986). One of the earliest and perhaps most dramatic demonstrations of the influence of qualitative research on nursing practice was the 4-year study of dying conducted by Glaser and Strauss (1965, 1968, 1971), which initiated the use of grounded theory research methods for health-related studies. At the time Glaser and Strauss were conducting their studies, the traditional view of dying was that people could not cope with knowing that they were terminally ill. For example, cancer patients were not told they had cancer, because a diagnosis of cancer was essentially a death sentence. People with cancer were kept in the hospital until they died. There were no resources in the community to provide care outside of the hospital. The environment of care in the hospital was designed to protect patients from the knowledge that they were dying. Glaser and Strauss described the social environment of dying patients in hospitals and reported their findings in three books: *Awareness of Dying* (Glaser & Strauss, 1965), *Time for Dying* (Glaser & Strauss, 1968), and *Status Passage* (Glaser & Strauss, 1971). They examined what that protective social environment meant for the patient. This study changed the perception of nurses, who began to recognize that the traditional care of dying patients created loneliness and isolation, rather than protection. Nurses began to see the patient in a new light and changed their methods of patient care. Kübler-Ross (1969), perhaps influenced by the work of Glaser and Strauss, began her studies of dying patients, using an approach similar to that of phenomenology. These findings from the perspective of dying patients resulted in the development of hospice and palliative care.

Gestalt

The concept of Gestalt is closely related to holism and proposes that knowledge about a particular phenomenon is organized into a cluster of linked ideas, a gestalt. A theory is a form of gestalt. If we are trying to understand something new and are offered a theory that explains it, our reaction may be, "Now that makes sense" or, "Oh, I see." The concept has "come together" for us. You may have experienced this the first time you provided care to a person living with heart failure. The pathophysiology, symptoms, and treatments were disjointed facts until you cared for a person with heart failure and the picture of the illness came together in the context of a human being.

One disadvantage of this process is that once we understand a phenomenon through the interpretation of a particular theory, it is difficult for us to "see" the phenomenon outside the meaning given to it by that particular theory. For example, the next time you encountered a person with edema, weight gain, and shortness of breath, you may have assumed the person had heart failure, only to learn that the person had renal failure or fluid overload. Therefore, in addition to giving meaning, a theory or "big picture" can limit meaning. Another example is Selye's theory of stress, which is very familiar to us as nurses. Our knowledge of that theory can make it difficult to examine the phenomenon of stress without using Selye's perspective and concepts.

Through the process of developing a qualitative study, researchers become familiar with published theories and research related to the phenomenon they are studying. These perspectives have shaped the researchers' initial "seeing" of the phenomenon. To move beyond the initial view, qualitative researchers must remain open to different pictures or gestalts of the phenomenon during data analysis and interpretation. Rigorous qualitative methods can encourage the researcher to maintain an open perspective on the phenomenon being studied.

Rigor in Qualitative Research

Scientific rigor is valued because the findings of rigorous studies are seen as being more credible and of greater worth. Studies are critically appraised as a means of judging rigor. Rigor is defined differently for qualitative research because the desired outcome is different from that in quantitative research (Burns, 1989; Denzin & Lincoln, 2005; Dzurec, 1989; Morse, 1989; Patton, 2002; Sandelowski, 1986, 1993; Sandelowski & Barroso, 2007). Evaluation of the rigor of a qualitative study is based in part on the logic of the emerging theory and the clarity with which it sheds light on the studied phenomenon. Rigor is assessed in relation to the detail built into the design of the qualitative study, the carefulness of data collection, and the thoroughness of analysis. Qualitative researchers are expected to be aware of their own subjectivity and acknowledge their interaction with the participants and the data (Bradbury-Jones, 2007). The qualitative researcher is expected to provide sufficient information in the published report to allow a thorough critical appraisal of these characteristics of the study.

Qualitative Research Approaches

Each of these four approaches is based on a philosophical orientation that influences the interpretation of the data. Thus, it is critical to understand the philosophy on which the method is based. Each approach is discussed in relation to its philosophical orientation and intended outcome. A nursing study is provided to illustrate each methodology.

Phenomenological Research

Philosophical Orientation

Phenomena are the world of experience. Phenomena occur only when a person experiences them. An experience is considered unique to the individual. Phenomenology refers to both a philosophy and a group of research methods congruent with the philosophy (Finlay, 2004).

Phenomenologists view the person as integrated with the environment. The world shapes the self, and the self shapes the world. The broad research question that phenomenologists ask is, "What is the meaning of one's lived experience?" Being a person is self-interpreting; therefore, the only reliable source of information to answer this question is the person (Mapp, 2008). Understanding human behavior or experience, which is a central concern of nursing, requires that the person interpret the action or experience for the researcher; the researcher must then interpret the explanation provided by the person.

Phenomenologists differ in their philosophical beliefs. Nursing phenomenological researchers most commonly base their study design on either Husserl or Heidegger, whose views of the person and the world in which that person exists differ (Johnson, 2000). Each of these philosophical perspectives supports a specific type of phenomenological research.

Husserl's view is that the focus is on the phenomenon itself and the meaning-laden statements in the data that capture the essence of what is perceived and experienced by the participant (Kleiman, 2004; Mapp, 2008). The meaning-laden statements are analyzed to discover the structure within the phenomenon. Husserl's philosophy supports descriptive phenomenological research, whose purpose is to describe experiences as they are lived, or in phenomenological terms, to capture the "lived experience" of study participants. To describe it, the researcher must experience the phenomenon in a naïve way (Kvigne, Gjengedal, & Kirkevold, 2002; Sadala & Adorno, 2002).

Heidegger's view is that the researcher interprets the data, creating a strong, insightful text that "brings to mind the phenomenon described" (Kleiman, 2004, p. 8) and gives insights into the meaning of the phenomenon. The interpretative approach, consistent with Heidegger's philosophy, involves analyzing the data and presenting a rich word picture of the phenomenon as interpreted by the researcher.

Hermeneutics is one type of interpretive phenomenological research method that is congruent with Heidegger's philosophical perspective and is being used by nurse researchers. Hermeneutics uses textual analysis as its primary research approach. Transcripts of interviews and published documents are usually the texts analyzed by nurse researchers. Textual analysis "emphasizes the social and historic influences on qualitative interpretation" (Byrne, 2001, p. 968) and exposes hidden meanings. Hermeneutics is used in nursing research to increase the understanding of human nature (Byrne, 2001; Cohen & Kahn, 2000). The method also has been adopted by some feminist researchers (Ceci, 2003; Finch, 2004; Fleming, Gaidys, & Robb, 2003; Mitchell, 2004).

 RESEARCH EXAMPLE Phenomenological Study

As oncology nurses, Wilson and Woodgate (2007) took care of children who were undergoing bone marrow transplants (BMT) as part of their cancer treatment. They became interested in the lived experience of being a sibling, some of whom donated bone marrow and some who did not. Data were collected from seven participants. Interviews were guided by statements such as, "Tell me what it was like for you when you were tested to see if your bone marrow was a match for your brother or sister" and, "Tell what it was like for you on the day of the transplant" (p. E30). Each participant was interviewed twice, with the second interview providing an opportunity for further description and clarification. Wilson and Woodgate found the essence of the lived experience to be "an interruption in family life" (p. E31), with participants describing feeling as if their lives had been put on hold. "It was like it was not really happening ... I knew it was happening. But it took me a while for me to realize everything" (p. E31).

Four themes were identified: Life goes on; Feeling more or less a part of the family; Faith in God that things would be okay; and Feelings around families (p. E31). Consistent with hermeneutic (interpretive) phenomenology, the researchers developed an illustrative statement for each theme found in the data. For example, for the theme of "feeling more or less a part of the family" (p. 31), Wilson and Woodgate interpreted the data with following statements:

- Belonging to the family is important.
- Being a part of the BMT experience helped increase siblings' sense of belonging.
- Understanding what was happening in their families helped siblings get through the BMT experience.
- Siblings needed to do whatever they could to help recipients get better (p. E31).

CRITICAL APPRAISAL

Wilson and Woodgate (2007) have made a significant contribution to family-centered care during BMT. The analysis of the data was not described in detail, however, and the rigor of the study is difficult to ascertain.

IMPLICATIONS FOR PRACTICE

The researchers concluded that siblings of BMT recipients had a range of feelings about the experience and needed to be part of the process. Because siblings were an integral part of the family and the experience, nurses needed to acknowledge their involvement in the treatment process.

A bibliography of more recent phenomenological studies in nursing can be found on the Evolve website. If you are using CINAHL, type the search terms *phenomenological* and *study* to search for current phenomenological studies, many of which are available in full text.

Grounded Theory Research

Grounded theory research is an inductive technique that emerged from the discipline of sociology. The term *grounded* means that the theory that developed from the research has its roots in the data from which it was derived. Grounded theory is based on symbolic interaction theory, which holds many views in common with phenomenology. George Herbert Mead (1934), a social psychologist, was a leader in the development of symbolic interaction theory. This theory explores how people define reality and how their beliefs are related to their actions. Reality is created by attaching meanings to situations. Meaning is expressed in such symbols as words, religious objects, and clothing. These symbolic meanings are the basis for actions and interactions. However, symbolic meanings are different for each individual, and we cannot completely know the symbolic meanings for another individual. In social life, meanings are shared by groups and are communicated to new members through socialization processes. Group life is based on consensus and shared meanings. Interaction may lead to redefinition and new meanings and can result in the redefinition of self (Jeon, 2004). The grounded theory researcher seeks to understand the interaction between self and group from the perspective of those involved.

Grounded theory has been used most frequently to study areas in which little previous research has been conducted and gain a new viewpoint in familiar areas of research. The work of Glaser and Strauss (1965, 1967, 1968, 1971) and Strauss et al. (1984) have attracted nurses to the idea of conducting grounded theory research.

Fully developed grounded theory studies result in a theoretical framework and usually a diagram displaying the interactions among the social processes that were identified. More than 20 years ago, Artinian (1988) recognized that not all grounded theory achieved this ideal result and these studies still contributed to nursing knowledge. She identified four qualitative modes of nursing inquiry within grounded theory: descriptive mode, discovery mode, emergent fit mode, and intervention mode. The descriptive mode provides rich detail and must precede all other modes. This mode, ideal for the beginning researcher, answers such questions as the following: "What is going on?" "How are activities organized?" "What roles are evident?" "What are the steps in a process?" "What does a patient do in a particular setting?" The discovery mode leads to the identification of patterns in a person's life experiences and relates the patterns to each other. Through this mode, a theory of social process, referred to as substantive theory, is developed; the theory explains a particular social world. The emergent fit mode is used when substantive theory has been developed to extend or refine this existing theory. This mode enables the researcher to focus on a selected portion of the theory, build on previous work, or establish a research program around a particular social process. The intervention mode is used to test the relationships in the substantive theory. The fundamental question for this mode is, "How can I make something happen in a way that brings about a new and desired state of affairs?" This mode demands deep involvement on the part of the researcher and practitioner.

RESEARCH EXAMPLE Grounded Theory Study

Slade, Molloy, and Keating (2009) conducted a grounded theory study in Australia to understand the processes shaping patients' experiences with exercise for non-specific, chronic, low-back pain (NSCLBP). The researchers collected data through three focus groups of six participants each. What the participants revealed about their experiences was rather unexpected. The basic social process was stigma. The researchers analyzed the data and developed a diagram showing the influences, processes, and outcomes of stigma in persons with NSCLBP.

The situations or norms that contributed to stigma were coded into six categories. Healthcare providers contributed to stigma by not believing patients when they said they had pain. Health-care providers tended to assume that the patients were imagining pain or were reporting pain to have an excuse not to work. One participant said, "the people running the program would get angry with me when I couldn't do the exercise correctly and so it didn't actually help. I felt guilty for a long time" (Slade et al., 2009, p. 147). Another said that healthcare providers "look at you as if you're silly and you don't know what you are talking about" (p. 147).

The chronic nature of their pain was reflected in the participants' desires for treatment to be provided in less clinical environments. Instead of treatment being from a sickness model, they preferred an approach that focused on wellness.

Another influencing factor on stigma was the reactions of the community, family, and friends. "... stigma that goes with back injuries is fairly nasty. I don't tell people I have a back injury. I'd rather tell them I was dying of something else than I've got a back injury" (p. 149).

A woman said that "people look at it [back pain] as a way, oh, they just want to get out of work" (p. 149). Another woman believed that the reactions of others could be attributed to the fact that "they can't see back pain. I don't have a cast on my arm, you know, if you cannot see the injury it's very difficult for people to understand" (p. 150). Being required to be on light duty at work was also viewed as causing stigma, even though poor workplace policies and training contributed to the injury. Among the participants was a nurse who said, "I trace my initial back injury back to my first year of my nursing ... we weren't taught properly and were unsupervised and lifted heavy people alone" (p. 150). Stigma was worse when imaging and other diagnostic tests did not provide evidence of the injury. Several of the participants stated that they felt relief when an x-ray or MRI revealed pathology.

Slade et al. (2009) found that the stigma experienced by persons with NSCLBP was a negative influence on seeking treatment and participating in exercise. Near the end of the focus groups, the participants were asked for their suggestions about how to decrease the stigma. Their suggestions included educating healthcare providers and communities; improving communication among patients, providers, families, and friends; forming support groups; and sharing success stories. These actions to decrease stigma were connected on the theory diagram to improved healthcare outcomes for persons with NSCLBP.

CRITICAL APPRAISAL

The researchers described a rigorous process of data analyses involving rounds of independent analysis followed by discussion and validation in a team meeting. Extensive quotations allowed the reader to hear the voices of the participants. The straightforward, simple diagram of the process of stigma enhanced the clarity of the written description and provided instructions to healthcare providers to decrease stigma.

IMPLICATIONS FOR PRACTICE

As you read this article, you may reflect on your own reactions to persons with back pain in clinical and social settings. The values of health care providers were evident to the participants with NSCLBP through the providers' demeaning and biased words and actions. Hearing the words of the persons who had been the target of such words and actions motivates us to examine our own attitudes and promote a positive environment in which persons can feel comfortable seeking care.

A bibliography of more recent grounded theory studies in nursing can be found on the Evolve website. If you are using CINAHL, type the search terms *grounded theory* and *study* to search for current grounded theory studies, many of which are available in full text.

Ethnographic Research

Ethnographic research was developed by anthropologists as a method to study cultures through immersion in the culture for a significant period of time. The word *ethnography* means "portrait of a people." Anthropologists study a people's origins, past ways of living, and ways of surviving through time. Early ethnography researchers studied primitive, foreign, or remote cultures. Such studies enabled the researcher to acquire new perspectives beyond his or her own ethnocentric perspective as a means to understand people, including their ways of living, believing, and adapting to changing environmental circumstances. Culture, the concept most central to anthropology, is "a way of life belonging to a designated group of people … a blueprint for living which guides a particular group's thoughts, actions, and sentiments … all the accumulated ways a group of people solve problems, which are reflected in the people's language, dress, food, and a number of accumulated traditions and customs" (Leininger, 1970, pp. 48-49). Current examples of ethnography include a study conducted by Weine, Bahromov, and Mirzoev (2008) to explore the social environment of male migrant workers from the nation of Tajikistan living in Moscow. The purpose of this study was to gain understanding of the contextual factors related to HIV/AIDS risk for these men. Tran and Garcia (2009) described their method for studying health behaviors of young Mexican adults as being focused ethnography.

The philosophical perspective of ethnographic research recognizes that culture is both material and nonmaterial. Material culture consists of all created objects associated with a given group. Nonmaterial culture consists of other aspects of culture, such as symbolic referents, the network of social relations, and the beliefs reflected in social and political institutions. Symbolic meaning, social customs, and beliefs—components of the nonmaterial culture—may be apparent in a different culture only over time, but they are essential elements of cultures. Cultures also have ideals that people hold as desirable, even though they do not always live up to these standards. Anthropologists seek to discover the many parts of a whole culture and how these parts are interrelated so that a picture of the wholeness of the culture evolves. There are two basic research approaches in anthropology: emic and etic. The **emic approach** involves studying behaviors from within the culture; the **etic approach** involves studying behavior from outside the culture and examining similarities and differences across cultures. Most current ethnographic research in nursing is now studying behaviors from within the culture (Roper & Shapiro, 2000).

Some nurses involved in ethnography obtained their doctoral preparation in anthropology and have used anthropological techniques to examine cultural issues of interest in nursing. The most well-known of these is Madeline Leininger, a nurse who lived in Papua, New Guinea as part of her doctoral education in anthropology. Her field work provided the basis for her Sunshine Model of Transcultural Nursing Care (Leininger, 1988). Although originated as the research methodology for the discipline of anthropology, ethnography is now a part of the cultural research conducted by a number of other disciplines, including social psychology, sociology, political science, education, and nursing, and also is used in feminist research.

Today, in nursing, the emphasis of ethnography has shifted to include obtaining cultural knowledge within the society to which a nurse researcher belongs (Munhall, 2007). For example, an ethnographic study may examine the culture of hospital units and other settings in which nurses provide care and how the culture influences patient perceptions of their care. In an adolescent ward in a hospital in Australia, Hutton (2007) conducted an ethnographic study to examine the environment and how space was used. She learned that the nurses had rules about how the ward should function and the role of patients in the work environment.

A group of nurse scientists influenced by Leininger's Theory of Transcultural Nursing, (Leininger, 2002) has developed an ethnographic research strategy for nursing. They refer to this strategy as **ethnonursing research**. Ethnonursing "focuses mainly on observing and documenting interactions with people of how these daily life conditions and patterns are influencing human care, health, and nursing care practices" (Leininger, 1985, p. 238). However, a number of nurse anthropologists not associated with the ethnonursing orientation also are providing important contributions to the nursing body of knowledge (Roper & Shapiro, 2000).

RESEARCH EXAMPLE Ethnographic Research

A study of family presence and surveillance during weaning from prolonged mechanical ventilation will be used as an example of an ethnographic study (Happ et al., 2007). You will also encounter this study as an example in Chapter 5. Here, we will be examining it from the perspective of research method.

The purpose of the study was to describe care and communication processes during weaning from long-term mechanical ventilation (LTMV). Although the researchers also collected quantitative data, we will be examining the qualitative elements of the study. Qualitative data were collected using field notes while observing the family, the patient, and the nurses interact during the weaning process. The nurse's behavior was also observed from the perspective of care processes. Patients, family members, and nurse clinicians were interviewed and the medical record was reviewed. Thirty patients with family and nurses were observed and interviewed during a 2-year time period. Family members were present during 46% of the weaning trials. Nurses categorized the presence of the family members as being helpful, not helpful, or having no effect.

CRITICAL APPRAISAL

The study was thorough and had a sufficient sample size to obtain a variation in interactions among the participants. Using multiple methods of obtaining data (observations, interviews, and examination of medical records) allowed for comparisons of data and cross-checking of results.

IMPLICATIONS FOR PRACTICE

The results of the study can be used by nurses to enable family members to assist a patient in the process of weaning. Detailed information within the field notes could be used to develop a program to teach family members how they can be most helpful to their patient.

A bibliography of more recent ethnographic studies in nursing can be found on the Evolve website. If you are using CINAHL, type the search terms *ethnographic* and *study* to search for current ethnographic studies, many of which are available in full text.

Historical Research

Historical research examines events of the past. Many historians believe that the greatest value of historical knowledge is increased self-understanding; in addition, historical knowledge provides nurses with an increased understanding of their profession. The three primary questions of history are the following: "Where have we come from?" "Who are we?" and "Where are we going?" Although the questions do not change, the answers do.

"There is nothing new under the sun." As a major assumption of historical philosophy, this statement provides the rationale for the foundation idea of historical research: We can learn from the past. Historians study the past through oral and written reports and artifacts, searching for patterns that can lead to generalizations. For example, to answer the question, "What causes wars?," a historian could search throughout history for commonalities in various wars and develop a theoretical explanation of the causes of wars. The philosophy of history is a search for wisdom in which the historian examines what has been, what is, and what ought to be. Historical philosophers have attempted to identify a developmental scheme for history to explain events and structures as elements of the same social process.

Nursing as a profession has a history that must be transmitted to those entering the profession. Christy (1978) asks, "[H]ow can we in nursing today possibly plan where we are going when we don't know where we have been … [or] how we got here?" (p. 9). Until recently, historical nursing research has not been a valued activity, and few nurse researchers had the skills or desire to conduct it. Therefore our knowledge of our past is sketchy. As nurses have recognized that current issues in nursing are not new, historical studies have been developed to explore relevant topics such as assessing knowledge of nursing students (Wood, 2009) and disaster management (Leifer & Glass, 2008).

The methods for historical research are unique to this type of research. As is true with all study designs, the research questions must be congruent with the method. For historical studies, the research questions or objectives are directed toward exploring, describing, and analyzing a process or event during a specific time period. The study conducted by Leifer and Glass (2008) will be used as an example.

 RESEARCH EXAMPLE Historical Nursing Research

Leifer and Glass (2008) examine mass causality preparation and the role of a specific nurse during the Cold War, designated as the 1950s and the 1960s. Their study objectives were:

- To analyze nurses' involvement in research and mass disaster preparations during the Cold War era and
- To describe the role of Harriet H. Werley and the Army Nurse Corps (p. 237).

The researchers identified primary sources of data to include "memos, speeches, letters, reports, photos, and publications in the Harriet H. Werley Papers" (p. 238) in a specific library at the University of Wisconsin-Milwaukee. A primary source is material most likely to shed true light on the information the researcher seeks. For example, material written by a person who experienced an event and letters and other mementos saved by the person being studied are primary source material. Data were also extracted from secondary sources, which included government records and documentation of mass causality and disaster planning educational programs and research projects in which Major Werley was involved. A secondary source is written by someone who previously read and summarized the primary source material. History books and textbooks are secondary source materials. Primary sources are considered to be more credible and consistent with the qualitative research perspective of seeking to understand phenomena from the perspective of the people most directly affected.

The findings of the study are presented as the story of what happened with details added that provide a glimpse into Major Werley's perspectives on the events. As nurse major, she was offered an administrative level position at the Walter Reed Army Institute of Research (WRAIR). She wrote in her memoirs (a primary source of data) that she hesitated to take the position, because she believed a doctorally prepared nurse was needed. Her appointment to the position received significant press coverage in 1955. Leifer and Glass (2008) also included excerpts from congratulatory notes she received from other nurses. The WRAIR, recognizing the potential impact of nuclear war on the health of members of the military and the general public, created the Department of Atomic Causalities Studies (DAC) and Major Werley was appointed to this department.

The events in the chronology of Major Werley and the DAC were placed in the social context of the response of the American people to the threat of nuclear war; the development of nursing research and graduate programs; the need to disseminate disaster management information through conferences and publications; and collaboration with nursing professional organizations. Leifer and Glass (2008) concluded their article by summarizing the leadership and accomplishment of Major Werley.

CRITICAL APPRAISAL

The description of Major Werley's professional contributions and the development of disaster management nursing as a specialty was rich with details and frequent references to the sources from which the details were extracted. The integration of findings and sources increased the credibility (believability) of the report. The report did not include the methods used to inventory the sources and determine the authenticity of the sources, which if used, would have strengthened the credibility of the study. Leifer and Glass (2008) demonstrated the relevance of the study by relating the events to more recent terrorist attacks in the United States and around the world.

IMPLICATIONS FOR PRACTICE

You can gain insight into the influence that nurse leaders have had on public policy and examine your own leadership potential in the profession. From the study, you may also realize the interactions among people, prior events, and current events and analyze similar elements as you consider the political and social environment for health care today.

If you are using CINAHL, type the search terms *historical* and *study* to search for current historical studies, many of which are available in full text.

Qualitative Research Methods

This section presents a detailed description of the methods commonly used in conducting qualitative studies. In some ways, the methods used are no different from those used in quantitative studies. The researcher must select a topic; state the problem or question; justify the significance of the study; design the study; identify sources of data, such as subjects; gain access to those sources of data; recruit subjects; gather data; describe, analyze, and interpret the data; and develop a written report of the results. There are, however, methods unique to qualitative studies and sometimes to specific types of qualitative research. An understanding of some of the unique methods used by qualitative researchers will help you appreciate the work involved in conducting such a study.

This section describes how participants (subjects) are selected, and how data are collected, managed, and analyzed. The methods used to ensure rigor in qualitative research also are explored.

Selection of Participants

Subjects in qualitative studies are referred to as **participants** because the researcher and the participants cooperatively carry out the study. Participants provide assistance and guidance to the researcher, who could not be successful in carrying out the study without their help. Participants are recruited by the researcher to participate in a study because of their particular knowledge, experience, or views related to the study. Roche-Fahy and Dowling (2009) conducted a phenomenological study of the lived experience of nurses providing palliative care. They publicized the study and its purpose by posting a memorandum about the study in an acute care hospital. Nurses who provided palliative care volunteered to participate.

Researcher-Participant Relationships

One of the important differences between quantitative and qualitative research lies in the degree of involvement of the researcher with the participants of the study. This involvement, considered a source of bias in quantitative research, is thought by qualitative researchers to be a critical element of the research process. The nature of the **researcher-participant relationship** has an impact on the collection and interpretation of data. The researcher creates a respectful relationship with each participant that includes being honest and open about the purpose and methods of the study. The researcher's aims and means need to be acceptable to the participants and honor their perspectives and values (Burns & Grove, 2009; Denzin & Lincoln, 2005; Marshall & Rossman, 2006; Mason, 2002; Munhall, 2007). Morse and Richards (2002) posit that data are made, not collected, in the interaction of the researcher with the topic and the participants. In various degrees, the researcher influences the people being studied and, in turn, is influenced by them. Thus, the researcher must have the support and confidence of these persons to complete the research. The researcher's personality is a key factor in qualitative research. Skills in empathy and intuition are cultivated; the researcher must become closely involved in the subject's experience to interpret it. It is necessary for the researcher to be open to the perceptions of the participants, rather than to attach his or her own meaning to the experience.

Researcher-participant relationships in qualitative studies may be brief when data collection occurs one time in an interview or focus group. Phenomenology and grounded theory studies may involve one or two interviews, although researcher-participant relationships may extend over time when the study design involves repeated interviews to study a lived experience or process over time.

Ethnographic studies require special attention to the researcher-participant relationship. The ethnographic researcher observes behavior, communication, and patterns within groups in specific cultures. The researcher may form close bonds with participants who are key informants, persons with extensive knowledge and influence in a culture. The relationships among the researcher and participants can become complex, especially in ethnography studies in which the researcher lives for an extended period of time in the culture being studied.

The ethnographic researcher must become very familiar with the culture being studied by active participation in it and extensive questioning of participants. The process of becoming **immersed** in the culture involves gaining increasing familiarity with aspects of the culture, such as language, sociocultural norms, traditions, and other social dimensions, including family, communication patterns (verbal and nonverbal), religion, work patterns, and expression of emotion. Immersion also involves gradually increasing acceptance of the researcher into the culture. Although ethnographic researchers must be actively involved in the culture they are studying, they must avoid "going native," which will interfere with both data collection and analysis. In **going native**, the researcher becomes a part of the culture and loses the ability to observe clearly (Roberts, 2009).

Data Collection Methods

The most common data collection methods used in the types of qualitative studies discussed in this chapter are interviewing participants, conducting focus groups, observing participants, and examining written text. These methods, as they are used in qualitative studies, are described in the following sections in some detail and an example from the literature is provided. Other types of qualitative studies, such as narrative inquiry, may involve collecting constructing life stories or developing case studies. Brief descriptions of these methods are also included.

Interviews

Differences exist between interviews conducted for a qualitative study and those conducted for a quantitative study. In quantitative studies, interviews are used to collect subject responses to questionnaires or surveys. Interviews in qualitative studies range from **semi-structured** (fixed set of questions, no fixed responses) to unstructured (open-ended questions with probes). **Probes** are queries made by the researcher to obtain more information from the participant about a particular interview question (Burns & Grove, 2009; Marshall & Rossman, 2006; Mason, 2002; Munhall, 2007). In qualitative studies, the interview format is more likely to be **open-ended interviews**. Although the researcher defines the focus of the interview, there may be no fixed sequence of questions. The questions addressed in interviews tend to change as the researcher gains insights from previous interviews and observations. Respondents are allowed, and even encouraged, to raise important issues not addressed by the researcher.

The researcher's goal is to obtain an authentic insight into the participant's experiences. Although data may be collected in a single interview, dialogue between researcher and participant may continue at intervals across weeks or months and provide rich data for analysis. Use of recurring interviews allows the researcher to explore an evolving process (Salander, 2007) and can help to decrease the problems associated with fleeting relationships, in which respondents may have little commitment to the study or may provide only the information they believe the researcher wishes to hear (Silverman, 1993).

Wimpenny and Gass (2000) compared the interviewing process in phenomenological and grounded theory research, to determine differences in interview technique. They examined interview methods used in both approaches to qualitative research in studies published between 1995 and 1998. They found that many qualitative researchers did not explicitly describe their data collection methods. This is still true today, making critical appraisal of data collection processes difficult.

Historical researchers may interview people who were participants in or observers of events that occurred in the past. The focus of the interview may be to validate available information about the event, uncover heretofore unknown details about the event, or obtain views about the event from persons who were not heard from previously. Historical events generally are considered to be constructed truths rather than factual. The individual perspectives on an event that emerge during an interview may provide additional insight into the constructed truths. The individual perspectives are not expected to provide the truth of an event, which will never be known (and perhaps does not exist). Interviews can also be used to construct the participants' biographies. The personal histories of a number of persons can be used to understand the evolving history of a region or institution.

Some strategies used to record information from interviews include writing notes during the interview, writing detailed notes immediately after the interview, and recording the interview on tape or digitally. Video may be recorded as well as audio. For example, Scheckel and Hedrick-Erickson (2009) recorded the interviews they conducted with RN-BSN students in their phenomenological study of interpretive pedagogies in patient education. The purpose of the study was to explore how the students learned to provide patient education. The interview of one subject was provided as follows:

> After I took the course—even teaching someone about Coumadin before they go home—we plug in the video, we have them watch the video, we give them the written material and say, can you read this, okay. If you have any questions we're here to answer them and it's just so impersonal. And I would stand and talk to them. Me just standing up there, the figure [saying] here's the stuff you need to know. More of a methodological approach, you know? … And the next time I went to go do that [Coumadin teaching], I actually pulled up a chair, sat eye-level with the patient and talked about it first. I asked him, 'can you tell me, did you ever have Coumadin before? 'What were your experiences with it?' I need to understand where the patient is at in his or her life, what's going on in their life, who's involved in their life and things like that. Just sitting down with them and having that conversation and asking an open ended question. What are their difficulties and what are their challenges? Instead of bringing out something with a list of things to do and saying this is what you need to know. … (Scheckel & Hedrick-Erickson, 2009, p. 60)

CRITICAL APPRAISAL

This is an excellent study in which the author provides text from a recorded interview. The interview text was provided to illustrate a point the authors were attempting to make. You can envision the scene and understand the effectiveness of teaching the patient by interacting with him or her personally, and thereby increasing the relevance of the teaching to the patient's life.

IMPLICATIONS FOR PRACTICE

The authors have demonstrated the increased effectiveness of teaching in dialogue with a patient rather than teaching at a patient. The recorded text makes the point much more strongly than saying in text that nurses should teach by talking with the patient.

Focus Groups

Focus groups were designed to obtain the participants' perceptions of a specific topic in a setting that is permissive and nonthreatening. One of the assumptions underlying the use of focus groups is that group dynamics can help people to express and clarify their views in ways that are less likely to occur in a one-to-one interview. The group may give a sense of "safety in numbers" to those wary of researchers or those who are anxious.

Focus groups were used initially in nursing in the late 1980s. However, they have been used in other fields for a long time. The technique serves a variety of purposes, from seeking patient (customer) perceptions of a specific hospital to develop a marketing strategy to analyzing a policy being implemented in a state health department. For qualitative research, focus groups are used to collect data to fulfill the purpose of the study.

The following assumptions underlie focus groups (Morrison & Peoples, 1999):

1. A homogeneous group provides the participants with freedom to express thoughts, feelings, and behaviors candidly.
2. Individuals are important resources of information.
3. People are able to report and verbalize their thoughts and feelings.
4. A group's dynamics can generate authentic information.
5. Data provided by a group are needed to achieve the study purpose.
6. The facilitator can help people recover forgotten information by focusing the group interaction.

Focus groups are usually conducted by a **moderator or facilitator** with the entire interaction audio-recorded, and some cases, video-recorded. In addition to the recording, often observers take notes of the proceedings. The context of the focus group such as time and environment are also critical elements to be documented because of their potential effect on the group (Halcomb et al., 2007; Vicsec, 2007). Integrating her personal experiences in conducting focus groups with the recommendations in the literature, Gray (2009) proposes that focus groups be conducted in natural settings, but notes that the researcher must plan ahead to protect the confidentiality and comfort of the participants. Participants may be less comfortable describing difficulties they have in communicating with their providers when the focus group is conducted in the clinic. In contrast, a focus group on the topic conducted in a meeting room in a library or church may result in richer dialogue and data. Researchers may elicit the help of moderators who share common characteristics with the participants. An example would be the urban researcher who hires a health professional who grew up on a farm to moderate a focus group on the subject of prevention of agricultural injuries. Gray

(2009) argues for thorough training for moderators to ensure that they follow the procedures or script developed by the researcher.

Researchers studying obesity in adolescence conducted eight focus groups with seventh and eighth graders, parents, and teachers (Power et al., 2010). Power and colleagues conducted separate groups for teachers, parents, and students using "standard focus group procedures" (p. 14). The researchers, outsiders to the schools, facilitated the focus groups and used similar questions in each group. The groups lasted one hour and had an average of four participants. "Ground rules for the focus groups were discussed (e.g., value the comment of all and allow all to speak) … that their responses would be kept confidential" (p. 14). The researchers included information about the process of obtaining assent from the underage students and parental consent for the students, in addition to securing informed consent from the parent and teacher participants.

CRITICAL APPRAISAL

Power et al. (2010) did not provide their rationale for using focus groups. They did, however, include in the report the detailed focus group questions. They provided adequate information about the setting and protection of human subjects. The small size of the focus groups may have limited the findings, but was compensated for, to some degree, by having eight groups.

IMPLICATIONS FOR PRACTICE

Adolescents in the focus groups made food choices based on taste and whether or not a food was filling, a finding that should be considered when developing nutrition teaching for adolescents. Adolescents were clear on the relationships among eating habits, physical activity, and short-term health outcomes, but did not mention long-term consequences of obesity. Nurses working with this age group should recognize developmental factors such as perceptions of time when developing interventions to prevent obesity.

Observation

Observation is a fundamental method of gathering data for qualitative studies, especially ethnography studies. The aim is to gather firsthand information in a naturally occurring situation. The researcher functions in the learning mode to answer the question, "What is going on here?" It is important for the researcher to look carefully and listen. In most cases, the activities being observed are routine for the participants. The researcher focuses on the details of the routine. The process of activities may be as important to note as the discrete events. Unexpected events occurring during routine activities may be significant and are carefully noted. As in any observation process, the qualitative researcher will attend to some aspects of the situation while disregarding others. The researcher's focus on particular aspects of the situation may increase as insights about "what is going on" occur (Carnevale et al., 2008; Silverman, 1993).

Various strategies may be used to record information about the observations. In some cases, the researcher will take detailed handwritten notes while observing. Observations recorded during the observation are called **field notes**. In other cases the researcher may focus entirely on the observational experience to avoid missing something meaningful and may wait until after the observation period to make detailed notes. Another useful strategy is to videotape the events, so that careful observations and detailed notes can be taken at a later time.

Foust (2007) conducted a study of discharge planning as part of daily nursing practice. Her purpose was to examine nurses' discharge planning efforts as they occurred in practice. She observed and interviewed eight nurses. Following are the researcher's comments about the observations:

"Participant observation was conducted to capture the flow of information (e.g., listening to shift reports), nurse-patient interactions (e.g., initial morning assessments), and unit activities (e.g., discharge, planning rounds)" (p. 74). The author states under major findings "Participant observations uncovered how nurses integrated patient teaching into their interactions with patients as they monitored their postoperative recovery" (p. 74). Later the author reports "documentation of ongoing discharge planning efforts was scarce. More typically, patient records contained nurses' assessments of physical care. Similarly, patient teaching flow sheets indicated typical instructions related to postoperative care that did not include discharge teaching. Discharge instructions were typically completed on the day of discharge, and a copy was sent home with the patients. The richness of nurses' discharge teaching and planning was missing from written documentation" (Foust, 2007, p. 76).

CRITICAL APPRAISAL

The problem that led to the study was a question of how nurses integrated patient teaching into their interactions with patients as they monitored their postoperative recovery. This question did not change during the course of the study. The study was feasible to conduct. The methods involved observing the provision of nursing teaching in interactions with patients and examining patient records for documentation of patient teaching. The findings addressed the purpose of the study. Interpretations of data were backed up by the data collected. The data appeared to be sufficiently analyzed. The researcher did not address variations in the findings. The author found that there is very little documentation of patient teaching, even on the day of discharge, when most teaching is conducted. There was a coherent logic to the statement of findings.

Foust's (2007) major finding was that nurses compared patients' progress with their own general expectations about how patients recover following gynecologic surgery. The nurses' expectations "guided their ongoing efforts to monitor their patients' progress, provide patient teaching, and communicate with other professionals. The nurses integrated many of these components into their daily practice with a specific discharge plan that evolved as their patient recovered" (p. 74).

Although nurses communicated specific assessment findings indicating progress or the lack thereof with each other during shift report, their "communication with other providers and documentation in medical records were less visible aspects of discharge planning" (p. 74).

Continued

IMPLICATIONS FOR PRACTICE

From this observational study in one hospital, it appears that nurses were not documenting the patient teaching they were doing. Patient teaching is a very important element of nursing practice and one for which nurses are accountable to the patient, the hospital, and the law. This finding should be explored in other hospitals and, if the failure to document is extensive, actions should be taken by nurses to emphasize and enforce this documentation.

Text as a Source of Qualitative Data

In qualitative studies, text is considered a rich source of data. The researcher may ask participants to write about a particular topic. In some cases, these written narratives may be solicited by mail or e-mail rather than in person. Text provided by participants may be a component of a larger study using a variety of sources of data. Text developed for other purposes, such as patient records or procedure manuals, can be accessed for qualitative analysis. Published text from newspaper articles, magazine articles, books, or the Internet also can be used as qualitative data. Transcriptions of recorded interviews are commonly used in qualitative studies. In historical research, written descriptions of historical events, letters, and documents related to the event may be accessed for text analysis. A historical study might examine the changing pattern of nursing practice in a selected area or of a nursing procedure by examining nursing textbooks and journal articles that describe a particular practice at different times. Notes taken during the reading of documents are important to the analysis process. For an example of text analysis, see Lusk (1997) who analyzed text from a variety of archival sources (p. 277).

Other Qualitative Methods of Data Collection

Collecting Stories

Stories can help researchers to understand a phenomenon of interest. In narrative inquiry, a qualitative method, the focus of the research may be the gathering of stories. Gathering of stories can enable healthcare providers to develop storytelling as a powerful means to increase insight and promote health behavior in clients. For example, Elliott (2010) explored the relationships between fathers and their daughters in recovery from anorexia nervosa. The study revealed the vulnerability of the daughters during developmental transitions.

Tales of success or tales of key leaders/personalities are familiar genres with which to maintain a collective sense of the culture of an organization. The use of atrocity stories and morality fables is also well documented within organizational and occupational settings. Tales of professional incompetence are used to give warning of "what not to do" and what will happen if you commit mistakes. Narratives are also a common genre from which to retell or come to terms with particularly sensitive or traumatic times and events (Coffey & Atkinson, 1996, p. 56; Gallia & Pines, 2009). Nwoga (1997, 2000) studied how African American mothers use storytelling to guide their adolescent daughters regarding sexual behavior. The stories could assist other mothers who are struggling to help their daughters with sexuality issues.

Constructing Life Stories

A life story is designed to reconstruct and interpret the life of an ordinary person. The methodology, which emerged from history, anthropology, and more recently phenomenology, has been described by a number of scholars (Clark, 2006; Davidson, 2004; DiCicco-Bloom & Crabtree, 2006; Foster, McAllister, & O'Brien, 2006; Hardy, Gregory, & Ramjeet, 2009; Keady & Williams, 2007; Kelly & Howie, 2007; Larem, 2008; Lovell, 2006; Wicks & Whiteford, 2006). The life story can be used to clarify meanings of various states of health, chronic illness, and disability in the lives of patients, their families, and other caregivers. These stories can help us understand the meaning to patients of their health behavior, lifestyles, illnesses, or impairments; the meaning of symptoms; their experiences of treatment; how they adapt; and their hopes and possibilities of reconstructing their lives. Interviews are tape recorded and transcribed. Notes from observations may be important, and personal documents such as diaries or historical records may be used. Analysis involves more than just stringing events together; events should be linked in an interpretation through which the researcher can create theoretical sense.

Materials are organized and analyzed according to theoretical interests. Constructing a life story often requires a long-term contact and extensive collaboration with the participant (Frank, 2000; Larson & Fanchiang, 1996; Mallinson, Kielhofner, & Mattingly, 1996).

Devault et al. (2008) conducted a study examining life stories of vulnerable young fathers to explore determinants of parenting from the perspective of Belsky's model. Belsky's model recognizes the influence of a parent's own developmental history and life experiences on the development of their children. Hearing the story of the person who has lived it allows the meaning given to the life events to emerge. The researcher is able "to compare different life stories and discover common themes that emerge within the identified group" (p. 231). The fathers told of their involvement in the lives of the children and their perception of being a father. Second interviews, conducted approximately 8 months later, focused on "the fathers' individual history in their family of origin" (p. 231). Questions focused on learning more about the fathers' own experiences as children and any traumatic life events they had experienced. The second interview also provided an opportunity for the researchers to probe for "details about aspects considered incomplete following the analysis of the first interview and inquired about changes in the participants' lives as fathers since the first meeting" (pp. 231-232).

CRITICAL APPRAISAL

The researchers are interested in the meaning given by the father to being a father and the degree to which the father plans to be involved with the child he parented. These are not questions generally asked of an unmarried father, and yet they are questions that may be important to ask. The questions may prompt the father to consider a degree of involvement that he may not have considered or may not feel is available to him. It is a well-designed study, interviewing the father twice, first early in the pregnancy and again later in the pregnancy.

Continued

IMPLICATIONS FOR PRACTICE

The information gained by this study is important to any provider involved in the care of fathers and mothers in an unwed pregnancy. Including the father in the care and encouraging involvement during the pregnancy and in the care of the child after the birth may make a considerable difference in the father's involvement as the child develops. These understandings can dramatically affect the welfare and mental health of the child for the rest of his or her life. Hearing the stories of unwed fathers may increase the nurse's commitment to including them in care more than reading statements from a text might.

Case Studies

A **case study** examines a single unit within the context of its real-life environment. The unit may be a person, a family, a nursing unit, or an organization. In the early twentieth century, the most common nursing study was a case study. Medical case studies were also common. Nursing case studies were published in the *American Journal of Nursing* and initiated a variety of nursing studies of patient care. As nursing research began to use more rigorous methods, the case study fell into disrepute. However, the importance of information from case studies is again being recognized. Case studies can use quantitative, qualitative, or mixed methods of data collection. It is important for the researcher to consider the multiple aspects that affect a particular case and include this essential information in the plan for data collection and analysis. Wardell, Rintala, and Tan (2008) used the case study method to analyze the effect of healing touch with veterans experiencing chronic neuropathic pain following spinal cord injury. Seven cases of beneficial or equivocal experiences were selected for analysis by the researchers. Clinical notes of certified health touch practitioners, narrative comments from veteran interviews, and pain assessments were analyzed to construct descriptions of a less familiar intervention for pain.

CRITICAL APPRAISAL

The researchers provide detailed information about an intervention for pain that is little known to most nurses. The type of pain experienced by the patients is not easily relieved by traditional methods. The authors go into great detail to help the reader understand the patient's situation and the treatment that is provided. The response to the treatment varies with the patient, and this difference in response is clearly illustrated in the study.

IMPLICATIONS FOR PRACTICE

Nurses are often reluctant to encourage treatments such as those described in the study because the treatments may not have a sufficient scientific basis. But for persons with long-term pain that is not relieved by traditional means, the nurse must consider whether or not they are worth encouraging the patient to try the treatment.

Data Management

Qualitative data analysis occurs concurrently with data collection, rather than sequentially as in quantitative research. Therefore, the researcher is attempting to simultaneously gather, manage, and interpret a growing bulk of data. Volumes of data are gathered during a qualitative study. The researcher must develop means of storing the data in an organized manner. Some data may be recorded as handwritten notes, but will be transferred to a word processing program for electronic storage as soon as possible, carefully dated, and with adequate notation to document where and when the data were collected. Keeping track of connections between various bits of data requires meticulous record keeping. The researchers will read, reread, and analyze the data over time to maintain a close link with—or become immersed in—the data being analyzed. Using the computer can promote creativity, facilitate documentation without the researcher losing touch with the data (Anderson, 1987; Miles & Huberman, 1994; Pateman, 1998; St. John & Johnson, 2000; Taft, 1993), and support researcher access to data being analyzed as a team.

Transcribing Interviews

Audio-recorded interviews generally are transcribed word for word. Morse and Field (1995) provide the following instructions for transcribing a recorded interview.

> Pauses should be indicated by using dashes, and ellipses should indicate gaps or prolonged pauses. All expressions, including exclamations, laughter, crying, and expletives, are included in the text and separated from the verbal text with square brackets. Type the interviews single-spaced with a blank line between each speaker. A generous margin on both sides of the page permits the left margin to be used for coding and the researcher's own critique of the interview style, and the right margin to be used for comments regarding the content. … Ensure that all pages are numbered sequentially and that each page is coded with the interview number and the participant number. (p. 131)

Listening to recordings as soon as possible after an interview is recommended. Voice tone, inflection, and pauses of the researcher and the participant are important to note. After the interview is transcribed, the researcher is advised to listen to the recording and read the written transcript of the tape simultaneously, making notations of observations on the transcript (Morse & Field, 1995).

Although data preparation is a distinctive stage in qualitative work in which data are put into a form that will permit analysis, a rudimentary kind of analysis often begins when the researcher proofs transcripts against the audiotaped interviews from which they were prepared. Indeed, the proofing process is often the first time a researcher gets a sense of the interview as a whole. It is occasionally the first time investigators hear something said, even though they conducted the interview. During the proofing process, researchers often underline key phrases, simply because they make some as yet amorphous impression on them. They may jot down ideas in the margins next to the text that triggered them, just because they do not want to lose some line of thinking.

The elements of transforming raw data into a meaningful picture of the phenomenon, process, or perspective being studied will be described as steps in a process; however, the steps are iterative and more circular than linear. These steps include immersion, data reduction, analysis, and interpretation.

Immersion in the Data

Data collected during a qualitative study may include narrative descriptions of observations, transcripts from audio recording of interviews, entries in the researcher's journal reflecting on the dynamics of the setting, or notes taken while reading written documents. In the initial phases of data analysis, the researcher needs to become familiar with the data as it is gathered. This process may involve reading and rereading notes and transcripts, recalling observations and experiences, listening to audio recordings, and viewing video recordings until the researcher has become immersed in the data. The recordings contain more than words; they contain feeling, emphasis, and nonverbal communications that provide the researcher clues about the participant's feelings and emphasis. These aspects are at least as important to the communication as are the words. In phenomenology, this immersion in the data is referred to as **dwelling with the data**. The initial purpose of this immersion is to address the question, "What is going on?" Writing about initial impressions of the data and talking about the data to other qualitative researchers are ways to start the process of analysis.

Data Reduction

Because of the volumes of data acquired in a qualitative study, initial efforts at analysis focus on reducing the volume of data so that the researcher can more effectively examine them, a process referred to as **data reduction**. During data reduction, the researcher begins to *tentatively* attach meaning to elements in the data. For example, the researcher might consider ways that things, persons, and events can be classified. In some cases, the researcher may identify a classification scheme within the data in the words used by participants. Other qualitative researchers may have developed a study based on a particular theoretical perspective and may begin to reduce the data according to the concepts within this perspective.

Data Analysis

Data analysis is a rigorous process. Because published qualitative studies may not contain the methodology in detail, many professionals believe that qualitative research is a freewheeling process with little structure. Creativity and deep thought may produce innovative views of the data, but the process requires discipline to develop data analysis plans that are consistent with the specific philosophical method of the study.

For example, researchers conducting grounded theory studies use the constant comparative process, in which emerging concepts and themes are compared with previously analyzed data and integrated into the analysis of data being considered for the first time. In grounded theory, the analysis begins with the first participant interview so that ideas from that participant can be integrated into questions and probes in subsequent interviews.

Codes and Coding

Coding is the process of reading the data, breaking text down into sub-parts, and giving a label to that part of the text. Morse and Richards (2002) note that, although coding is used by all qualitative researchers, the sequence and purpose of coding varies according to the type of qualitative study. When coding data for a phenomenological study, the researcher will first label shifts in meaning in the flow of the transcript (Liamputtong, 2009). A grounded theory researcher first codes using open codes to compare the data. These labels provide a way for the researcher to begin to identify patterns in the data, because sections of text that were coded the same way can be compared for similarities and differences.

A code is a symbol or abbreviation used to classify words or phrases in the data. Codes may be handwritten on a printed transcript or indicated by highlighting a section of text and making a comment in the margin within a word processing program. Some qualitative researchers may develop a numbered list of codes as they analyze the data and use the numbers to indicate how a section of text is coded. Others will use a computerized data management program that allows the researchers to retrieve all the participant statements that were coding with the same word.

Organizing data, selecting specific elements of the data for categories, and naming these categories reflect the philosophical base of the study. Codes may result in themes, processes, or exemplars of the phenomenon being studied. A descriptive qualitative study about pain experiences of surgical patients may result in a taxonomy of types of pain, activities that resulted in pain, and types of pain relief strategies. In study from a grounded theory perspective of medication adherence, participants mentioned clocks, schedules, hours, and doses that the researcher coded as "time." As the researcher continued the analysis, he or she searched and compiled all the statements coded as being related to time.

The researcher should provide information on the codes used in the study in the research report. In critically appraising a study, you need to judge whether or not you consider the codes to be appropriate and adequate for the study.

During data analysis, a dynamic interaction occurs between the researcher and his or her experience of the data, whether the data are communicated orally or in writing. During this process, referred to as **reflexive thought**, the researcher explores personal feelings and experiences that may influence the study and integrates this understanding into the study. The process requires a conscious self-awareness and documenting one's thinking about the data and decisions made about coding in the journal being kept by the researcher.

Thus, an important part of writing a report of a qualitative study is a description of the analysis process of the researcher. As you review qualitative studies, you will critically appraise the description of the analysis for logic and congruence with the study method.

 RESEARCH EXAMPLE Qualitative Analysis

A recurrence of breast cancer can cause an emotional upheaval and precipitate a search for life's meaning. Sarenmalm and colleagues (2009) described coding the data collected during a grounded theory study to include several steps.

> Data collection and analysis was a simultaneous process, with the emerging results directing further data collection. We used the constant comparative analysis method to identify similarities and differences across participant data. Starting with open inductive coding line-by-line, we combined analytical procedures for explicit coding and constant comparison. When codes continually reappeared, we used focused coding to cluster these codes into subcategories. (p. 118)

The researchers also describe how these codes became categories and, eventually, a core category and conceptual framework. The researchers' description made it possible to determine that they used a logical process that was congruent with grounded theory methodology.

Reflection

Qualitative studies require interaction between the researcher and the data. In some phenomenological research this critical thinking leads to bracketing, which is used to help the researcher avoid misinterpreting the phenomenon as it is being experienced by the participants. Bracketing is suspending or laying aside what the researcher knows about the experience being studied (Oiler, 1982). Other phenomenologists, especially those using Heideggerian phenomenology, do not bracket, but they do identify beliefs, assumptions, and preconceptions about the research topic. These are put in writing at the beginning of the study for self-reflection and external review. These procedures are intended to facilitate openness and new insights (Munhall, 2007).

Identifying Themes

Themes are developed from codes. Codes tend to be descriptive and more closely related to transcribed text, whereas themes are inferred from codes. Although themes have been used in qualitative data analysis for some time, specific strategies for developing themes and their role in data analysis has not been clearly specified. However, recently, scholars have provided more detailed directions for developing and using themes in the analysis process (Braun & Clarke, 2006; Fereday & Muir-Cochrane, 2006; Hayes, 2000a,b; Joffe & Yardley, 2004; Patton, 2002; Smith & Dunworth, 2003; Smith, Jarman, & Osborn, 1999; Ziebland & McPherson, 2006).

Codes tend to be developed for transcribed textual data. It is easy to show how the codes are linked to the data from participants. However, themes are not as closely linked to the textual data. Themes are derived from codes that are linked to data from participants. Sometimes there are several layers of themes, each layer further from the initial codes. Making links between these themes and the original data is sometimes difficult. The rigor and clarity of the linking is of great importance, and it is the researcher who must remain rigorous in showing the links from the themes back to the original data. When you read qualitative studies that have used themes, search for evidence of links back to the original data. If you are critically appraising a qualitative study that uses themes, identify the themes and judge whether they seem sufficient and adequate for the study. Are the themes clearly linked to the codes?

Analysis of Focus Group Data

Reports of focus groups tend to address primarily the formation of the groups, the questions addressed by the groups, and the general sense of conclusions reached by the group, if any. Little space in the report addresses the analysis of data. This is because analysis of focus group data is complex. It involves recorded and transcribed data from individuals and, in most cases, data from individuals attending one of several groups. The individuals in a group are influenced in the things they say by the group. Individuals in one group would likely be influenced differently than those in another group. Thus, analyzing the remarks of individuals alone is not sufficient in interpreting the meanings in the data.

There has been no generally accepted approach to analyzing focus group data. Many researchers ignore the group situation and discuss only individual remarks. Vicsec (2007) proposes a scheme for analyzing focus group data that includes both individual and group data. She proposes that situational factors such as interactional factors, the environment, time factors, the content, personal characteristics, manifestations of group influence, and characteristics of the moderator be included in the analysis. Thus, she recommends a situational analysis and a thematic analysis that are conducted simultaneously.

In critically appraising a focus group study, it is important for you to note what analysis has been done as well as who composed the focus group and how it was conducted. The researcher who reports very little about the data analysis leaves the question of rigor unanswered.

Interpretation

Identifying themes or writing a description of the lived experiences begins the process of interpretation in most qualitative studies. During interpretation, the researcher places the findings in a larger context and may link different themes or factors in the findings to each other. The researcher is answering the questions, "What do the findings mean?" Interpretation may focus on the usefulness of the findings for clinical practice or may move toward theorizing.

KEY CONCEPTS

- Qualitative research is a systematic, subjective approach used to describe life experiences and give them meaning using words, instead of numbers.
- Qualitative researchers set aside their own values and experiences to allow the multiple realities of the persons experiencing a phenomenon to emerge.
- Rigor in qualitative research requires scrupulous adherence to a philosophical perspective, thoroughness in collecting, analyzing, and interpreting the data, and transparency in the description of the methods.
- Phenomenological researchers provide descriptions of a specific experience from the perspective of the persons who have lived the experience.
- Grounded theory researchers explore underlying social processes and describe the meaning of an event as expressed through the symbols of language, religion, relationships, and clothing. A theoretical framework may result.
- Ethnographic researchers spend time in a culture to understand the environment, people, power relations, and communication patterns of a work setting, community, or ethnic group.
- Historical researchers explore past events to gain insight into causes and factors surrounding the event.
- Data collection in qualitative studies occurs in the context of the relationship between the participant and the researcher.
- Data in qualitative studies are collected through interviews, focus groups, observation, and review of documents.
- Data management, analysis, and interpretation require clear procedures to ensure methodological rigor and credibility of the findings.

REFERENCES

Anderson, N. L. R. (1987). Computer-assisted analysis of textual field note data. *Western Journal of Nursing Research*, *9*(4), 626-630.

Artinian, B. A. (1988). Qualitative modes of inquiry. *Western Journal of Nursing Research*, *10*(2), 138-149.

Ayres, L., & Poirier, S. (1996). Focus on qualitative methods: Virtual text and the growth of meaning in qualitative research. *Research in Nursing & Health*, *19*(2), 163-169.

Bradbury-Jones, C. (2007). Enhancing rigour in qualitative health research: Exploring subjectivity through Peshkin's I's. *Journal of Advanced Nursing Research*, *59*(30), 290-298.

Braun, V., & Clarke, V. (2006). Using thematic analysis in psychology. *Qualitative Research in Psychology*, *3*, 77-101.

Burns, N. (1989). Standards for qualitative research. *Nursing Science Quarterly*, *2*(1), 44-52.

Burns, N., & Grove, S. (2009). *The practice of nursing research*. Philadelphia: Saunders.

Byrne, M. (2001). Hermeneutics as a methodology for textual analysis. *AORN Journal*, *73*(5), 968-970.

Carnevale, F. A., Macdonald, M. E., Bluebond-Langner, M., & McKeever, P. (2008). Using participant observation in pediatric health care settings: Ethical challenges and solutions. *Journal of Child Health Care*, *12*(1), 18-32.

Ceci, C. (2003). Midnight reckonings: On a question of knowledge and nursing. *Nursing Philosophy*, *4*(1), 61-76.

Christy, T. E. (1978). The hope of history. In M. L. Fitzpatrick (Ed.), *Historical studies in nursing* (pp. 3-11). New York: Teachers College Press.

Clark, A. (2006). Qualitative interviewing: Encountering ethical issues and challenges. *Nurse Researcher*, *3*(4), 19-29.

Coffey, A., & Atkinson, P. (1996). *Making sense of qualitative data*. Thousand Oaks, CA: Sage.

Cohen, M. Z., & Kahn, D. L. (2000). *Hermaneutic phenomenological research: A practical guide for nurse researchers*. Thousand Oaks, CA: Sage.

Davidson, J. (2004). Dilemmas in research: Issues of vulnerability and empowerment for the social worker/researcher. *Journal of Social Work Practice*, *18*(3), 379-393.

Denzin, N. K., & Lincoln, Y. S. (2005). *The Sage handbook of qualitative research* (3rd ed.). Thousand Oaks, CA: Sage.

Devault, A., Milcent, M-P., Ouellet, F., Laurin, I., Jauron, M., & Lacharit, E. (2008). Life stories of young fathers in contexts of vulnerability. *Fathering*, *6*(3), 226-248.

DiCicco-Bloom, B., & Crabtree, B. F. (2006). The qualitative research interview. *Medical Education*, *40*(4), 314-321.

Dzurec, L. C. (1989). The necessity for and evolution of multiple paradigms for nursing research: A poststructuralist perspective. *Advances in Nursing Science*, *11*(4), 69-77.

Elliott, J. C. (2010). Fathers, daughters, and anorexia nervosa. *Perspectives in Psychiatric Care*, *46*(1), 37-47.

Fereday, J., & Muir-Cochrane, E. (2006). Demonstrating rigor using thematic analysis: A hybrid approach of inductive and deductive coding and theme development. *International Journal of Qualitative Methods*, *5*(1), 1-11.

Finch, L. P. (2004). Understanding patients' lived experiences: The interrelationships of rhetoric and hermeneutics. *Nursing Philosophy*, *5*(3), 251-257.

Finlay, L. (2004). Exploring lived experience: Principles and practice of phenomenological research. *International Journal of Theory and Rehabilitation*, *16*(9), 474-481.

Fleming, V., Gaidys, U., & Robb, Y. (2003). Hermeneutic research in nursing: Developing a Gadamerian-based research method. *Nursing Inquiry*, *19*(2), 113-120.

Foster, K., McAllister, M., & O'Brien, L. (2006). Extending the boundaries of autoethnography as an emergent method in mental health nursing research. *International Journal of Mental Health Nursing*, *5*(1), 44-53.

Foust, J. B. (2007). Discharge planning as part of daily nursing practice. *Applied Nursing Research*, *20*, 72-77.

Frank, A. W. (2000). The standpoint of storyteller. *Qualitative Health Research*, *10*(3), 354-365.

Gallia, K. S., & Pines, E. W. (2009). Narrative identity and spirituality of African American churchwomen surviving breast cancer. *Journal of Cultural Diversity*, *16*(2), 50-55.

Glaser, B. G., & Strauss, A. (1965). *Awareness of dying*. Chicago: Aldine.

Glaser, B. G., & Strauss, A. (1967). *The discovery of grounded theory: Strategies for qualitative research*. Chicago: Aldine.

Glaser, B. G., & Strauss, A. (1968). *Time for dying*. Chicago: Aldine.

Glaser, B. G., & Strauss, A. (1971). *Status passage*. London: Routledge & Kegan Paul.

Grace, J. T., & Powers, B. A. (2009). Claiming our core: Appraising qualitative evidence for nursing questions about human response and meaning. *Nursing Outlook*, *57*, 27-34.

Gray, J. (2009). Rooms, recordings, and responsibilities: The logistics of focus groups. *Southern Online Journal of Nursing Research*, *9*(1). Available at http://www.snrs.org/publications/journal.html

Halcomb, E. J., Gholizadeh, L., DiGiacomo, M., Phillips, J., & Davidson, P. M. (2007). Literature review: Considerations in undertaking focus group research with culturally and linguistically diverse groups. *Journal of Clinical Nursing*, *16*, 1000-1011.

Happ, M. B., Swigart, V. A., Tate, J. A., Arnold, R. M., Sereika, S. M., & Hoffman, L. A. (2007). Family presence and surveillance during weaning from prolonged mechanical ventilation. *Heart & Lung: The Journal of Acute and Critical Care*, *36*(1), 47-57.

Hardy, S., Gregory, S., & Ramjeet, J. (2009). An exploration of intent for normative methods of inquiry. *Nurse Researcher*, *16*(4), 7-19.

Haverkamp, B. E., & Young, R. A. (2007). Paradigms, purpose, and the role of the literature: Formulating a rationale for qualitative investigations. *The Counseling Psychologist*, *35*, 265-294.

Hayes, N. (2000a). *Doing psychological research: Gathering and analysing data*. Buckingham, UK: OU Press.

Hayes, N. (2000b). *Doing psychological research*. London: Sage.

Hutton, A. (2007). An adolescent ward: 'In name only?' *Journal of Clinical Nursing*, *17*, 3142-3149.

Jeon, Y. (2004). The application of grounded theory and symbolic interactionism. *Scandinavian Journal of Caring Science, 18*, 249-256.

Joffe, H., & Yardley, I. (2004). Content and thematic analysis, pp. 56-68. In: Marks, D. F. (Ed.), *Research methods for clinical and health psychology*. London: Sage.

Johnson, M. E. (2000). Heidegger and meaning: Implications for phenomenological research. *Nursing Philosophy, 1*(2), 134-146.

Keady, J., & Williams, S. (2007). Co-constructing inquiry: A new approach to generating, disseminating and discovering knowledge in qualitative research. *Quality in Ageing, 8*(2), 27-36.

Kelly, J., & Howie, L. (2007). Working with stories in nursing research: Procedures used in narrative analysis. *International Journal of Mental Health Nursing, 6*(3), 136-144.

Kleiman, S. (2004). Phenomenology: To wonder and search for meanings. *Nurse Researcher, 11*(4), 7-19.

Kübler-Ross, E. (1969). *On death and dying*. New York: Macmillan.

Kvigne, K., Gjengedal, E., & Kirkevold, M. (2002). Gaining access to the life-world of women suffering from stroke: Methodological issues in empirical phenomenological studies. *Journal of Advanced Nursing, 40*(1), 61-68.

Larem, G. F. (2008). Making sense of stories: The use of patient narratives with mental health research. *Nursing Philosophy, 9*(1), 62-71.

Larson, E. A., & Fanchiang, S. C. (1996). Life history and narrative research: Generating a humanistic knowledge base for occupational therapy. *American Journal of Occupational Therapy, 50*(4), 247-250.

Leifer, S. L., & Glass, L. K. (2008). Planning for mass disaster in the 1950s. *Nursing Research, 57*(4), 237-244.

Leininger, M. M. (1970). *Nursing and anthropology: Two worlds to blend*. New York: Wiley.

Leininger, M. M. (1985). *Qualitative research methods in nursing*. Orlando, FL: Grune & Stratton.

Leininger, M. M. (1988). Leininger's theory of nursing: Cultural care diversity and universality. *Nursing Science Quarterly, 1*, 152-160.

Leininger, M. M. (2002). Culture care theory: A major contribution to advance transcultural nursing knowledge and practice. *Journal of Transcultural Nursing, 13*(3), 189-192.

Liamputtong, P. (2009). *Qualitative research methods* (3rd ed.). South Melbourne, Australia: Oxford University Press.

Lincoln, Y. S., & Guba, E. G. (1985). *Naturalistic inquiry*. Beverly Hills, CA: Sage.

Lovell, A. (2006). Research methodology. Daniel's story: Self-injury and the case study as method. *British Journal of Nursing, 15*(3), 166-170.

Lusk, B. (1997). Historical methodology for nursing research. *Image: The Journal of Nursing Scholarship, 29*(4), 355-359.

Mallinson, T., Kielhofner, G., & Mattingly, C. (1996). Metaphor and meaning in a clinical interview. *American Journal of Occupational Therapy, 50*(5), 338-346.

Mapp, T. (2008). Understanding phenomenology: The lived experience. *British Journal of Midwifery, 16*(5), 308-311.

Marshall, C., & Rossman, G. B. (2006). *Designing qualitative research* (4th ed.). Thousand Oaks, CA: Sage.

Mason, J. (2002). *Qualitative researching*. Thousand Oaks, CA: Sage.

Mead, G. H. (1934). *Mind, self and society*. Chicago: University of Chicago Press.

Miles, M. B., & Huberman, A. M. (1994). *Qualitative data analysis: An expanded sourcebook* (2nd ed.). Thousand Oaks, CA: Sage.

Mitchell, G. J. (2004). An emerging framework for human becoming criticism. *Nursing Science Quarterly, 17*(2), 103-109.

Morrison, R. S., & Peoples, L. (1999). Using focus group methodology in nursing. *Journal of Continuing Education in Nursing, 30*(2), 62-65.

Morse, J. M. (1989). Qualitative nursing research: A free-for-all? In J. M. Morse (Ed.), *Qualitative nursing research: A contemporary dialogue* (pp. 14-22). Rockville, MD: Aspen.

Morse, J. M., & Field, P. A. (1995). *Qualitative research methods for health professionals* (2nd ed.). Thousand Oaks, CA: Sage.

Morse, J. M., & Richards, L. (2002). *Read me first for a user's guide to qualitative methods*. Thousand Oaks, CA: Sage.

Munhall, P. L. (Ed.). (2007). *Nursing research: A qualitative perspective* (4th ed.). Sudbury, MA: Jones & Bartlett.

Nicholls, D. (2009). Qualitative research: Part one- philosophies. *International Journal of Therapy and Rehabilitation, 16*(10), 526-533.

Nwoga, I. (1997). *Mother-daughter conversations related to sex-role socialization and adolescent pregnancy*. Ph.D. dissertation, The University of Florida.

Nwoga, I. (2000). African American mothers use stories for family sexuality education. *MCN, American Journal of Maternal Child Nursing, 25*(1), 31-36.

Oiler, C. (1982). The phenomenological approach in nursing research. *Nursing Research, 31*(3), 178-181.

Pateman, B. (1998). Computer-aided qualitative data analysis: The value of NUD*IST and other programs. *Nurse Researcher, 5*(3), 77-89.

Patton, M. Q. (2002). *Qualitative evaluation and research methods* (3rd ed.). Newbury Park, CA: Sage.

Power, T. G., Bindler, R. C., Goetz, S., & Daratha, K. B. (2010). Obesity prevention in early adolescence: Student, parent, and teacher views. *Journal of School Health, 80*(1), 13-19.

Roberts, T. (2009). Understanding ethnography. *British Journal of Midwifery, 17*(5), 291-294.

Roche-Fahy, V., & Dowling, M. (2009). Providing comfort to patients in their palliative care trajectory: Experiences of female nurses working in an acute setting. *International Journal of Palliative Nursing, 15*(3), 134-141.

Roper, J. M., & Shapiro, J. (2000). *Ethnography in nursing research*. Thousand Oaks, CA: Sage.

Sadala, M. L., & Adorno, R. C. (2002). Phenomenology as a method to investigate the experience lived: A perspective from Husserl and Merleau Polty's thought. *Journal of Advanced Nursing, 37*(3), 282-293.

Salander, P. (2007). Atributions of lung cancer: My own illness is hardly caused by smoking. *Psycho-Oncology, 16*, 587-592.

Sandelowski, M. (1986). The problem of rigor in qualitative research. *Advances in Nursing Science, 8*(3), 27-37.

Sandelowski, M. (1993). Rigor or rigor mortis: The problem of rigor in qualitative research revisited. *Advances in Nursing Science, 16*(2), 1-8.

Sandelowski, M., & Barroso, J. (2007). *Handbook for synthesizing qualitative research.* New York: Springer.

Sarenmalm, E. K., Thoren-Jonsson, A. L., Gaston-Johansson, F., & Ohlen, J. (2009). Making sense of living under the shadow of death: Adjusting to a recurrent breast cancer illness. *Qualitative Health Research, 19,* 1116-1130.

Scheckel, M., & Hedrick-Erickson, J. (2009). Decentering resources: A phenomenological study of interpretive pedagogies in patient education. *Journal of Professional Nursing, 25*(1), 57-64.

Schwartz-Barcott, D., & Kim, H. S. (1986). A hybrid model for concept development. In P. L. Chinn (Ed.), *Nursing research methodology: Issues and implementation* (pp. 91-101). Rockville, MD: Aspen.

Silverman, D. (1993). *Interpreting qualitative data: Methods for analyzing talk, text and interaction.* Thousand Oaks, CA: Sage.

Slade, S. C., Molloy, E., & Keating, J. L. (2009). Stigma experienced by people with nonspecific chronic low back pain: A qualitative study. *Pain Medicine, 10*(1), 143-154.

Smith, J. A., & Dunworth, F. (2003). Qualitative methods in the study of development. In K. Connolly, & J. Valsiner (Eds.), *The handbook of developmental psychology.* London: Sage.

Smith, J. A., Jarman, M., & Osborn, M. (1999). Doing interpretative phenomenological analysis. In M. Murray, & K. Chamberlain (Eds.), *Qualitative health psychology: Theories and methods.* London: Sage.

St. John, W., & Johnson, P. (2000). The pros and cons of data analysis software for qualitative research. *Journal of Nursing Scholarship, 32*(4), 393-397.

Strauss, A. L., Corbin, J., Fagerhaugh, S., Glaser, B. G., Maines, D., Suczek, B., et al. (1984). *Chronic illness and the quality of life* (2nd ed.). St. Louis: Mosby.

Taft, L. B. (1993). Computer-assisted qualitative research. *Research in Nursing & Health, 16*(5), 379-383.

Tran, P. D., & Garcia, K. (2009). An international study of health knowledge, behaviors, and cultural perceptions of young Mexican adults. *Hispanic Health Care International, 7*(1), 5-10.

Vicsec, L. (2007). A scheme for analyzing the results of focus groups. *International Journal of Qualitative Methods, 6*(4), 20-34.

Wardell, D. W., Rintala, D., & Tan, G. (2008). Study descriptions of healing touch with veterans experiencing chronic neuropathic pain from spinal cord injury. *Explore, 4*(3), 187-195.

Weine, S., Bahromov, M., & Mirzoev, A. (2008). Unprotected Tajik male migrant workers in Moscow at risk for HIV/AIDS. *Journal of Immigrant and Minority Health, 10,* 461-468.

Wicks, A., & Whiteford, G. (2006). Conceptual and practical issues in good iterative research: Reflections on a life-history study. *Scandinavian Journal of Occupational Therapy, 13*(2), 94-100.

Wilson, K. L. & Woodgate, R. L. (2007). An interruption in family life: Siblings' lived experience as they transition through the pediatric bone marrow transplant trajectory. *Oncology Nursing Forum, 34*(2), E28-E35.

Wimpenny, P., & Gass, J. (2000). Interviewing in phenomenology and grounded theory: Is there a difference? *Journal of Advanced Nursing, 31*(6), 1485-1492.

Wood, P. J. (2009). The enduring issue of assessing nursing knowledge: Surgical nursing final examination in Australia and New Zealand, 1905-1930. *Contemporary Nurse, 32*(1-2), 109-122.

Ziebland, S., & McPherson, A. (2004). Making sense of qualitative data analysis: An introduction with illustrations from DIPEx (personal experiences of health and illness.) *Medical Education, 40,* 405-414.

Examining Ethics in Nursing Research

Chapter Overview

Historical Events Influencing the Development of Ethical Codes and Regulations   104
Nazi Medical Experiments   104
Nuremberg Code   104
Declaration of Helsinki   105
Tuskegee Syphilis Study   106
Willowbrook Study   106
Jewish Chronic Disease Hospital Study   107
Department of Health, Education, and Welfare 1973 Regulations for the Protection of Human Research Subjects   107
National Commission for the Protection of Human Subjects of Biomedical and Behavioral Research   107
Current Federal Regulations for the Protection of Human Subjects   108
Protecting Human Rights   110
Right to Self-Determination   110
Right to Privacy   114
Right to Anonymity and Confidentiality   117
Right to Fair Treatment   118
Right to Protection from Discomfort and Harm   118
Critical Appraisal Guidelines to Examine Protection of Human Rights in Studies   120

Understanding Informed Consent   122
Essential Information for Consent   122
Comprehension of Consent Information   123
Competence to Give Consent   124
Voluntary Consent   125
Documentation of Informed Consent   125
Critical Appraisal Guidelines to Examine Informed Consent in Studies   128
Understanding Institutional Review   130
Levels of Reviews Conducted by Institutional Review Boards   131
Influence of HIPAA Privacy Rule on Institutional Review Boards   133
Examining the Benefit-Risk Ratio of a Study   134
Critical Appraisal Guidelines for Examining the Ethical Aspects of Studies   136
Understanding Research Misconduct   137
Role of the Office of Research Integrity in Promoting the Conduct of Ethical Research   138
Examining the Use of Animals in Research   139

Learning Outcomes

After completing this chapter, you should be able to:

1. Identify the historical events influencing the development of ethical codes and regulations for research.
2. Identify the ethical principles that are important in conducting research on human subjects.
3. Describe the human rights that require protection in research.
4. Critically appraise the informed consent and institutional review processes in published studies.
5. Examine the benefit-risk ratio of published studies.
6. Describe the types of possible scientific misconduct in the conduct, reporting, and publication of healthcare research.

Key Terms

Anonymity, p. 117

Assent to participate in research, p. 112

Autonomous agents, p. 110

Benefit-risk ratio, p. 134

Breach of confidentiality, p. 117

Coercion, p. 110

Confidentiality, p. 117

Consent form, p. 123

Covered entities, p. 115

Covert data collection, p. 110

Data use agreement, p. 117

Deception, p. 110

Diminished autonomy, p. 111

Discomfort and harm, p. 118

Ethical principles, p. 107

   Principle of beneficence, p. 107

   Principle of justice, p. 107

   Principle of respect for person(s), p. 107

Fabrication, p. 137

Falsification, p. 137

Human rights, p. 110

Individually identifiable health information, p. 115

Informed consent, p. 122

Institutional review, p. 130

   Complete review, p. 133

Exempt from review, p. 131

Expedited review, p. 131

Institutional review board (IRB), p. 130

Invasion of privacy, p. 114

Minimal risk, p. 131

Nontherapeutic research, p. 105

Permission to participate in research, p. 112

Plagiarism, p. 137

Privacy, p. 114

Research misconduct, p. 137

Therapeutic research, p. 105

Voluntary consent, p. 125

STUDY TOOLS

Be sure to visit *http://elsevier.com/evolve/Burns/understanding* for additional examples and self-tests. Also, a review of this chapter's concepts and practice exercises can be found in Chapter 4 of the Study Guide for *Understanding Nursing Research: Building an Evidence-Based Practice*, 5th edition.

Ethical research is essential for generating sound empirical knowledge for evidenced-based practice, but what does ethical conduct of research involve? This is a question that researchers, philosophers, lawyers, and politicians have debated for many years. The debate continues, probably because of the complexity of human rights issues; the focus of research in new, challenging arenas of technology and genetics; the complex ethical codes and regulations governing research; and the various interpretations of these codes and regulations. This chapter introduces you to the national and international codes and regulations developed to promote the ethical conduct of research.

You might think that unethical studies that violate subjects' rights are a thing of the past but this is not the case. There are still incidences where researchers do not protect the subjects' privacy adequately or the study participants are not treated as fairly as they should be during a study. Another serious ethical problem that has increased over the last 25 years is research misconduct. This misconduct includes incidences of fabrication, falsification, or plagiarism in the process of conducting and reporting research in nursing and other health-care disciplines (Office of Research Integrity [ORI], 2009). Thus, the ethical aspects of published studies and of research conducted in clinical agencies need to be critically appraised. Most published studies include ethical information about subject selection and treatment of subjects during data collection in the Methods section of the report. Institutional review boards (IRBs) in universities and clinical agencies have been organized to examine the ethical aspects of studies before they are conducted. Nurses often are members of IRBs and participate in the review of research for conduct in clinical agencies.

To provide a background for examining ethical aspects of studies, this chapter describes the ethical codes and regulations that currently guide the conduct of biomedical and behavioral research. The following elements of ethical research are detailed: (1) protecting human rights, (2) understanding informed consent, (3) understanding institutional review of research, and (4) examining the balance of benefits and risks in a study. The chapter provides critical appraisal guidelines for examining the ethical aspects of published studies and research proposed for conduct in clinical agencies. The chapter concludes with a discussion of two additional important ethical issues: research misconduct and the use of animals in research.

Historical Events Influencing the Development of Ethical Codes and Regulations

Since the 1940s four experimental projects have been highly publicized for their unethical treatment of human subjects: the Nazi medical experiments, the Tuskegee Syphilis Study, the Willowbrook Study, and the Jewish Chronic Disease Hospital Study (Berger, 1990; Levine, 1986). Although these were biomedical studies and the primary investigators were physicians, the evidence suggests that nurses understood the nature of the research, identified potential research subjects, delivered treatments to the subjects, and served as data collectors. These unethical studies demonstrate the importance of ethical conduct for nurses while they are reviewing, participating in, or conducting nursing or biomedical research (Havens, 2004; Veatch, Haddad, & English, 2009). These studies also influenced the formulation of ethical codes and regulations that currently direct the conduct of research.

Nazi Medical Experiments

From 1933 to 1945 the Third Reich in Europe performed atrocious unethical medical activities. The programs of the Nazi regime included sterilization, euthanasia, and medical experimentation for the purpose of producing a population of "racially pure" Germans who were destined to rule the world. The medical experiments were conducted on prisoners of war and persons considered to be racially valueless, such as Jews, who were confined in concentration camps. The experiments involved exposing subjects to high altitudes, freezing temperatures, malaria, poisons, spotted fever (typhus), or untested drugs and performing surgical procedures, usually without any form of anesthesia for the subjects. Extensive examination of the records from some of these studies indicated that they were poorly conceived and conducted. Thus, this research was not only unethical but also generated little if any useful scientific knowledge (Berger, 1990; Steinfels & Levine, 1976).

The Nazi experiments violated numerous rights of the research subjects as subjects and as human beings. The selection of subjects for these studies was racially based and unfair, and the subjects had no choice: They were prisoners who were forced to participate. As a result of these experiments, subjects frequently were killed, or they sustained permanent physical, mental, and social damage (Levine, 1986).

Nuremberg Code

Those involved in the Nazi experiments were brought to trial before the Nuremberg Tribunals, and their unethical research received international attention. The mistreatment of human subjects in these studies led to the development of the Nuremberg Code in 1949.

Table 4–1	The Nuremberg Code

The voluntary consent of the human subject is absolutely essential. ...

The experiment should be such as to yield fruitful results for the good of society, unprocurable by other methods or means of study, and not random and unnecessary in nature.

The experiment should be so designed and based on the results of animal experimentation and a knowledge of the natural history of the disease or other problem under study that the anticipated results will justify the performance of the experiment.

The experiment should be so conducted as to avoid all unnecessary physical and mental suffering and injury.

No experiment should be conducted where there is an *a priori* reason to believe that death or disabling injury will occur, except, perhaps, in those experiments where the experimental physicians also serve as subjects.

The degree of risk to be taken should never exceed that determined by the humanitarian importance of the problem to be solved by the experiment.

Proper preparations should be made and adequate facilities provided to protect the experimental subject against even remote possibilities of injury, disability, or death.

The experiment should be conducted only by scientifically qualified persons. The highest degree of skill and care should be required through all stages of the experiment of those who conduct or engage in the experiment.

During the course of the experiment the human subject should be at liberty to bring the experiment to an end if he has reached the physical or mental state where continuation of the experiment seems to him to be impossible.

During the course of the experiment the scientist in charge must be prepared to terminate the experiment at any stage, if he has probable cause to believe, in the exercise of the good faith, superior skill and careful judgment required of him that a continuation of the experiment is likely to result in injury, disability, or death to the experimental subject.

Nuremberg Code. (1949). *Trials of war criminals before the Nuremberg Military Tribunals under Control Council Law*, 2(1), 181-182. Washington, D.C.: U.S. Government Printing Office. Retrieved April 1, 2009, from *http://www.hhs.gov/ohrp/references/nurcode.htm*

Table 4–1 presents this code. The code includes guidelines that should help you evaluate the consent process, the protection of subjects from harm, and the balance of benefits and risks in a study (Nuremberg Code, 1949).

Declaration of Helsinki

The Nuremberg Code provided the basis for the development of the Declaration of Helsinki, which was adopted in 1964 and revised seven times with the most recent in 2004 by the World Medical Association. A major focus of the initial document was the differentiation of therapeutic research from nontherapeutic research. **Therapeutic research** provides patients with an opportunity to receive an experimental treatment that might have beneficial results. **Nontherapeutic research** is conducted to generate knowledge for a discipline; the results of the study might benefit future patients but probably will not benefit those acting as research subjects.

The Declaration of Helsinki includes the following ethical principles: (1) the investigator should protect the life, health, privacy, and dignity of human subjects; (2) the investigator should exercise greater care to protect subjects from harm in nontherapeutic research; and (3) the investigator should conduct research only when the importance of the objective outweighs the inherent risks and burdens to the subjects. The most recent addition to the Declaration of Helsinki is that researchers must use extreme caution in studies where participants receive a placebo, which means they receive a "sugar pill," not a specific drug treatment. Researchers must provide these participants access to proven diagnostic and therapeutic procedures after the study (World Medical Association, 2004). The ethical principles of the Declaration of Helsinki are available online at *http://ohsr.od.nih.gov/guidelines/helsinki.html.* Most institutions conducting clinical research adopted the Nuremberg Code and Declaration of Helsinki; however, episodes of unethical research related to selection and treatment of subjects continued to occur in biomedical and behavioral research.

Tuskegee Syphilis Study

In 1932, the U.S. Public Health Service initiated a study of syphilis in African American men in the small rural town of Tuskegee, Alabama (Levine, 1986; Rothman, 1982). The study, which continued for 40 years, was conducted to determine the natural course of syphilis in African American men. Many of the subjects who consented to participate in the study were not informed about the purpose and procedures of the research. Some were unaware that they were subjects in a study. By 1936 it was apparent that the men with syphilis had developed more complications than those observed in the men in the control group. Ten years later the death rate among those with syphilis was twice as high as it was for the control group. The subjects were examined periodically but were not treated for syphilis, even when penicillin was determined to be an effective treatment for the disease in the 1940s. Information about an effective treatment for syphilis was withheld from the subjects, and deliberate steps were taken to deprive them of treatment (Brandt, 1978).

Published reports of the Tuskegee Syphilis Study started appearing in 1936, and additional papers were published every 4 to 6 years. No effort was made to stop the study; in fact, in 1969 the Centers for Disease Control and Prevention (then called the Center for Disease Control) decided that the study should continue. In 1972, an account of the study in the *Washington Star* sparked public outrage; only then did the Department of Health, Education, and Welfare (DHEW) stop the study. The study was investigated and found to be ethically unjustified (Brandt, 1978).

Willowbrook Study

From the mid-1950s to the early 1970s, Dr. Saul Krugman conducted research on hepatitis at Willowbrook, an institution for the mentally retarded in Staten Island, New York (Rothman, 1982). The subjects were children who were deliberately infected with the hepatitis virus. During the 20-year study, Willowbrook closed its doors to new inmates because of overcrowded conditions. However, the research ward continued to admit new inmates, and parents had to give permission for their child to be in the study to gain admission to the institution (Levine, 1986).

From the late 1950s to the early 1970s, Krugman's research team published several articles describing the study protocol and findings. In 1966, Beecher cited the Willowbrook Study in *The New England Journal of Medicine* as an example of unethical research. The investigators defended injecting the children with the hepatitis virus because they believed most of the children would acquire the infection on admission to the institution. They also stressed the benefits the subjects received, which were a cleaner environment, better supervision, and a higher nurse-patient ratio on the research ward (Rothman, 1982). Despite the controversy, this unethical study continued until the early 1970s.

Jewish Chronic Disease Hospital Study

Another highly publicized unethical study was conducted at the Jewish Chronic Disease Hospital in New York in the 1960s. The purpose of this study was to determine patients' rejection responses to live cancer cells. Twenty-two patients were injected with a suspension containing live cancer cells that had been generated from human cancer tissue (Levine, 1986). Because researchers did not inform these patients that they were taking part in research or that the injections they received were live cancer cells, their rights were not protected. In addition, the study was never presented for review to the research committee of the Jewish Chronic Disease Hospital, and the physicians caring for the patients were unaware that the study was being conducted. The physician directing the research was an employee of the Sloan-Kettering Institute for Cancer Research, and there was no indication that this institution had conducted a review of the research project (Hershey & Miller, 1976). This unethical study was conducted without the informed consent of the subjects and without institutional review and had the potential to injure, disable, or cause the death of the human subjects. The study was stopped immediately and steps were taken to ensure proper care for the patients exposed to the cancer cells and the review of all future research to be conducted in this agency.

Department of Health, Education, and Welfare 1973 Regulations for the Protection of Human Research Subjects

The continued conduct of harmful, unethical research from the 1960s to the 1970s made additional controls necessary. In 1973, the DHEW published its first set of regulations for the protection of human research subjects. These regulations also provided protection for persons having limited capacity to consent, such as people who are ill, mentally impaired, or dying (Levine, 1986). According to the DHEW regulations, all research involving human subjects had to undergo full institutional review, which increased the protection of human subjects. However, reviewing all studies without regard for the degree of risk involved greatly increased the time for study approval and reduced the number of studies conducted.

National Commission for the Protection of Human Subjects of Biomedical and Behavioral Research

Because the DHEW regulations did not resolve the issue of protecting human subjects in research, the National Commission for the Protection of Human Subjects of Biomedical and Behavioral Research (1978) was formed. This commission was established by the National Research Act (Public Law 93-348), which was passed in 1974. The commission identified three ethical principles that are relevant to the conduct of research involving human subjects: respect for persons, beneficence, and justice. The principle of respect for persons indicates that people should be treated as autonomous agents with the right to self-determination and the freedom to participate or not participate in research. Those persons with diminished autonomy, such as children, people who are terminally or mentally ill, and prisoners, are entitled to additional protection. The principle of beneficence encourages the researcher to do good and "above all, do no harm." The principle of justice states that human subjects should be treated fairly in terms of the benefits and the risks of research. Before it was dissolved in 1978, the commission developed ethical research guidelines based on these three principles and made recommendations to the U.S. Department of Health and Human Services (DHHS) in the *Belmont Report*. (Information on this report and the three ethical principles—respect for persons, beneficence, and justice—are available online at *http://ohsr.od.nih.gov/guidelines/belmont.html.*)

Current Federal Regulations for the Protection of Human Subjects

In response to the commission's recommendations, the U.S. DHHS developed a set of federal regulations for the protection of human research subjects in 1981, and these regulations were revised in 1983, 1991, 2001, and 2005 (U.S. DHHS, 1981, 1983, 1991, 2001, 2005). The 2005 regulations are part of the *Code of Federal Regulations* (CFR), Title 45 Part 46 Protection of Human Subjects. These regulations provide direction for (1) protection of human subjects in research, with additional protection for pregnant women, human fetuses, neonates, children, and prisoners; (2) documentation of informed consent; and (3) implementation of the IRB process. You can access these regulations online at *http://ohsr.od.nih.gov/guidelines/45cfr46.html.*

The DHHS Protection of Human Subjects Regulations (U.S. DHHS, 2005) and the U.S. Food and Drug Administration govern most of the biomedical and behavioral research conducted in the United States (FDA, 2002; online at *http://www.access.gpo.gov/nara/cfr/waisidx_02/21cfr50_02.html*). The FDA, within the DHHS, manages the CFR Title 21 Food and Drugs, Part 50 Protection of Human Subjects (FDA, 2002) and Part 56 Institutional Review Boards (2009). The FDA has additional human subject protection regulations that apply to clinical investigations involving products regulated by the FDA under the Federal Food, Drug, and Cosmetic Act and research that supports applications for research or marketing permits for these products. Thus, these regulations apply to studies of drugs for humans, medical devices for human use, biological products for human use, human dietary supplements, and electronic products (FDA, 2004; online at *http://www.fda.gov/opacom/laws/default.htm*). The physician and nurse researchers conducting clinical trials to generate new drugs and refine existing drug treatments must comply with these FDA regulations. Table 4–2 clarifies the focus of the U.S. DHHS and FDA Protection of Human Subjects Regulations.

The U.S. DHHS and FDA regulations provide guidelines for the protection of subjects in federally and privately funded research to ensure their privacy and the confidentiality of the information obtained through research. With the mechanisms for the electronic access and transfer of individuals' information, however, the public became concerned about the potential abuses of the health information of persons in all circumstances, including research projects. Thus, a federal regulation—the Health Insurance Portability and Accountability Act (HIPAA), or Public Law 104-191—was enacted in August, 1996, and implemented in April, 2003, to protect people's private health information (U.S. DHHS, 2003). (HIPAA regulations are available online at *http://privacyruleandresearch.nih.gov.*) Table 4–2 clarifies the focus of HIPAA regulations as compared with the DHHS and FDA regulations (U.S. DHHS, 2007, February 2c).

The DHHS developed regulations entitled the *Standards for Privacy of Individually Identifiable Health Information*, and compliance with these regulations is known as the Privacy Rule (U.S. DHHS, 2003, 45 CFR Parts 160 and 164). The HIPAA Privacy Rule established

Table 4-2	Clarification of the Focus of Federal Regulations and Impact on Research		
Area of Distinction	HIPAA Privacy Rule	DHHS Protection of Human Subjects Regulations Title 45 CFR Part 46	FDA Protection of Human Subjects Regulations Title 21 CFR Parts 50 & 56
Overall Objective	Establish a federal floor of privacy protections for most individually identifiable health information by establishing conditions for its use and disclosure by certain healthcare providers, health plans, and healthcare clearinghouses	To protect the rights and welfare of human subjects involved in research conducted or supported by DHHS Not specifically a privacy regulation	To protect the rights, safety, and welfare of subjects involved in clinical investigations regulated by the FDA Not specifically a privacy regulation
Applicability	Applies to HIPAA-defined covered entities, regardless of the source of funding	Applies to human subjects' research conducted or supported by DHHS and research with private funding	Applies to research involving products regulated by the FDA Federal support is not necessary for FDA regulations to be applicable When research subject to FDA jurisdiction is federally funded, both the DHHS Protection of Human Subjects Regulations and FDA Protection of Human Subjects Regulations apply

From U.S. Department of Health and Human Services. (2007, February 2c). How do other privacy protections interact with the privacy rule? *HIPAA privacy rule: Information for researchers*. Retrieved April 7, 2009, from *http://privacyruleandresearch.nih. gov/pr_05.asp*

DHHS, Department of Health and Human Services; *FDA*, Food and Drug Administration; *HIPAA*, Health Insurance Portability and Accountability Act.

a category entitled protective health information (PHI), which allows covered entities, such as health plans, healthcare clearinghouses, and healthcare providers that transmit health information, to use or disclose PHI to others only in certain situations. These situations are discussed later in this chapter.

The HIPAA Privacy Rule has an impact not only on the healthcare environment, but also on the research conducted in this environment. A person must provide his or her signed permission, or authorization, before that person's PHI can be used or disclosed for research purposes. Researchers must develop their research projects to comply with the HIPAA Privacy Rule. The DHHS has a website entitled "HIPAA Privacy Rule: Information for Researchers" to address the impact of this rule on the informed consent and IRB processes in research and to answer common questions about HIPAA (available at *http://privacyruleand research.nih.gov/*) (U.S. DHHD, 2007, February 2a). The HIPAA Privacy Rule has had a negative affect on researchers' abilities to conduct studies and the Institute of Medicine and other professional organizations are encouraging lessening the impact or removing research from the HIPAA regulation (Infectious Diseases Society of America, 2009).

Protecting Human Rights

What are human rights? How are these rights protected during research? Human rights are claims and demands that have been justified in the eyes of an individual or by the consensus of a group of people. Nurses who critically appraise published studies, review research for conduct in their agencies, or assist with data collection for a study have an ethical responsibility to determine whether the rights of the research subjects or participants are protected. The human rights that require protection in research are the rights to (1) self-determination, (2) privacy, (3) anonymity and confidentiality, (4) fair treatment, and (5) protection from discomfort and harm (American Nurses Association, 2001; American Psychological Association, 2002).

Right to Self-Determination

The right to self-determination is based on the ethical principle of respect for persons, and it indicates that humans are capable of controlling their own destiny. Thus, humans should be treated as autonomous agents, who have the freedom to conduct their lives as they choose without external controls. Researchers treat subjects as autonomous agents in a study if the researcher has (1) informed them about the study, (2) allowed them to choose whether to participate, and (3) allowed them to withdraw from the study at any time without penalty (Levine, 1986).

Violation of the Right to Self-Determination

A subject's right to self-determination can be violated through the use of coercion, covert data collection, and deception. Coercion occurs when one person intentionally presents an overt threat of harm or an excessive reward to another to obtain compliance. Some subjects are coerced (forced) to participate in research because they fear harm or discomfort if they do not participate. For example, some patients feel that their medical and nursing care will be negatively affected if they do not agree to be research subjects. Other subjects are coerced to participate in studies because they believe that they cannot refuse the excessive rewards offered, such as large sums of money, special privileges, or jobs (Emanuel, 2004; U.S. DHHS, 2005).

With covert data collection, subjects are unaware that research data are being collected (Reynolds, 1979). For example, in the Jewish Chronic Disease Hospital Study, most of the patients and their physicians were unaware of the study. The subjects were informed that they were receiving an injection of cells, but the word "cancer" was omitted (Beecher, 1966).

The use of deception, the actual misinforming of subjects for research purposes, also can violate a subject's right to self-determination (Kelman, 1967). A classic example of deception is seen in the Milgram (1963) study, in which the subjects thought they were administering electric shocks to another person, but the person was really a professional actor who pretended to feel the shocks. If deception is used in a study, the research report should indicate how the subjects were deceived and that the subjects were informed of the actual research activities and the findings at the end of the study.

Persons with Diminished Autonomy

Persons have diminished autonomy when they are vulnerable and less advantaged because of legal or mental incompetence, terminal illness, or confinement to an institution (U.S. DHHS, 2005). These persons require additional protection of their right to self-determination because of their decreased ability or inability to give informed consent. In addition, these persons are vulnerable to coercion and deception. The research report should include justification for the use of subjects with diminished autonomy, and the need for justification increases as the subjects' risks and vulnerability increase.

Legal and Mental Limitations of Those Consenting to Research

Minors (neonates and children), pregnant women and fetuses, mentally impaired persons, and unconscious patients are legally and/or mentally unable to give informed consent. These individuals often lack the ability to comprehend information about a study and/or to make decisions about participating in or withdrawing from the study. These persons have a range of vulnerability from minimal to absolute. The use of persons with diminished autonomy as research subjects is more acceptable if the following are true: (1) the research is therapeutic, that is, the subjects might benefit from the experimental process; (2) the researcher is willing to use both vulnerable and nonvulnerable people as subjects; (3) the risk is minimized in the study; and (4) the consent process is strictly followed to ensure the rights of the prospective subjects (U.S. DHHS, 2005).

Neonates

A neonate is defined as a newborn and is identified as either viable or nonviable on delivery. Viable neonates are able to survive after delivery, if given the benefit of available medical therapy, and can independently maintain a heartbeat and respiration. "A nonviable neonate means that a newborn after delivery, although living, is not viable" (U.S. DHHS, 2005, 45 CFR Section 46.202). Neonates are extremely vulnerable and require extra protection to determine their involvement in research. However, viable neonates, neonates of uncertain viability, and nonviable neonates may be involved in research if the following conditions are met: (1) the study is scientifically appropriate and the preclinical and clinical studies have been conducted and provide data for assessing the potential risks to the neonates; (2) the study provides important biomedical knowledge, which researchers cannot obtain by other means, and will not add risk to the neonate; (3) the research holds out the prospect of enhancing the probability of survival of the neonate; (4) both parents are fully informed about the research during the consent process; and (5) researchers will have no part in determining the viability of a neonate. In addition, for "nonviable neonates, the vital functions of the neonate should not be artificially maintained because of the research and the research should not terminate the heartbeat or respiration of the neonate" (U.S. DHHS, 2005, 45 CFR Section 46.205).

Children

The laws defining the minor status of a child are statutory and vary from state to state. Often a child's competence to give consent depends on his or her age, with incompetence being irrefutable up to age 7 (Broome, 1999; Thompson, 1987). However, by age 7 children can think in terms of concrete operations and can provide meaningful assent to participation as research subjects. With advancing age and maturity the child can play a stronger role in the consent process.

The DHHS regulations require "soliciting the assent of the children (when capable) and the permission of their parents or guardians. **Assent to participate in research** means a child's affirmative agreement to participate in research. ... **Permission to participate in research** means the agreement of parent(s) or guardian to the participation of their child or ward in research" (U.S. DHHS, 2005, Section 46.402). The therapeutic nature of the research and the risks versus benefits also influence the decision about using children as research subjects. Thompson (1987) developed a guide for obtaining informed consent based on the child's level of competence, the therapeutic nature of the research, and the risks versus benefits (Table 4–3). Table 4–4 presents an example assent form for children 6 to 12 years of age developed by Broome (1999). During a study, researchers need to give the child an option to ask questions and to withdraw from the study if he or she desires.

There is an increased need for ethical research with children and adolescents as subjects. Researchers are being urged to conduct clinical trials with children to determine the effectiveness of selected pharmacological and nonpharmacological treatments for various age groups (Rosato, 2000). Thus, the U.S. Congress enacted the Pediatric Research Equity Act (2003) to promote the inclusion of children and adolescents in clinical research. However, it is important that parents be actively involved with their children in the research process to promote the increased participation of young people in research (Hadley, Smith, Gallo, Angst, & Knafl, 2007). It is better to contact children and their parents directly rather than by phone or mail to increase their participation. Also the approval process by the IRB is more complex in conducting research on children (Savage & McCarron, 2009).

Table 4–3	Guide to Obtaining Informed Consent, Based on the Relationship between a Child's Level of Competence, the Therapeutic Nature of the Research, and Risk versus Benefits*			
	Nontherapeutic		Therapeutic	
	MMR-LB	MR-LB	MR-HB	MMR-HB
Child, incompetent (generally 0-7 yr)				
Parents' consent	Necessary	Necessary	Sufficient*	Sufficient
Child's assent	Optional[†]	Optional[†]	Optional	Optional
Child, relatively competent (7 yr and older)				
Parents' consent	Necessary	Necessary	Sufficient[‡]	Recommended
Child's assent	Necessary	Necessary	Sufficient[§]	Sufficient

HB, high benefit; *LB*, low benefit; *MMR*, more than minimal risk; *MR*, minimal risk.

*A parent's refusal can be superseded by the principle that a parent has no power to forbid the saving of a child's life.

[†]Children making a "deliberate objection" would be precluded from participation by most researchers.

[‡]In cases not involving the privacy rights of a "mature minor."

[§]In cases involving the privacy rights of a "mature minor."

Table 4-4	Sample Assent Form for Children Ages 6 to 12 Years: Pain Interventions for Children with Cancer

Oral Explanation:

I am a nurse who would like to know if relaxation, special ways of breathing, and using your mind to think pleasant things help children like you to feel less afraid and feel less hurt when the doctor has to do a bone marrow aspiration or spinal tap. Today, and the next five times you and your parent come to the clinic, I would like for you to answer some questions about the things in the clinic that scare you. I would also like you to tell me about how much pain you felt during the bone marrow or spinal tap. In addition, I would like to videotape (take pictures of) you and your mom and/or dad during the tests. The second time you visit the clinic I would like to meet with you and teach you special ways to relax, breathe, and use your mind to imagine pleasant things. You can use the special imagining and breathing then during your visits to the clinic. I would ask you and your parents to practice the things I teach you at home between your visits to the clinic. At any time you could change your mind and not be in the study anymore.

To child:

I want to learn special ways to relax, breathe, and imagine.

I want to answer questions about things children may be afraid of when they come to the clinic.

I want to tell you how much pain I feel during the tests I have.

I will let you videotape me while the doctor does the tests (bone marrow and spinal taps).

If the child says YES, have him/her put an "X" here:

If the child says NO, have him/her put an "X" here:

Date:

Child's signature:

From Broome, M. E. (1999). Consent (assent) for research with pediatric patients. *Seminars in Oncology Nursing, 15*(2), 101.

Pregnant Women and Fetuses

Pregnant women require additional protection in research because of the presence of the fetus. Federal regulations define pregnancy as encompassing the period of time from implantation until delivery. "A woman is assumed to be pregnant if she exhibits any of the pertinent presumptive signs of pregnancy, such as missed menses, until the results of a pregnancy test are negative or until delivery" (U.S. DHHS, 2005, 45 CFR section 46.202). Research conducted with pregnant women should have the potential to directly benefit the woman or the fetus. If the investigation provides a direct benefit just to the fetus, then researchers need to obtain the consent of the pregnant woman and the father. Studies with "pregnant women should include no inducements to terminate the pregnancy and the researcher should have no part in any decision to terminate a pregnancy" (U.S. DHHS, 2005, 45 CFR Section 46.204).

Persons with Mental Illness or Cognitive Impairment

Certain persons, because of mental illness, cognitive impairment, or a comatose state, are incompetent and incapable of giving informed consent. Persons are said to be incompetent if, in the judgment of a qualified clinician, they have those attributes that ordinarily provide the grounds for designating incompetence (Levine, 1986). Incompetence can be temporary (e.g., with inebriation), permanent (e.g., with advanced senile dementia), or subjective or transitory (e.g., with behavior or symptoms of psychosis). If a person is judged incompetent and incapable of giving consent, the researcher must seek approval from the prospective subject and his or her legally authorized representative. A legally authorized representative is a person or another body authorized under applicable law to consent on behalf of a pro-spective subject to the subject's participation in the research procedure(s) (U.S. DHHS, 2005).

Terminally Ill Subjects

Participating in research may carry increased risks with minimal or no benefits for terminally ill subjects. In addition, the dying subject's condition potentially may affect the study results, leading the researcher to misinterpret the findings. Cancer patients are an example of an overstudied population. It is not unusual that the majority of procedures performed on cancer patients is a result of research protocols that include blood work, bone marrow aspirations, body scans, lumbar punctures, and biopsies. These biomedical research treatments can easily compromise the care of these patients, which poses ethical dilemmas for clinical nurses. More nurses will be responsible for ensuring adherence to ethical standards in research as they participate in institutional review of research and serve as patient advocates in the clinical setting (Havens, 2004; Njie & Thomas, 2001; Stone, 2003; U.S. DHHS, 2005).

Persons Confined to Institutions

Prisoners are people who are confined to institutions and are designated as having diminished autonomy by federal law (U.S. DHHS, 2005). Prison inmates may feel coerced to participate in research because they fear harm or desire the benefits of early release, special treatment, or monetary gain.

Hospitalized patients are a vulnerable population but are not designated as having dimin-ished autonomy by law. Patients are vulnerable because they are ill and are confined in set-tings that are controlled by healthcare personnel. Some hospitalized patients feel obligated to be research subjects because they want to assist a particular nurse or physician with his or her research. Others feel coerced to participate because they fear that their care will be adversely affected if they refuse. Thus, researchers should be cautious about protecting the rights of patients in healthcare agencies who participate in research.

Right to Privacy

Privacy is the freedom people have to determine the time, extent, and general circumstances under which their private information will be shared with or withheld from others. Private information includes that concerning a person's attitudes, beliefs, behaviors, opinions, and records. The research subject's privacy is protected if the subject is informed, consents to participate in a study, and voluntarily shares private information with a researcher. An **inva-sion of privacy** occurs when private information is shared without a person's knowledge or against his or her will. The invasion of subjects' right to privacy brought about the Privacy Act of 1974. As a result of this act, people now have the right to provide or prevent access of others to their records (Levine, 1986; Veatch et al., 2009). A research report often will indicate that the subjects' privacy was protected and may include the details of how this was accomplished.

The HIPAA Privacy Rule expanded the protection of a person's privacy—specifically, his or her protected, individually identifiable health information—and described the ways in which covered entities can use or disclose this information. Covered entities are healthcare providers, health plans, employers, and healthcare clearinghouses (public or private entities that process or facilitate the processing of health information). Individually identifiable health information (IIHI) means

> ... any information, including demographic information collected from an individual that is created or received by healthcare provider, health plan, or healthcare clearinghouse; and related to past, present, or future physical or mental health or condition of an individual, the provision of health care to an individual, or the past, present, or future payment for the provision of health care to an individual, and identifies the individual; or with respect to which there is a reasonable basis to believe that the information can be used to identify the individual. (U.S. DHHS, 2003, 45 CFR, Section 160.103)

According to the HIPAA Privacy Rule, the IIHI is protected health information (PHI) that is transmitted by electronic media, maintained in electronic media, or transmitted or maintained in any other form or medium. Thus, the HIPAA privacy regulations affect nursing research in the following areas:

1. Accessing data from a covered entity, such as reviewing a patient's medical record in clinics or hospitals;
2. Developing health information, such as the data developed when an intervention is implemented in a study to improve a subject's health; and
3. Disclosing data from a study to a colleague in another institution, such as sharing data from a study to facilitative development of an instrument or scale (Frank-Stromborg, 2004; Olsen, 2003).

The DHHS developed guidelines to assist researchers, healthcare organizations, and healthcare providers determine when they can use and disclose IIHI. IIHI can be used or disclosed to a researcher in the following situations:

- The protected health information (PHI) has been de-identified under the HIPAA Privacy Rule.
- The data are part of a limited data set and a data use agreement with the researcher(s) is in place.
- The person who is a potential subject for a study provides authorization for the researcher to use and disclose his or her PHI.
- A waiver or alteration of the authorization requirement is obtained from an IRB or privacy board. (U.S. DHHS, 2007, February 2b)

The first two items are discussed in this section of the text. The section "Understanding Informed Consent," discusses the authorization process, and the section "Understanding Institutional Review" covers the waiver or alteration of authorization requirement.

De-identifying Protected Health Information under the Privacy Rule

Covered entities, such as healthcare providers and agencies, can allow researchers access to health information if the information has been de-identified. De-identifying health data involves removing the elements that could identify a specific person or that person's relatives, employer, or household members. You need to be aware of these elements to ensure patients'

PHI are kept confidential in healthcare agencies in which you are a student or work. The elements that require de-identifying are:

- Names
- All geographic subdivisions smaller than a state, including street address, city, county, precinct, ZIP code, and their equivalent geographical codes, except for the initial three digits of a ZIP code if, according to the current publicly available data from the Bureau of the Census
- The geographic unit formed by combining all ZIP codes with the same three initial digits contains more than 20,000 people
- The initial three digits of a ZIP code for all such geographic units containing 20,000 or fewer people are changed to 000
- All elements of dates (except year) for dates directly related to an individual, including birth date, admission date, discharge date, date of death; and all ages over 89 and all elements of dates (including year) indicative of such age, except that such ages and elements may be aggregated into a single category of age 90 or older
- Telephone numbers
- Facsimile numbers
- Electronic mail addresses
- Social security numbers
- Medical record numbers
- Health plan beneficiary numbers
- Account numbers
- Certificate/license numbers
- Vehicle identifiers and serial numbers, including license plate numbers
- Device identifiers and serial numbers
- Web universal resource locators (URLs)
- Internet protocol (IP) address numbers
- Biometric identifiers, including fingerprints and voiceprints
- Full-face photographic images and any comparable images
- Any other unique identifying number, characteristic, or code, unless otherwise permitted by the Privacy Rule for re-identification. (U.S. DHHS, 2007, February 2b; online at *http://privacyruleandresearch.nih.gov/pr_08.asp*)

A person's health information also can be de-identified using statistical methods. However, the covered entity and the researcher must ensure that the individual subject cannot be identified, or that there is a very small risk that the subject could be identified from the information used. The statistical method used for de-identification of the health data must be documented, and the study must certify that the elements for identification have been removed or revised to prevent identification of a specific person. This certification information must be kept for a period of six years by the researcher.

Limited Data Set and Data Use Agreement

Covered entities—healthcare provider, health plan, and healthcare clearinghouse—may use and disclose a limited data set to a researcher for a study without an individual subject's authorization or an IRB waiver. However, a limited data set is considered PHI, and the covered entity and the researcher need to have a data use agreement. The data use agreement limits how the data set may be used and how it will be protected. The HIPAA Privacy Rule requires that the following information be included in a data use agreement:

- Specifies the permitted uses and disclosures of the limited data set
- Identifies the researcher who is permitted to use or receive the limited data set
- Stipulates that the recipient (researcher) will:
  - Not use or disclose the information other than permitted by the agreement
  - Use appropriate safeguards to prevent the use or disclosure of the information, except as provided for in the agreement
  - Hold any other person (co-researchers, statisticians, or data collectors) to the standards, restrictions, and conditions stated in the data use agreement with respect to the health information
  - Not identify the information or contact the individuals whose data are in the limited data set. (U.S. DHHS, 2007, February 2b; online at *http://privacyruleandresearch.nih. gov/pr_08.asp*)

Right to Anonymity and Confidentiality

On the basis of the right to privacy, the research subject has the right to anonymity and the right to assume that the data collected will be kept confidential. Complete anonymity exists when the subject's identity cannot be linked, even by the researcher, with his or her individual responses (American Nurses Association, 2001).

In most studies, researchers know the identity of their subjects, and they promise the subjects that their identity will be kept anonymous from others and that the research data will be kept confidential. Confidentiality is the researcher's management of private information shared by a subject or participant. The researcher must refrain from sharing that information without the authorization of the subject. Confidentiality is grounded in the following premises:

(1) Individuals can share personal information to the extent they wish and are entitled to have secrets; (2) one can choose with whom to share personal information; (3) those accepting information in confidence have an obligation to maintain confidentiality; and (4) professionals, such as researchers, have a duty to maintain confidentiality that goes beyond ordinary loyalty. (Levine, 1986, p. 164)

A breach of confidentiality can occur when a researcher, by accident or direct action, allows an unauthorized person to gain access to the raw data of a study. Confidentiality also can be breached in reporting or publishing a study if a participant's identity is accidentally revealed, violating his or her right to anonymity (Ramos, 1989). Breach of confidentiality is of special concern in qualitative studies that have few study participants and involve the reporting of long quotes made by those participants. In addition, qualitative researchers and participants often have relationships in which detailed stories of the participants' lives are shared requiring careful management of study data to ensure confidentiality (Eide & Kahn, 2008). Breaches of confidentiality that can be especially harmful to participants include those regarding religious preferences; sexual practices; income; racial prejudices; drug use; child abuse; and personal attributes such as intelligence, honesty, and courage. Thus, research reports need to be examined closely for evidence that the participants' confidentiality was maintained during data collection and analysis (Munhall, 2007a; Sandelowski, 1994). In addition, the research findings should be reported so that a participant or group of participants cannot be identified by their responses.

Right to Fair Treatment

The right to fair treatment is based on the ethical principle of justice. According to this principle, people must be treated fairly and receive what they are due or owed. The research report needs to indicate that the selection of subjects and their treatment during the study were fair.

Fair Selection and Treatment of Subjects

In the past, injustice in subject selection resulted from social, cultural, racial, and sexual biases in society. For many years, research was conducted on categories of people who were thought to be especially suitable as research subjects, such as persons living in poverty, charity patients, prisoners, slaves, peasants, dying persons, and others who were considered undesirable (Reynolds, 1979). Researchers often treated these subjects carelessly and had little regard for the harm and discomfort they experienced. The Nazi medical experiments, the Tuskegee Syphilis Study, the Willowbrook Study, and the Jewish Chronic Disease Hospital Study all exemplify unfair subject selection.

Another concern with subject selection is that some researchers select subjects because they like them and want them to receive the specific benefits of a study. Other researchers have been swayed by power or money to make certain patients subjects so these patients can receive potentially beneficial treatments. Random selection of subjects can eliminate some of the researchers' biases that may influence subject selection.

Each study must include a specific researcher-subject agreement regarding the researcher's role and the subject's participation in a study (American Psychological Association, 2002; U.S. DHHS, 2005). While conducting the study, the researcher must treat the subjects fairly and respect that agreement. For example, the activities or procedures that subjects are to perform should not be changed without the subjects' consent. The benefits promised to the subjects should be provided. In addition, subjects who participate in studies should receive equal benefits regardless of age, race, or socioeconomic level.

The research report needs to indicate that the selection and treatment of the subjects were fair. Subjects must have been selected for reasons directly related to the problem being studied and not for their easy availability, compromised position, manipulability, or friendship with the researcher (National Commission for the Protection of Human Subjects of Biomedical and Behavioral Research, 1978). In addition, the "Procedures" section of the research report must indicate fair and equal treatment of the subjects during data collection.

Right to Protection from Discomfort and Harm

The right to protection from discomfort and harm from a study is based on the ethical principle of beneficence, which states that one should do good and, above all, do no harm. According to this principle, members of society must take an active role in preventing discomfort and harm and promoting good in the world around them. In research, discomfort and harm can be physical, emotional, social, or economic, or any combination of these four

(Weijer, 2000). Reynolds (1972) identified five categories of studies based on levels of discomfort and harm: no anticipated effects, temporary discomfort, unusual levels of temporary discomfort, risk of permanent damage, and certainty of permanent damage.

No Anticipated Effects

In some studies, no positive or negative effects are expected for the subjects. For example, studies that involve reviewing patients' records, students' files, pathology reports, or other documents have no anticipated effects on the research subjects. In this type of study, the researcher does not interact directly with the subjects. However, there is still a potential risk of invading a subject's privacy. With the HIPAA regulations, a subject's IIHI must be protected during data collection and analysis and in publication of the final report (U.S. DHHS, 2003).

Temporary Discomfort

Studies that cause temporary discomfort are described as minimal-risk studies, in which the discomfort is similar to what the subject would encounter in his or her daily life and is temporary, ending with termination of the experiment (U.S. DHHS, 2005). Many nursing studies require the completion of questionnaires or participation in interviews, which usually involve minimal risk or are a mere inconvenience for the subjects. The physical discomfort may include fatigue, headache, or muscle tension. The emotional and social risks may include anxiety or embarrassment associated with answering certain questions. The economic risks may include the time commitment for the study or travel costs to the study site.

Most clinical nursing studies examining the effect of a treatment involve minimal risk. For example, a study may involve examining the effects of exercise on the blood glucose levels of diabetic subjects. For the study, the subjects are asked to test their blood glucose level one extra time per day. Discomfort occurs when the blood is obtained, and there is a potential risk of physical changes that may occur with exercise. The subjects also may feel anxiety and fear associated with the additional blood testing, and the testing may be an added expense. The diabetic subjects in this study will encounter similar discomforts in their daily lives, however, and the discomfort will cease with the termination of the study.

Unusual Levels of Temporary Discomfort

In studies that involve unusual levels of temporary discomfort, subjects frequently have discomfort both during the study and after they have completed it. For example, subjects may have prolonged muscle weakness, joint pain, and dizziness after participating in a study that required them to be confined to bed for 10 days to determine the effects of immobility. Studies that require subjects to experience failure, extreme fear, or threats to their identity or to act in unnatural ways involve unusual levels of temporary discomfort. In some qualitative studies, researchers ask participants questions that open old wounds or involve reliving traumatic events (Eide & Kahn, 2008; Ford & Reuter, 1990). For example, asking participants to describe their rape experience could precipitate feelings of extreme anger, fear, sadness, or any combination of these emotions. In such studies, investigators need to indicate in the research report that they were vigilant in assessing the participants' discomfort and referred them as necessary for appropriate professional intervention.

Risk of Permanent Damage

In some studies, the possibility exists for subjects to sustain permanent damage; this is more common in biomedical research than in nursing research. For example, new drugs and surgical procedures being tested in medical studies have the potential to cause subjects permanent physical damage. Some topics investigated by nurses have the potential to permanently damage subjects emotionally and socially. Studies examining sensitive information, such as sexual behavior, child abuse, AIDS/HIV status, or drug use, can be very risky for subjects. These studies have the potential to cause permanent damage to a subject's personality or reputation. There also are potential economic risks, such as those resulting from a decrease in job performance or loss of employment.

Certainty of Permanent Damage

In some research, such as the Nazi medical experiments and the Tuskegee Syphilis Study, the subjects have a certainty of experiencing permanent damage. Conducting research that has a certainty of causing permanent damage to study subjects is highly questionable, regardless of the benefits that will be gained. Frequently the benefits gained from such a study are experienced not by the research subjects, but by others in society. Studies causing permanent damage to subjects violate the fifth principle of the Nuremberg Code and probably should not be conducted (see Table 4–1).

Critical Appraisal Guidelines to Examine Protection of Human Rights in Studies

The guidelines that follow will assist you in critically appraising a study to ensure protection of human rights. The human rights that require protection in research include the rights to: (1) self-determination, (2) privacy, (3) confidentiality, (4) fair selection and treatment, and (5) protection from discomfort and harm. These guidelines are followed by an example from a qualitative study that is critically appraised with a discussion of the study's implications for practice.

CRITICAL APPRAISAL GUIDELINES

Protection of Human Rights

When critically appraising studies, evaluate whether the participants' human rights are protected by asking questions such as the following:

1. Did the study participants or subjects have diminished autonomy because of legal or mental incompetence, terminal illness, or confinement to an institution? If they did, were special precautions taken in obtaining consent from these participants and their parents or guardians?
2. Were the participants' right to privacy protected? Was the individually identifiable health information protected according to the HIPAA Privacy Rule (U.S. DHHS, 2003)?
3. Were the participants selected in a fair way for the study?
4. Were the participants treated in a fair way during the conduct of the study?
5. Were the participants protected from discomfort or harm?

RESEARCH EXAMPLE Ethical Conduct of Research with Adolescents

Wickman, Anderson, and Greenberg (2008) conducted a phenomenological study of adolescents' perception of invincibility and its influence on teen acceptance of health promotion strategies. The ethical aspects of the study were described as follows.

Method

Sample and setting.

Participants (*N* = 10) were recruited at a military treatment facility (MTF) providing healthcare services to Armed Forces members and their families. The MTF offers a specialty clinic for teens that provides health maintenance and acute care services to approximately 1000 adolescents per month. Teens were selected to obtain diversity of participants in regard to gender and ethnicity within an age range of 14-17 [right to fair selection] …

Procedures

Approval was obtained from the university Office of Protection of Research Subjects and the Committee for the Protection of Human Subjects at the MTF [IRB approvals]. When participants checked in for their clinical appointment, they were given an invitation letter that explained relevant details about the study [right to self-determination]. If the participants indicated interest in hearing more about the study, the teen and parent were approached and given further information [right to privacy, self-determination, and fair selection]. If they agreed to participate, the written assent/consent process was initiated [consent process]. Referral procedures were established with clinical personnel in the event that participants' comments or behaviors suggested the need for mental or physical health interventions(s)" [right to fair treatment and protection from discomfort and harm] (Wickman et al., 2008, pp. 461-462).

CRITICAL APPRAISAL

Wickman et al. (2008) described their sampling process, which indicated a fair selection of study participants who reflected diversity in gender and ethnicity within the adolescent age range of 14 to 17 years. The researchers also recognized that adolescents have diminished autonomy because they are less than the adult age of 18. Thus, they explained the study to both the adolescents and their parents and obtained assent of the adolescents and the consent of the parents to participate in the study. The researchers provided a letter explaining the study and asking individuals to participate, which protected potential participants' right to self-determination. Only those interested in participating were contacted and provided additional information indicating a protection of the right to privacy and fair selection of potential participants. The adolescents and their parents' rights to self-determination, privacy, confidentiality, fair selection and treatment, and protection from discomfort and harm were protected by the informed consent process. The informed consent process outlines the protection of participants' human rights within a study and this process is presented in the next section. The researchers set up a referral system to ensure the study participants could receive the mental and physical care needed during the study, which reflects fair treatment of the study participants and reduces the potential for discomfort or harm. The researchers also obtained IRB approval for their study from both the university and the MTF where the adolescents and parents came for clinical appointments. All of these activities protected the rights of the study participants and promoted the ethical conduct of this study according to the DHHS regulations (FDA, 2002; U.S.

Continued

CRITICAL APPRAISAL—cont'd

DHHS, 2005). However, the ethical discussion of the study would have been strengthened by a discussion of compliance with the HIPAA Privacy Rule and the protection of participants' protected health information (U.S. DHHS, 2003).

IMPLICATIONS FOR PRACTICE

In this study, the adolescents believed they were invincible, which means they thought they could take risks and would be protected from harm. In addition, they believed they could handle risks and could get away with risky behaviors. Wickman et al. (2008, p. 467) concluded that "Understanding adolescent's perception of invincibility helps healthcare providers target appropriate approaches and interventions to reduce risky behaviors and promote adolescent health." Additional research is needed to test interventions that might be effective in encouraging adolescents to recognize their limitations, decrease their risky behaviors, and increase their acceptance of health promotion strategies.

Understanding Informed Consent

What is informed consent? How is informed consent obtained from research subjects and documented in the research report? "Informing" is the transmission of essential ideas and content from the investigator to the prospective subject. "Consent" is the prospective subject's agreement to participate in a study as a subject. Every prospective subject, to the degree that he or she is capable, should have the opportunity to choose whether to participate in research (FDA, 1998; U.S. DHHS, 2005). Informed consent includes four elements: (1) disclosure of essential study information to the study participant or subject, (2) comprehension of this information by the subject, (3) competence of the subject to give consent, and (4) voluntary consent of the subject to participate in the study.

Essential Information for Consent

Informed consent requires the researcher to disclose specific information to all prospective subjects. The following information is essential for obtaining informed consent from research subjects (FDA, 1998; U.S. DHHS, 2005):

1. *Introduction of research activities.* The initial information presented to prospective subjects clearly indicates that a study is to be conducted and that they are being asked to participate as subjects.
2. *Statement of the research purpose.* The researcher states the immediate purpose of the research and any long-range goals related to the study.
3. *Selection of research subjects.* The researcher explains to prospective subjects why they were selected to participate in the study.

4. *Explanation of procedures.* Prospective subjects receive a complete description of the procedures to be followed and identification of any procedures that are experimental in the study (U.S. DHHS, 2005, Section 46.116a).

5. *Description of risks and discomforts.* Prospective subjects are informed of any reasonably foreseeable risks or discomforts (physical, emotional, social, and economic) that might result from the study.

6. *Description of benefits.* The investigator describes any benefits to the subjects or to other people or future patients that may reasonably be expected from the research, including any financial advantages or other rewards for participating in the study.

7. *Disclosure of alternatives.* The investigator discloses the appropriate alternative procedures or courses of treatment, if any, that might be advantageous to the subjects (FDA, 1998; U.S. DHHS, 2005). For example, the researchers of the Tuskegee Syphilis Study should have informed the subjects with syphilis that penicillin was an effective treatment for the disease.

8. *Assurance of anonymity and confidentiality.* Prospective subjects should know the extent to which their responses and records will be kept confidential. Subjects are promised that their identity will remain anonymous in reports and publications of the study.

9. *Offer to answer questions.* The researcher offers to answer any questions the prospective subjects may have.

10. *Voluntary participation.* Consent form includes a statement that participation is voluntary and that refusal to participate will involve no penalty or loss of benefits to which the subject is otherwise entitled.

11. *Option to withdraw.* Subjects are informed that they may discontinue participation (withdraw from a study) at any time without penalty or loss of benefits (U.S. DHHS, 2005, Section 46.116a).

12. *Consent to incomplete disclosure.* In some studies, subjects are not completely informed of the study purpose because that knowledge would alter their actions. However, prospective subjects must be told when certain information is being withheld deliberately.

A **consent form** is a written document that includes the elements of informed consent required by the DHHS Regulations (U.S. DHHS, 2005) and FDA (1998) Regulations. In addition, a consent form may include other information required by the institution where the study is to be conducted or by the agency funding the study. An example of a consent form is in Figure 4–1. The boldface terms indicate the essential consent information.

Comprehension of Consent Information

Informed consent implies not only that the researcher has imparted information to the subjects, but also that the prospective subjects have comprehended that information. The researcher must take the time to teach the subjects about the study. The amount of information to be taught depends on the subjects' knowledge of research and the specific research topic. Researchers need to discuss the benefits and risks of a study in detail, with examples that the potential subject can understand. Nurses often serve as patient advocates in clinical agencies and need to assess whether patients involved in research understand the purpose and the potential risks and benefits of their participation in a study (Veatch et al., 2009).

Study title: The Needs of Family Members of Critically Ill Adults
Investigator: Linda L. Norris, R.N.

Ms. Norris is a registered nurse studying the emotional and social needs of family members of patients in the Intensive Care Units **(research purpose)**. Although the study will not benefit you directly, it will provide information that might enable nurses to identify family members' needs and to assist family members with those needs **(potential benefits)**.

The study and its procedures have been approved by the appropriate people and review boards at The University of Texas at Arlington and X hospital **(IRB approval)**. The study procedures might cause fatigue for you or your family **(potential risks)**. The procedures include: (1) responding to a questionnaire about the needs of family members of critically ill patients and (2) completing a demographic data sheet **(explanation of procedures)**. Participation in this study will take approximately 20 minutes **(time commitment)**. You are free to ask any questions about the study or about being a subject and you may call Ms. Norris at (999) 999-9999 (work) or (999) 999-9999 (home) if you have further questions **(offer to answer questions)**.

Your participation in this study is voluntary; you are under no obligation to participate **(alternative option and voluntary consent)**. You have the right to withdraw at any time and the care of your family member and your relationship with the healthcare team will not be affected **(option to withdraw)**.

The study data will be coded so they will not be linked to your name. Your identity will not be revealed while the study is being conducted or when the study is reported or published. All study data will be collected by Ms. Norris, stored in a secure place, and not shared with any other person without your permission **(assurance of anonymity and confidentiality)**.

I have read this consent form and voluntarily consent to participate in this study.

(If Appropriate)

_____   _____
Subject's Signature   Date   Legal Representative   Date

I have explained this study to the above subject and to have sought his/her understanding for informed consent.

_____
Investigator's Signature   Date

Figure 4–1. Sample consent form.

Competence to Give Consent

Autonomous persons, who are capable of understanding the benefits and risks of a proposed study, are competent to give consent. Persons with diminished autonomy because of legal or mental incompetence, terminal illness, or confinement to an institution frequently are not legally competent to consent to participate in research (see Right to Self-Determination). Frequently, the researcher determines the competence of the subject (Douglas & Larson, 1986). In the research report the investigator needs to indicate the competence of the subjects and the process that was used for obtaining informed consent (FDA, 1998, 2002; U.S. DHHS, 2005).

Voluntary Consent

Voluntary consent means that the prospective subject has decided to take part in a study of his or her own volition without coercion or any undue influence (U.S. DHHS, 2005). Researchers obtain voluntary consent after the prospective subject receives the essential information about the study and has demonstrated comprehension of this information. All of these elements of informed consent need to be documented in a consent form.

Documentation of Informed Consent

The documentation of informed consent depends on (1) the level of risk involved in the study and (2) the discretion of the researcher and those reviewing the study for institutional approval. Most studies require a written consent form, although in some studies, the requirement for written consent is waived. Nurses may be asked to identify subjects for studies, obtain consent forms for studies, collect study data, or participate in an IRB to review the ethics of a study. Thus, they need to be aware of the process for documenting informed consent in research.

Written Consent Waived

The requirements for written consent may be waived in research that "presents no more than minimal risk of harm to subjects and involves no procedures for which written consent is normally required outside of the research context" (U.S. DHHS, 2005, 45 CFR Section 46.117c). For example, researchers using questionnaires to collect relatively harmless data do not need to obtain a signed consent form from the subjects. The subject's completion of the questionnaire may serve as consent. The top of the questionnaire might contain a statement such as, "Your completion of this questionnaire indicates your consent to participate in this study."

Written consent also is waived in a situation in which "the only record linking the subject and the research would be the consent document and the principal risk would be potential harm resulting from a breach of confidentiality. Each subject will be asked whether the subject wants documentation linking the subject with the research, and the subject's wishes will govern" (U.S. DHHS, 2005, 45 CFR Section 46.117c). Thus, in this situation, subjects are given the option to sign or not sign a consent form that links them to the research. The four elements of consent—disclosure, comprehension, competency, and voluntariness—are essential in all studies, whether written consent is waived or required.

Written Consent Documents

The short form consent document includes the following statement: "The elements of informed consent required by Section 46.116 [see "Information Essential for Consent"] have been presented orally to the subject or the subject's legally authorized representative" (U.S. DHHS, 2005, 45 CFR Section 46.117a). The researcher must develop a written summary of what is to be said to the subject in the oral presentation, and an IRB must approve the summary. When the researcher makes the oral presentation to the subject or to the subject's representative, a witness is required. The subject or the representative must sign the short form consent document. "The witness shall sign both the short form and a copy of the summary, and the person actually obtaining consent shall sign a copy of the summary" (U.S. DHHS, 2005, 45 CFR Section 46.117a). Copies of the summary and short form are given to the subject and the witness, and the researcher retains the original documents. The researcher must keep these documents for three years. The short form written consent documents typically are used in studies that present minimal or moderate risk to the subjects.

The formal written consent document includes the elements of informed consent required by the DHHS (U.S. DHHS, 2005) and FDA (1998) regulations (see Information Essential for Consent). In addition, a consent form may include other information required by the institution where the study is to be conducted or by the agency funding the study. Figure 4–1, p. 124 presents a sample consent form with descriptors of the essential consent information. The consent form can be read by the subject or read to the subject by the researcher; however, it is wise also to explain the study to the subject. The form is signed by the subject and is witnessed by the investigator or research assistant collecting the data. This type of consent can be used for any type of study, from minimal risk to high risk. All persons signing the consent form—including the subject, researcher, and any witnesses—must receive a copy of it. The original consent form is kept by the researcher for a period of three years.

Studies that involve subjects with diminished autonomy require a written consent form. If these prospective subjects have some comprehension of the study and agree to participate as subjects, they must sign the consent form. However, the form also must be signed by the subject's legally authorized representative. The representative indicates his or her relationship with the subject under the signature (see Figure 4–1). Sometimes nurses are asked to sign a consent form as a witness for a biomedical study. They must know the study purpose and procedures and the subject's comprehension of the study before signing the form. It is really best if the nurse and others involved in the consent process be educated to ensure the consistent implementation of the consent process. Larson, Cohn, Meyer, and Boden-Albala (2009) identified problems with the lack of standardization of the informed consent process in health-related studies that leads to disparities in those participating in studies. Certain individuals elect not to participate in research because of the way the study is presented to them during the consent process. Larson et al. (2009, p. 95) recommended a formal educational program for researchers and those involved in the consent process "to reduce disparities in research participation by improving communication between research staff and potential participants." You can obtain more information on education for the research consent process from the Health Resources and Services Administration (HRSA) website entitled "Protecting Human Subjects Training" at *http://www.hrsa.gov/humansubjects/default. htm*.

HIPAA Privacy Rule: Authorization for Research Uses and Disclosure

The HIPAA Privacy Rule provides people, as research subjects, the right to authorize covered entities (healthcare provider, health plan, and healthcare clearinghouse) to use or disclose their PHI for research purposes (U.S. DHHS, 2004, July 1). HIPAA regulates this authorization in addition to the informed consent that the DHHS regulates (U.S. DHHS, 2005, CFR 45 Part 46) and the FDA (1998, CFR 21 Part 50). The authorization focuses on the privacy risks and states how, why, and to whom the PHI will be shared. The

REQUIRED ELEMENTS:

If you sign this document, you give permission to [name or other identification of specific health care provider(s) or description of classes of persons, e.g., all doctors, all healthcare providers] at [name of covered entity or entities] to use or disclose (release) your health information that identifies you for the research study described below:
[Provide a description of the research study, such as the title and purpose of the research.]

The health information that we may use or disclose (release) for this research includes [complete as appropriate]:
[Provide a description of information to be used or disclosed for the research project. This may include, for example, all information in a medical record, results of physical examinations, medical history, lab tests, or certain health information indicating or relating to a particular condition.]
The health information listed above may be used by and/or disclosed (released) to:
[Name or class of persons involved in the research; i.e., researchers and their staff**]

[Name of covered entity] is required by law to protect your health information. By signing this document, you authorize [name of covered entity] to use and/or disclose (release) your health information for this research. Those persons who receive your health information may not be required by Federal privacy laws (such as the Privacy Rule) to protect it and may share your information with others without your permission, if permitted by laws governing them.

Please note that [include the appropriate statement]:
- You do not have to sign this Authorization, but if you do not, you may not receive research-related treatment.
  (When the research involves treatment and is conducted by the covered entity or when the covered entity provides health care solely for the purpose of creating protected health information to disclose to a researcher)

- [Name of covered entity] may not condition (withhold or refuse) treating you on whether you sign this Authorization.
  (When the research does not involve research-related treatment by the covered entity or when the covered entity is not providing health care solely for the purpose of creating protected health information to disclose to a researcher)

Please note that [include the appropriate statement]
- You may change your mind and revoke (take back) this Authorization at any time, except to the extent that [name of covered entity(ies)] has already acted based on this Authorization. To revoke this Authorization, you must write to: [name of the covered entity(ies) and contact information].
  (Where the research study is conducted by an entity other than the covered entity)

- You may change your mind and revoke (take back) this Authorization at any time. Even if you revoke this Authorization, [name or class of persons at the covered entity involved in the research] may still use or disclose health information they already have obtained about you as necessary to maintain the integrity or reliability of the current research. To revoke this Authorization, you must write to: [name of the covered entity(ies) and contact information].
  (Where the research study is conducted by the covered entity)

| Signature of participant or participant's personal representative | Date |

| Printed name of participant or participant's personal representative | If applicable, a description of the personal representative's authority to sign for the participant |

**Where a covered entity conducts the research study, the Authorization must list ALL names or other identification, or ALL classes, of persons who will have access through the covered entity to the protected health information (PHI) for the research study (e.g., research collaborators, sponsors, and others who will have access to data that includes PHI). Examples may include, but are not limited to the following:

- Data coordinating centers that will receive and process PHI;
- Sponsors who want access to PHI or who will actually own the research data; and/or
- Institutional Review Boards or Data Safety and Monitoring Boards.

If the research study is conducted by an entity other than the covered entity, the authorization need only list the name or other identification of the outside researcher (or class of researchers) and any other entity to whom the covered entity is expected to make the disclosure.

Figure 4–2. The Authorization to Use or Disclose (Release) Health Information That Identifies You for a Research Study. (From U.S. Department of Health and Human Services. (2004, July 1). Information for covered entities and researchers on authorizations for research uses or disclosures of protected health information. HIPAA Privacy Rule: Information for Researchers. Available at *privacyruleandresearch.nih.gov/authorization.rtf*.

authorization "Core Elements" can be found online at *http://privacyruleandresearch.nih.gov/authorization.asp* (U.S. DHHS, 2004, July 1). The authorization information can be included as part of the consent form, but it probably is best to have two separate forms (Olsen, 2003; U.S. DHHS, 2003). The DHHS has developed a sample authorization form, presented in Figure 4–2.

Yehle, Sands, Rhynders, and Newton (2009) conducted a quasi-experimental study to determine the effect of shared medical visits on knowledge and self-care in patients with heart failure (HF). These researchers clearly described how they complied with the HIPAA Privacy Rule (U.S. DDHS, 2003) and maintained confidentiality of subjects' protected health information.

> Patients interested in the study were asked for permission for their name and telephone number to be provided so they could be contacted about participation in the study by the primary investigator or the clinic's nurse practitioner. At the next clinic visit with the nurse practitioner, the primary investigator described the study and obtained consent. The primary investigator obtained an 'Authorization for Release or Use of Protected Health Information for Research Purposes' at the time of consent to participate in the study and screened the medical records. (Yehle et al., 2009, p. 27)

Critical Appraisal Guidelines to Examine Informed Consent in Studies

All studies require the obtaining of informed consent from the study participants or subjects. The consent process must meet the DHHS (U.S. DHHS, 2005), FDA (2002), and HIPAA (U.S. DHHS, 2003) regulations for the conduct of ethical research with human subjects. Research reports often discuss the consent process and identify some of the essential consent information that was provided to the potential subjects. Some mention of the consent process for that study is required, but the depth of the discussion will vary according to the research purpose and the types of participants or subjects included in the study. The consent process is usually presented in the "Methods" section under a discussion of study procedures or data collection process. The following critical appraisal guidelines will assist you in examining the consent process of a published study or for a study to be conducted in your clinical agency. The guidelines are followed by an example of the ethical aspects of a quantitative study that was conducted by Bryanton, Gagnon, Hatem, and Johnston (2009).

CRITICAL APPRAISAL GUIDELINES

Examining Informed Consent Process

Consider the following questions when critically appraising the consent process of a study.

1. Was informed consent obtained from the subjects or participants?
2. Was the information that was essential for consent provided?
3. Were the subjects capable of comprehending the information? Did the researcher take any action to promote the subjects' comprehension of the consent process?
4. Were the subjects competent to give consent? If the subjects were not competent to give consent, who acted as their legally authorized representatives?
5. Did it seem that the subjects participated voluntarily in the study?

RESEARCH EXAMPLE

Informed Consent

Bryanton and colleagues (2009) conducted a quantitative correlational study to determine if perception of the childbirth experience was a predictor of women's early parenting behaviors. The following excerpt documents the process for obtaining informed consent from the women in this study.

Ethical Considerations

Ethics approval was secured from two university and two hospital research ethics boards [IRB approvals]. When recruiting, the research assistants emphasized that participation was voluntary and women could choose not to answer questions or withdraw from the study without their or their infants' care being affected. They emphasized that there would be no way to identify individual women in the results and that their information would remain confidential. Participants were informed that the results may contribute to better care for mothers and infants in the future and that there were no known risks in participating. Written consent was obtained in hospital and consent was re-confirmed verbally before the in-home data collection (Bryanton et al., 2009, pp. 194-196).

CRITICAL APPRAISAL

Bryanton and colleagues (2009) identified the essential elements of the informed consent process for this type of study in their research report. The researchers indicated that the study participants (women with infants) were provided information about the study and asked to sign a consent form. The research assistants also verbally emphasized the essential elements of the consent process (voluntary, right not to answer questions, right to withdraw from the study without their care or their infants' care being affected, and confidentiality of data). The consent process also included a discussion of the benefits and risks of the study. The study subjects were women with new infants who were competent to consent to participate in this type of study. Because the study data were collected in both the hospital and home, the written consent was obtained in the hospital and the consent was re-confirmed in the participants' homes. These steps increased the study subjects' comprehension of the consent process and allowed them an option to voluntarily participate in this study. Bryanton et al. (2009) clearly described their consent process, which was in compliance with the DHHS regulations (U.S. DHHS, 2005).

IMPLICATIONS FOR PRACTICE

Bryanton et al. (2009, p. 191) found that "women's birth experience did not predict early parenting behaviors, however being better educated and having a vaginal birth did. Excellent partner support and maternal mental health were also significantly associated with positive parenting at one month." The researchers recommended that nurses assess women for possible risks of parenting difficulties based on the predictors identified in this study. Additional research is needed to identify the most effective interventions to use to support and enhance parenting behaviors.

Understanding Institutional Review

In institutional review, a study is examined for ethical concerns by a committee of the researcher's peers. The first federal policy statement on protection of human subjects by institutional review was issued by the Public Health Services (PHS) in 1966. The statement required that research involving human subjects must be reviewed by a committee of peers or associates to confirm that (1) the rights and welfare of the persons involved were protected, (2) the appropriate methods were used to secure informed consent, and (3) the potential benefits of the investigation were greater than the risks (Levine, 1986).

In 1974, DHEW passed the National Research Act, which required that all research involving human subjects undergo institutional review. The DHHS reviewed and revised these guidelines five times with the last revision in 2005 (45 CFR Sections 46.107-46.115; online at *http://ohsr.od.nih.gov/guidelines/45cfr46.html*). The FDA (2009, 21 CFR Part 56; online at *http://edocket.access.gpo.gov/2009/E9-682.htm*) also has very similar guidelines for institutional review of research. The regulations describe the membership, functions, and operations of the body responsible for institutional review. An institutional review board (IRB) is a committee that reviews research to ensure that the investigator is conducting the research ethically. Universities, hospitals, corporations, and many managed care centers have IRBs to promote the conduct of ethical research and protect the rights of prospective subjects at their institutions (Veatch et al., 2009).

Each IRB has at least five members of varying backgrounds (cultural, economic, educational, gender, racial) to promote complete, scholarly, and fair review of research that is commonly conducted in an institution. If an institution regularly reviews studies with vulnerable subjects, such as children, neonates, pregnant women, prisoners, and the mentally disabled, the IRB must include one or more members with knowledge about and experience in working with these subjects. The members must have sufficient experience and expertise to review a variety of studies, including quantitative, qualitative, and outcomes research (Burns & Grove, 2009; Munhall, 2007b). The IRB members must not have a conflicting interest related to a study conducted in an institution. Any member having a conflict of interest with a research project being reviewed must excuse himself or herself from the review process, except to provide information requested by the IRB. The IRB also must include one member whose primary concern is nonscientific, such as an ethicist, lawyer, or minister. At least one of the IRB members must be someone who is not affiliated with the institution (FDA, 2009; U.S. DHHS, 2005). The IRBs in hospitals often are composed of physicians, nurses, lawyers, scientists, clergy, and community lay persons.

In 2009, the FDA regulations were revised to require all IRBs to register through a system maintained by the Department of Health and Human Services. "The registration information includes contact information, (such as addresses and telephone numbers), the number of active protocols involving FDA-regulated products reviewed during the preceding 12 months, and a description of the types of FDA-regulated products involved in the protocols reviewed" (FDA, 2009, 21 CFR Section 56.106). The IRB registration requirement was implemented to make it easier for the FDA to inspect IRBs and communicate information to them. This rule was made effective July 14, 2009.

Levels of Reviews Conducted by Institutional Review Boards

The functions and operations of an IRB involve the review of research at three different levels: (1) exempt from review, (2) expedited review, and (3) complete review. The IRB chairperson and/or committee, not the researcher, decide the level of the review required for each study. Studies usually are **exempt from review** if they pose no apparent risks for the research subjects. Table 4–5 lists the studies that typically are considered exempt from review by the federal regulations. Nursing studies that carry no foreseeable risks or involve procedures posing a mere inconvenience for subjects usually are identified as exempt from review by the chairperson of the IRB committee.

Studies that carry some risks, which are viewed as minimal, qualify for an **expedited review**. **Minimal risk** means that "the probability of and magnitude of harm or discomfort

Table 4–5	Research Qualifying for Exemption from Review

Unless otherwise required by department or agency heads, research activities in which the only involvement of human subjects will be in one or more of the following categories are exempt from review.

- Research conducted in established or commonly accepted educational settings, involving normal educational practices, such as (i) research on regular and special education instructional strategies, or (ii) research on the effectiveness of or the comparison among instructional techniques, curricula, or classroom management methods.
- Research involving the use of educational tests (cognitive, diagnostic, aptitude, achievement), survey procedures, interview procedures or observation of public behavior, unless: (i) information obtained is recorded in such a manner that human subjects can be identified, directly or through identifiers linked to the subjects; and (ii) any disclosure of the human subjects' responses outside the research could reasonably place the subjects at risk of criminal or civil liability or be damaging to the subjects' financial standing, employability, or reputation.
- Research involving the use of educational tests (cognitive, diagnostic, aptitude, achievement), survey procedures, interview procedures, or observation of public behavior that is not exempt under paragraph (b)(2) of this section, if: (i) the human subjects are elected or appointed public officials or candidates for public office; or (ii) Federal statute(s) require(s) without exception that the confidentiality of the personally identifiable information will be maintained throughout the research and thereafter.
- Research involving the collection or study of existing data, documents, records, pathological specimens, or diagnostic specimens, if these sources are publicly available or if the information is recorded by the investigator in such a manner that subjects cannot be identified, directly or through identifiers linked to the subjects.
- Research and demonstration projects which are conducted by or subject to the approval of Department or Agency heads, and which are designed to study, evaluate, or otherwise examine: (i) Public benefit or service programs; (ii) procedures for obtaining benefits or services under those programs; (iii) possible changes in or alternatives to those programs or procedures; or (iv) possible changes in methods or levels of payment for benefits or services under those programs.
- Taste and food quality evaluation and consumer acceptance studies, (i) if wholesome foods without additives are consumed or (ii) if a food is consumed that contains a food ingredient at or below the level and for a use found to be safe, or agricultural chemical or environmental contaminant at or below the level found to be safe, by the Food and Drug Administration or approved by the Environmental Protection Agency or the Food Safety and Inspection Service of the U.S. Department of Agriculture.

From U.S. Department of Health and Human Services. (2005, June 23). Protection of human subjects. *Code of Federal Regulations*, Title 45, Part 46. Retrieved April 7, 2009, from *http://www.hhs.gov/ohrp/humansubjects/guidance/45cfr46.htm*.

anticipated in the research are not greater in and of themselves than those ordinarily encountered in daily life or during the performance of routine physical or psychological examinations or tests" (U.S. DHHS, 2005, 45 CFR Section 46.102i). Expedited review procedures also can be used to review minor changes in previously approved research. Under expedited review procedures, the review may be carried out by the IRB chairperson or one or more experienced reviewers designated by the chairperson from among members of the IRB. In reviewing the research, the reviewers may exercise all of the authorities of the IRB except disapproval of the research. A research activity may be disapproved only after a complete review of the IRB (FDA, 2009; U.S. DHHS, 2005).

Table 4–6 identifies research that usually qualifies for expedited review. Donahue and colleagues (2008) conducted a quantitative descriptive correlational study to examine the relationships between nurses' perceptions of empowerment and patient satisfaction. The IRBs determined that the Donahue et al. study had minimal risk for the study subjects. The researchers described their approval process as follows.

Table 4-6	Research Qualifying for Expedited Institutional Review Board Review

Expedited review (by committee chairpersons or designated members) for the following research involving no more than minimal risk is authorized:

- Collection of hair and nail clippings, in a nondisfiguring manner; deciduous teeth and permanent teeth if patient care indicates a need for extraction.
- Collection of excreta and external secretions including sweat, uncannulated saliva, placenta removed at delivery, and amniotic fluid at the time of rupture of the membrane before or during labor.
- Recording of data from subjects 18 years of age or older using noninvasive procedures routinely employed in clinical practice. This includes the use of physical sensors that are applied either to the surface of the body or at a distance and do not involve input of matter or significant amounts of energy into the subject or an invasion of the subject's privacy. It also includes such procedures as weighing, testing sensory acuity, electrocardiography, electroencephalography, thermography, detection of naturally occurring radioactivity, diagnostic echography, and electroretinography. It does not include exposure to electromagnetic radiation outside the visible range (for example, x-rays, microwaves).
- Collection of blood samples by venipuncture, in amounts not exceeding 450 ml in an 8-week period and no more than two times per week, from subjects 18 years of age or older and who are in good health and not pregnant.
- Collection of both supragingival and subgingival dental plaque and calculus, provided the procedure is not more invasive than routine prophylactic scaling of the teeth and the process is accomplished in accordance with accepted prophylactic techniques.
- Voice recordings made for research purposes such as investigations of speech defects.
- Moderate exercise by healthy volunteers.
- The study of existing data, documents, records, pathological specimens, or diagnostic specimens.
- Research on individual or group behavior or characteristics of individuals, such as studies of perception, cognition, game theory, or test development, where the investigator does not manipulate subjects' behavior and research will not involve stress to subjects.
- Research on drugs or devices for which an investigational new drug exemption or an investigational device exemption is not required.

From U.S. Department of Health and Human Services. (2005, June 23). Protection of human subjects. *Code of Federal Regulations*, Title 45, Part 46. Retrieved April 7, 2009 from *http://www.hhs.gov/ohrp/humansubjects/guidance/45cfr46.htm*.

This research study involved no more than a minimal risk to the subjects (nurse subjects and patients) and involved no procedures for which written consent is normally required outside the research context. Institutional review board approvals were obtained. Nurses' and patients' consent for participation in this study were indicated by the return of the question-naire or survey" (Donahue et al., 2008, p. 4).

A study that carries greater than minimal risks must receive a **complete review** by an IRB. To obtain IRB approval, researchers must ensure that

(1) risks to subjects are minimized, (2) risks to subjects are reasonable in relation to anticipated benefits, (3) selection of subjects is equitable, (4) informed consent will be sought from each prospective subject or the subject's legally authorized representative, (5) informed consent will be appropriately documented, (6) the research plan makes adequate provision for monitoring data collection for subjects' safety, and (7) adequate provisions are made to protect the privacy of subjects and to maintain the confidentiality of data. (FDA, 2009, 21 CFR 56.111; U.S. DHHS, 2005, 45 CFR Section 46.111)

Most studies indicate that IRB approval was obtained, but do not indicate whether the study was exempt from review, expedited review, or complete review. If a researcher is affiliated with a university, then the study needs to be approved by the IRB of that university before seeking IRB approval from a clinical agency where the study is to be conducted. If a study is conducted in more than one clinical agency, then researchers must obtain IRB approval from all clinical sites where the study is to be conducted. A research report needs to clearly identify the IRBs that reviewed and approved a study for implementation. For example Bryanton et al. (2009) indicated that IRB approval was sought from two university and two hospital research boards before the study was conducted.

Influence of HIPAA Privacy Rule on Institutional Review Boards

Under the HIPAA Privacy Rule, an IRB or institutional established privacy board can act on requests for a waiver or an alteration of the authorization requirement for a research project. If an IRB and privacy board both exist in an agency, the approval of only one board is required, and it probably will be the IRB for research projects. Researchers can choose to obtain a signed authorization form from potential subjects or can ask for a waiver or an alteration of the authorization requirement. An altered authorization requirement occurs when an IRB approves a request that some but not all of the required 18 elements be removed from health information that is to be used in research. The researcher also can request a partial or complete waiver of the authorization requirement from the IRB. The partial waiver involves the researcher's obtaining PHI to contact and recruit potential subjects for a study. An IRB can give a researcher a complete waiver of authorization in studies in which the informed consent requirements also might be waived (U.S. DHHS, 2004, July 8). (The HIPAA regulations related to IRBs can be found online at *http://privacyruleandresearch.nih.gov/irbandprivacyrule.asp*).

The HIPAA Privacy Rule does not change the IRB membership and functions that are designated under the DHHS (2005) and FDA (2009) IRB regulations. For clarification, Table 4–7 outlines the responsibilities of the IRB/privacy board for HIPAA (U.S. DHHS, 2004, July 8) and the responsibilities of the IRBs under the DHHS (U.S. DHHS, 2005) and FDA (2002, 2009).

Table 4–7	Comparison of IRB/Privacy Board Responsibilities for HIPAA, DHHS, and FDA		
Area of Distinction	HIPAA Privacy Rule	DHHS Protection of Human Subjects Regulations Title 45 CFR Part 46	FDA Protection of Human Subjects Regulations Title 21 CFR Parts 50 & 56
Permissions for research IRB/privacy board responsibilities	Authorization Requires the covered entity to obtain authorization for research use or disclosure of PHI unless a regulatory permission applies. Because of this, the IRB or privacy board would see only requests to waive or alter the authorization requirement. In exercising Privacy Rule authority, the IRB or privacy board does not review the authorization form	Informed consent and authorization Requires the covered entity to obtain authorization for research use or disclosure of PHI unless a regulatory permission applies. Because of this, the IRB or privacy board would only see requests to waive or alter the authorization requirement. In exercising Privacy Rule authority, the IRB or privacy board does not review the authorization form.	Informed consent and authorization The IRB must ensure that informed consent will be sought from, and documented for, each prospective subject or the subject's legally authorized representative, in accordance with, and to the extent required by, FDA regulations. If specified criteria are met, the requirements for either obtaining informed consent or documenting informed consent may be waived. The IRB must review and approve the authorization form if it is combined with the informed consent document. Privacy boards have no authority under the FDA Protection of Human Subjects Regulations.

U.S. Department of Health and Human Services. (2007, February 2b). How can covered entities use and disclose protected health information for research and comply with the Privacy Rule? HIPAA Privacy Rule: Information for Researchers. Retrieved online April 7, 2009, from *http://privacyruleandresearch.nih.gov/pr_08.asp*.
DHHS, Department of Health and Human Services; *FDA*, Food and Drug Administration; *HIPAA*, Health Insurance Portability and Accountability Act; *IRB*, institutional review board; *PHI*, protected health information.

Examining the Benefit-Risk Ratio of a Study

Nurses who serve on an IRB for their agencies, serve as patient advocate when research is conducted in their agencies, or are asked to collect data for a study should examine the balance of benefits and risks in studies. To determine this balance, or benefit-risk ratio, assess the benefits and risks associated with the sampling method, consent process, procedures, and potential outcomes of the study (Figure 4–3). Informed consent must be obtained from subjects, and selection and treatment of subjects during the study must be fair. An important outcome of research is the development and refinement of knowledge. The type of knowledge that might be obtained from the study and who will be influenced by the knowledge also must be identified.

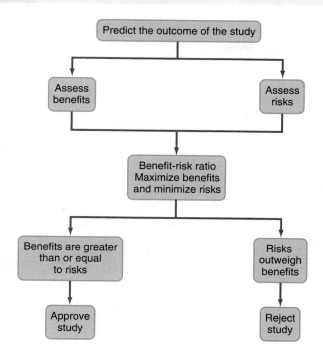

Figure 4–3. Balancing benefits and risks for a study.

The type of research conducted—therapeutic or nontherapeutic—affects the potential benefits for the subjects. In therapeutic research, subjects might benefit from the study procedures in areas such as skin care, range of motion, touch, and other nursing interventions. The benefits might include improved physical condition, which could facilitate emotional and social benefits. Some researchers have noted that participation in qualitative research has encouraged subjects to process and disclose thoughts regarding life-altering events, and that these actions have been beneficial to the subjects' health and well-being (Eide & Kahn, 2008). Nontherapeutic nursing research does not benefit subjects directly, but it is important because it generates and refines nursing knowledge for future patients, the nursing profession, and society (King, 2000). Most subjects involved in a study do benefit by having an increased understanding of the research process and knowing the findings from a particular study.

Examining the benefit-risk ratio also involves assessing the type, degree, and number of risks that subjects might encounter while participating in a study. The risks involved depend on the purpose of the study and the procedures used to conduct the study. Risks can be physical, emotional, social, or economic and can range in level from no anticipated risk or mere inconvenience to certain risk of permanent damage (see Right to Protection from Discomfort and Harm) (Levine, 1986; Reynolds, 1972). If the risks outweigh the benefits, the study probably is unethical and should not be conducted. If the benefits outweigh the risks, the study probably is ethical and has the potential to add to nursing's knowledge base (see Figure 4–3) (Burns & Grove, 2009).

Critical Appraisal Guidelines for Examining the Ethical Aspects of Studies

The following guidelines can be used to critically appraise the ethical aspects of a study, which includes an examination of the benefit-risk ratio of the study, IRB approval, informed consent, and protection of subjects' human rights. This information needs to be included in published studies. Steele and Porche (2005) conducted a quantitative study to predict women's likelihood of getting a mammogram. The ethical aspects of this study are presented as an example.

CRITICAL APPRAISAL GUIDELINES

Examining the Ethical Aspects of a Study

When conducting a study, researchers must meet the DHHS (U.S. DHHS, 2005), FDA (2002, 2009), and HIPAA (U.S. DHHS, 2003) regulations for the conduct of ethical research with human subjects. Consider the following questions when critically appraising the ethical aspects of a study.

1. Was the benefit-risk ratio of the study acceptable? Was the level of risk reasonable for the study and did the benefits outweigh the risks? (Use Figure 4–3 to examine the benefit-risk ratio of the study.)
2. Was the study approved by the appropriate IRB(s)?
3. Was informed consent obtained from the subjects?
4. Were the rights of the subjects protected during the study?

 RESEARCH EXAMPLE Determining the Ethics of a Study

Steele and Porche (2005) conducted their study to test the Theory of Planned Behavior to predict the intentions of rural women in Southeastern Louisiana to obtain a mammogram. The researchers described the following ethical aspects of their study.

Procedure

The institutional review board [IRB] at Louisiana State University Health Sciences Center approved the study. Upon obtaining written permission to collect data within the agencies, participants were recruited by posting flyers in rural churches, health clinics, hospitals, senior centers, and school employee lunchrooms. Women who accessed the rural community-based organization during the study period, attended briefing sessions, and met the eligibility requirements were asked to participate [right to self-determination and fair subject selection]. The researcher discussed the purpose of the study with each participant, answered any questions, and allowed time for them to review and sign the consent form [informed consent with protection of human rights]. ... The informational incentive consisted of a pamphlet specifically designed by the National Cancer Institute for low-literacy multicultural populations. The content included information concerning the importance of annual mammography, pictures describing the mammography process, and information on how to obtain mammography. A financial incentive of a $10 gift certificate was given to all participants who completed the questionnaire [fair treatment of subjects with balanced benefit-risk ratio] (Steele & Porche, 2005, p. 335).

CRITICAL APPRAISAL

Steele and Porche (2005) presented the essential content that documents the ethical aspects of a study. The study was presented to IRB committees and approved for conduct in a rural town in Louisiana. The subjects were fairly selected because fliers were placed in numerous sites and participants who met the eligibility criteria were invited to participate. Thus subjects' right to self-determination was protected since they had a choice to participate or not in the study. Steele and Porche followed the elements of informed consent because they provided subjects with an explanation of the study and allowed questions before the subjects signed a written consent form that provided for a protection of their rights. The subjects were offered important informational rewards to promote their obtaining a mammogram and a small financial incentive of a $10 gift certificate to encourage their participation in the study. The financial incentive was probably not large enough for people to feel that they had to participate just to receive the money. Thus, the benefit-risk ratio of this study was acceptable since the risk level of completing questionnaires is minimal and the benefit of encouraging the women to get mammograms might result in early detection of breast cancer.

IMPLICATIONS FOR PRACTICE

The study provided support for the use of the Theory of Planned Behavior to predict the likelihood of women in a rural town to obtain a mammogram. The perceived behavior control was the strongest predictor of mammography intention. However, more research is needed to explain the women's attitudes toward mammography and their motivation to get a mammogram. This additional knowledge is needed before an intervention can be developed to increase mammography intention and use (Steele & Porche, 2005).

Understanding Research Misconduct

The goal of research is to generate sound scientific knowledge, which is possible only through the honest conduct, reporting, and publication of quality research. However, during the last 25 years an increasing number of fraudulent studies have been published in prestigious scientific journals. "**Research misconduct** means fabrication, falsification, or plagiarism in processing, performing, or reviewing research, or in reporting research results. It does not include honest error or differences in opinion" (ORI, 2007, 42 CFR Section 93.103). **Fabrication** is the making up of results and recording or reporting them. **Falsification** is manipulating research materials, equipment, or processes, or changing or omitting data or results such that the research is not accurately represented in the research record. **Plagiarism** is the appropriation of another person's ideas, processes, results, or words without giving appropriate credit, including those obtained through confidential review of others' research proposals and manuscripts.

Research misconduct became a public issue in 1981 when the House of Representatives began holding public hearings. In 1986, Congress passed the Health Research Extension Act that provided for a process to report and review incidences of research misconduct. In 1989, two new federal agencies were organized for reporting and investigating scientific misconduct. The Office of Scientific Integrity Review (OSIR) was established to manage scientific misconduct by grant recipients. The Office of Scientific Integrity (OSI) supervised the implementation of the rules and regulations related to scientific misconduct and managed any investigations (Hawley & Jeffers, 1992; U.S. DHHS, 1989). The investigations by the OSIR and the OSI revealed a variety of fraudulent behaviors. In some instances, the fraudulent studies were never conducted, and the researchers fabricated the data and study results. In other cases, the findings were consciously distorted. In 1992, the OSIR and the OSI were consolidated into the Office of Research Integrity (ORI) (ORI, 2008).

An example of scientific misconduct was evident in the publications of Dr. Robert Slutsky, a heart specialist at the University of California, San Diego, School of Medicine. He resigned in 1986 when confronted with inconsistencies in his research publications. His publications contained "statistical anomalies that raised the question of data fabrication" (Friedman, 1990, p. 1416). In six years, Slutsky published 161 articles, and during one period he was completing an article every 10 days. Eighteen of the articles were found to be fraudulent and now have retraction notations, and 60 articles were questionable (Friedman, 1990).

Dr. Stephen Breuning, a psychologist at the University of Pittsburgh, engaged in deceptive and misleading practices in reporting his research on retarded children. He used his fraudulent research to obtain more than $300,000 in federal grants. In 1988 he was criminally charged with research fraud. He pleaded guilty, was fined $20,000, and faced up to 10 years in prison (Chop & Silva, 1991). Evidence of research misconduct has occurred in all disciplines of healthcare research, including nursing (Rankin & Esteves, 1997).

Role of the Office of Research Integrity in Promoting the Conduct of Ethical Research

Currently, the ORI promotes the integrity of biomedical and behavioral research in about 4000 institutions worldwide (ORI, 2009; online at *http://ori.dhhs.gov/*). The ORI protects the integrity of the Public Health Services' extramural and intramural research programs. The extramural program provides funding to research institutions, and the intramural program provides funding for research conducted within the federal government. The current functions of the ORI are as follows:

- Developing policies, procedures and regulations related to the detection, investigation, and prevention of research misconduct and the responsible conduct of research;
- Reviewing and monitoring research misconduct investigations conducted by applicant and awardee institutions, intramural research programs, and the Office of Inspector General in the Department of Health and Human Services (DHHS);
- Recommending research misconduct findings and administrative actions to the Assistant Secretary for Health for decision, subject to appeal;
- Assisting the Office of the General Counsel (OGC) to present cases before the HHS Departmental Appeals Board;
- Providing technical assistance to institutions that respond to allegations of research misconduct;
- Implementing activities and programs to teach the responsible conduct of research, promote research integrity, prevent research misconduct, and improve the handling of allegations of research misconduct;

- Conducting policy analyses, evaluations, and research to build the knowledge base in research misconduct, research integrity, and prevention and to improve DHHS research integrity policies and procedures;
- Administering programs for: maintaining institutional assurances, responding to allegations of retaliation against whistleblowers, approving intramural and extramural policies and procedures, and responding to Freedom of Information Act and Privacy Act requests (ORI, 2007; online at *http://ori.dhhs.gov/misconduct*).

Over the last 10 years, ORI has had a major role in the investigation of allegations of misconduct in research within several institutions The ORI classifies research misconduct as (1) an act that involves a significant departure from the acceptable practice of the scientific community for maintaining the integrity of the research record; (2) an act that was committed intentionally; and (3) an allegation that can be proved by a preponderance of evidence. ORI has a section on their website entitled "Handling Misconduct" that includes a summary of the allegations and investigations managed by its office (ORI, 2007). The most common sites for the investigations were medical schools (68%), hospitals (11%), and research institutes (10%). The individuals charged with misconduct were primarily males holding a PhD or medical degree (MD) and were mostly associate professors, professors, and postdoctoral fellows. When research misconduct was documented, the actions taken against the researchers or agencies might have included: debarred from receiving federal funding for periods ranging from 18 months to eight years; prohibition from U.S. PHS advisory service; and other actions requiring supervised research, certification of data, certification of sources, and correction or retraction of articles. The regulations governing ORI (2009) and the current investigations and activities of ORI are available online at *http://ori.dhhs.gov/*.

Examining the Use of Animals in Research

The use of animals as research subjects is a controversial issue of growing concern to nurse researchers (Burns & Grove, 2009). A small but increasing number of nurse scientists are conducting physiological studies that require the use of animals. Many scientists, especially physicians, believe the current animal rights movement could threaten the future of healthcare research. Animal rights groups are active in anti-research campaigns that have cost research centers in the billions of dollars to manage. Some of these groups are trying to raise the consciousness of researchers and society to ensure that animals are used wisely in the conduct of research and are treated humanely.

Two important questions should be addressed: (1) Should animals be used as subjects in research? (2) If animals are used in research, what mechanisms ensure that they are treated humanely? The type of research project influences the selection of subjects. Animals are just one of a variety of subjects used in research; others include human beings, plants, and computer data sets. If possible, most researchers use non-animal subjects because this approach generally is less expensive. If the studies are low risk, which most nursing studies are, human beings frequently are used as subjects. However, some studies require the use of animals to answer the research question. Approximately 25 million animals are used in research each year, and 90% of them are rodents. The combined percentage of dogs and cats used in research is only 1% to 2% (Goodwin & Morrison, 2000).

Because animals are deemed valuable subjects for selected research projects, what mechanisms ensure that animals are treated humanely? At least five separate types of regulations exist to protect research animals from mistreatment. The federal government, state governments, independent accreditation organizations, professional societies, and individual institutions work to ensure that research animals are used only when necessary and only under humane conditions. At the federal level, animal research is conducted according to the guidelines of the PHS Policy on Humane Care and Use of Laboratory Animals, which was adopted in 1986 and reprinted essentially unchanged in 1996. These guidelines are available on the Office of Laboratory Animal Welfare (OLAW) website at *http://grants.nih.gov/grants/olaw/olaw.htm* (OLAW, 2009).

The Humane Care and Use of Laboratory Animals Regulations define *animal* as any live, vertebrate animal used or intended for use in research, research training, experimentation, or biological testing or for related purposes. Any institution proposing research involving animals must have a written Animal Welfare Assurance statement acceptable to the U.S. PHS that documents compliance with the U.S. PHS policy. The National Institutes of Health's Office for Protection from Research Risks (OPRR) evaluates every assurance statement to determine the adequacy of the institution's proposed program for the care and use of animals in activities conducted or supported by the U.S. PHS (OLAW, 2009).

Institutions' assurance statements about compliance with the U.S. PHS policy have promoted the humane care and treatment of animals in research. In addition, more than 700 institutions conducting health-related research have sought accreditation by the American Association for Accreditation of Laboratory Animal Care (AAALAC), which was developed to ensure the humane treatment of animals in research. In critically appraising studies, you must ensure that animals were the appropriate subjects for a study and that they were treated humanely during the conduct of the study (OLAW, 2009).

Yamakage and colleagues (2009) conducted a study to clarify the effects of beta-1 selective adrenergic antagonist on hyperactive airways of guinea pigs and described their ethical protection of the research animals as follows.

> The experimental protocol was approved by the Animal Care and Use Committee of our institution. The care and handling of the animals were in accord with National Institutes of Health guidelines. (Department of Health and Human Services Publication No. 85-23, 1985; Yamakage et al., 2009, p. 49)

KEY CONCEPTS

- Four experimental projects have been highly publicized for their unethical treatment of human subjects: (1) the Nazi medical experiments, (2) the Tuskegee Syphilis Study, (3) the Willowbrook Study, and (4) the Jewish Chronic Disease Hospital Study.
- Two historical documents, the Nuremberg Code and the Declaration of Helsinki, have had a strong impact on the conduct of research.
- The DHHS (1981, 1983, 1991, 2001, 2005) and the FDA (1998, 2002, 2009) passed regulations to promote ethical conduct in research, including (1) general requirements for informed consent and (2) guidelines for IRB review of research.

- The HIPAA Privacy Rule was enacted in 2003 to protect the privacy of people's health information.
- The human rights that require protection in research are (1) self-determination, (2) privacy, (3) anonymity and confidentiality, (4) fair treatment, and (5) protection from discomfort and harm.
- Informed consent involves (1) transmission of essential study information to the potential subject, (2) comprehension of that information by the potential subject, (3) competence of the potential subject to give consent, and (4) voluntary consent by the potential subject to participate in the study.
- An institutional review board consists of a committee of peers who examine studies for ethical concerns with three levels of review: exempt, expedited, and complete.
- To balance the benefits and risks of a study, the type, degree, and number of risks are examined, and the potential benefits are identified.
- Scientific misconduct is a serious ethical problem of the last few decades, with the conducting, reporting, and publication of fraudulent research.
- Animals are important subjects to use for certain studies and they must be treated humanely during the conduct of the study.

REFERENCES

American Nurses Association. (2001). *Code of ethics for nurses with interpretive statements.* Washington, DC: Author. Copy available for viewing only. Retrieved March 25, 2009 from *http://www.nursingworld.org/MainMenuCategories/ThePracticeofProfessionalNursing/EthicsStandards/CodeofEthics.aspx.*

American Psychological Association. (2002). *Ethical principles of psychologists and code of conduct.* Washington, DC: Author. Retrieved March 25, 2009 from *http://www.apa.org/ethics/code/index.aspx.*

Beecher, H. K. (1966). Ethics and clinical research. *The New England Journal of Medicine, 274*(24), 1354-1360.

Berger, R. L. (1990). Nazi science: The Dachau hypothermia experiments. *The New England Journal of Medicine, 322*(20), 1435-1440.

Brandt, A. M. (1978). Racism and research: The case of the Tuskegee syphilis study. *Hastings Center Report, 8*(6), 21-29.

Broome, M. E. (1999). Consent (assent) for research with pediatric patients. *Seminars in Oncology Nursing, 15*(2), 96-103.

Bryanton, J. B., Gagnon, A. J., Hatem, M., & Johnston, C. (2009). Does perception of the childbirth experience predict women's early parenting behaviors? *Research in Nursing & Health, 32*(2), 191-203.

Burns, N., & Grove, S. K. (2009). *The practice of nursing research: Appraisal, synthesis, and generation of evidence* (6th ed.). Philadelphia: Saunders.

Chop, R. M., & Silva, M. C. (1991). Scientific fraud: Definitions, policies, and implications for nursing research. *Journal of Professional Nursing, 7*(3), 166-171.

Donahue, M. O., Piazza, I. M., Griffin, M. Q., Dykes, P. C., & Fitzpatrick, J. J. (2008). The relationship between nurses' perceptions of empowerment and patient satisfaction. *Applied Nursing Research, 21*(1), 2-7.

Douglas, S., & Larson, E. (1986). There's more to informed consent than information. *Focus on Critical Care, 13*(2), 43-47.

Eide, P., & Kahn, D. (2008). Ethical issues in the qualitative researcher-participant relationship. *Nursing Ethics, 15*(2), 199-207.

Emanuel, E. J. (2004). Ending concerns about undue inducement. *The Journal of Law, Medicine & Ethics: A Journal of the American Society of Law, Medicine & Ethics, 32*(1), 100-105.

Food and Drug Administration. (1998). A guide to informed consent. Code of Federal Regulations, Title 21 Part 50. Retrieved April 7, 2009 from *http://www.fda.gov/oc/ohrt/irbs/informedconsent.html.*

Food and Drug Administration. (2002, April 1). Protection of human subjects. *Code of Federal Regulations, Title 21 Part 50.* Retrieved April 7, 2009 from *http://www.access.gpo.gov/nara/cfr/waisidx_02/21cfr50_02.html.*

Food and Drug Administration. (2004, December 31). Laws enforced by the FDA and other statues. *Code of Federal Regulations, Title 21.* Retrieved April 7, 2009 from *http://www.fda.gov/opacom/laws/default.htm.*

Food and Drug Administration. (2009, January 15). Institutional review boards. *Code of Federal Regulations, Title 21 Part 56.* Retrieved April 7, 2009 from *http://www.accessdata.fda.gov/scripts/cdrh/cfdocs/cfcfr/CFRsearch.cfm?CFRPart=56.*

Ford, J. S., & Reuter, L. I. (1990). Ethical dilemmas associated with small samples. *Journal of Advanced Nursing, 15*(2), 187-191.

Frank-Stromborg, M. (2004). They're real and they're here: The new federally regulated privacy rules under HIPAA. *Dermatology Nursing, 16*(1), 13-25.

Friedman, P. J. (1990). Correcting the literature following fraudulent publication. *Journal of the American Medical Association, 263*(10), 1416-1419.

Goodwin, F. K., & Morrison, A. R. (2000). Science and self-doubt. *Reason, 32*(5), 22-28.

Hadley, E. K., Smith, C. A., Gallo, A. M., Angst, D. B., & Knafl, K. A. (2007). Parents' perspectives on having their children interviewed for research. *Research in Nursing & Health, 31*(1), 4-11.

Havens, G. A. (2004). Ethical implications for the professional nurse of research involving human subjects. *Journal of Vascular Nursing, 22*(1), 19-23.

Hawley, D. J., & Jeffers, J. M. (1992). Scientific misconduct as a dilemma for nursing. *Image-The Journal of Nursing Scholarship, 24*(1), 51-55.

Hershey, N., & Miller, R. D. (1976). *Human experimentation and the law.* Rockville, MD: Aspen.

Infectious Diseases Society of America. (2009). Grinding to a halt: The effects of the increasing regulatory burden on research and quality improvement efforts. *Clinical Infectious Diseases, 49*(3),328-335.

Kelman, H. C. (1967). Human use of human subjects: The problem of deception in social psychological experiments. *Psychological Bulletin, 67*(1), 1-11.

King, N. M. (2000). Defining and describing benefit appropriately in clinical trials. *The Journal of Law, Medicine & Ethics: A Journal of the American Society of Law, Medicine & Ethics, 28*(4), 332-343.

Larson, E. L., Cohn, E. G., Meyer, D. D., & Boden-Albala, B. (2009). Consent administrator training to reduce disparities in research participation. *Journal of Nursing Scholarship, 41*(1), 95-103.

Levine, R. J. (1986). *Ethics and regulation of clinical research* (2nd ed.). Baltimore: Urban & Schwarzenberg.

Milgram, S. (1963). Behavioral study of obedience. *Journal of Abnormal and Social Psychology, 67*(4), 371-378.

Munhall, P. L. (2007a). Ethical considerations in qualitative research. In P. L. Munhall (Ed.), *Nursing research: A qualitative perspective* (4th ed., pp. 501-513). Sudbury, MA: Jones & Bartlett.

Munhall, P. L. (2007b). Institutional review of qualitative research proposals: A task of no small consequence. In P. L. Munhall (Ed.), *Nursing research: A qualitative perspective* (4th ed., pp. 515-527). Sudbury, MA: Jones & Bartlett.

National Commission for the Protection of Human Subjects of Biomedical and Behavioral Research. (1978). *Belmont report: Ethical principles and guidelines for research involving human subjects.* DHEW Publication No. (05) 78-0012. Washington, DC: U.S. Government Printing Office.

Njie, V. P., & Thomas, A. C. (2001). Quality issues in clinical research and the implications on health policy (QICRHP). *Journal of Professional Nursing, 17*(5), 233-242.

Nuremberg Code. (1949). *Trials of War Criminals before the Nuremberg Military Tribunals under Control Council Law, 2*(1), 181-182. Washington, D.C.: U.S. Government Printing Office. Retrieved April 1, 2009 from *http://www.hhs.gov/ohrp/references/nurcode.htm.*

Office of Laboratory Animal Welfare (2009). Public Health Service policy on humane care and use of laboratory animals. Retrieved April 7, 2009 from *http://grants.nih.gov/grants/olaw/olaw.htm.*

Office of Research Integrity. (2007, June 20). Handling misconduct. Retrieved April 1, 2009 from *http://ori.dhhs.gov/misconduct.*

Office of Research Integrity. (2008). About the Office of Research Integrity-History. Retrieved April 1, 2009 from *http://ori.dhhs.gov/about/history.shtml.*

Office of Research Integrity. (2009). Welcome to the Office of Research Integrity. Retrieved April 1, 2009 from *http://ori.dhhs.gov/.*

Olsen, D. P. (2003). Methods: HIPAA privacy regulations and nursing research. *Nursing Research, 52*(5), 344-348.

Pediatric Research Equity Act. (2003). 108th Congress. Retrieved April 1, 2009 from *http://frwebgate.access.gpo.gov/cgi-bin/getdoc.cgi?dbname=108_cong_public_laws&docid=f:publ155.108.*

Ramos, M. C. (1989). Some ethical implications of qualitative research. *Research in Nursing & Health, 12*(1), 57-63.

Rankin, M., & Esteves, M. D. (1997). Perceptions of scientific misconduct in nursing. *Nursing Research, 46*(5), 270-276.

Reynolds, P. D. (1972). On the protection of human subjects and social science. *International Social Science Journal, 24*(4), 693-719.

Reynolds, P. D. (1979). *Ethical dilemmas and social science research.* San Francisco: Jossey-Bass.

Rosato, J. (2000). The ethics of clinical trials: A child's view. *The Journal of Law, Medicine & Ethics: A Journal of the American Society of Law, Medicine & Ethics, 28*(4), 362-378.

Rothman, D. J. (1982). Were Tuskegee and Willowbrook "studies in nature"? *Hastings Center Report, 12*(2), 5-7.

Sandelowski, M. (1994). Focus on qualitative methods: The use of quotes in qualitative research. *Research in Nursing & Health, 17*(6), 479-482.

Savage, E., & McCarron, S. (2009). Research access to adolescents and young adults. *Applied Nursing Research, 22*(1), 63-67.

Steele, S. K., & Porche, D. J. (2005). Testing the theory of planned behavior to predict mammography intention. *Nursing Research, 54*(5), 332-338.

Steinfels, P., & Levine, C. (1976). Biomedical ethics and the shadow of Nazism. *Hastings Center Report, 6*(4), 1-20.

Stone, P. W. (2003). Ask an expert: HIPAA in 2003 and its meaning for nurse researchers. *Applied Nursing Research, 16*(4), 291-293.

Strauman, J. J., & Cotanch, P. H. (1988). Oncology nurse research issues: Over-studied populations. *Oncology Nursing Forum, 15*(5), 665-667.

Thompson, P. J. (1987). Protection of the rights of children as subjects for research. *Journal of Pediatric Nursing, 2*(6), 392-399.

U.S. Department of Health and Human Services. (1981, January 26). Final regulations amending basic HHS policy for the protection of human research subjects. Code of Federal Regulations, Title 45 Part 46.

U.S. Department of Health and Human Services. (1983, March 8). Protection of human subjects. Code of Federal Regulations, Title 45 Part 46.

U.S. Department of Health and Human Services. (1989). Final rule: Responsibilities of awardee and applicant institutions for dealing with and reporting possible misconduct in science. *Federal Register, 54*, 32446-32451.

U.S. Department of Health and Human Services. (1991, June 18). Protection of human subjects. Code of Federal Regulations, Title 45 Part 46.

U.S. Department of Health and Human Services. (2001, November 13). Protection of human subjects. Code of Federal Regulations, Title 45 Part 46.

U.S. Department of Health and Human Services. (2003, April 14). Standards for privacy of individually identifiable health information; final rule. Code of Federal Regulations, Title 45 Public Welfare, Parts 160 and 164. Retrieved March 23, 2009 from *http://privacyruleandresearch.nih.gov/pr_02.asp*.

U.S. Department of Health and Human Services. (2004, July 1). Information for covered entities and researchers on authorizations for research uses or disclosures of protected health information. HIPAA Privacy Rule: Information for Researchers. Retrieved March 23, 2009 from *http://privacyruleandresearch.nih.gov/authorization.asp*.

U.S. Department of Health and Human Services. (2004, July 8). Institutional review boards and the HIPAA Privacy Rule. HIPAA Privacy Rule: Information for Researchers. Retrieved March 23, 2009 from *http://privacyruleandresearch.nih.gov/irbandprivacyrule.asp*.

U.S. Department of Health and Human Services. (2005, June 23). Protection of human subjects. Code of Federal Regulations, Title 45 Part 46. Retrieved April 7, 2009 from *http://www.hhs.gov/ohrp/humansubjects/guidance/45cfr46.htm*.

U.S. Department of Health and Human Services. (2007, February 2a). HIPAA Privacy Rule: Information for Researchers. Retrieved April 7, 2009 from *http://privacyruleandresearch.nih.gov*.

U.S. Department of Health and Human Services. (2007, February 2b). How can covered entities use and disclose protected health information for research and comply with the Privacy Rule? HIPAA Privacy Rule: Information for Researchers. Retrieved April 7, 2009 from *http://privacyruleandresearch.nih.gov/pr_08.asp*.

U.S. Department of Health and Human Services. (2007, February 2c). How do other privacy protections interact with the privacy rule? HIPAA Privacy Rule: Information for Researchers. Retrieved April 7, 2009 from *http://privacyruleandresearch.nih.gov/pr_05.asp*.

Veatch, R. M., Haddad, A., & English, D. D. (2009). *Case studies in biomedical ethics: Decision making, principles, and cases.* Oxford University Press.

Weijer, C. (2000). The ethical analysis of risk. *The Journal of Law, Medicine & Ethics: A Journal of the American Society of Law, Medicine & Ethics, 28*(4), 344-361.

Wickman, M. E., Anderson, N. L., & Greenberg, C. S. (2008). The adolescent perception of invincibility and its influence on teen acceptance of health promotion strategies. *Journal of Pediatric Nursing, 23*(6), 460-468.

World Medical Association. (2004). Regulations and ethical guidelines. *World Medical Association Declaration of Helsinki.* Retrieved March 23, 2009 from *http://www.wma.net/en/30publications/10policies/b3/index.html*.

Yamakage, M., Iwasaki, S., Jeong, S., Satoh, J., & Namiki, A. (2009). Beta-1 selective adrenergic antagonist landiolol and esmolol can be safely used in patients with airway hyperactivity. *Heart & Lung, 38*(1), 48-55.

Yehle, K. S., Sands, L. P., Rhynders, P. A., & Newton, G. D. (2009). The effect of shared medical visits on knowledge and self-care in patients with heart failure: A pilot study. *Heart & Lung, 38*(1), 25-33.

Research Problems, Purposes, and Hypotheses

Chapter Overview

What Are Research Problems and Purposes? 146

Identifying the Problem and Purpose in Quantitative, Qualitative, and Outcomes Studies 148

Problems and Purposes in Types of Quantitative Studies 148

Problems and Purposes in Types of Qualitative Studies 151

Problems and Purposes in Outcomes Research 154

Determining the Significance of a Study Problem and Purpose 155

Influences Nursing Practice 155

Builds on Previous Research 155

Promotes Theory Testing or Development 155

Addresses Nursing Research Priorities 156

Examining the Feasibility of a Problem and Purpose 158

Researcher Expertise 158

Money Commitment 158

Availability of Subjects, Facilities, and Equipment 159

Ethical Considerations 159

Examining Research Objectives, Questions, and Hypotheses in Research Reports 159

Research Objectives or Aims Implemented in Quantitative Studies 160

Research Objectives or Aims Implemented in Qualitative Studies 161

Research Questions Implemented in Quantitative Studies 163

Research Questions Implemented in Qualitative Studies 165

Hypotheses 167

Understanding Study Variables and Research Concepts 176

Types of Variables in Quantitative Research 176

Conceptual and Operational Definitions of Variables in Quantitative Research 178

Research Concepts Investigated in Qualitative Research 181

Demographic Variables 182

Learning Outcomes

After completing this chapter, you should be able to:

1. Identify research topics, problems, and purposes in published quantitative, qualitative, and outcomes studies.

2. Critically appraise the significance of research problems and purposes in published studies.

3. Critically appraise the feasibility of a study problem and purpose by examining the researcher's expertise; money commitment; availability of subjects, facilities, and equipment; and the study's ethical considerations.

4. Differentiate among the types of hypotheses (simple versus complex, nondirectional versus directional, associative versus causal, and statistical versus research) in published studies.

5. Critically appraise the quality of objectives, questions, and hypotheses presented in published studies.

6. Differentiate the types of variables in published studies.

7. Critically appraise the conceptual and operational definitions of variables in published studies.

Key Terms

Associative hypothesis,
    p. 167
Background for a problem,
    p. 146
Causal hypothesis, p. 170
Complex hypothesis, p. 172
Conceptual definition, p. 178
Confounding variables,
    p. 177
Demographic variables,
    p. 182
Dependent (response or
    outcome) variable, p. 176
Directional hypothesis,
    p. 174

Environmental variables,
    p. 177
Extraneous variables, p. 177
Hypothesis, p. 167
Independent (treatment or
    experimental) variable,
    p. 176
Nondirectional hypothesis,
    p. 173
Null (statistical) hypothesis,
    p. 174
Operational definition, p. 178
Problem statement, p. 146
Research concepts, p. 181
Research hypothesis, p. 175

Research objective, p. 160
Research problem, p. 146
Research purpose, p. 146
Research question, p. 163
Research topic, p. 145
Research variables, p. 176
Sample characteristics,
    p. 182
Significance of a research
    problem, p. 146
Simple hypothesis, p. 172
Statistical hypothesis, p. 174
Testable hypothesis, p. 175
Variables, p. 176

STUDY TOOLS

Be sure to visit http://evolve.elsevier.com/Burns/understanding/ for additional examples and self-tests. Also, a review of this chapter's concepts and practice exercises can be found in Chapter 5 of the Study Guide for *Understanding Nursing Research: Building an Evidence-Based Practice*, 5th edition.

We are constantly asking questions to gain a better understanding of ourselves and the world around us. This human ability to wonder and ask creative questions is the first step in the research process. By asking questions, clinical nurses and nurse researchers are able to identify significant research topics and problems that will generate research findings that can ultimately be used to make evidence-based changes in practice. A **research topic** is a concept or broad issue that is important to nursing, such as acute pain, chronic pain management, coping with illness, or health promotion. Each topic contains numerous potential research problems to guide quantitative, qualitative, and outcomes studies. For example, chronic pain management is a research topic that includes such potential problems as, "What is chronic pain?" and, "What is it like to live with chronic pain?" Qualitative research might be used to investigate these problems or areas of concern in nursing. Quantitative research might be used to study such problems as, "What is the most accurate way to assess chronic pain?" and, "What are effective interventions for managing chronic pain?" Outcomes research methodologies might be used to examine patient outcomes and the cost effectiveness of care provided in a chronic pain management clinic.

The problem or area of concern provides the basis for developing the research purpose using a variety of methodologies, quantitative, qualitative, and outcomes research. The purpose or goal of a study guides the development of the objectives, questions, or hypotheses in quantitative and outcomes studies. The objectives, questions, or hypotheses bridge the gap between the more abstractly stated problem and purpose and the detailed design for conducting the study. Objectives, questions, and hypotheses include the variables, the relationships among the variables, and often the population to be studied. In qualitative research, the purpose and often broadly stated research questions guide the study of selected research concepts.

This chapter includes content that will assist you in differentiating a problem from a purpose in published quantitative, qualitative, and outcomes studies. Objectives, questions, and hypotheses are discussed, and the different types of study variables are introduced. Also presented are guidelines that will assist you in critically appraising the problems, purposes, objectives, questions, hypotheses, and variables or concepts in published quantitative, qualitative, and outcomes studies.

What Are Research Problems and Purposes?

A **research problem** is an area of concern in which there is a gap in the knowledge base needed for nursing practice. Research is required to generate essential knowledge to address the practice concern, with the ultimate goal of providing evidence-based nursing care (Brown, 2009; Craig & Smyth, 2007; Cullum, Ciliska, Haynes, & Marks, 2008). In a study, the research problem (1) identifies an area of concern for a particular population, (2) indicates the significance of the problem, (3) provides a background for the problem, and (4) outlines the need for additional study in a problem statement. The **significance of a research problem** indicates the importance of the problem to nursing and health care and to the health of individuals, families, and communities. The **background for a problem** briefly identifies what we know about the problem area, and the **problem statement** identifies the specific gap in the knowledge needed for practice. Not all published studies include a clearly expressed problem, but the problem usually can be identified in the first page of the paper. The **research purpose** is a clear, concise statement of the specific goal or focus of a study. In quantitative and outcomes studies, the goal of a study might be to identify, describe, or explain a situation; examine the effectiveness of an intervention; or determine outcomes of health care. The purpose also includes the variables, the population, and often the setting for the study. A clearly stated research purpose can capture the essence of a study in a single sentence and is essential for directing the remaining steps of the research process. The research problem and purpose from Schultz and colleagues' (2008) study of the effectiveness of gel pillows for reducing bilateral head flattening in preterm infants are presented as an example. This research example is critically appraised using the following questions.

CRITICAL APPRAISAL GUIDELINES

Problems and Purposes in Studies
1. Is the problem clearly and concisely expressed early in the study?
2. Does the problem include significance, background, and problem statement?
3. Is the problem significant to study to generate essential knowledge for practice?
4. Does the purpose clearly express the goal or focus of the study?
5. Does the purpose identify the variables or concepts and population for the study?

RESEARCH EXAMPLE Problem and Purpose of a Quantitative Study

Problem Significance

Survival rates for very low birth weight (VLBW) infants, defined as infants weighing <1500 g [grams] at birth, continue to rise (Kenner, Lott, & Flandermeyer, 1997). In the 1990s, an alarming rise in the number of premature infants presenting with plagiocephaly without synostosis (i.e., head flattening without fusion of normally separate bones, due in part to head molding) has been reported by several craniofacial centers (Argenta, 2004; Najarian, 1999). This increasing incidence has been linked to the American Academy of Pediatrics' (1996) recommendation regarding sleep positions (supine and side lying) to prevent sudden infant death syndrome and to the increase in the survival of VLBW infants ... (Schultz et al., 2008, p. 191)

Problem Background

Although this outcome [head molding] has been minimized with some success by repositioning, in very tiny infants with delayed motor development, the head may retain the abnormal shape for a much longer period, even into adulthood ... (Shin & Pershing, 2003) ... Studies have been conducted to examine the effectiveness of various surfaces, pillows, and turning protocols designed to reduce bilateral head molding in preterm infants. ... (Schultz et al., 2008, pp. 191-192)

Problem Statement

Early studies suggest that water pillows and air-filled mattresses are effective for preventing undesirable bilateral head molding in preterm infants; however, no studies measuring the effectiveness of gel pillows, a newer product on the market, for reducing bilateral head molding have been found. (Schultz et al., 2008, p. 193)

Research Purpose

The study purpose was to examine the effectiveness of gel pillows for reducing bilateral head molding (plagiocephaly) in preterm infants, as determined by the cephalic index (CI). (Schultz et al., 2008, p. 191)

CRITICAL APPRAISAL

Research Problem

Schultz and colleagues (2008) presented a clear, concise research problem or area of concern and included the following parts of the problem: (1) significance, (2) background, and (3) problem statement. In this study, the first paragraph clearly identified the area of concern (plagiocephaly or bilateral head flattening caused by head molding) for a particular population (preterm infants). Head molding is a significant problem because it is increasing with the survival of more VLBW infants and the positioning of infants in supine and side-lying positions during sleep. In addition, the abnormal shape of the head can continue into adulthood. The second paragraph provided a concise background indicating various interventions have been studied to determine their effectiveness in preventing or reducing head molding.

The discussion of the problem concluded with a concise problem statement that indicated the gap in the knowledge needed for practice and provided a basis for the study conducted by Schultz and colleagues. Each problem provides the basis for generating a variety of research purposes; and in this study, the knowledge gap regarding the effectiveness of gel pillows on head molding provides clear direction for the formulation of the research purpose.

Continued

RESEARCH PURPOSE

In a published study, the purpose frequently is reflected in the title of the study, stated in the study abstract, and restated after the literature review. Schultz et al. (2008) included the purpose of their study in all three places. The goal of this quasi-experimental study was to examine the effectiveness of the nursing intervention gel pillows (independent variable) in reducing bilateral head molding (dependent variables) for preterm infants (population). The purpose was clearly stated, indicated the type of study conducted (quasi-experimental), included the study variables and population, and inferred the study was conducted in a neonatal intensive care unit (NICU) (setting).

(This critical appraisal was based on the Critical Appraisal Guidelines in the previous box on page 146.)

IMPLICATIONS FOR PRACTICE

The findings from the Schultz et al. (2008, p. 191) study indicated "the trend was toward less molding over time for smaller infants on gel pillows who were hospitalized longer; however, the sample size was too small to detect statistical significance." Thus, additional research with a larger sample is needed to determine if gel pillows are effective in reducing head molding in preterm infants before this product is purchased for use in NICUs.

Identifying the Problem and Purpose in Quantitative, Qualitative, and Outcomes Studies

Quantitative, qualitative, and outcomes research approaches enable nurses to investigate a variety of research problems and purposes. Examples of research topics, problems, and purposes for different types of quantitative, qualitative, and outcomes studies are presented in this section.

Problems and Purposes in Types of Quantitative Studies

Example research topics, problems, and purposes for the different types of quantitative research (descriptive, correlational, quasi-experimental, and experimental) are presented in Table 5–1. If little is known about a topic, the researcher usually starts with a descriptive study and progresses to quasi-experimental and experimental studies. An examination of the problems and purposes in Table 5–1 will reveal the differences and similarities among the types of quantitative research. The research purpose usually reflects the type of study that was conducted (Burns & Grove, 2009). The purpose of descriptive research is to identify and describe concepts or variables, identify possible relationships among variables, and delineate differences between or among existing groups, such as males and females or different ethnic groups.

Rambur, McIntosh, Palumbo, and Reinier (2005) conducted a descriptive study to compare job satisfaction and career retention for registered nurses (RNs) whose highest degree was Associate Degree in Nursing (ADN) or Bachelor of Science in Nursing (BSN).

The RNs with a BSN had "significantly higher job satisfaction related to: (a) opportunity for autonomy and growth, (b) job stress and physical demands, and (c) job and organizational security" (Rambur et al., p. 185). Thus, these findings support the preparation of RNs with a BSN versus an ADN for greater individual and social return on the educational investment.

The purpose of correlational research is to examine the type (positive or negative) and strength of relationships among variables. In their correlational study, Howell, Rice, Carmon, and Hauber (2007) examined the relationships among anxiety, anger, and blood pressure (BP) in children (see Table 5–1). "This study supports the belief that certain modifiable risk factors [anger expression, anxiety, height, and weight] for hypertension are present at an early age" (Howell et al., 2007, p. 22). Thus, the researchers recommended the BP should be monitored at all scheduled physical exams for every child age three and older.

Table 5–1	Quantitative Research: Topics, Problems, and Purposes	
Type of Research	**Research Topic**	**Research Problem and Purpose**
Descriptive research	Educational preparation, associate degree prepared nurse, baccalaureate degree prepared nurse, registered nurses, individual (job satisfaction), social return on investment (career retention)	*Title of study:* "Education as a determinant of career retention and job satisfaction among registered nurses" (Rambur, McIntosh, Palumbo, & Reinier, 2005, p. 185) *Problem:* "As the current nursing shortage increases concerns about staff of healthcare facilities' ability to provide high quality care (Aiken, Clarke, Sloan, Sochalski, & Silber, 2002), many initiatives are being aimed at the recruitment and retention of the nursing workforce. The pressing need to educate more nurses should stimulate reconsideration of how limited resources for nursing education are spent as educational capacity is increased. ... Although many studies have been aimed toward understanding the outcomes of baccalaureate and associate degree education for nurses, few studies have been focused on education as an individual or social return on investment or in years contributed to the profession" (Rambur et al., 2005, pp. 185–186). *Purpose:* The purpose of this study was "to compare job satisfaction and career retention in two cohorts of RNs, those whose highest degrees were the associate's degree (AD) or the bachelor's degree (BS) in nursing" (Rambur et al., 2005, p. 185).
Correlational research	Hypertension, blood pressure, psychosocial factors, biological factors	*Title of study:* "The relationships among anxiety, anger, and blood pressure in children" (Howell, Rice, Carmon, & Hauber, 2007, p. 17). *Problem:* "Hypertension affects over 50 million Americans aged 6 and over and is a recognized risk factor for the development of cardiovascular disease (American Heart Association, 2004). Although few children have hypertension or cardiovascular disease, biological and psychosocial risk factors for the development of hypertension in adulthood are estimated to be present in children by the age of 8 (Solomon & Matthews, 1999). ... Although the contribution of these factors to the development of hypertension has been investigated in adults and adolescents. ... much less research has been done with children (Hauber et al., 1998; Howell et al., 2007, p. 17). *Purpose:* "The purpose of this study was to determine the relationships between trait anxiety, trait anger, height, weight, patterns of anger expression, and blood pressure in a group of elementary school children" (Howell et al., 2007, p. 18).

Continued

Table 5-1	Quantitative Research: Topics, Problems, and Purposes—cont'd	
Type of Research	Research Topic	Research Problem and Purpose
Quasi-experimental research	Nurse-case-managed intervention, hepatitis A and B vaccine completion, sociodemographic factors, risk behaviors, and homeless adults	*Title of study:* "Effects of a nurse-managed program on hepatitis A and B vaccine completion among homeless adults" (Nyamathi et al., 2009, p. 13). *Problem:* "Hepatitis B virus (HBV) infection poses a serious threat to public health in the United States. Recent estimates place the true prevalence of chronic HBV in the United States at approximately 1.6 cases per 100,000 persons (Centers for Disease Control & Prevention [CDC], 2008). It is estimated that there were 51,000 new cases of HBV infection in 2005 (Wasley, Miller, & Finelli, 2007), a financial burden reaching $1 billion annually (Cohen et al., 2007). … Homeless populations are at particularly high risk of HBV infection due to high rates of unprotected sexual behavior and sharing of needles and other IDU [injection drug user] paraphernalia. Previous studies have reported that HBV infection rates among homeless populations range from 17% to 31% (i.e., from 17,000 to 31,000 per 100,000…) compared with 2.1 per 100,000 in the general United States population (CDC, 2006b) … Vaccination is the most effective way to prevent HBV infection (CDC, 2006a) … Improving vaccination adherence rates among homeless persons is an important step toward reducing the high prevalence of HBV infection in this population. … Thus, little is known about adherence to HBV vaccination among community samples of urban homeless person[s] or about the effect of stronger interventions to incorporate additional strategies, such as nurse case management and targeted HBV education along with client tracking" (Nyamathi et al., 2009, pp. 13-14). *Purpose:* The purpose of this study was to determine the "effectiveness of a nurse-case-managed intervention compared with that of two standard programs on completion of the combined hepatitis A virus (HAV) and HBV vaccine series among homeless adults and to assess socio-demographic factors and risk behaviors related to the vaccine completion" (Nyamathi et al., 2009, p. 13).
Experimental research	Pain management, analgesics, morphine, beta-endorphin (BE), circadian rhythm, animals	*Title of study:* "Effects of morphine and time of day on pain and beta-endorphin (BE)" (Rasmussen & Farr, 2003, p. 105). *Problem:* "Although narcotics have been used as analgesics for many years, clients still are experiencing pain. … Morphine is an important pharmacological modulator of pain and initiator of analgesia. … Circadian (approximately 24 hours) rhythms influence the expression of pain and the body's responsiveness to analgesic mediations. … Endogenous opioids, such as morphine, activate the descending pain control system. … Currently, the timing of the administration of morphine is not based on its circadian effects. Both PLRL [paw-licking response latency in mice] and BE are known to exhibit a circadian rhythm, or a rhythm that repeats once in a 24-hour period. Yet no well-controlled, time-based studies have been conducted to test the effects of morphine on pain response (PLRL) and plasma BE when administered at different times of day" (Rasmussen & Farr, 2003, pp. 105-107). *Purpose:* "The purpose of the study … was to investigate whether there were time-of-day differences in the effects of morphine on the pain tolerance threshold and the circadian plasma BE response to pain" (Rasmussen & Farr, 2003, p. 107).

Quasi-experimental studies are conducted to determine the effect of a treatment or independent variable on designated dependent or outcome variables. Nyamathi and colleagues (2009) conducted a quasi-experimental study to examine the effectiveness of a nurse-case-managed intervention on hepatitis A and B vaccine completion among homeless adults. The research topics, problem, and purpose for this study are presented in Table 5–1. The findings from this study "revealed that a culturally sensitive comprehensive program, which included nurse case management plus targeted hepatitis education, incentives, and client tracking, performed significantly better than did a usual care program" (Nyamathi et al., 2009, p. 21). Thus, the researchers recommended that public health program planners and funders use this type of program to promote increased completion of hepatitis A and B vaccinations with high risk groups.

Experimental studies are conducted in highly controlled settings, using a highly structured design to determine the effect of one or more independent variables on one or more dependent variables. Rasmussen and Farr (2003) conducted an experimental study of the effects of morphine and time of day on pain and beta-endorphin (BE) in groups of mice in a laboratory setting (see Table 5–1). In this basic research, the investigators found that morphine abolishes the BE response to pain but does not inhibit pain equally at all times of the day. Thus, morphine doses should be titrated to maximize pain control, with less medication. Additional research in humans is needed, however, before the findings will have implications for nursing practice.

Problems and Purposes in Types of Qualitative Studies

The problems formulated for qualitative research identify areas of concern that require investigation to gain new insights, expand understanding, and improve comprehension of the whole (Munhall, 2007). The purpose of a qualitative study indicates the focus of the study, which may be a concept such as pain, an event such as loss of a child, or a facet of a culture such as the healing practices of a specific Native American Indian tribe. In addition, the purpose often indicates the qualitative approach used to conduct the study. The basic assumptions for this approach are discussed in the research report (Creswell, 2008). Examples of research topics, problems, and purposes for the types of qualitative research—phenomenological, grounded theory, ethnographic, and historical—commonly conducted in nursing are presented in Table 5–2.

Phenomenological research is conducted to promote a deeper understanding of complex human experiences as they have been lived by the study participants (Munhall, 2007). The study by Cashin, Small, and Solberg (2008) entitled "The Lived Experience of Fathers Who Have Children with Asthma: A Phenomenological Study" is presented as an example (see Table 5–2). Cashin and colleagues (2008, p. 372) identified five themes important to fathers: "feeling relief in knowing the diagnosis, learning the ropes, being vigilant, living with concern, and being comfortable with asthma management. Understanding the experience of fathers who have children with asthma and gaining insight into their needs and concerns are essential first steps to providing supportive nursing care."

In grounded theory research, the problem identifies the area of concern and the purpose indicates the focus of the theory to be developed to account for a pattern of behavior for those involved in the study (Wuest, 2007). For example, El-Mallakh (2007) investigated the poverty and self-care among individuals with schizophrenia and diabetes mellitus. The

Table 5-2	Qualitative Research: Topics, Problems, and Purposes	
Type of Research	Research Topic	Research Problem and Purpose
Phenomenological research	Lived experience of fathers, understanding childhood asthma, chronic illness	*Title of study:* "The lived experience of fathers who have children with asthma: A phenomenological study" (Cashin, Small, & Solberg, 2008, p. 327). *Problem:* "Asthma is an inflammatory disorder of the airways characterized by paroxysmal or persistent symptoms such as shortness of breath, chest tightness, wheezing, and cough (Becker et al., 2005). It is a common chronic illness of childhood ... and a major cause of school absenteeism (Global Initiative for Asthma, 2006). It impacts various functional domains, including the physical, social, and psychological (Halfon & Newacheck, 2000) ... Although there is a growing body of knowledge concerning parenting children who have asthma, the research had predominantly been about mothers, with fathers' perspectives receiving little attention. The same has been noted within the vast body of literature concerning parents and childhood chronic illness in general in that much of the research had focused on mothers, not fathers" (Cashin et al., 2008, p. 327). *Purpose:* "The purpose of this study was, therefore, to attain an understanding of what it is like to be the father of a child with asthma" (Cashin et al., 2008, p. 372).
Grounded theory research	Self-care, poverty, schizophrenia, diabetes mellitus	*Title of study:* "Doing my best: Poverty and self-care among individuals with schizophrenia and diabetes mellitus" (El-Mallakh, 2007, p. 49). *Problem:* "Mental health clinicians and researchers increasingly recognize that individuals with schizophrenia have a high risk of developing diabetes mellitus (DM) (Bushe & Holt, 2004). Whereas rates of diabetes in the general populations range from 2% to 6%, prevalence rates of diabetes among individuals with schizophrenia range from 15% to 18%, and up to 30% have impaired glucose tolerance (Bushe & Holt, 2004; Schizophrenia and Diabetes Expert Consensus Group, 2004). ... The recent mental health literature has focused on the screening, diagnosis, and treatment of diabetes in this population, including discussions of the risks and benefits of atypical antipsychotic use. ... However, few researchers have investigated the influence of social and demographic characteristics on diabetic self-care among individuals with schizophrenia and diabetes" (El-Mallakh, 2007, pp. 49-50). *Purpose:* "A grounded theory study was conducted to examine several aspects of diabetic self-care in individuals with schizophrenia and DM" (El-Mallakh, 2007, p. 50).
Ethnographic research	Critical illness, mechanical ventilation, weaning, family presence	*Title of study:* "Family presence and surveillance during weaning from prolonged mechanical ventilation" (Happ, Swigart, Tate, Arnold, Sereika, & Hoffman, 2007, p. 47). *Problem:* "During critical illness, mechanical ventilation imposes physical and communication barriers between family members and their critically ill loved ones. ... Most studies of family members in the intensive care unit (ICU) have focused on families' needs for information, access to the patient, and participation in decisions to withdraw or withhold life-sustaining treatment. ... Although numerous studies have been conducted of patient experiences with short- and long-term mechanical ventilation (LTMV), research has not focused on family interactions with patients during weaning from mechanical ventilation. Moreover, the importance of family members' bedside presence and clinicians' interpretation of family behaviors at the bedside have not been critically examined" (Happ et al., 2007, pp. 47-48). *Purpose:* "With the use of data from an ethnographic study of the care and communication processes during weaning from LTMV, we sought to describe how family members interact with the patients and respond to the ventilator and associated ICU bedside equipment during LTMV weaning" (Happ et al., 2007, p. 48).

Table 5–2	Qualitative Research: Topics, Problems, and Purposes—cont'd	
Type of Research	**Research Topic**	**Research Problem and Purpose**
Historical research	History, Cold War, mass disaster, nursing research, 1950s, Harriet H. Werley, Army Nurse Corps	*Title of study:* "Planning for mass disaster in the 1950s: Harriet H. Werley and nursing research" (Leifer & Glass, 2008, p. 237) *Problem:* "Americans were continually aware of the potential for nuclear disaster during the Cold War era. … Because the fear of nuclear war was ever present, military and civil defence programs were developed to help Americans prepare for disaster. … Military and civilian healthcare personnel were mobilized to prepare for any mass casualties caused by a nuclear attack. In the 21st century, world events remind nurses of the need to be prepared to respond to disaster. Since the events of September 11, 2001; the Southeast Asian tsunami in 2004; and the Gulf Coast hurricanes in 2005, there has been an increased emphasis on preparedness and response planning for man-made or natural disaster. … During the turbulent Cold War era, Harriet H. Werley, an Army Nurse Corps (ANC) major, was a pioneer in mass disaster education and nursing research. She served as the first nursing consultant in the newly formed Department of Atomic Casualties Studies (DACS) from 1955-1958. … When working with military officials in Washington, DC, including the ANC, the Office of the Surgeon General, the Army Institute of Research, and the Walter Reed Army Hospital, Werley shared her vision of an evolving role for nurses that included increased opportunities for leadership, research, and expanded practice. … Primary and secondary sources regarding Werley's work in the DACS and the field of disaster nursing were examined to obtain data for this historical study" (Leifer & Glass, 2008, pp. 237-238). *Purpose:* The purpose of this historical study "was to analyze nurses" involvement in research and mass disaster preparations during the Cold War era and to describe the role of Harriet H. Werley and the Army Nurse Corps" (Leifer & Glass, 2008, p. 237).

research topics, problem, and purpose for this study are presented in Table 5–2. Based on the findings from this grounded theory study, El-Mallakh (2007, p. 49) developed a "model, Evolving Self-Care, that describes the process by which respondents developed health beliefs about self-care of dual illnesses. One subcategory of the model, Doing My Best, was further analyzed to examine the social context of respondents' diabetic self-care."

In ethnographic research, the problem and purpose identify the culture and the specific attributes of the culture that are to be examined, described, analyzed, and interpreted to reveal the social actions, beliefs, values, and norms of the culture (Wolf, 2007). Happ, Swigart, Tate, Arnold, Sereika, and Hoffman (2007) conducted an ethnographic study of family presence and surveillance during weaning of their family member from a ventilator. Table 5–2 includes the research topics, problem, and purpose for this study. These researchers concluded that "this study provided a potentially useful conceptual framework of family behaviors with long-term critically ill patients that could enhance the dialogue about family-centered care and guide future research on family presence in the intensive care unit" (Happ et al., 2007, p. 47).

The problem and purpose in historical research focus on a specific individual, a characteristic of society, an event, or a situation in the past and usually identifies the time period in the past that was examined by the study (Fitzpatrick, 2007). For example, Leifer and Glass (2008, p. 237) conducted a historical study entitled "Planning for Mass Disaster in the 1950s:

Harriet H. Werley and Nursing Research" (see Table 5–2). Harriet Werley had a vision for nursing research and was a strong advocate for research-based disaster management in the 1950s. Werley's "actions influenced the nursing community to consider its professional responsibility as a key provider in disaster management and partner in interdisciplinary research" (Leifer & Glass, 2008, p. 237). The work of Werley provides a basis for understanding what faces nursing professionals in meeting the demands and challenges involved in disaster management preparations for the twenty-first century. The problems and purposes investigated in qualitative research are discussed in greater detail in Chapter 3.

Problems and Purposes in Outcomes Research

Outcomes research is conducted to examine the end results of care. Table 5–3 includes the topics, problem, and purpose from an outcomes study by Rudy, Daly, Douglas, Montenegro, Song, and Dyer (1995). This study was conducted to determine the outcomes for patients who are chronically critically ill in the special care unit (SCU) compared with the intensive care unit (ICU). Common health outcomes—cost, patient satisfaction, length of stay, complications, and readmissions—were examined to determine the impact of care in these two units on the patients and the healthcare system. The findings from this 4-year study demonstrated that nurse case managers in an SCU setting can produce patient outcomes as good as or better than those obtained in the traditional ICU environment, for long-term critically ill patients. In addition, caring for patients in the SCU was more cost effective than caring for those in the ICU.

Table 5-3	Outcomes Research: Topics, Problem, and Purpose	
Type of Research	**Research Topic**	**Research Problem and Purpose**
Outcomes research	Patient outcomes, special care unit, intensive care unit, chronically critically ill	*Title of study:* "Patient outcomes for the chronically critically ill: Special care unit versus intensive care unit" (^Rudy, Daly, Douglas, Montenegro, Song, & Dyer, 1995) *Problem:* "The original purpose of intensive care units (ICUs) was to locate groups of patients together who had similar needs for specialized monitoring and care so that highly trained healthcare personnel would be available to meet these specialized needs. As the success of ICUs has grown and expanded, the assumption that a typical ICU patient will require only a short length of stay in the unit during the most acute phase of an illness has given way to the recognition that stays of more than one month are not uncommon. ... These long-stay ICU patients represent a challenge to the current system, not only because of costs, but also because of concern for patient outcomes. ... While ample evidence confirms that this subpopulation of ICU patients represents a drain on hospital resources, few studies have attempted to evaluate the effects of a care delivery system outside the ICU setting on patient outcomes, costs, and nurse outcomes" (^Rudy et al., 1995, p. 324). *Purpose:* "The purpose of this study was to compare the effects of a low–technology environment of care and a nurse case management care delivery system (specific care unit, SCU) with the traditional high–technology environment (ICU) and primary nursing care delivery system on the patient outcomes of length of stay, mortality, readmission, complications, satisfaction, and cost" (^Rudy et al., 1995, p. 324).

Determining the Significance of a Study Problem and Purpose

A research problem is significant in nursing when it has the potential to generate or refine relevant knowledge for practice (Brown, 2009). When critically appraising the significance of the problem and purpose in a published study, you need to determine whether the knowledge generated in the study (1) influences nursing practice, (2) builds on previous research, (3) promotes theory testing or development, and/or (4) addresses current concerns or priorities in nursing (Burns & Grove, 2009).

Influences Nursing Practice

The practice of nursing needs to be evidence-based or built on empirical knowledge that is generated through research (Craig & Smyth, 2007; Melnyk & Fineout-Overholt, 2005). Thus, studies that address clinical concerns and generate findings to improve nursing practice are considered significant. Several research problems and purposes have focused on the effects of nursing interventions or on ways to improve these interventions. For example, researchers have examined the effects of (1) hygienic hand washing on infection control (Celik & Kocasli, 2008); (2) gel pillows for reducing bilateral head flattening in preterm infants (Schultz et al., 2008); and (3) guided health imagery to promote smoking cessation (Wynd, 2005). Intervention-focused studies generate significant empirical knowledge that moves nursing toward evidence-based practice and the delivery of quality care for patients and their families.

Builds on Previous Research

A significant study problem and purpose are based on previous research. In a research article, the Introduction and Literature Review sections include relevant studies that provide a basis for the current study. Often, a summary of the current literature indicates what is known and not known in the area being studied. The gaps in the current knowledge base provide support for and document the significance of the study's purpose. The study by Schultz and colleagues (2008), introduced earlier in this chapter, indicated what was known about the effectiveness of selected interventions (bed surfaces, pillows, and turning protocols) on bilateral head flattening. What was not known was the effectiveness of a new product, gel pillows, on head flattening in preterm infants. Schultz et al. (2008) built on previous research in conducting their study, identified the initial effectiveness of gel pillows, and indicated the need for additional research before these pillows are used in NICU.

Promotes Theory Testing or Development

Significant problems and purposes are supported by theory, and the study may focus on either testing or developing theory (Chinn & Kramer, 2008). For example, Steele and Porche (2005) conducted a study to test the theory of planned behavior by Ajzen (2002). A model of Ajzen's theory is presented in Figure 5–1. This theory was used to predict the intentions of rural southeastern Louisiana women to obtain a mammogram. The model indicates that behavioral belief strength influences attitude, normative belief strength influences subjective norm, and control belief strength influences perceived behavior control. Attitude, subjective norm, and

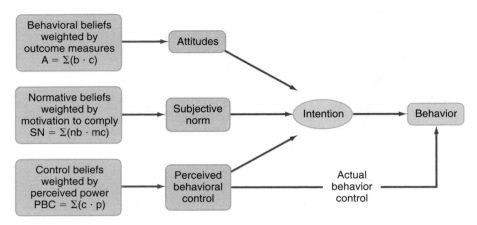

Figure 5–1. The theory of planned behavior (Ajzen, 2002).

perceived behavioral control are predictive of a person's intention, and intention is predictive of behavior. The researchers found that perceived behavior control was the most predictive of a woman's intention to get a mammogram, and attitude was the second greatest predictor. The woman's intention to get a mammogram was predictive of her behavior of obtaining the mammogram. Thus, Ajzen's theory was supported by the conduct of this study, and it can be used to explain the mammography intentions of rural women (Steele & Porche, 2005). Ajzen's theory and the findings from this study can be used to develop educational programs to encourage rural women to get mammograms.

Addresses Nursing Research Priorities

For the last 30 years, nurse leaders, professional nursing organizations, and federal institutes and agencies have developed research priorities and agendas to identify the significant research needed to build an evidence-based practice for nursing. The first research priorities were developed in 1975 for clinical practice under the leadership of Dr. Lindeman. These research priorities included nursing interventions focused on care of the elderly, patient education, and pain management, which continue to be important areas for research today.

Many professional organizations have identified research priorities that are communicated through their websites. For example, the American Association of Critical-Care Nurses (AACN) published its most current research priorities on its website (*http://www.aacn.org* and search for Research Priorities). The AACN (2009) identified five broad research areas: (1) effective and appropriate use of technology to achieve optimal patient assessment, management, and/or outcomes; (2) creation of a healing, humane environment; (3) processes and systems that foster the optimal contribution of critical care nurses; (4) effective approaches to symptom management; and (5) prevention and management of complications.

The Oncology Nursing Society (ONS) conducted a study of their membership in 2008 to determine the research priorities for oncology nursing (Doorenbos et al., 2008). The ONS identified their top 20 research priorities, which will be used in the development of the 2009-2013 ONS Research Agenda. The top five research priorities identified were: (1) quality of life, (2) pain, (3) late effects of treatment, (4) access to care, and (5) palliative care. The ONS Research Agenda and research priorities can be viewed on the ONS website at http://www.ons.org/Research/.

The American Organization of Nurse Executives (AONE) established their 2009 Education and Research Priorities and provided it on their website at *http://www.aone.org/aone/edandcareer/priorities.html*. The priorities were organized into four major areas of (1) design of future patient care delivery systems, (2) healthful practice environments, (3) leadership, and (4) positioning nurse leaders as valued healthcare executives and managers. These four general areas included 30 different priorities that can be viewed online (AONE, 2009).

A significant funding agency for nursing research is the National Institute of Nursing Research (NINR). A major initiative of NINR is the development of a national nursing research agenda that will involve identifying nursing research priorities, outlining a plan for implementing priority studies, and obtaining resources to support these priority projects. NINR (2009) developed four strategies for building the science of nursing for 2006-2010: (1) "Integrating biological and behavior science for better health; (2) adopting, adapting, and generating new technologies for better health care; (3) improving methods for future scientific discoveries; and (4) developing scientists for today and tomorrow." The areas of research emphasis for 2006-2010 include: (1) Promoting health and preventing disease, (2) improving quality of life, (3) eliminating health disparities, and (4) setting directions for end-of-life research (NINR, 2009). Specific research priorities were identified for each of these four areas of research emphasis and included in the *NINR Strategic Plan for 2006-2010*. Details about the NINR mission, strategic plan, and research priorities are available on their website at *http://www.nih.gov/ninr/*.

Another important federal agency involved in funding healthcare research is the Agency for Healthcare Research and Quality (AHRQ), formerly the Agency for Health Care Policy and Research (AHCPR). The purpose of the AHRQ (2009) is to enhance the quality, appropriateness, and effectiveness of healthcare services, as well as the access to such services, through the establishment of a broad base of scientific research and the promotion of improvements in clinical practice and in the organization, financing, and delivery of healthcare services. Some of the current funding priorities are research focused on prevention; health information technology; patient safety; long-term care; pharmaceutical outcomes; system capacity and emergency preparedness; and cost, organization, and socioeconomics of health care. For a complete list of funding opportunities and grant announcements, see the AHRQ website at *http://www.ahrq.gov/*.

Expert researchers, professional organizations, and federal agencies have identified research priorities to direct the future conduct of healthcare research. When conducting a critical appraisal of a study, you need to determine whether the problem and purpose are based on previous research, theory, and current research priorities. Whether the study findings will influence nursing practice also needs to be determined. These four elements, discussed in this section, document the significance of the study in developing and refining nursing knowledge to build an evidence-based practice for nursing (Brown, 2009; Craig & Smyth, 2007).

Examining the Feasibility of a Problem and Purpose

A critical appraisal of research begins by determining the feasibility of the problem and purpose of the study. The feasibility of a study is determined by examining the researchers' expertise; money commitment; availability of subjects, facilities, and equipment; and the study's ethical considerations (Rogers, 1987). The feasibility of Schultz and colleagues' (2008) study of the effectiveness of gel pillows on bilateral head flattening in preterm infants is critically appraised and presented as an example. The critical appraisal involved answering the following questions: Was it feasible for the researchers to study the problem and purpose identified? Did the researchers have the expertise to conduct the study? Did they have adequate money, subjects, setting, and equipment to conduct the study? Was the purpose of the study ethical?

Researcher Expertise

The research problem and purpose studied need to be within the area of expertise of the researchers. Research reports usually identify the education of the researchers and their current positions, which indicate their expertise to conduct a study. Also examine the reference list to determine if the researchers have conducted additional studies in this area. If you desire more information, you can search the web for the researchers' accomplishments and involvement in research (Burns & Grove, 2009). Schultz, for example, has a doctoral degree and is part of the Center for the Advancement of Evidence-Based Practice at Arizona State University. Her educational preparation and academic position support her research expertise. Goodwin, Jesseman, and Toews are nurses employed in the neonatal intensive care unit at Barbara Bush Children's Hospital at Maine Medical Center, which supports the strength of their clinical expertise in managing preterm infants. In addition, Jesseman is a neonatal nurse practitioner (NNP), which indicates educational preparation with specialization in the care of preterm infants. Lane is a family nurse practitioner at Maine Centers for Healthcare, and Smith is employed by the Visiting Nurse Association of Brooklyn. The two nurse practitioners also have research expertise in implementing evidenced-based practice for their patients. Thus, Schultz and her co-authors have strong research and clinical expertise to conduct this study. The study would have been strengthened if the researchers had conducted additional research in this area.

Money Commitment

The problem and purpose studied are influenced by the amount of money available to the researchers. The cost of a research project can range from a few dollars for a student's small study to hundreds of thousands and even millions of dollars for complex projects. In critically appraising a study, you must determine if the researchers had adequate financial resources to complete their study. Sources of funding for a study usually are identified in the article. For example, a study may have been funded by a federal research grant from the NINR or a professional organization such as Sigma Theta Tau or the AACN.

The researchers may have received financial assistance from companies that provided necessary equipment or support from the agency where they work. Receiving funding for a study indicates that it was reviewed by peers who chose to support the research financially. Schultz et al. (2008, p. 198) indicated their study "was supported, in part, by Children's

Medical ventures, which donated the gel pillows." Nurses at the Barbara Bush Children's Hospital participated in this study as part of their employment in the neonatal intensive care unit (NICU), indicating agency financial support of the study.

Availability of Subjects, Facilities, and Equipment

Researchers need to have adequate sample size, facilities, and equipment to implement their study. Most published studies indicate the sample size and setting(s) in the Methods section of the research report. Often nursing studies are conducted in natural or partially controlled settings, such as a home, hospital unit, or clinic. Many of these facilities are easy to access, and the hospitals and clinics provide access to large numbers of patients. Schultz and colleagues' (2008, p. 194) study included 52 neonates who were obtained from "a tertiary level III NICU that averages more than 600 admissions annually." The researchers recognized the small sample size as a study limitation and a possible cause of the nonsignificant findings. The enrollment of infants was limited to the time that the researchers were available in the NICU; thus, only 81 infants were enrolled in the study. In addition, the attrition in the study by five weeks was high (35%) because of discharge, transfer, and scheduling errors. In this study, an adequate number of subjects were available but because of other circumstances the sample completing the study was small.

A review of the Methods section of the research article will determine if adequate, accurate equipment was available. Nursing studies frequently require a limited amount of equipment, such as a tape or video recorder for interviews, or physiological instruments, such as an electrocardiogram (ECG) or thermometer. Schultz et al. (2008) conducted a quasi-experimental study that examined the effectiveness of gel pillows (independent variable) on head flattening in preterm infants and a company provided the pillows for the study. Head molding (dependent variable) was measured with digital calipers that were available in the NICU. Thus, the researchers had adequate support to implement the independent variable and measure the dependent variable in their study.

Ethical Considerations

The purpose selected for investigation must be ethical, which means that the subjects' rights and the rights of others in the setting are protected (Burns & Grove, 2009). An ethical study confers more benefits than risks in its conduct and will generate useful knowledge for practice. The Schultz et al. (2008) study carried limited potential risk of increased head molding with the gel pillows and a great potential benefit of reduced head flattening. The researchers obtained Institutional Review Board approval from their clinical agency and informed consent from the parents of the infants. Thus, this is an ethical study that protected the rights of the subjects and has a potential to improve preterm infants' outcomes.

Examining Research Objectives, Questions, and Hypotheses in Research Reports

Research objectives, questions, and hypotheses evolve from the problem, purpose, literature review, and study framework, and direct the remaining steps of the research process. In a published study the objectives, questions, or hypotheses usually are presented after the

Literature Review section and right before the Methods section. The content in this section is provided to assist you in identifying and critically appraising the objectives, questions, and hypotheses in published studies.

Research Objectives or Aims Implemented in Quantitative Studies

A **research objective** is a clear, concise, declarative statement that is expressed in the present tense. The objectives are sometimes referred to as aims and are used most often in descriptive and correlational quantitative studies. For clarity, an objective or aim usually focuses on one or two variables and indicates whether they are to be identified or described. Sometimes the purpose of objectives is to identify relationships among variables or to determine differences between two or more existing groups regarding selected variables. Duffy, Reeves, Hermann, Karvonen, and Smith (2008) conducted a descriptive study to determine the wants and needs of Veteran Affairs (VA) patients and staff for in-hospital smoking cessation programs. This study demonstrates the logical flow from research problem and purpose to research objectives in a quantitative study. The following questions are used to conduct a critical appraisal of this research example.

CRITICAL APPRAISAL GUIDELINES

Research Objectives in Studies
1. Are the objectives clearly and concisely expressed in the study?
2. Are the study objectives based on the purpose?
3. Is the focus of each objective clearly presented?

RESEARCH EXAMPLE Problem, Purpose, and Objectives from a Quantitative

Research Problem

Tobacco use is the leading cause of mortality in the United States, with an estimated 18.1% of total deaths in the year 2000 attributed to Tobacco (Mokdad, Marks, Stroup, & Gerberding, 2004). Smoking rates are higher in the veteran populations (33% vs. 22% of nonveterans) (Center for Disease Control, 2003b; Office of Quality and Performance, 2001). Psychiatric comorbidities, which are associated with smoking and are common among veterans, may contribute to elevated mortality rates from cancer, cardiovascular disease, and hepatic disorders [problem significance]. ... The majority of smoking services in the VA are provided by outpatient programs. Although efficacious, outpatient smoking cessation programs are poorly attended, and few smokers are reached (Cromwell et al., 1997). In contrast, inpatient programs, compared to outpatient programs, enroll a higher percentage of patients who smoke and result in higher cessation [problem background]. ... However, inconsistent or minimal cessation services are provided to inpatients in the VA system. ... In preparation for delivering an inpatient smoking cessation intervention, veteran inpatient smokers and their staff caregivers at two Michigan VAs were surveyed and interviewed. [problem statement] (Duffy et al., 2008, pp. 199-200)

Research Purpose

The purpose of this study was to determine the motivation of veterans to quit smoking and to identify facilitators and barriers to inpatient staff delivery of inpatient cessation services. (Duffy et al., 2008, p. 199)

Research Objectives

The objectives of the study were to: (1) determine the motivation of inpatient veterans to quit smoking and the types of services they would prefer; (2) determine facilitators and barriers to inpatient staff delivery of inpatient cessation services; and (3) seek suggestions and insight from inpatients and staff about what would be important to include in an inpatient smoking cessation program. (Duffy et al., 2008, p. 200)

CRITICAL APPRAISAL

Duffy and colleagues (2008) identified a significant problem of smoking or nicotine addiction that can be linked to cancer, cardiovascular disease, and hepatic disorders. They also provided a background for the problem that indicated what was known in this problem area. The problem statement clearly indicates what is not known and provides a basis for the purpose and objectives of this study. The purpose clearly indicates this is a descriptive study that is focused on a population of inpatient veterans who smoke to determine their motivation to quit smoking and the facilitators and barriers to conducting smoking cessation services (research variables). The study objectives build on the problem and purpose and provide more clarity regarding the focus of the study. All three objectives focused on description, with the first objective focused on describing inpatient veterans' motivation to quit. The second objective focused on describing the facilitators and barriers to smoking cessation services. The third objective focused on describing what to include in the smoking cessation program. Thus, this study identified a significant problem and a feasible purpose for research. In addition, the study objectives provided clear direction for the conduct of the study and the interpretation of the study results.

This critical appraisal is based on the Critical Appraisal Guidelines for Research Objectives in Studies presented in the previous box on page 160.

IMPLICATIONS FOR PRACTICE

Duffy et al. (2008) found that two thirds of the veterans surveyed were motivated to quit smoking and were able to identify many benefits associated with smoking cessation. Barriers to conducting smoking cessation programs were identified by the staff, but also they noted the importance of developing inpatient smoking cessation services to meet the specific needs of veterans. This descriptive study provides a background for the development of an inpatient smoking cessation program that could be tested in future studies to determine if it improves smoking cessation for veterans.

Research Objectives or Aims Implemented in Qualitative Studies

Qualitative research is most appropriate when the focus of the study is to obtain a personal perspective of a situation, experience, or event (Hale, Treharne, & Kitas, 2007). The research objectives or aims formulated for quantitative and qualitative studies have some similarities because they focus on exploration, description, and determination of relationships. However, the objectives directing qualitative studies commonly are broader in focus and include concepts that are more complex and abstract than those of quantitative studies. The aims or objectives focus on obtaining a holistic, comprehensive understanding of the area of study (Creswell, 2008; Munhall, 2007). A qualitative study by Wickman, Anderson, and Greenberg (2008) demonstrates the logical flow from the research problem and purpose to the study aims or objectives. This phenomenological study focuses on adolescent perception of invincibility and how it influences teens' acceptance of health promotion strategies.

RESEARCH EXAMPLE Problem, Purpose, and Aims in a Qualitative Study

Research Problem

Behavioral patterns begun during adolescence have a long-term impact on health and well-being. The common adolescent belief of invincibility, however, leads to the perception that somehow the consequences of high-risk behavior will not happen to them. … Morbidity and mortality statistics in teens indicate otherwise. High-risk behaviors have significant adverse outcomes for teens including infection with sexually transmitted infections (STIs), HIV, temporary and permanent injury and disability, and even death. … (Centers for Disease Control and Prevention, 2003a, 2006b) [problem significance]. … Although community and school-based programs have enhanced awareness of these problems, teen involvement in risk behaviors continues to be challenging because of the physical, social, and cognitive development capabilities of this age-group. … (Erikson, 1968)

Although quantitative studies clearly reinforce increased vulnerability to risk outcomes for the teen who believes he or she is invincible, these studies typically focus on the frequency of risk-taking behaviors [problem background]. … A lack of research in this area reinforces the need to learn more about the meaning of invincibility and risk perception for this age-group to intervene most effectively with the teen who believes he or she is invincible. [problem statement] (Wickman et al., 2008, pp. 460-461)

Research Purpose

The purposes of this study were to explore the phenomenon of invincibility and to identify key factors contributing to risk behavior involvement in teens. (Wickman et al., 2008, p. 460)

Research Aims or Objectives

Specific aims of this study were to:

1. define the concept of invincibility from the teen perspective
2. identify the characteristics of adolescent thinking that typify invincibility
3. explore the relationship between invincibility and risk behavior involvement
4. identify strategies for working with teens that take into consideration developmental characteristics of teen thinking (Wickman et al., 2008, p. 461)

CRITICAL APPRAISAL

In this phenomenological study, the problem significance, background, and statement provide a basis for the purpose of this study, which is to gain an understanding of adolescents' perception of invincibility.

The stated aims or objectives further clarify the purpose or focus of this qualitative study. The first aim focused on defining invincibility (study concept), and the second aim focused on identification of adolescent characteristics of thinking that typify invincibility. The third aim focused on exploring relationships between invincibility and risk behavior involvement (study concept), and the fourth aim focused on identification of strategies for working with teens (study concept). This study is concerned with complex, abstract concepts, rather than variables, to promote understanding of adolescent invincibility. Thus, Wickman and colleagues' (2008) problem provided a basis for identifying a feasible, focused qualitative study purpose, and the aims provided additional clarification of the study focus.

IMPLICATIONS FOR PRACTICE

Wickman and colleagues (2008) found that spending time with teens and sharing personal stories made the experiences about risk behaviors more real.

> Focusing on the here and now versus teaching about long-term health consequences of risk behaviors is an important guiding principle in health teaching mentioned by participants. ... These findings provide direction for public policy and reinforce the need for programs that empower both teens and parents in creating relationships that 'bridge the gap' between parents, teens, and society. Programs targeting risk behaviors can optimally empower teens by recognizing and building on teen strengths and maximizing protective factors in the teen's environment. (Wickman et al., 2008, p. 466)

This study also provides the basis for conducting quantitative studies to examine the effectiveness of teen programs to manage risk behaviors.

Research Questions Implemented in Quantitative Studies

A **research question** is a clear, concise interrogative statement that is worded in the present tense, includes one or more variables, and is expressed to guide the implementation of quantitative studies. The foci of research questions are description of variable(s), examination of relationships among variables, and determination of differences between two or more groups regarding selected variable(s). The research questions for quantitative studies are usually concisely and narrowly focused and inclusive of the study variables and population. It is really a matter of choice whether researchers identify objectives or questions for their study. Celik and Kocasli (2008) conducted a comparative descriptive study of the hygienic hand washing activities among nursing students in a hospital setting. Research questions were developed to direct the conduct of this study. The flow from research problem and purpose to research questions is demonstrated in the following excerpts from this study. The following questions are used to conduct a critical appraisal of this research example.

CRITICAL APPRAISAL GUIDELINES

Research Questions in Studies

1. Are the research questions clearly and concisely expressed in the study?
2. Are the study questions based on the purpose?
3. Is the focus of each question clearly presented?

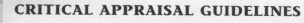

RESEARCH EXAMPLE Problem, Purpose, and Questions from a Quantitative Study

Research Problem

Hospital infections develop in 5% to 15% of patients. These infections are a major source of mortality and morbidity and contribute to high costs of health care [problem significance]. ... Nurses are sources of contamination in their nursing roles, which include getting patients out of bed, taking pulse rates, measuring arterial blood pressure and body temperature, performing various invasive interventions, as well as dressing and feeding patients (French & Friedman, 2003). Hygienic hand washing before and after these procedures is a simple, cheap, and applicable key component of the reduction and prevention of infections during patient care (Jumaa, 2005). ... A review of previous studies on hand washing shows that these studies have primarily been conducted with healthcare professionals and school children [problem background]. However, not much is known about hand washing among nursing students. [problem statement] (Celik & Kocasli, 2008, p. 207)

Research Purpose

The purpose of this study was to determine the application status of hand washing information given within the context of infection control measures in practice areas among nursing students. (Celik & Kocasli, 2008, p. 207)

Research Questions

The research questions were as follows:

1. In what situations do the students wash their hands in clinical areas?
2. Is there a significant difference between the number of patient care activities of students in clinical areas and the frequency of hand washing?
3. Do they wash their hands for a sufficient period?
4. What are the agents that they use for hand washing? (Celik & Kocasli, 2008, p. 208)

CRITICAL APPRAISAL

Celik and Kocasli (2008) provide a clearly stated, significant problem of hand washing by nursing students in a hospital setting. The problem statement indicated what was not known and provided the basis for the research purpose. The four research questions provided clear direction for the conduct of the study. Question 1 focused on identification of the situations for hand washing. Question 2 focused on the difference between the number of care activities and hand washing frequency. Questions 3 and 4 focused on description of hand washing time period and types of agents used. These questions were presented immediately before the Methods section of the research report and were used to direct the implementation of the study procedures, organize data analysis, and facilitate the interpretation of the findings.

(This critical appraisal was based on the Critical Appraisal Guidelines for Research Questions in Studies presented in the previous box on page 163.)

IMPLICATIONS FOR PRACTICE

Celik and Kocasli (2008) found that the student responses indicated they had knowledge about hand washing; however, their practice of hand washing in the clinical setting was inadequate and careless. The researchers stressed the importance of faculty in serving as role models for hand washing and that they need to provide frequent feedback to the students to increase their rate of hand washing. Further quasi-experimental studies are needed to determine the most effective strategies for faculty to implement to promote quality hand washing behaviors of students in clinical settings.

Research Questions Implemented in Qualitative Studies

The research questions directing qualitative studies are often limited in number, broadly focused, and inclusive of variables or concepts that are more complex and abstract than those of quantitative studies. Marshall and Rossman (2006) indicate that questions developed to direct qualitative research might be theoretical ones, which can be studied with different populations or in a variety of sites, or the questions could be focused on a particular population or setting. The specific study questions formulated are very important for the selection of the qualitative research method to be used to conduct the study (Hale et al., 2007). Polzer (2007) conducted a qualitative study to describe African Americans with type 2 diabetes perceptions of the spiritual role of health care providers (HCPs) and the effects of that role on their self-management of their diabetes. The problem, purpose, and research questions used to direct this study are presented in the following excerpts.

RESEARCH EXAMPLE Problem, Purpose, and Questions from a Qualitative Study

Research Problem

The establishment of quality patient/provider relationships is paramount in empowering patients to manage chronic illnesses. ... Type 2 diabetes mellitus is a major health problem for African Americans, and is one of the primary causes of morbidity and mortality in this population (Center for Disease Control [CDC], 2005) [problem significance]. ... For many African Americans, spirituality is a source of support in managing diabetes. ... Some, however, may also turn their self-management practices over to God in lieu of following health provider recommendations. ... In a recent grounded theory study (Polzer & Miles, 2007; parent study), the researchers examined how spirituality affected self-management of diabetes in African Americans. The core construct identified in this study was self-management through a relationship with God. Based on their views, participants fell into one of three typologies: Relationship and Responsibility: God is in the Background; Relationship and Responsibility: God is in the Forefront; and Relationship and Relinquishing of Self-Management: God is Healer. ... The three typologies shed light on how African Americans viewed their relationship with God, its impact on self-management, and how these perceptions

Continued

RESEARCH EXAMPLE—cont'd

affected their beliefs about HCPs helping them manage their diabetes [problem background]. Knowledge of these perceptions of spiritual care is important as there is little information related to spiritual interventions for African Americans. [problem statement] (Polzer, 2007, pp. 164-166)

Research Purpose

Based on the grounded theory study [Polzer & Miles, 2007], a qualitative descriptive study was conducted to examine these perceptions of spiritual care, and further extend the three typologies. (Polzer, 2007, p. 166)

Research Questions

The research questions addressed in this analysis were:
(1) What are the perceptions of African Americans with diabetes regarding how, if, and when nurses and other HCPs should address spirituality in their care?
(2) How do these perceptions differ by typology of self-management through a relationship with God? (Polzer, 2007, p. 166)

CRITICAL APPRAISAL

Polzer (2007) identified a significant problem of determining how HCPs should address spirituality in their care and how African Americans' self-management of their type 2 diabetes is influenced by their relationships with God. The problem statement indicated what was not known and provided the basis for the research purpose. The research questions provided clear direction for the conduct of this qualitative study. The first study question focused on description of African Americans' (population) perceptions of the complex concept of HCPs addressing spirituality in their care. The second question focused on examining differences in the African Americans' perceptions based on their relationship with God.

(Critical Appraisal is based on Critical Appraisal Guidelines for Research Questions in Studies presented in the box on page 163.)

IMPLICATIONS FOR PRACTICE

Based on her study findings, Polzer (2007) identified the following implications for practice: "The model of the three typologies may help health providers understand the importance of spiritual care for some African Americans, as well as how this care can affect self-management. This information also may assist in developing culturally sensitive interventions to improve self-management of diabetes among African Americans" (p. 173).

Hypotheses

A **hypothesis** is a formal statement of the expected relationship(s) between two or more variables in a specified population. The hypothesis translates the research problem and purpose into a clear explanation or prediction of the expected results or outcomes of selected quantitative and outcome studies. A clearly stated hypothesis includes the variables to be manipulated or measured, identifies the population to be examined, and indicates the proposed outcomes for the study. Hypotheses also influence the study design, sampling method, data collection and analysis process, and interpretation of findings. Quasi-experimental and experimental quantitative studies are conducted to test the effectiveness of a treatment or intervention, and these types of studies should include hypotheses to predict the study outcomes. In this section, types of hypotheses are described and the elements of a testable hypothesis are discussed.

Types of Hypotheses

Different types of relationships and numbers of variables are identified in hypotheses. A study might have one, four, or more hypotheses, depending on its complexity. The type of hypothesis developed is based on the purpose of the study. Hypotheses can be described using four categories: (1) associative versus causal, (2) simple versus complex, (3) nondirectional versus directional and (4) null versus research.

Associative versus Causal Hypotheses

The relationships identified in hypotheses are associative or causal. An **associative hypothesis** proposes relationships among variables that occur or exist together in the real world, so that when one variable changes, the other changes (Reynolds, 2007). Associative hypotheses usually are expressed using one of the following formats:

- Variable X is related to variables Y and Z in a specified population (predicts relationships among variables but does not indicate the types of relationships).
- An increase in variable X is associated with an increase in variable Y in a specified population (predicts a positive relationship).
- A decrease in variable X is associated with a decrease in variable Y in a specified population (predicts a positive relationship).
- An increase in variable X is associated with a decrease in variable Y in a specified population (predicts a negative relationship).
- Variables X and Y can be used to predict variable Z in a study (independent variables used to predict a dependent variable in a predictive correlational study).

Associative hypotheses identify relationships among variables in a study but do not indicate that one variable causes an effect on another variable.

Reishtein (2005) conducted a quantitative, predictive correlational study to predict if the symptoms of dyspnea, fatigue, and sleep difficulty were predictive of the functional performance of individuals with chronic obstructive pulmonary disease (COPD). The research problem, purpose, and associative hypotheses from this study are presented as an example. The following questions were used to critically appraise this research example.

CRITICAL APPRAISAL GUIDELINES

Hypotheses in Studies

1. Are the hypotheses formally stated in the study? If the study is quasi-experimental or experimental, hypotheses are needed to direct the study.
2. Do the hypotheses clearly identify the relationships among variables of the study?
3. Do the hypotheses clearly predict the outcomes of the study?
4. Are the hypotheses associative or causal, simple or complex, directional or nondirectional, and research or null?

RESEARCH EXAMPLE Associative Hypotheses

Research Problem

COPD has been estimated to affect 14 million people in the United States, limiting activity in 1,310,000 individuals. As the population ages, the prevalence of COPD is predicted to increase. ... Researchers have examined the link between symptoms and function. ... Two components of affected performance, physical performance and role performance, together can be considered aspects of functional performance. ... No researchers have explored the collective impact of the symptoms dyspnea, fatigue, and sleep difficulty on functional performance in patients with COPD. (Reishtein, 2005, pp. 39-40)

Research Purpose

Thus, the purpose of this study was to use the Theory of Unpleasant Symptoms to determine the interrelationships and relative contributions of three symptoms [dyspnea, fatigue, and sleep difficulty] to functional performance in people with COPD. (Reishtein, 2005, p. 40)

Hypotheses

Reishtein (2005) tested three associate hypotheses in her study that are identified below:

(1) Positive relationships exist among dyspnea, fatigue, and sleep difficulty in people with COPD;
(2) Dyspnea, fatigue, and sleep difficulty are related to functional performance; and
(3) Dyspnea, fatigue, and sleep difficulty, taken together, will explain more of the variance in functional performance in people with COPD than any of these symptoms alone. (Reishtein, 2005, p. 40)

CRITICAL APPRAISAL

The research problem stated by Reishtein (2005) is significant because many individuals have COPD and their quality of life is affected by their functional performance (physical and role performance). The problem identifies an area of concern and the purpose of the study is clearly focused on addressing that concern. The hypotheses build on the problem and purpose and clearly predict the outcomes of the study. Associate hypotheses are appropriate to direct predictive correlational studies (Burns & Grove, 2009).

Hypothesis 1 predicts positive relationships or associations among the three variables dyspnea, fatigue, and sleep difficulty for patients with COPD. A positive relationship means that the variables change together; thus, they will all increase together in value or all decrease together. These relationships are depicted in the following diagram.

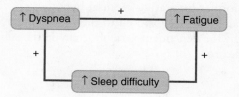

Hypothesis 2 predicts relationships between three variables—dyspnea, fatigue, and sleep difficulty—and the variable functional performance but does not identify the type of relationship. These associative relationships are shown in the following diagram.

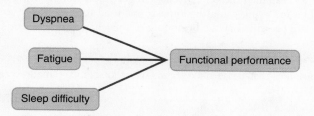

Hypothesis 3 uses the independent variables dyspnea, fatigue, and sleep difficulty to predict the functional performance of COPD patients. This relationship can be diagrammed as follows.

Dyspnea + Fatigue + Sleep difficulty ⟶ Functional performance

These hypotheses provide clear direction for the study by indicating what is to be examined in the study and the expected outcomes. In addition, these hypotheses clearly identify the study independent variables (dyspnea, fatigue, and sleep difficulty), dependent or outcome variable (functional performance), and population (COPD patients).

This critical appraisal is based on the Critical Appraisal Guidelines for Hypotheses in Studies presented in the box on page 168.

IMPLICATIONS FOR PRACTICE

The results from the study only partially supported the hypotheses. Only dyspnea was related to the other symptoms of fatigue and sleep difficulty and to functional performance. Thus, managing dyspnea may be the best way to improve symptoms and functional performance in patients with COPD. Additional research is needed to recognize other symptoms that might be predictive of performance function in COPD patients and direct future management of this disease (Reishtein, 2005).

A **causal hypothesis** proposes a cause-and-effect interaction between two or more variables, which are referred to as independent and dependent variables. The independent variable (treatment or experimental variable) is manipulated by the researcher to cause an effect on the dependent variable. The researcher then measures the dependent variable (outcome or criterion variable) to examine the effect created by the independent variable (Reynolds, 2007). A format for stating a causal hypothesis is the following: The subjects in the experimental group, who are exposed to the independent variable, demonstrate greater change, as measured by the dependent variable, than do the subjects in the comparison group who receive standard care.

RESEARCH EXAMPLE Causal Hypothesis

Schultz et al. (2008, p. 191) studied the "effectiveness of gel pillows for reducing bilateral head flattening in preterm infants." The following causal hypothesis was used to direct their study. The problem and purpose for this study are presented at the beginning of this chapter in the section identifying research problems and purposes.

The hypothesis was that infants in the experimental group (on gel pillows) would demonstrate significantly less head molding over time than those in the control group (on standard mattresses) by 5 weeks postbirth. (Schultz et al., 2008, p. 194)

CRITICAL APPRAISAL

Schultz et al. (2008) conducted a quasi-experimental study so it is important that a hypothesis was stated to predict the outcome of this study. This causal hypothesis clearly identifies the independent variable (gel pillows) that was implemented to determine its effect on the dependent variable (head holding). The study has two groups and the experimental group is exposed to the gel pillows and the control group receives standard care of mattresses. The population is identified as infants, but the study really was conducted on preterm infants, who are most likely to experience head molding after birth. This hypothesis is diagrammed in the following figure, in which a causal arrow (→) is used to show the causal relationship between the independent and dependent variables. This hypothesis expresses a negative relationship in that the more gel pillows are used, the less the head molding. Thus, the variables are moving in opposite directions or a negative relationship.

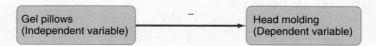

IMPLICATIONS FOR PRACTICE

The findings from this study were not significant and thus did not support the hypothesis that gel pillows would reduce head molding. However, the results were moving in the direction of significance, but the study lacked adequate sample size to achieve significant results. The researchers did indicate that the study findings had clinical significance and demonstrated this with a picture of the heads of two preterm infants (Figure 5–2). The infant in the top picture is using the gel pillow and does appear to have less head flattening or molding than the infant below it on a standard mattress. However, additional research is needed with a larger sample size to determine the effectiveness of the gel pillows on preterm infant head molding.

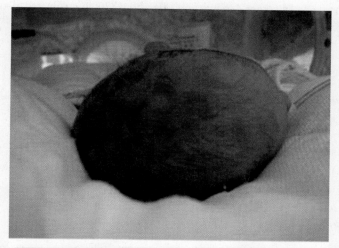

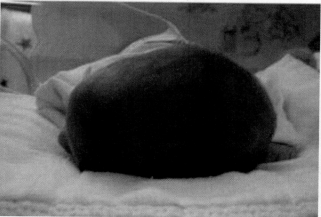

Figure 5–2. Clinical significance. From Schultz, A. A., Goodwin, P. A., Jesseman, C., Toews, H. G., Lane, M., & Smith, C. (2008). Evaluating the effectiveness of gel pillows for reducing bilateral head flattening in preterm infants: A randomized controlled pilot study. *Applied Nursing Research, 21*(4), p. 197.

Simple versus Complex Hypotheses

A simple hypothesis states the relationship (associative or causal) between two variables. A complex hypothesis states the relationships (associative or causal) among three or more variables.

RESEARCH EXAMPLE Simple Hypothesis

Epstein, Tsaras, Amoateng-Adjepong, Greiner, and Manthous (2009) conducted a study to determine if race affected the readmission rate to the hospital after a critical illness. These researchers stated the following simple hypothesis to direct their study:

> we hypothesized that racial status is a risk factor for early (within 7 days) hospital readmission after initial recovery from critical illness and respiratory failure. (Epstein et al., 2009, p. 66)

CRITICAL APPRAISAL

This hypothesis is a clearly stated simple, associative hypothesis. This hypothesis states a positive relationship between two variables (racial status as a risk factor and early hospital readmission), as shown in the following diagram.

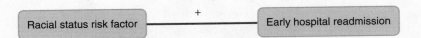

This hypothesis clearly indicates the expected outcome of the study and identifies the study variables and population (patients recovering from critical illness and respiratory failure).

IMPLICATIONS FOR PRACTICE

The study findings did not support this hypothesis since race was not associated with rapid readmission or mortality of critically ill patients. In this study, 20.6% of the Hispanics and 16.5% of the Caucasians ($p = 0.3$, nonsignificant result) were readmitted within 7 days. Epstein and colleagues (2009) found that rapid readmission was linked to those patients who were mechanically ventilated beyond 29 days and were sent to acute rehabilitation or skilled nursing facilities after hospitalization. However, the researchers indicated that further study was needed to determine if these findings are generalizable or unique to this clinical agency.

RESEARCH EXAMPLE Complex Hypothesis

A complex hypothesis predicts the relationship (associative or causal) among three or more variables. Polman, de Castro, and van Aken (2007) conducted a study of the effects of playing versus watching violent video games on children's aggressive behavior. These researchers developed a complex hypothesis to direct the conduct of their study. Their hypothesis was as follows:

> It was hypothesized that playing a violent video game will lead to higher levels of aggression than watching a violent video game or playing a non-violent game. (Polman, et al., 2007, p. 257)

CRITICAL APPRAISAL

Polman et al. (2007) conducted a quasi-experimental study to examine the effects of three independent variables or treatments (playing violent video game, watching a violent video game, and playing a non-violent game) on the dependent variable level of aggression. Thus, it was appropriate that a hypothesis was developed to direct this study. This hypothesis clearly identifies the variables but not the population, which included children (boys and girls) in this study. The study included three groups and each group included both boys and girls, who were exposed to one of the interventions or independent variables. The causal relationships examined in this study are presented in the following diagrams.

Group 1
   Playing a violent video game → Level of aggression

Group 2
   Watching a violent video game → Level of aggression

Group 3
   Playing a non-violent game → Level of aggression

IMPLICATIONS FOR PRACTICE

This hypothesis was supported by the study findings for boys but not for girls. Polman and colleagues (2007) found that boys who played violent video games were more aggressive than if they watched violent video games. However, there was no relationship between game conditions and aggressive behavior in girls. The researchers recommend additional studies with larger samples and to investigate not only whether violent video games lead to aggression, but why. Polman and colleagues also recommend that parents and caregivers pay special attention to the regulation of violent video game play by boys.

Nondirectional versus Directional Hypotheses

A **nondirectional hypothesis** states that a relationship exists but does not predict the nature of the relationship. If the direction of the relationship being studied is not clear in clinical practice or the theoretical or empirical literature, the researcher has no clear indication of the nature of the relationship. Under these circumstances, nondirectional hypotheses are developed, such as the one by Reishtein (2005, p. 40) identified earlier in this section: "(2) Dyspnea, fatigue, and sleep difficulty are related to functional performance." This is an associative, complex, nondirectional hypothesis. It is associative because it predicts a relationship; complex because there are four variables (dyspnea, fatigue, sleep difficulty, and functional performance); and nondirectional because the nature of the relationships (positive or negative) among the variables is not indicated.

A directional hypothesis states the nature (positive or negative) of the interaction between two or more variables. The use of terms such as *positive*, *negative*, *less*, *more*, *increase*, *decrease*, *greater*, *higher*, or *lower* in a hypothesis indicates the direction of the relationship. Directional hypotheses are developed from theoretical statements (propositions), findings of previous studies, and clinical experience. As the knowledge on which a study is based increases, the researcher is able to make a prediction about the direction of a relationship between the variables being studied. For example, Reishtein stated a directional hypothesis: "…Positive relationships exist among dyspnea, fatigue, and sleep difficulty in people with COPD" (2005, p. 40). This is an associative, complex, directional hypothesis. It is associative because it predicts a relationship; complex because there are three variables (dyspnea, fatigue, and sleep difficulty); and directional because a positive relationship is predicted. A positive relationship indicates that the variables change together and can either increase or decrease together.

A causal hypothesis predicts the effect of an independent variable on a dependent variable, specifying the direction of the relationship. The independent variable either increases or decreases each dependent variable. Thus, all causal hypotheses are directional. Polman et al. (2007) conducted their study to test a complex, causal, directional hypothesis to guide their study. They predicted that playing violent video games would cause higher levels of aggression, which was supported for boys but not for girls.

Null versus Research Hypotheses

The null hypothesis (H_0), also referred to as a statistical hypothesis, is used for statistical testing and for interpreting statistical outcomes. Even if the null hypothesis is not stated, it is implied, because it is the converse of the research hypothesis (Kerlinger & Lee, 2000). Some researchers state the null hypothesis because it is more easily interpreted on the basis of the results of statistical analyses. The null hypothesis also is used when the researcher believes there is no relationship between two variables and when theoretical or empirical information is inadequate to state a research hypothesis.

A null hypothesis can be simple or complex and associative or causal. An example of a simple, associative, null hypothesis is the following: "There is no relationship between the number of experiences performing a developmental assessment skill and learning of the skill" (Koniak, 1985, p. 85).

Schultz, Drew, and Hewitt (2002) conducted a quasi-experimental study to determine the effectiveness of heparinized and normal saline flushes in maintaining the patency of 24-gauge (G) intermittent peripheral intravenous (IV) catheters in neonates in intensive care. "The hypothesis stated that there would be no significant difference in the duration of patency of a 24 G IV lock in a neonatal patient when flushed with 0.5 mL [millimeters] of heparinized saline (2U/mL), our standard practice, compared with 0.5 mL of 0.9% normal saline" (Schultz et al., 2002, p. 30).

This is a simple, null hypothesis with one independent variable (0.9% normal saline flush) and one dependent variable (patency of 24 G IV catheter). The comparison group received standard care of heparinized saline flush, and the population was neonates in an intensive care setting. The findings of the study did not support the null hypothesis because the catheters flushed with heparinized saline were patent significantly longer than the catheters flushed with normal saline. Thus, the researchers recommended continuing the use of heparinized saline as the standard for flushing 24 G catheters in infants.

A research hypothesis is the alternative hypothesis (H_1 or H_A) to the null hypothesis and states that a relationship exists between two or more variables. All of the hypotheses stated in previous sections of this chapter have been research hypotheses, except for the two null hypotheses given in the previous paragraph. Research hypotheses can be simple or complex, nondirectional or directional, and associative or causal.

Testable Hypothesis

The value of a hypothesis ultimately is derived from whether it is testable in the real world. A testable hypothesis is one that clearly predicts the relationships among variables and contains variables that are measurable or able to be manipulated in a study. Thus, the independent variable must be clearly defined, often by a protocol, so that it can be implemented precisely and consistently as a treatment in the study. The dependent variable must be clearly defined to indicate how it will be precisely and accurately measured.

A testable hypothesis also needs to predict a relationship that can be "supported" or "not supported" as indicated by the data collected and analyzed. If the hypothesis states an associative relationship, correlational analyses are conducted on the data to determine the existence, type, and strength of the relationship between the variables studied. The hypothesis that states a causal link between the independent and dependent variables is evaluated using statistics that examine differences between the experimental and comparison or control groups, such as the *t*-test or ANOVA. It is the null hypothesis (stated or implied) that is tested to determine whether the independent variable produced a significant effect on the dependent variable (Burns & Grove, 2009).

Hypotheses are clearer without specifying the presence or absence of a "significant difference," because determination of the level of significance is only a statistical technique applied to sample data. Thus, the hypothesis stated by Schultz et al. (2008) presented earlier in this section would have been stronger if the term "significantly" was omitted.

In addition, hypotheses should not identify methodological points, such as techniques of sampling, measurement, and data analysis (Kerlinger & Lee, 2000). Therefore, such phrases as "measured by," "in a random sample of," and "using ANOVA" (analysis of variance) are inappropriate because they limit the hypothesis to the measurement methods, sample, or analysis techniques identified for one study. In addition, hypotheses need to reflect the variables and population outlined in the research purpose and are expressed in the present tense, not the future tense. Expressing hypotheses in the present tense does not limit them to the study being conducted and enables them to be used in additional research.

In summary, the research objectives, questions, and hypotheses must be clearly focused and concisely expressed in studies. Both objectives and questions are used in qualitative studies and descriptive and correlational quantitative studies, but questions are more common. Some correlational studies focus on predicting relationships and may include hypotheses. Quasi-experimental and experimental studies should be directed by hypotheses.

Understanding Study Variables and Research Concepts

The research purpose and objectives, questions, and hypotheses include the variables or concepts to be examined in a study. Variables are qualities, properties, or characteristics of persons, things, or situations that change or vary. Variables should be concisely defined to promote their measurement or manipulation within quantitative or outcomes studies (Chinn & Kramer, 2008). Research concepts are studied in qualitative research and are at higher levels of abstraction than variables. In this section different types of variables are described, and conceptual and operational definitions of variables are discussed. The research concepts investigated in qualitative research are discussed with their conceptual definitions.

Types of Variables in Quantitative Research

Variables are classified into a variety of types to explain their use in research. Some variables are manipulated; others are controlled. Some variables are identified but not measured; others are measured with refined measurement devices. The types of variables presented in this section include independent, dependent, research, and extraneous (Reynolds, 2007).

Independent and Dependent Variables

The relationship between independent and dependent variables is the basis for formulating hypotheses for correlational, quasi-experimental, and experimental studies. An independent variable is a stimulus or activity that is manipulated or varied by the researcher to create an effect on the dependent variable. The independent variable is also called a treatment or experimental variable. A dependent variable is the outcome or response that the researcher wants to predict or explain. Changes in the dependent variable are presumed to be caused by the independent variable. Schultz and colleagues (2008) conducted a quasi-experimental study that examined the effect of the independent variable gel pillows on the dependent variable of head molding in preterm infants. The discussion of this study was introduced earlier in this chapter.

In predictive correlational studies, the variables measured to predict a single dependent variable are also called independent variables (Burns & Grove, 2009). Reishtein (2005) conducted a predictive correlational study that was introduced earlier in this chapter under the hypothesis section. In this study, Reishtein measured the independent variables dyspnea, fatigue, and sleep difficulty to predict the dependent variable functional performance in patients with COPD. The researcher found that only dyspnea was predictive of functional performance in COPD patients.

Research Variables

Descriptive and correlational quantitative studies involve the investigation of research variables. Research variables are the qualities, properties, or characteristics identified in the research purpose and objectives or questions that are observed or measured in a study. Research variables are used when the intent of the study is to observe or measure variables as they exist in a natural setting without the implementation of a treatment. Thus no independent variables are manipulated, and no cause-and-effect relationships are examined.

Extraneous Variables

Extraneous variables exist in all studies and can affect the measurement of study variables and the relationships among these variables. Extraneous variables are of primary concern in quantitative studies because they can interfere with obtaining a clear understanding of the relational or causal dynamics within these studies. These variables are classified as recognized or unrecognized and controlled or uncontrolled. Some extraneous variables are not recognized until the study is in progress or is completed, but their presence influences the study outcome.

Researchers attempt to recognize and control as many extraneous variables as possible in quasi-experimental and experimental studies, and specific designs and sample criteria have been developed to control the influence of extraneous variables that might influence the outcomes of studies. Schultz et al. (2008, p. 194), in their quasi-experiment study of the use of gel pillows to reduce head molding, identified the following inclusion and exclusion sample criteria for their study: "Infants were potentially eligible for the study if they were = 34 weeks of age and weighed = 1500 g. Exclusion criteria included hydrocephaly, microcephaly, cranial deformities, or central nervous system abnormalities." These sample criteria ensured that the subjects were preterm infants of a select size and the exclusion criteria removed the impact of extraneous variables that might have been associated with infants who have the congenital defects identified. The removal of extraneous variables from a study increases the ability of the researcher to determine the true effect of the independent variable on the dependent variable.

The extraneous variables that are not recognized until the study is in process, or are recognized before the study is initiated but cannot be controlled, are referred to as confounding variables. Sometimes extraneous variables can be measured during the study and controlled statistically during analysis. However, extraneous variables that cannot be controlled or measured are a design weakness and can hinder the interpretation of findings (see Chapter 8). As control in correlational, quasi-experimental and experimental studies decreases, the potential influence of confounding variables increases.

Environmental variables are a type of extraneous variable composing the setting in which the study is conducted. Examples of these variables include climate, family, healthcare system, and governmental organizations. If a researcher is studying humans in an uncontrolled or natural setting, it is impossible and undesirable to control all the extraneous variables. In qualitative and some quantitative (descriptive and correlational) studies, little or no attempt is made to control extraneous variables. The intent is to study subjects in their natural environment without controlling or altering that setting or situation (Munhall, 2007). The environmental variables in quasi-experimental and experimental research can be controlled by using a laboratory setting or a specially constructed research unit in a hospital. Environmental control is an extremely important part of conducting an experimental study. For example, Rasmussen and Farr (2003) conducted an experimental study using rats in a laboratory setting. (See Table 5–1 for the problem and purpose of this study.) The laboratory controlled for many of the environmental variables, so they did not have an impact on the study outcome.

Conceptual and Operational Definitions of Variables in Quantitative Research

A variable is operationalized in a study by the development of conceptual and operational definitions. A conceptual definition provides the theoretical meaning of a variable (Chinn & Kramer, 2008) and often is derived from a theorist's definition of a related concept. In a published study, the framework includes concepts and their definitions, and the variables are selected to represent the concepts. Thus, the variables are conceptually defined, indicating the link with the concepts in the framework. An operational definition is derived from a set of procedures or progressive acts that a researcher performs to receive sensory impressions (such as sound, visual, or tactile impressions) that indicate the existence or degree of existence of a variable (Reynolds, 2007). Operational definitions need to be independent of time and setting so that variables can be investigated at different times and in different settings using the same operational definitions. An operational definition is developed so that a variable can be measured or manipulated in a concrete situation, and the knowledge gained from studying the variable will increase the understanding of the theoretical concept that this variable represents.

The two variables from the Schultz et al. (2008) study, which examined the effect of gel pillows on bilateral head molding or flattening, are operationalized as an example. This quasi-experimental study had an independent variable of gel pillows and a dependent variable of head molding. The conceptual and operational definitions for these two variables are presented in the following research example. The questions identified in the Box were used to critically appraise the variables and their definitions in Schultz et al. (2008) study.

CRITICAL APPRAISAL GUIDELINES

Study Variables
1. Are the variables clearly identified in the study purpose and/or research objectives, questions, or hypotheses?
2. What types of variables are examined in the study? Are independent and dependent variables or research variables or concepts examined in the study?
3. Are the variables conceptually defined?
4. Are the variables operationally defined?

RESEARCH EXAMPLE Conceptual and Operational Definitions of Variables

Independent Variable: Gel Pillow

Conceptual Definition

The gel pillow is a therapeutic or care factor implemented to promote quality outcomes for preterm infants (Schultz et al., 2008).

Operational Definition

The Gel-E Donut manufactured by Children's Medical Ventures (Wallingford, CT) is 3/8 inches thick and 7 inches in diameter (see Figure 5–3). The pillow is a nontoxic carboxy vinyl bag filled with a combination of water and antibacterial agent. It is designed to reduce pressure while providing support. The pillow was placed under the mattress sheet at the head of the bed. (Schultz et al., 2008, p. 195)

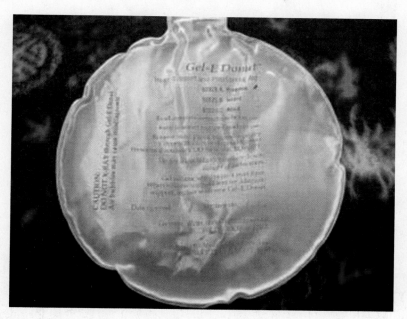

Figure 5–3. Gel pillow. From Schultz, A. A., Goodwin, P. A., Jesseman, C., Toews, H. G., Lane, M., & Smith, C. (2008). Evaluating the effectiveness of gel pillows for reducing bilateral head flattening in preterm infants: A randomized controlled pilot study. *Applied Nursing Research, 21*(4), p. 194.

Dependent Variable: Head Molding or Flattening

Conceptual Definition

Bilateral head molding or flattening is an undesirable outcome in preterm infants and healthcare professionals attempt to prevent this outcome with therapeutic interventions or care factors (Schultz et al., 2008).

Operational Definition

The degree of head flattening was expressed as the AP:BP [anterior-posterior:biparietal] ratio or the CI [cephalic index]. The AP and BP diameters were measured using a 6-inch Digimatic caliper (700-113 MyCal Lite; see Figure 5–4) manufactured by Mitutoya (Suzhou, PR China). (Schultz et al., 2008, p. 195)

Continued

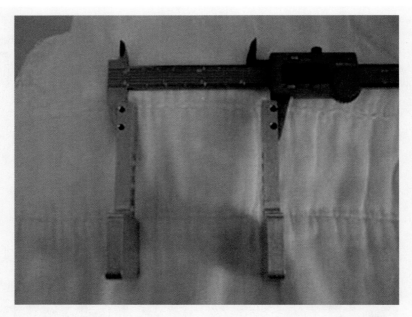

Figure 5–4. Digital calipers. From Schultz, A. A., Goodwin, P. A., Jesseman, C., Toews, H. G., Lane, M., & Smith, C. (2008). Evaluating the effectiveness of gel pillows for reducing bilateral head flattening in preterm infants: A randomized controlled pilot study. *Applied Nursing Research, 21*(4), p. 195.

 ## CRITICAL APPRAISAL

The variables in the Schultz et al. (2008) study were clearly identified and defined. The independent and dependent variables were identified in the study purpose and hypothesis. The conceptual definitions for gel pillow and head molding were found in the framework section of the article so there was a clear link between the concepts in the framework and the study variables. The operational definitions were found in the methods section of the research report. The gel pillow was clearly described and a picture of the pillow was provided in the article. The degree of head flattening was measured with digital calipers, which were also pictured in the article. The conceptual definitions based on the framework provided direction for the development of the gel pillow intervention and the measurement of the dependent variable head molding. Findings from this study are presented earlier in this chapter.

Research Concepts Investigated in Qualitative Research

The variables in quasi-experimental and experimental research are narrow and specific in focus and can be quantified (converted to numbers) or manipulated using specified steps that are often developed into a protocol. In addition, the variables are objectively defined to decrease researcher bias, as indicated in the previous section. Qualitative research is more abstract, subjective, and holistic than quantitative research and involves the investigation of research concepts versus research variables. Research concepts include the ideas, experiences, situations, or events that are investigated in qualitative research. For example, Wickman et al. (2008, p. 460) conducted a qualitative study to "explore the phenomenon of invincibility and to identify key factors contributing to risk behavior involvement in teens." The problem, purpose, and aims for this study were presented earlier in this chapter. The research concepts explored in this study were "invincibility" and "risk behavior involvement." In many qualitative studies, the focus of the study is to define the concept(s) being studied. Thus, the conceptual definition of the concept is often presented in the findings section of the study. For example, Cashin et al. (2008) conducted a phenomenological study to explore the lived experience of fathers who have children with asthma. This study was introduced earlier in this chapter and the study topics, problem, and purpose are presented in Table 5–2. The conceptual definition for the research concept explored in this study is presented as follows. Guidelines are provided to direct you in critically appraising the research concepts and conceptual definitions in qualitative studies.

CRITICAL APPRAISAL GUIDELINES

Research Concepts

1. Are the research concepts clearly identified in the study purpose and/or research aims or questions?
2. Are the research concepts conceptually defined in the study?

RESEARCH EXAMPLE Research Concept and Conceptual Definition

Research Concept: Lived Experience of Fathers with Asthmatic Children

Conceptual Definition

The lived experience of the fathers with asthmatic children was conceptually defined by the five themes generated from the study findings that included: "feeling relief in knowing the diagnosis, learning the ropes, being vigilant, living with concern, and being comfortable with asthma management" (Cashin et al., 2008, p. 376).

Continued

RESEARCH EXAMPLE—cont'd

The conceptual definition was developed using phenomenological methodology. Van Manen's (1994) method was used to "pursue the human science research that uses hermeneutic phenomenology and consists of the following six research activities: 1. Turning to a phenomenon which seriously interests us and commits us to the world. … 2. Investigating experience as we live it rather than as we conceptualize it. … 3. Reflecting on the essential themes which characterize the phenomenon. … 4. Describing the phenomenon through the art of writing and rewriting it. … 5. Maintaining a strong and orientated relation. … 6. Balancing the research context by considering parts and whole" (Cashin et al., 2008, pp. 374-375).

CRITICAL APPRAISAL

The study purpose clearly identified the research concept to be described in this study (see Table 5–2). In addition, the research concept of the lived experience of fathers with asthmatic children was conceptually defined in the research report. The conceptual definition was in the Discussion section of the study because the focus was on describing the experience for the fathers. The conceptual definition in this study was developed using the philosophy of Van Manen (1994), whose human science approach is well recognized for conducting phenomenological research. More details on the types of qualitative research are provided in Chapter 3.

Demographic Variables

Demographic variables are attributes of subjects that are collected to describe the sample. The demographic variables are identified by the researcher when a proposal is developed for conducting a study. Some common demographic variables are age, education, gender, ethnic origin (race), marital status, income, job classification, and medical diagnosis. Once data are collected from the study subjects on these demographic variables and analyzed, the results are called **sample characteristics** that are used to describe the sample. A study's sample characteristics can be presented in table format or narrative. As discussed earlier in this chapter, Duffy et al. (2008) conducted a descriptive study identifying the need for in-hospital smoking cessation programs for VA patients. The demographic variables examined in this study included: age, gender, race, marital status, education, reason for admission, comorbidities, significant depressive symptoms, and alcohol use. Table 5–4 presents the demographic information or profile of the subjects in this study; this profile is also referred to as the sample characteristics for the study.

Sample characteristics can also be presented in narrative format in the research report. For example, Celik and Kocasli (2008) studied the hand washing by nursing students in a hospital and described their sample using a narrative format. The demographic variables for this study were gender, age, and status in nursing educational program. These researchers described their sample characteristics as follows:

> Most of the nursing students (99.1%) were female. Among the students, 61.2% were enrolled at the College of Nursing, 35.6% were second-year students, and 25.1% were taking a medical nursing course. Most of the students (69.8%) were between 20 and 22 years old (20 ± 1.58 years). (Celik & Kocasli, 2008, p. 209)

Table 5-4	VA Inpatient Survey Results: Demographic Information

Characteristics	Values
Age in years (n = 87) [M (range) (SD)]	59 (40-82) (9)
Male gender (n = 87) [n (%)]	84 (97)
Race/ethnicity (n = 86) [n (%)]	
White	63 (73)
Non-white	23 (27)
Marital status (n = 85) [n (%)]	
Married	24 (28)
Widowed	8 (9)
Divorced/separated	37 (44)
Never married	16 (19)
Education (n = 85) [n (%)]	
High school or less	47 (55)
Some college	29 (34)
4-Year degree or more	9 (11)
Reason for admission (n = 85) [n (%)]	
Cancer	8 (9)
Lung disease	7 (8)
Heart disease	19 (22)
Stroke	4 (5)
Diabetes	4 (5)
Arthritis/orthopedic	10 (12)
Wound care	8 (9)
Characteristics	
Surgery	6 (7)
Vascular	3 (4)
Other	16 (19)
Comorbidities [n (%)]	
Cancer (n = 72)	12 (17)
Lung disease (n = 74)	23 (31)
Heart disease (n = 79)	37 (47)
Stroke (n = 72)	11 (15)
Psychiatric problems (n = 75)	30 (40)
Diabetes (n = 72)	14 (19)
Arthritis/orthopedic (n = 69)	29 (42)
Significant depressive symptoms (n = 71) [n (%)]	40 (56)
Alcohol use (n = 84) [n (%)]	
Currently drinks alcohol	28 (33)
Quit last month	8 (10)
Quit last year	12 (14)
Quit more than a year ago	28 (33)
Never drank alcohol	8 (10)
Alcohol problem (n = 84) (AUDIT score ≥8)	26 (31)

From Duffy, S. A., Reeves, P., Hermann, C., Karvonen, C., & Smith, P. (2008). In-hospital smoking cessation programs: What do VA patients and staff want and need? *Applied Nursing Research, 21*(4), p. 201.

KEY CONCEPTS

- The research problem is an area of concern in which there is a gap in the knowledge base needed for nursing practice. The problem includes significance, background, and problem statement.
- The research purpose is a concise, clear statement of the specific goal or focus of the study.
- A significant problem and purpose influence nursing practice, build on previous research, promote theory development, and/or address current concerns or priorities in nursing.
- Study feasibility is evaluated by examining the researchers' expertise; money commitments; availability of subjects, facilities, and equipment; and the study's ethical considerations.
- Research objectives, questions, or hypotheses are formulated to bridge the gap between the more abstractly stated research problem and purpose and the detailed quantitative design and data analysis.
- Qualitative study often includes problem, purpose, and research questions or aims to direct the study.
- A hypothesis is the formal statement of the expected relationship(s) between two or more variables in a specified population in a quantitative or outcomes study.
- Hypotheses can be described using four categories: (1) associative versus causal, (2) simple versus complex, (3) nondirectional versus directional, and (4) null versus research.
- Variables are qualities, properties, or characteristics of persons, things, or situations that change or vary.
- An independent variable is an intervention or treatment that is manipulated or varied by the researcher to create an effect on the dependent variable.
- A dependent variable is the response, behavior, or outcome that the researcher wants to predict or explain.
- Research variables are the qualities, properties, or characteristics that are observed or measured in descriptive and correlational studies.
- A variable is operationalized in a study by developing conceptual and operational definitions.
- A conceptual definition provides the theoretical meaning of a variable and is derived from a theorist's definition of a related concept.
- Operational definitions indicate how a treatment or independent variable will be implemented and how the dependent or outcome variable will be measured.
- Research concepts include the ideas, experiences, situations, or events that are investigated in qualitative research.
- Research concepts are conceptually defined during the conduct of a qualitative study.
- Demographic variables are characteristics or attributes of the subjects that are collected and analyzed to describe the study sample.

REFERENCES

Agency for Healthcare Research and Quality (AHRQ) (2009). *AHRQ research funding priorities.* Retrieved March 5, 2009 from *http://www.ahrq.gov/.*

Aiken, L. H., Clarke, S. P., Sloan, D. M., Sochalski, J., & Silber, J. H. (2002). Hospital nurse staffing and patient mortality, nurse burnout, and job dissatisfaction. *Journal of the American Medical Association, 288*(16), 1987-1993.

Ajzen, I. (2002). The theory of planned behavior: Home page. Retrieved October 21, 2005 from *http://www-unix. oit.umass.edu/~aizen/index.html.*

American Academy of Pediatrics. (1996). Task force on infant positions and SIDS. Position and sudden infant death syndrome (SIDS): Update. *Pediatrics, 98,* 1216-1218.

American Association of Critical Care Nurses (AACN) (2009). *Research priorities.* Retrieved March 9, 2009 from *http://www.aacn.org* and search for Research Priorities.

American Heart Association. (2004). *Statistical supplement.* Retrieved August 10, 2004 from *http://americanheart.org.*

American Organization of Nurse Executives (AONE) (2009). *AONE 2009 education and research priorities.* Retrieved March 5, 2009 from *http://www.aone.org/.*

Argenta, L. (2004). Clinical classification of positional plagiocephaly. *Journal of Craniofacial Surgery, 15*(3), 368-372.

Becker, A., Berbue, D., Chad, Z., Dolovich, M., Ducharme, F., D'Urzo, T., et al. (2005). Canadian pediatric asthma consensus guidelines, 2003 (updated to December 2004). *Canadian Medical Association Journal, 173*(Suppl. 6), S12-S55.

Brown, S. J. (2009). *Evidence-based nursing: The research-practice connection.* Sudbury, MA: Jones & Bartlett.

Burns, N., & Grove, S. K. (2009). *The practice of nursing research: Appraisal, synthesis, and generation of evidence* (6th ed.). Philadelphia: Saunders.

Bushe, C., & Holt, R. (2004). Prevalence of diabetes and impaired glucose tolerance in patients with schizophrenia. *British Journal of Psychiatry, 184*(Suppl 47), S67-S71.

Cashin, G. H., Small, S. P., & Solberg, S. M. (2008). The lived experience of fathers who have children with asthma: A phenomenological study. *Journal of Pediatric Nursing, 23*(5), 372-385.

Celik, S., & Kocasli, S. (2008). Hygienic hand washing among nursing students in Turkey. *Applied Nursing Research, 21*(4), 207-211.

Center for Disease Control and Prevention. (2005). *Diabetes surveillance report.* Department of Health and Human Services. Retrieved November 26, 2005 from *http://www.cdc. gov/diabetes/statistics/prevalence_national.htm.*

Centers for Disease Control and Prevention. (2003a). Buckle up America week: Focus on teens and young adults. *Morbidity and Mortality Weekly Report, 52.* Retrieved February 5, 2008 from *http://www.cdc.gov/mmwr/preview/mmwrhtml/ mm5219a9.htm.*

Centers for Disease Control and Prevention. (2003b). Cigarette smoking among adults—United States 2001. *Morbidity and Mortality Weekly Report, 52*(40), 953-956.

Centers for Disease Control and Prevention. (2006a). A comprehensive immunization strategy to eliminate transmission of hepatitis B virus infection in the United States. *Morbidity and Mortality Weekly Report, 55*(RR-16), 1-25.

Centers for Disease Control and Prevention. (2006b). Trends in HIV-related risk behaviors among high school students—United States, 1991-2005. *Morbidity and Mortality Weekly Report, 55,* 851-854.

Centers for Disease Control and Prevention. (2008). Surveillance for acute viral hepatitis—United States, 2006. *Morbidity and Mortality Weekly Report, 57*(SS02), 1-24.

Chinn, P. L., & Kramer, M. K. (2008). *Theory and nursing: Integrated knowledge development* (7th ed.). St. Louis: Mosby.

Cohen, C. A., London, W. T., Evans, A. A., Block, J., Conti, M. C., & Block, T. (2007). *Underestimation of chronic hepatitis B in APIs: A call for advocacy and action* [Abstract 149577]. Paper presented at the 135th American Public Health Association Annual Meeting & Exposition.

Craig, J. V., & Smyth, R. L. (2007). *The evidence-based practice manual for nurses* (2nd ed.). Edinburgh: Churchill Livingstone, Elsevier.

Creswell, J. W. (2008). *Research design: Qualitative, quantitative, and mixed method approaches* (3rd ed.). Thousand Oaks, CA: Sage.

Cromwell, J., Bartosch, W. J., Fiore, M. C., Hasselbald, V., & Baker, T. (1997). Cost-effectiveness of the clinical practice recommendations in the AHCPR guideline for smoking cessation. Agency for Health Care Policy and Research. *JAMA, 278*(21), 1759-1766.

Cullum, N., Ciliska, D., Haynes, R. B., & Marks, S. (2008). *Evidence-based nursing: An introduction.* Boston: Blackwell.

Doorenbos, A. Z., Berger, A. M., Brohard-Holbert, C., Eaton, L., Kozachik, S., LoBindo-Wood, G., et al. (2008). 2008 ONS research priorities survey. *Oncology Nursing Forum, 35*(6), E100-E107.

Duffy, S. A., Reeves, P., Hermann, C., Karvonen, C., & Smith, P. (2008). In-hospital smoking cessation programs: What do VA patients and staff want and need? *Applied Nursing Research, 21*(4), 199-206.

El-Mallakh, P. (2007). Doing my best: Poverty and self-care among individuals with schizophrenia and diabetes mellitus. *Archives of Psychiatric Nursing, 21*(1), 49-60.

Epstein, C. D., Tsaras, G., Amoateng-Adjepong, Y., Greiner, P. A., & Manthous, C. (2009). Issues in administration: Does race affect readmission to hospital after critical illness? *Heart & Lung, 38*(1), 66-76.

Erikson, E. (1968). *Identity: Youth and crises.* New York: Norton.

Fitzpatrick, M. L. (2007). Historical research: The method. In P. L. Munhall (Ed.), *Nursing research: A qualitative perspective* (4th ed., pp. 375-386). Sudbury, MA: Jones & Bartlett.

French, G., & Friedman, C. (Eds.). (2003). *Infection control: Basic concept and training* (2nd ed., pp. 25-35). United Kingdom: International Federation of Infection Control.

Global Initiative for Asthma. (2006). *Global strategy for asthma management and prevention.* Retrieved February 4,

2007 from *http://www.ginasthma.org/Guidelineitem.asp? 11=2&12=1&intld=60.*

Hale, E. D., Treharne, G. J., & Kitas, G. D. (2007). Qualitative methodologies I: Asking research questions with reflexive insight. *Musculoskeletal Care, 5*(3), 139-147.

Halfon, N., & Newacheck, P. W. (2000). Characterizing the social impact of asthma in children. In K. B. Weiss, A. S., Buist, & S. D. Sullivan (Eds.), *Asthmas' impact on society: The social and economic burden* (pp. 23-35). New York: Marcel & Dekker.

Happ, M. B., Swigart, V. A., Tate, J. A., Arnold, R. M., Sereika, S. M., & Hoffman, L. A. (2007). Family presence and surveillance during weaning from prolonged mechanical ventilation. *Heart & Lung, 36*(1), 47-57.

Hauber, R. P., Rice, M. H., Howell, C. C., & Carmon, M. (1998). Anger and blood pressure readings in children. *Psychosomatic Medicine, 11*(1), 2-11.

Howell, C. C., Rice, M. H., Carmon, M., & Hauber, R. P. (2007). The relationships among anxiety, anger, and blood pressure in children. *Applied Nursing Research 20*(1), 17-23.

Jumaa, P. A. (2005). Hand hygiene: Simple and complex. *International Journal of Infectious Diseases, 9*(1), 3-14.

Kenner, C., Lott, J. W., & Flandermeyer, A. A. (1997). *Comprehensive neonatal nursing: A physiologic perspective.* Philadelphia: Saunders.

Kerlinger, F. N., & Lee, H. B. (2000). *Foundations of behavioral research* (4th ed.). Atworth, TX: Harcourt College.

Koniak, D. (1985). Autotutorial and lecture-demonstration instruction: A comparative analysis of the effects upon students' learning of a developmental assessment skill. *Western Journal of Nursing Research, 7*(1), 80-100.

Leifer, S. L., & Glass, L. K. (2008). Planning for mass disaster in the 1950s: Harriet H. Werley and nursing research. *Nursing Research, 57*(4), 237-244.

Lindeman, C. A. (1975). Delphi survey of priorities in clinical nursing research. *Nursing Research, 24*(6), 434-441.

Marshall, D., & Rossman, G. B. (2006). *Designing qualitative research* (4th ed.). Thousand Oaks, CA: Sage.

Melnyk, B. M., & Fineout-Overholt, E. (2005). *Evidence-based practice in nursing & healthcare: A guide to best practice.* Philadelphia: Lippincott Williams & Wilkins.

Mokdad, A. H., Marks, J. S., Stroup, D. F., & Gerberding, J. L. (2004). Actual causes of death in the United States, 2000. *JAMA, 291*(10), 1238-1245.

Munhall, P. L. (2007). *Nursing research: A qualitative perspective* (4th ed.). Sudbury, MA: Jones & Bartlett.

Najarian, S. P. (1999). Infant cranial molding deformation and sleep position: Implications for primary care. *Journal of Pediatric Health Care, 13*(4), 173-177.

National Institute of Nursing Research (NINR) (2009). Mission and strategic plan. Retrieved March 1, 2009 from *http://www.ninr.nih.gov/.*

Nyamathi, A., Liu, Y., Marfisee, M., Shoptaw, S., Gregerson, P., Saab, S., et al. (2009). Effects of a nurse-managed program on hepatitis A and B vaccine completion among homeless adults. *Nursing Research, 58*(1), 13-22.

Office of Quality and Performance. (2001). *Health behaviors of veterans in the VHA: Tobacco use. 1999 Large health survey of enrollees.* Washington, DC: Veterans Health Administration.

Polman, H., de Castro, B. O., & van Aken, M. A. (2007). Experimental study of the differential effects of playing versus watching violent video games on children's aggressive behavior. *Aggressive Behavior, 34,* 256-264. Retrieved March 12, 2009 from *www.interscience.wiley.com.*

Polzer, R. L. (2007). African Americans and diabetes: Spiritual role of the health care provider in self-management. *Research in Nursing & Health, 30*(2), 164-174.

Polzer, R. L., & Miles, M. S. (2007). Spirituality in African Americans with diabetes: Self-management through a relationship with God. *Qualitative Health Research, 17*(2), 176-188.

Rambur, B., McIntosh, B., Palumbo, M.V., & Reinier, K. (2005). Education as a determinant of career retention and job satisfaction among registered nurses. *Journal of Nursing Scholarship, 37*(2), 185-192.

Rasmussen, N. A., & Farr, L. A. (2003). Effects of morphine and time of day on pain and beta-endorphin. *Biological Research for Nursing, 5*(2), 105-116.

Reishtein, J. L. (2005). Relationship between symptoms and functional performance in COPD. *Research in Nursing & Health, 28*(1), 39-47.

Reynolds, P. D. (2007). *A primer in theory construction.* Boston: Allyn & Bacon Classics.

Rogers, B. (1987). Research corner: Is the research project feasible? *American Association of Occupational Health Nurses Journal, 35*(7), 327-328.

Rudy, E. B., Daly, B. J., Douglas, S., Montenegro, H. D., Song, R., & Dyer, M. A. (1995). Patient outcomes for the chronically critically ill: Special care unit versus intensive care unit. *Nursing Research, 44*(6), 324-331.

Schizophrenia and Diabetes Expert Consensus Group. (2004). Consensus summary. *British Journal of Psychiatry, 47*(2), S112-S114.

Schultz, A. A., Goodwin, P. A., Jesseman, C., Toews, H. G., Lane, M., & Smith, C. (2008). Evaluating the effectiveness of gel pillows for reducing bilateral head flattening in preterm infants: A randomized controlled pilot study. *Applied Nursing Research, 21*(4), 191-198.

Schultz, A. A., Drew, D., & Hewitt, H. (2002). Comparison of normal saline and heparinized saline for patency of IV locks in neonates. *Applied Nursing Research, 15*(1), 28-34.

Shin, J. H., & Pershing, J. (2003). Asymmetric skull shapes: Diagnosis and management of posterior plagiocephaly. *Journal of Craniofacial Surgery, 14*(6), 696-699.

Solomon, K., & Matthews, K. (1999, March). Paper presented at the American Psychosomatic Society Annual Meeting. Vancouver, BC, Canada.

Steele, S. K., & Porche, D. J. (2005). Testing the theory of planned behavior to predict mammography intention. *Nursing Research, 54*(5), 332-338.

Van Manen, M. (1994). *Researching lived experience: Human science for an action sensitive pedagogy.* London, ON: The Althouse Press.

Wasley, A., Miller, J. T., & Finelli, L. (2007). Surveillance for acute viral hepatitis-United States, 2005. *Morbidity and Mortality Weekly Report. CDC Surveillance Summaries, 56*(3), 1-24.

Wickman, M. E., Anderson, N. L., & Greenberg, C. S. (2008). The adolescent perception of invincibility and its influence on teen acceptance of health promotion strategies. *Journal of Pediatric Nursing, 23*(6), 460-468.

Wolf, Z. R. (2007). Ethnography: The method. In P. L. Munhall (Ed.), *Nursing research: A qualitative perspective* (4th ed., pp. 293-330). Sudbury, MA: Jones & Bartlett.

Wuest, J. (2007). Grounded theory: The method. In P. L. Munhall (Ed.), *Nursing research: A qualitative perspective* (4th ed., pp. 239-271). Sudbury, MA: Jones & Bartlett.

Wynd, C. A. (2005). Guided health imagery for smoking cessation and long-term abstinence. *Journal of Nursing Scholarship, 37*(3), 245-250.

Understanding the Literature Review in Published Studies

Chapter Overview

Reviewing the Literature 189
  Sources Included in a Literature Review 190
  Purpose of the Literature Review in Quantitative
    Research 192
  Purpose of the Literature Review in Qualitative
    Research 192
**Critically Appraising the Literature Review in
a Published Study** 193
  Guidelines for Conducting a Critical
    Appraisal 194
  A Sample Critical Appraisal of a Quantitative
    Study 195
  A Sample Critical Appraisal of a Qualitative
    Study 202
Performing a Literature Review 208
Using the Library 208
Identifying Relevant Research Sources 210

Selecting Databases to Search 210
Selecting Keywords 211
Using Reference Management Software 212
Locating Relevant Literature 213
  Performing Complex Searches 213
  Limiting the Search 214
  Selecting Search Fields 216
  Linking 217
  Searching Electronic Journals 217
  Searching the Internet 218
  Systematically Recording References 219
**Clarifying Evidence for Best Practices
through Literature Reviews** 220
  Integrated Literature Reviews: State of the
    Science 220
  Meta-analyses 222
Writing a Review of Literature 222

Learning Outcomes

After completing this chapter, you should be able to:

1. Critically appraise the literature review section of a published study.
2. Conduct a computerized search of the literature.
3. Write a literature review to promote the use of evidence-based knowledge in nursing practice.

Key Terms

Academic library, p. 208
Article, p. 190
Benchmarking, p. 222
Bibliographical database,
  p. 210

Citation, p. 190
Clustered, p. 220
Complex search, p. 213
Current sources, p. 190
Data-based literature, p. 190

Dissertation, p. 191
Electronic journal,
  p. 217
Evidence for best practices,
  p. 220

Integrative review of
   research, p. 220
Interlibrary loan department,
   p. 208
Keywords, p. 211
Landmark studies, p. 194
Library sources, p. 209
Linking, p. 217

Meta-analyses, p. 222
Monograph, p. 190
Paraphrasing, p. 220
Peer reviewed, p. 190
Periodical, p. 190
Primary source, p. 191
Public library, p. 208
Relevant studies, p. 190

Review of literature, p. 189
Search field, p. 216
Secondary source, p. 192
Special library, p. 208
Surfing the Web, p. 219
Synthesis of sources, p. 220
Theoretical literature, p. 190
Thesis, p. 191

STUDY TOOLS

Be sure to visit http://evolve.elsevier.com/Burns/understanding/ for additional examples and self-tests. Also, a review of this chapter's concepts and practice exercises can be found in Chapter 6 of the Study Guide for *Understanding Nursing Research: Building an Evidence-Based Practice,* 5th edition.

A wealth of information from nursing studies is available in the literature for clinicians and researchers. More research information appears every day. The number of nursing journals also is increasing dramatically, and a multitude of nursing research reports is available in full text electronically, as well as in print form. Thus, conducting a literature review is much more enlightening now than in the past.

A **review of literature** provides you with the current theoretical and scientific knowledge about a particular problem, enabling you to synthesize what is known and not known. You may keep current in your practice by regularly searching the literature for information on topics of particular interest. Increasingly, nurses in clinical practice are conducting small studies on their own units. If you plan to conduct such a study, however, be sure to first examine the literature for information about previous studies relevant to the clinical problem. Literature searching is also necessary to keep current in your clinical practice—to base your practice on the current evidence base.

Although the Internet has made literature searching relatively easy, using bibliographic databases allow an efficiency and precision unavailable from general search engines such as Google, Google Scholar, or Yahoo. You can conduct a literature review for information about clinical problems, synthesize the knowledge you have gathered in a written summary, and share it with your colleagues. This chapter provides essential information to assist you in searching the literature, critically appraising the literature review sections of quantitative and qualitative studies, and synthesizing research evidence to guide practice.

Reviewing the Literature

Literature reviews in published studies provide a background for the problem studied. Such reviews include (1) a description of the current knowledge of a practice problem, (2) identification of the gaps in this knowledge base, and (3) the contribution of the present study to the building of knowledge in this area. The scope of a literature review must be both broad enough to allow the reader to become familiar with the research problem and narrow enough to include only the most relevant sources. Sources used need to be relevant and current. Relevant studies are those with a direct bearing on the problem of concern. Current sources are those published within 5 years before acceptance of the manuscript for publication.

To increase your understanding of the literature reviews presented in published studies, the following areas are addressed in this section:

- Sources included in a literature review
- Purpose of the literature review in quantitative studies
- Purpose of the literature review in qualitative studies

Sources Included in a Literature Review

Two main types of sources are cited in the review of literature for research: (1) theoretical and (2) empirical. The word *empirical* in this context refers to knowledge derived from research. In other words, the knowledge is based on data from research (data-based). Other types of published information, such as descriptions of clinical situations, educational literature, and position papers, are examined by the researcher in the process of reviewing the literature, but are rarely cited in a research publication because of their subjectivity (Pinch, 1995). Sources in literature reviews may be either primary or secondary; as discussed later on, this is an important distinction. Citation is the act of quoting a source, using it as an example, or presenting it as support for a position taken. Citations also have a relationship to a reference. The reference is documentation of the origin of the cited quote or idea and provides enough information for the readers to locate the original material. This information is typically the original author's name, year and title of publication, and, when necessary, periodical, or monograph title, volume, pages, and other finding information as required by standard style writing manuals. An article is a piece of writing about a specific topic and may be published together with other articles on similar themes in journals (periodicals), encyclopedia, or edited books. As part of an edited book, articles may alternatively be called chapters. A periodical, such as a journal, is published over time and is numbered sequentially for the years published. This sequential numbering is seen in the year, volume, issue, and page numbering of a journal. A monograph, such as a book on a specific subject, a record of conference proceedings, or a pamphlet, usually is a one-time publication, and may be updated with a new edition. Periodicals and monographs are available in a variety of media, including on-line and print.

Theoretical and Data-Based Literature

Theoretical literature includes concept analyses, models, theories, and conceptual frameworks that support a selected research problem and purpose. Theoretical sources can be found in periodicals and monographs. In a published study, theoretical and conceptual sources are described and summarized to reflect the current understanding of the research problem and to provide a basis for the study framework. Data-based literature consists of reports of research and includes published studies, usually in journals or books, and unpublished studies, such as master theses and doctoral dissertations. Data-based publications are peer reviewed before being published. Peer reviewed means that scholars familiar with the

Table 6-1	Peer Reviewed Journals: How Can You Tell?

A journal becomes professionally respected based on how articles are accepted for publication. For many journals, authors have to justify the quality of original research or their interpretation of the ideas and research presented by others. These articles have an evaluation called a review before the article is accepted. The manuscripts are sent to several editors or reviewers to be judged for quality. This process can also be called a referee or peer review when the reviewers are also scholars of similar interests or expertise as the writer.

Use Clues

It can be difficult to determine if articles are quality resources if someone gave you a copy of a single article he or she thought was good or if the articles were obtained from a full text electronic source, like the Internet or a library's databases. Clues to quality include 1. where the article originates (from an indexing service, a research institution, etc.) and 2. if the article has references, how many and of what type. Just as you are citing your work, an article of any depth would mention other views of the issue under discussion. Once you think the article seems substantive, you can choose to find out more about the journal from which it comes.

Issue Is Available

If you have the book or print issue in hand, you can examine the front information to find a statement about how articles are accepted for publication or to see if the journal has an editorial board and a review or referee process. The individuals on a large listing of members of the editorial board or on a list of reviewers are typically associated with colleges and universities.

Issue Is Not Available

Sometimes only a copy of the article is available and there is no access to the whole issue or book. Sometimes you can find the journal acceptance information, board of editors, or list of reviewers by searching the book or journal's website. Libraries have directories listing journals by title with notes about referee/peer review. These directories include: *The Serials Directory, Ulrich's International Periodicals Directory* (Ulrichsweb), *Magazines For Libraries, Cabell's Directory of Publishing Opportunities*, or one of several indexing services such as CINAHL or other EBSCO databases which provide this information as part of their service.

Modified from Hough, H. (2008. February 25). *Academic Journals: How Can You Tell?* Retrieved April 20, 2009, from http://libguides.uta.edu/content.php?pid=4502.

topic of the research read the report and validate its accuracy and the appropriateness of the methodology used in the study. Thus, the paper is considered trustworthy. (See Table 6–1 for techniques to determine if a particular resource is peer reviewed.) A **thesis** is a report of a research project completed by a postgraduate student as part of the requirements for a master's degree. A **dissertation** is a report of an extensive, usually original research project that is completed as the final requirement for a doctoral degree. The data-based literature reviewed depends on the study problem and the type of research conducted. Research problems that have been studied frequently or are currently being investigated have a more extensive data-based literature than that available for new or unique problems.

Primary and Secondary Sources

The published literature includes primary and secondary sources. A **primary source** is written by the person who originated or is responsible for generating the ideas published. In data-based publications, a primary data-based source is written by the person(s) who conducted the research. A primary theoretical source is written by the theorist who developed the theory or conceptual content. A **secondary source** summarizes or quotes content from primary sources. Thus, authors of secondary sources paraphrase the works of researchers and theorists. The problem with secondary sources is that the author has interpreted the works of someone else, and the interpretation is influenced by this latter author's perception and bias. Sometimes errors and misinterpretations have been spread by authors using secondary sources rather than primary sources. Predominantly primary sources are cited in research reports. Secondary sources are used only if primary sources cannot be located or the secondary source provides creative ideas or a unique organization of information not found in a primary source.

Purpose of the Literature Review in Quantitative Research

The review of literature in quantitative research is conducted to direct the planning and execution of a study. The major literature review is performed at the beginning of the research process (before the study is conducted). A limited review is conducted after the study is completed to identify studies published since the original literature review. The results of both reviews are included in writing the research report. The purpose of the literature review is similar for the different types of quantitative studies—descriptive, correlational, quasi-experimental, and experimental.

A quantitative research report cites relevant sources in its Introduction, Methods, Results, and Discussion sections. The Introduction section uses relevant sources to summarize the background and significance of the research problem. The Review of Literature section includes both theoretical and data-based sources that document the current knowledge of the problem studied.

A quantitative study develops its Framework section (not always so labeled) from the theoretical literature and sometimes from data-based literature, depending on the focus of the study. The Methods section of the research report describes the design, sample, measurement methods, treatment, and data collection process. Information from the literature review may be cited in various parts of the Methods section to validate the methods used in the study. The Results section compares the analysis of the data in the present study with the results of previous studies. The Discussion section of the research report provides conclusions that are a synthesis of the findings from previous research and those from the present study.

Purpose of the Literature Review in Qualitative Research

In qualitative research the purpose and timing of the literature review vary according to the type of study to be conducted (Table 6–2). Phenomenologists believe that the literature should be reviewed *after* data collection and analysis, so that the information in the literature will not influence the researcher's openness (Munhall, 2007). For example, if a researcher decides to describe the phenomenon of dying, the review of literature will include Kübler-Ross' (1969) five stages of grieving. Knowing the details of these stages can influence the way the researcher views the phenomenon during data collection and analysis. If the literature review is delayed until after the data have been collected and analyzed, however, the information from the literature can be compared with findings from the present study to determine similarities and differences, without any bias from preknowledge.

Table 6-2	Purposes of the Literature Review in Qualitative Research
Type of Research	Specific Purpose
Phenomenological research	Compare and combine findings from the study with the literature to determine current knowledge of a phenomenon
Grounded theory research	Explain, support, and extend the theory generated in the study
Ethnographic research	Provide a background for conducting the study, as in quantitative research
Historical research	Develop research questions and provide a source of data in the study

Grounded theory researchers include a minimal review of relevant studies at the beginning of the research process. This review is merely a means of making the researcher aware of what studies have been conducted, but the information from these studies is not used to direct data collection or theory development for the current study. The researcher uses the literature primarily to explain, support, and extend the theory generated in the study (Munhall, 2007).

The review of literature in ethnographic research is similar to that in quantitative research. The literature is reviewed early in the research process to provide a general understanding of the variables to be examined in a selected culture. The literature usually is theoretical, because few studies typically have been conducted in the area of interest. From these sources a framework is developed for examining complex human situations in the selected culture (Munhall, 2007). The literature review also provides a background for conducting the study and interpreting the findings.

Historical researchers conduct an initial literature review to select a research topic and develop research questions. Then the investigator develops an inventory of sources, locates these sources, and examines them; thus, the literature constitutes a major source of data in historical research. Because historical research requires an extensive review of literature that is sometimes difficult to locate, the researcher can spend months and even years locating and examining sources. The information gained from the literature is analyzed and organized into a report to explain how an identified phenomenon has evolved over a particular time period (Munhall, 2007).

Critically Appraising the Literature Review in a Published Study

The Review of Literature section of a research report must be identified and critically appraised for quality. The literature review might be a clearly identified section in the report, part of the introduction, or part of the background. A good-quality literature review logically builds a case for the study being reported. Thus, reading the literature review provides a basic understanding of the study problem and evidence that the study conducted was appropriate as indicated by the current knowledge of this problem. This section provides guidelines for critically appraising the literature review in a published study and an example literature review appraisal.

Guidelines for Conducting a Critical Appraisal

Appraising the literature review of a published study involves examining the quality of the content and sources presented. A correctly prepared literature review includes what is known and not known about the study problem and identifies the focus of the present study. Thus, the review provides a basis for the study purpose and often is organized according to the variables in the purpose statement. The sources cited must be relevant and current for the problem and purpose of the study. The reviewer must locate and review the sources or respective abstracts to determine whether these sources are relevant. To judge whether all of the relevant sources are cited, the reviewer must search the literature to determine the relevant sources. This is very time consuming and usually is not done for appraisal of an article. However, you can review the reference list and determine the focus of the sources, the number of data-based and theoretical sources cited, and where and when the sources were published. Sources should be current up to the date the paper was accepted for publication. (Recall that a current source is one published within 5 years of the date accepted for publication.)

Sources cited should be comprehensive as well as current. How comprehensive the list of sources is depends on whether the problem studied has existed for years or is relatively new. Some problems have been studied for decades, and the literature review often includes landmark studies that were conducted years ago. Landmark studies are significant research projects that generate knowledge that influences a discipline and sometimes society as a whole. Such studies frequently are replicated or serve as the basis for the generation of additional studies. For example, Williams (1972) studied factors that contribute to skin breakdown, and the findings from this landmark study provided the basis for numerous studies on the prevention, care, and treatment of pressure ulcers. As of March 11, 2009, a CINAHL search using the keywords pressure ulcer and study yielded 1343 studies. Many of these studies have been synthesized to provide guidelines for the prediction, care, and prevention of pressure ulcers in clinical practice (Barczak, Barnett, Childs, & Bosley, 1997; Bergstrom et al., 1994; Clark, Sanders, Carlson, Blanche, & Jackson 2007; Cullum, Deeks, Sheldon, Song, & Fletcher, 2001; Harrison, Wells, Fisher, & Prince, 1996; Kottner, Raeder, Halfens, & Dassen, 2009; Lewis, Pearson, & Ward, 2003; National Pressure Ulcer Advisory Panel, 1989; Panel for the Prediction and Prevention of Pressure Ulcers in Adults, 1992; Pressure Ulcer Consensus Group, 2000; Rutledge, Donaldson, & Pravikoff, 2000; Stotts, 1999; Whittemore, 1998). These syntheses are the basis for evidence-based practice. As a nurse, you are held accountable for keeping up with current research-based knowledge in your area of practice.

The usefulness of a study for research-based knowledge depends on the quality of the study. This quality begins with the literature review. Appraising the literature review section of a published study often is difficult for students because they are less familiar with the topic than are the authors of the article. In addition, the literature review sections frequently are too concise to present the current knowledge on selected topics because the review often is reduced to comply with space limitations for publication (Downs, 1999a,b).

CRITICAL APPRAISAL GUIDELINES FOR QUANTITATIVE STUDIES

The Literature Review

Ask the following questions to assess the quality of a literature review in a quantitative study. Your instructor may provide additional questions to guide you in assignments requiring appraising a review of literature.

1. Focus: What is the focus of the present study?
2. Sources: Identify the primary data-based sources cited in the review. How did you determine that they are primary data-based sources? Are the references current? Which of these data-based sources are quantitative and which are qualitative? What references cited are primary sources but are not data-based? How did you determine that they are not data-based? Are secondary sources cited?
3. Relevance: Are relevant studies identified and described? What criteria did you use to determine whether the studies are relevant?
4. Relevance: Are relevant theories identified and described? What criteria did you use to determine whether the theories are relevant?
5. Relevance: Are relevant landmark studies described? How did you determine that the studies you identified are landmark studies?
6. Relevance: Are relevant studies appraised? Identify the appraisal statements made.
7. Paraphrasing: Are the sources paraphrased to promote the flow of the content presented or are there too many direct quotes? Quote three paraphrased statements from the article.
8. Currency: Is the current knowledge about the research problem described? (What is known?) How did you determine that the knowledge is current?
9. Gaps: Does the literature review identify the gap(s) in the knowledge base that provides a basis for the study conducted? (What is not known?) Provide the statements made by the author that identify the gap in knowledge.
10. Organization: Is the literature review clearly organized, logically developed, and concisely written? Justify your conclusion.
11. Logic: Does the literature review logically build a case for the study being reported? Why or why not?
12. Identify the disciplines of the authors of studies cited in this paper. Does it appear that the author searched databases outside of CINAHL for relevant studies?

Two literature reviews are provided as examples for critical appraisal, one quantitative and one qualitative.

A Sample Critical Appraisal of a Quantitative Study

The review of literature from Thomas et al. (2009) is presented as an example for use in performing a critical appraisal.

QUANTITATIVE RESEARCH EXAMPLE A Literature Review

Substantial evidence indicates that patients who receive implantable cardioverter defibrillators (ICDs) after arrhythmic events or sudden cardiac death (SCD) experience psychological distress, including depression, anxiety, and impaired social support (Burke, Hallas, Clark-Carter, White, & Connelly, 2003; Friedmann, Thomas, Liu, Morton, Chapa, & Gottlieb, 2006; Thomas, Friedmann, & Kelley, 2001).

In a recent cross-sectional study of patients who received ICDs for secondary prevention, psychological distress was correlated with time after implantation (Friedmann, Thomas, Inguito, Kao, Metcalf, Kelley, & Gottlieb, 2006). In contrast, in a prospective longitudinal study of 132 patients who received ICDs after SCD, anxiety and depression did not change over 1 year of follow up (Kamphuis, de Leeuw, Derksen, Hauer, & Winnubst, 2003).

A preponderance of evidence from cross-secondary studies of patients with ICDs for secondary prevention indicated that ICD discharges have negative psychosocial consequences. Discharges of ICDs were related to depression (Denollet & Brutsaert, 1998; Goodman & Hess, 1999; Schuster, Phillips, Dillon, & Tomich, 1998), anxiety (Carroll & Hamilton, 2005; Denollet & Brutsaert, 1998; Goodman & Hess, 1999; Keren, Aarons, & Veltri, 1991; Pauli, Wiedemann, Dengler, Blaumann-Benninghoff, & Kühlkamp, 1999; Schuster et al., 1998), anger (Denollet & Brutsaert, 1998), stress (Denollet & Brutsaert, 1998), psychosocial distress (Carroll & Hamilton, 2005), and fear of future shocks (Pauli et al., 1999). Dunbar and colleagues (Dunbar, Jenkins, Hawthorne, & Porter, 1996) found that patients who had experienced ICD shocks were less anxious about the ICD than those who had not been shocked. Kamphuis et al. (2003) reported that ICD recipients who had received shocks were less anxious about subsequent shocks. Longitudinal studies produced mixed results. In a prospective longitudinal secondary prevention study, depression over 1 year did not differ between patients who received and did not receive shocks, but anxiety was higher in patients who received shocks than those who did not (Kamphuis et al., 2003). Interview data suggested that ICD shocks may have reassured the patients who received shocks that the ICD was useful and would help save their lives (Dunbar et al., 1996).

The psychological and social impact of ICDs in patients who have not experienced an arrhythmic event or sudden cardiac arrest and the impact of shocks in these patients are unknown. One-year prospective longitudinal data for patients with HF who received ICDs for primary prevention found no significant change in mental health quality of life over the first year after implantation (Piotrowicz, Noyes, Lyness, McNitt, Andrews, Dick, et al., 2007). There was no change in mental health quality of life among patients who received appropriate shocks, but there was deterioration in physical health quality of life in that same time period (Piotrowicz et al., 2007).

Disruption in psychologic status can potentiate the pathologic processes that increase the risk of SCD in patients who receive ICDs (Thomas et al., 1997). The full benefits of ICDs can only be achieved when the patient's psychosocial status is maintained. Thus, it is important to understand the impact of living with an ICD and ICD shocks on the psychosocial status in patients with HF who receive them. The purpose of this study was to evaluate longitudinal changes in anxiety, depression, and social support in patients with HF who received ICDs and evaluate the impact of demographic and disease characteristics and of ICD shocks on these changes (Thomas et al., 2009, p. 110).

References

Burke, J. L., Hallas, C. N., Clark-Carter, D., White, D., & Connelly, D. (2003). The psychosocial impact of the implantable cardioverter defibrillator: A meta-analytic review. *British Journal of Health Psychology, 8*(Pt 2), 165-178.

Carroll, D. L., & Hamilton, G. A. (2005). Quality of life in implanted cardioverter defibrillator recipients: The impact of a device shock. *Heart & Lung, 34*(3), 169-178.

Denollet, J., & Brutsaert, D. L. (1998). Personality disease severity and the risk of long term cardiac events with decreased ejection fraction after myocardial infarction. *Circulation, 97*(2), 167-173.

Dunbar, S. B., Jenkins, L. S., Hawthorne, M., & Porter, L. S. (1996). Mood disturbance in patients with recurrent ventricular dysrhythmia before insertion of implantable cardioverter defibrillator. *Heart & Lung, 25*(4), 253-262.

Friedmann, E., Thomas, S. A., Inguito, P., Kao, C. W., Metcalf, M., Kelley, F. J., & Gottlieb, S. S. (2006). Quality of life and psychological status of patients with implantable cardioverter defibrillators. *Journal of Interventional Cardiac Electrophysiology, 17*(1), 65-72.

Friedmann, E., Thomas, S.A., Liu, F., Morton, P. G., Chapa, D., & Gottlieb, S. S. (2006). Relationship of depression, anxiety, and social isolation to chronic heart failure outpatient mortality. *American Heart Journal, 152*(5), 940-948.

Goodman, M., & Hess, B. (1999). Could implantable cardioverter defibrillators provide a human model supporting the learned helplessness theory of depression? *General Hospital Psychiatry, 21*(5), 382-385.

Kamphuis, H. C., de Leeuw, J. R., Derksen, R., Hauer, R. N., & Winnubst, J. A. (2003). Implantable cardioverter defibrillator recipients: Quality of life in recipients with and without ICD shock delivery: A prospective study. *Europace, 5*(4), 381-389.

Keren, R., Aarons, D., & Veltri, E. P. (1991). Anxiety and depression in patients with life-threatening ventricular arrhythmias: Impact of the implantable cardioverter-defibrillator. *Pacing Clinical Electrophysiology, 14*(2 Pt 1), 181-187.

Pauli, P., Wiedemann, G., Dengler, W., Blaumann-Benninghoff, G., & Kühlkamp, V. (1999). Anxiety in patients with an automatic implantable cardioverter defibrillator: What differentiates them from panic patients. *Psychosomatic Medicine, 61*(1), 69-76.

Piotrowicz, K., Noyes, K, Lyness, J. M., McNitt, S., Andrews, M. L., Dick, A., et al. (2007). Physical functioning and mental well-being in association with health outcome in patients enrolled in the Multicenter Automatic Defibrillator Implantation Trial II. *European Heart Journal, 28*(5), 601-607.

Schuster, P. M., Phillips, S., Dillon, D. L., & Tomich, P. L. (1998). The psychosocial and physiological experiences of patients with an implantable cardioverter defibrillator. *Rehabilitation Nursing, 23*(1), 30-37.

Thomas, S. A., Friedmann, E., & Kelley, F. H. (2001). Living with an implantable cardioverter defibrillator (ICD): A review of the current literature related to psychosocial factors. *AACN Clinical Issues in Critical Care Nursing, 12*(1), 156-163.

Thomas, S. A., Friedmann, E., Wimbush, F., & Schron, E. (1997). Psychological factors and survival in the cardiac arrhythmia suppression trial (CAST): A reexamination. *American Journal of Critical Care, 6*(2), 116-126.

CRITICAL APPRAISAL

1. Thomas and colleagues cited a number of primary data-based sources, including the following:

Carroll & Hamilton (2005). Quality of life in implanted cardioverter defibrillator recipients: The impact of a device shock. *Heart & Lung, 34*(3), 169-178.

The abstract indicates that this is a study.

Denollet & Brutsaert (1998). Personality disease severity and the risk of long term cardiac events with decreased ejection fraction after myocardial infarction. *Circulation, 97*(2), 167-173.

The abstract indicates that this is a study.

Dunbar, Jenkins, Hawthorne, & Porter (1996). Mood disturbance in patients with recurrent ventricular dysrhythmia before insertion of implantable cardioverter defibrillator. *Heart & Lung, 25*(4), 253-262.

The abstract indicates that this is a study.

Continued

CRITICAL APPRAISAL—cont'd

Friedmann, Thomas, Inguito, Kao, Metcalf, Kelley, & Gottlieb (2006). Quality of life and psychological status of patients with implantable cardioverter defibrillators. *Journal of Interventional Cardiac Electrophysiology, 17*(1), 65-72.

The abstract indicates that this is a study.

Friedmann, Thomas, Liu, Morton, Chapa, & Gottlieb (2006). Relationship of depression, anxiety, and social isolation to chronic heart failure outpatient mortality. *American Heart Journal, 152*(5), 940-948.

The CINAHL Publication Type classified the article as receiving Research Support from NIH

Goodman & Hess B (1999). Could implantable cardioverter defibrillators provide a human model supporting the learned helplessness theory of depression? *General Hospital Psychiatry, 21*(5), 382-385.

The MeSH Terms in CINAHL for this study listed Scales; Questionnaires; Regression Analysis; Retrospective Studies.

Kamphuis, de Leeuw, Derksen, Hauer, & Winnubst, (2003). Implantable cardioverter defibrillator recipients: Quality of life in recipients with and without ICD shock delivery: A prospective study. *Europace, 5*(4), 381-389.

The MeSH Terms in CINAHL for this paper included Studies.

Keren, Aarons, & Veltri, (1991). Anxiety and depression in patients with life-threatening ventricular arrhythmias: Impact of the implantable cardioverter-defibrillator. *Pacing Clinical Electrophysiology, 14*(2 Pt 1), 181-187.

The abstract indicates that it is a study.

Pauli, Wiedemann, Dengler, Blaumann-Benninghoff, & Kühlkamp (1999). Anxiety in patients with an automatic implantable cardioverter defibrillator: What differentiates them from panic patients. *Psychosomatic Medicine, 61*(1), 69-76.

The Publication Type classifies this as a Comparative Study.

Piotrowicz, Noyes, Lyness, McNitt, Andrews, Dick, et al. (2007). Physical functioning and mental well-being in association with health outcome in patients enrolled in the Multicenter Automatic Defibrillator Implantation Trial II. *European Heart Journal, 28*(5), 601-607.

The abstract indicates it as a study.

Schuster, Phillips, Dillon, & Tomich (1998). The psychosocial and physiological experiences of patients with an implantable cardioverter defibrillator. *Rehabilitation Nursing, 23*(1), 30-37.

The Publication Type in CINAHL classifies it as research

Thomas, Friedmann, Wimbush, & Schron (1997). Psychological factors and survival in the cardiac arrhythmia suppression trial (CAST): A reexamination. *American Journal of Critical Care, 6*(2), 116-126.

The Publication Type in CINAHL classifies it as a Clinical Trial.

Secondary Sources

Burke, Hallas, Clark-Carter, White, & Connelly (2003). The psychosocial impact of the implantable cardioverter defibrillator: A meta-analytic review. *British Journal of Health Psychology, 8*(Pt 2), 165-178.

Thomas, Friedmann, & Kelley (2001). Living with an implantable cardioverter defibrillator (ICD): A review of the current literature related to psychosocial factors. *AACN Clinical Issues in Critical Care Nursing, 12*(1), 156-163.

2. Are the references current?

It is not clear in the article when the paper was accepted for publication. However, most studies require one and one half to two years after submission before being published. We have estimated this at 2008. Current sources cited within 5 years of the date accepted for publication (estimated at 2008) would be 2003-2008. The articles meeting this criterion include:

Burke, Hallas, Clark-Carter, White, & Connelly (2003). The psychosocial impact of the implantable cardioverter defibrillator: A meta-analytic review. *British Journal of Health Psychology, 8*(Pt 2), 165-178.

Carroll & Hamilton (2005). Quality of life in implanted cardioverter defibrillator recipients: The impact of a device shock. *Heart & Lung, 34*(3), 169-178.

Denollet & Brutsaert (1998). Personality disease severity and the risk of long term cardiac events with decreased ejection fraction after myocardial infarction. *Circulation, 97*(2), 167-173.

Friedmann, Thomas, Inguito, Kao, Metcalf, Kelley, & Gottlieb (2006). Quality of life and psychological status of patients with implantable cardioverter defibrillators. *Journal of Interventional Cardiac Electrophysiology, 17*(1), 65-72.

Friedmann, Thomas, Liu, Morton, Chapa, & Gottlieb (2006). Relationship of depression, anxiety, and social isolation to chronic heart failure outpatient mortality. *American Heart Journal, 152*(5), 940-948.

Kamphuis, de Leeuw, Derksen, Hauer, & Winnubst (2003). Implantable cardioverter defibrillator recipients: Quality of life in recipients with and without ICD shock delivery: A prospective study. *Europace, 5*(4), 381-389.

Piotrowicz, Noyes, Lyness, McNitt, Andrews, Dick, et al. (2007). Physical functioning and mental well-being in association with health outcome in patients enrolled in the Multicenter Automatic Defibrillator Implantation Trial II. *European Heart Journal, 28*(5), 601-607.

3. Are relevant studies identified and described?

Yes, the studies are all relevant and addressed emotional reactions of patients who were cardioverter defibrillator recipients.

4. Are relevant theories identified and described?

Theories that explore the process "by which psychosocial and biological factors contribute to cardiac morbidity and SCD" are discussed. Such a model was presented by

Thomas, Friedmann, & Kelley (2001). Living with an implantable cardioverter defibrillator (ICD): A review of the current literature related to psychosocial factors. *AACN Clinical Issues in Critical Care Nursing, 12*(1), 156-163.

As indicated in the article, this theoretical work is based in the work of Engel, Audy, and the cardiovascular stress models, cited in the following:

Audy (1971). *Measurement and diagnosis of health. Environmental essays on the planet as home.* Boston, MA: Houghton Mifflin.

Engel (1971). Sudden and rapid death during psychological stress: Folklore or folk wisdom? *Annals of Internal Medicine, 74*(5), 771-782.

Continued

CRITICAL APPRAISAL—cont'd

Lown, Verrier, & Corbalan (1973). Psychological stress and thresholds of repetitive ventricular response. *Science, 182*(114), 834-836.

Selye (1956). *The stress of life.* New York: McGraw-Hill.

Skinner (1985). Regulation of cardiac vulnerability by the cerebral defense system. *Journal of the American College of Cardiology, 5*(6 Suppl), 88B-94B.

Skinner & Reed (1981). Blockade of frontocardial-brain stem pathway prevents ventricular fibrillation of ischemic heart. *American Journal of Physiology, 240*(2), H156-163.

5. Landmark studies have influenced a discipline and sometimes society. This influence may be that the study triggers the initiation of additional research and the building of knowledge that changes practice. Landmark studies are often the first study conducted to address a clinical concern. In this light, one study cited could be considered landmark study:

Luderitz, Jung, Deister, Marneras, & Manz (1993). Patient acceptance of the implantable cardioverter defibrillator in ventricular tachyarrhythmias. *Pacing Clinical Electrophysiology, 16*(9), 1815-1821.

6. Are relevant studies appraised? Identify the critique statements made.

There is an examination of the body of knowledge coming from these studies, but there is no critique of their methodology.

7. Are the sources paraphrased to promote the flow of content? There were no direct quotes from previous studies; neither were there paraphrased statements from studies. Rather, the study findings from all of the cited studies were synthesized. Thus, the authors did not discuss individual studies but instead merged the findings from all of the studies to identify what is currently known in this field of research.

8. Is the current knowledge about the research problem described? Yes, the current knowledge is described. We conducted a literature search to determine if there were other studies that were listed but found none.

9. Does the literature review identify the gap(s) in the knowledge base that provides a basis for the study conducted? Yes. An example is the following statement: "The psychologic and social impact of ICDs in patients who have not experienced an arrhythmic event or sudden cardiac arrest and the impact of shocks in these patients are unknown." (p. 110)

10. What is the focus of the study? The focus of the study is the psychological and social impact of ICDs.

11. Is the literature review clearly organized, logically developed, and concisely written? The literature review summarized a large body of research in the area of concern in the limited space allowed by the journal. The reader has a good understanding of the previous work, the building of knowledge, and what issues are still to be addressed.

12. Does the literature review logically build a case for the study being reported? Yes, the authors state: "Disruption in psychologic status can potentiate the pathologic processes that increase the risk of SCD in patients who receive IDSs. The full benefits of ICDs can only be achieved when the patient's psychosocial status is maintained. Thus, it is important to understand the impact of living with an ICD and ICD shocks on the psychosocial status in patients with HF who receive them. The purpose of this study was to evaluate longitudinal changes in anxiety, depression, and social support in patients with HF who received ICDs and to evaluate the impact of demographic and disease characteristics and of ICD shocks on these changes. ...

Our study ... was designed to evaluate longitudinal changes in depression, anxiety, and social support in patients with HF who received ICDs in SCD-HeFT and to evaluate the effects of ICD shocks, age, and NYHA class of these changes." (p. 110)

IMPLICATIONS FOR PRACTICE

A variety of interventions may be useful for decreasing psychosocial distress among ICD recipients. Few studies address strategies to mitigate psychosocial distress in patients who received ICDs for primary or secondary prevention, and none address those who received ICDs for primary prevention of SCD. In a small randomized trial of ICD recipients, cognitive behavioral therapy performed at follow-up visits was effective at reducing anxiety and depression and improving adjustment to the ICD among those who received ICD shocks, but not ICD recipients who did not receive ICD shocks (Kohn et al., 2000). A series of 8 weekly structured telephone nursing interventions were effective at reducing patients' anxiety up to 3 months and 1 year after ICD implantation for secondary prevention (Dougherty, Lewis, Thompson, et al., 2004; Dougherty, Thompson, & Lewis, 2005). Education to reduce ICD concerns may be effective for reducing anxiety and depression in ICD recipients. Anxiety and depression were correlated with ICD concerns an average of 55 months after ICD implantation. ICD recipients who had experienced ICD shocks had more concerns than those who did not receive ICD shocks (Pedersen, van Domburg, Theuns, Jordeans, & Erdman, 2005). Among both those who had and had not received ICD shocks, depression and anxiety were higher for those with higher ICD concerns than for those with lower concerns. Weekly educational intervention for the first 8 weeks after implantation was effective at decreasing patients' concerns and increasing their knowledge of sudden cardiac arrest among patients who received ICDs for secondary prevention (Dougherty et al., 2005).

Support groups or other interventions might be considered to prevent decreases in social support experienced by younger ICD recipients and to enhance low social support among those who are older. In addition to traditional support groups, social support via computer interface using modalities such as bulletin boards, chat rooms, and list serves also may be effective to maintain or improve social networks of ICD recipients (Kuhl, Sears, & Conti, 2006a,b). (pp. 117-118)

References of Interventions Designed to Address Psychosocial Reactions to IDCS

Dougherty, C. M., Lewis, F. M., Thompson, E. A., Baer, J. D., & Kim, W. (2004). Short-term efficacy of a telephone intervention by expert nurses after an implantable cardioverter defibrillator. *Pacing Clinical Electrophysiology, 27*(12), 1594-1602.

Dougherty, C. M., Thompson, E. A., & Lewis, F. M. (2005). Long-term outcomes of a telephone intervention after an ICD. *Pacing Clinical Electrophysiology, 28*(11), 1157-1167.

Kohn, C. S., Petrucci, R. J., Baessler, C., Soto, D. M., & Movsowitz, C. (2000). The effect of psychological intervention on patients' long-term adjustment to the ICD: A prospective study. *Pacing Clinical Electrophysiology, 23*(4 Pt 1), 450-456.

Kuhl, E. A., Sears, S. F., & Conti, J. B. (2006a). Internet-based behavioral change and psychosocial care for patients with cardiovascular disease: A review of cardiac disease-specific applications. *Heart & Lung, 35*(6), 374-382.

Kuhl, E. A., Sears, S. F., & Conti, J. B. (2006b). Using computers to improve the psychosocial care of implantable cardioverter defibrillator recipients. *Pacing Clinical Electrophysiology, 29*(12), 1426-1433.

Pedersen, S. S., van Domburg, R. T., Theuns, D. A., Jordaens, L., & Erdman, R. A. (2005). Concerns about the implantable cardioverter defibrillator: A determinant of anxiety and depressive symptoms independent of experienced shocks. *American Heart Journal, 149*(4), 664-669.

CRITICAL APPRAISAL GUIDELINES FOR QUALITATIVE STUDIES

The Literature Review

Ask the following questions to assess the quality of a literature review in a qualitative study. Your instructor may provide additional questions to guide you in assignments requiring appraising a review of literature.

1. Identify the primary data-based sources cited in the review. How did you determine that they are primary data-based sources? Which of these data-based sources are qualitative and which are quantitative? What references cited are primary sources but are not data-based? How did you determine that they are not data-based? Are secondary sources cited?
2. Are the references current? What years would be current for the study being critically appraised? Note: qualitative studies that are relevant to the current study may be much older than you might find in quantitative studies and still provide information important to the current study. So the 5-year limit for relevant studies does not apply in qualitative studies.
3. Are relevant studies identified and described? What criteria did you use to determine whether the studies are relevant?
4. What relevant studies did you find that were not cited by the author?
5. Are relevant theories identified and described? What criteria did you use to determine whether the theories are relevant?
6. Are relevant landmark studies described? How did you determine that the studies you identified are landmark studies?
7. Are relevant studies appraised? Identify the appraisal statements made.
8. Are the sources paraphrased to promote the flow of the content presented or are there too many direct quotes? Quote three paraphrased statements from the article.
9. Is the current knowledge about the research problem described? (What is known?) How did you determine that the knowledge is current?
10. Does the literature review identify the gap(s) in the knowledge base that provides a basis for the study conducted? (What is not known?) Provide the statements made by the author that identify the gap in knowledge.
11. What is the focus of the present study?
12. Is the literature review clearly organized, logically developed, and concisely written? Justify your conclusion.
13. Does the literature review logically build a case for the study being reported? Why or why not?
14. Identify the disciplines of the authors of studies cited in this paper. Does it appear that the author searched databases outside of CINAHL for relevant studies?

A Sample Critical Appraisal of a Qualitative Study

The review of literature from Meyerson and Kline (2009) "Qualitative analysis of a mutual goal-setting intervention in participants" is presented as an example for use in performing a critical appraisal. Often, in qualitative studies, the author does not provide the traditional literature review that is commonly found in quantitative studies. Rather, the literature is presented simultaneously with the study findings and results from the literature are compared with the study findings. As you will see, this is the case with the example provided in the following.

 QUALITATIVE RESEARCH Example Literature Review (2009)

Discussion

In the current analysis, participants involved in the Mutual Goal Setting (MGS) intervention identified numerous concerns in addition to HF (heart failure). Other studies have found similar themes revolving around a variety of complex issues related to and independent of HF. These included (1) adaptation to HF and psychological adjustment, (2) concerns about activity and quality of life, (3) learning about HF, and (4) doing whatever needed to be done to stay out of the hospital (Costello & Boblin, 2004; Mårtensson, Karlsson, & Fridlund, 1997). All of these themes were consistent with the four themes identified in this analysis.

Competing Priorities

Mutually setting goals with a nurse interventionist enhanced HF self-management for some participants in this analysis. At the same time, barriers emerged for other participants that prevented them from focusing on HF and its management or hindered goal attainment. Fundamentally, Sawyer and Aroni (2003) noted that self-management strategies are often "based on the expectations of patient behavioral change, with little reference to the social context in which the patient lives." The nurse interventionists in the MGS study not only acknowledged the social context in which these participants lived but also discovered barriers to self-management (i.e., competing priorities), many of which emerged as goals were set.

In a study of patients with HF by Strömberg, Broström, Dahlström, and Fridlund (1999), factors influencing self-management were categorized as inward (including the patient's personality and attitudes, disease process, and therapeutic regimen) and outward (e.g., psychosocial factors and healthcare professionals). Although HF controlled the lives of some of the patients in the study, others tried to live in such a way that HF would have the least possible impact on their lives. Both inward and outward factors, categorized as competing priorities, also emerged in the current analysis, including comorbidities (inward) and concern about family members (outward) (Strömberg et al., 1999).

Self-Efficacy Related to Heart Failure Self-Management

Many patients in the current analysis acknowledged a lack of confidence in HF self-management skills, such as their ability to monitor symptoms or follow dietary restrictions. Other studies have emphasized the need for nurses to educate patients about HF while acknowledging the influence of factors on self-management, corresponding to the self-efficacy theme identified in the current analysis. Although Wehby and Brenner (1999) posit that learning about HF is the foundation of self-management, the authors noted that shorter hospitalizations reduce the amount of education patients receive about HF. Costello and Boblin (2004) also identified confusion resulting from the lack of knowledge about HF as a theme in their analysis of men and women with HF.

Figård, Hermerén, and Herlitz (2004) found a limited understanding of HF among patients with HF and suggested modifying education on the basis of the patient's attitudes and ability to understand. Some patients in their study were accepting, some were indifferent, and some were unaware of their knowledge deficit concerning HF. Again, these conclusions are comparable to the findings in the current analysis.

Continued

QUALITATIVE RESEARCH—cont'd

Activity Level

Many participants in the current analysis described goals related to maintaining their independence and activity levels; this corresponds to one theme identified by Costello and Boblin (2004). They indicated that maintenance of independence refers to the need of patients with HF to control their environments as well as their health care, such as the patient who described himself as "very independent … if somebody tries to help me, they probably won't do it right, so I will do it myself." A participant in the current analysis echoed much the same sentiment when he stated that he simply wanted to stay out of the hospital and did not "want a nurse or doctor to tell me what to do."

A similar theme, feeling a sense of activity limitation, emerged in the Mårtensson et al. (1998) study. These authors found that fatigue was a dominant feeling in their analysis, causing social isolation and loneliness in women with HF. Feelings of loss and grief as a result of activity limitations in individuals with HF were also identified by Zambroski (2003). These feelings resonated with participants in the current analysis as they struggled to return to their usual activities, visit family members, and reconnect with others in their social circles.

Psychosocial Adaptation

Adjusting to the diagnosis of HF served as the basis for many goals revolving around psychosocial adaptation for the participants in the MGS intervention. Several studies have also examined the lived experiences of patients with HF, with findings comparable to the psychosocial adaptation theme that emerged in the current analysis. Mahoney (2001), in an ethnographic study of the illness experiences of patients living with HF, identified categories for themes similar to those categorized in this analysis. In her thematic analysis, Mahoney classified these themes as (1) struggling or "making sense of the illness experience"; (2) "participating in partnerships," such as those with family, friends, and God; (3) "finding purpose and meaning in the illness experience;' and (4) surrendering or "letting go, having peace that one can handle the illness." Mahoney's themes are congruent with the psychosocial adaptation theme that emerged from the current analysis, emphasizing the struggles that patients undergo in dealing with the diagnosis and management of HF.

Themes also emerged in a study conducted by Costello and Boblin (2004) which looked at the experience of both men and women with HF. Themes such as burden to others, frustration, loss, acceptance, and fear are similar to the psychosocial adaptation theme that emerged in the MGS intervention. Fatigue, maintenance of independence, and isolation are related to the activity level theme in the current analysis.

Mårtensson, Karlsson, and Fridlund (1997, 1998), using a phenomenological approach, examined male and female patients with HF in two separate studies. For male patients, six categories related to their conception of their life situation emerged: feeling a belief in the future, gaining awareness, feeling support from the environment, feeling limitation, feeling a lack of energy, and feeling resignation (Mårtensson et al., 1997). These differed somewhat from the themes that emerged from women with HF: feeling content, feeling a sense of support, feeling a sense of limitation, feeling anxiety, and feeling powerlessness (Mårtensson et al., 1998). Both studies, while examining gender differences in patients with HF, identified themes similar to those in the current analysis, such as anxiety and lack of energy. However, some of their themes were more positively oriented than those discovered in the current analysis, such as feeling content and a belief in the future.

Mutual Goal Setting

Goal attainment is essential for patients to meet their healthcare goals. Clark (2003), in her model of chronic disease management, identified goal attainment as an opportunity for success, recognizing a highly personal goal as the primary motivating factor for a patient. King (1999) described MGS as a transaction: "When the nurse and patient have established mutual understanding of events, mutually set goals to be achieved by the patient, and agree on goals to be achieved by the patient, and agree on means to achieve the goal, a transaction occurs." King's model, when practiced by nurses and patients, will theoretically lead to goal attainment.

Czar (1987) compared two processes of goal setting: (1) MGS and (2) nurse-determined goal setting. The author concluded that although "both goal-setting processes had a beneficial effect on an individual's degree of outcome behavioral change ... the change in the outcome behavior group was significantly greater in the MGS group." This study further validates MGS as a nursing intervention for patients facing critical life changes, and a diagnosis of HF would certainly qualify as a critical life change.

References

Clark, N. M. (2003). Management of chronic disease by patients. *Annual Review of Public Health, 24*, 289-331.

Costello, J., & Boblin, S. (2004). What is the experience of men and women with congestive heart failure? *Canadian Journal of Cardiovascular Nursing, 14*(3), 9-20.

Czar, M. (1987). Two methods of goal setting in middle-aged adults facing critical life changes. *Clinical Nurse Specialist, 1*(4), 171-177.

Figård, A., Hermerén, G., & Herlitz, J. (2004). When is a patient with heart failure adequately informed? A study of patients' knowledge of and attitudes toward medical information. *Heart & Lung, 33*(4), 219-226.

King, I. M. (1999). Theory of goal attainment: Philosophical and ethical implications. *Nursing Science Quarterly, 12*(4), 292-296.

Mahoney, J. S. (2001). An ethnographic approach to understanding the illness experiences of participants with congestive heart failure and their family members. *Heart & Lung, 30*(6), 429-436.

Mårtensson, J., Karlsson, J-E., & Fridlund, B. (1997). Male patients with congestive heart failure and their conception of the life situation. *Journal of Advanced Nursing, 25*(3), 579-586.

Mårtensson, J., Karlsson, J-E., & Fridlund, B. (1998). Female patients with congestive heart failure: How they conceive their life situation. *Journal of Advanced Nursing, 28*(6), 1216-1224.

Sawyer, S. M., & Aroni, R. A. (2003). Sticky issue of adherence. *Journal of Paediatric Child Health, 39*(1), 2-5.

Strömberg, A., Broström, A., Dahlström, U., & Fridlund, B. (1999). Factors influencing patient compliance with therapeutic regimens in chronic heart failure: A critical incident technique analysis. *Heart & Lung, 28*(5), 334-341.

Wehby, D., & Brenner, P. S. (1999). Perceived learning needs of patients with heart failure. *Heart & Lung, 28*(1), 31-40.

Zambroski, C. H. (2003). Qualitative analysis of living with heart failure. *Heart & Lung, 32*(1), 32-40.

STUDY CRITICAL APPRAISAL

1. Identify the primary data-based sources cited in the review. How did you determine that they are primary data-based sources? Which of these data-based sources are qualitative and which are quantitative? What references cited are primary sources but are not data-based? How did you determine that they are not data-based? Are secondary sources cited?

   Costello & Boblin (2004). What is the experience of men and women with congestive heart failure? *Canadian Journal of Cardiovascular Nursing, 14*(3), 9-20. Indicated as data-based source in Minor Subjects of abstract. **Qualitative Study**

   Czar (1987). Two methods of goal setting in middle-aged adults facing critical life changes. *Clinical Nurse Specialist, 1*(4), 171-177. Indicated as data-based source in abstract. **Quantitative Study**

Continued

STUDY CRITICAL APPRAISAL—cont'd

Figård, Hermerén, & Herlitz (2004). When is a patient with heart failure adequately informed? A study of patients' knowledge of and attitudes toward medical information. *Heart & Lung, 33*(4), 219-226. **Qualitative Study**

Mahoney (2001). An ethnographic approach to understanding the illness experiences of participants with congestive heart failure and their family members. *Heart & Lung, 30*(6), 429-436. Indicated as data-based source in Minor Subjects of abstract. **Qualitative Study**

Mårtensson, Karlsson, & Fridlund (1997). Male patients with congestive heart failure and their conception of the life situation. *Journal of Advanced Nursing, 25*(3), 579-586. Indicated as data-based source in Minor Subjects of abstract. **Qualitative Study**

Mårtensson, Karlsson, & Fridlund (1998). Female patients with congestive heart failure: How they conceive their life situation. *Journal of Advanced Nursing, 28*(6), 1216-1224. Indicated as data-based source in Minor Subjects of abstract. **Qualitative Study**

Strömberg, Broström, Dahlström, & Fridlund (1999). Factors influencing patient compliance with therapeutic regimens in chronic heart failure: A critical incident technique analysis. *Heart & Lung, 28*(5), 334-341. Indicated as data-based source in Minor Subjects of abstract. **Qualitative Study**

Wehby & Brenner (1999). Perceived learning needs of patients with heart failure. *Heart & Lung, 28*(1), 31-40. Indicated as data-based source in Minor Subjects of abstract. **Quantitative Study**

Zambroski (2003). Qualitative analysis of living with heart failure. *Heart & Lung, 32*(1), 32-40. Indicated as data-based source in Minor Subjects of abstract. **Quantitative Study**

Primary Sources but Not Data-Based

King (1999). Theory of goal attainment: Philosophical and ethical implications. *Nursing Science Quarterly, 12*(4), 292-296.

Theory Paper

Sawyer & Aroni (2003). Sticky issue of adherence. *Journal of Paediatric Child Health, 39*(1), 2-5.

Concept Paper

Clark (2003). Management of chronic disease by patients. *Annual Review of Public Health, 24*, 289-331. **Literature Synthesis, Secondary Source**

2. Are the references current? What years would be current for the study being critiqued? Note: Qualitative studies that are relevant to the current study may be much older than you might find in quantitative studies and still provide information important to the current study. So the 5-year limit for relevant studies does not apply in qualitative studies.

References are acceptably current for a qualitative study.

3. Are relevant studies identified and described? What criteria did you use to determine whether the studies are relevant?

All of the studies cited were relevant to the focus of the study. Relevance was determined based on patients who were experiencing heart failure and their responses to their life situation.

4. What relevant studies did you find that were not cited by the author?

The study likely was accepted for publication in 2007. The oldest study cited was published in 1987. Therefore, a search was conducted for studies published from 1987 to 2007. Searches were limited to CINAHL. Search results were compared to the reference list from Meyerson and Kline (2009). The following terms (taken from the literature review) were used as search terms: heart failure and self-management. A search of the literature using these terms yielded 75 citations in the selected time period. Examining the abstracts of the listed studies, one could surmise that the use of available literature was inadequate. A second search was performed specifically for qualitative studies. Available qualitative studies were also inadequately represented.

A second literature search is expected to be conducted after the analysis of data and before submission of the paper for publication. This search is expected to be specific to the findings of the study and the search results compared with the study findings. This was clearly not done for the present study.

5. Are relevant theories identified and described? What criteria did you use to determine whether the theories are relevant? King and Pajares were theorists who were identified.

6. Are relevant landmark studies described? How did you determine that the studies you identified are landmark studies? No landmark studies were identified.

7. Are relevant studies appraised? Identify the appraisal statements made. Relevant studies were included but were not appraised.

8. Are the sources paraphrased to promote the flow of the content presented or are there too many direct quotes? Quote three paraphrased statements from the article.

   The literature review is included in the findings. Below are the paraphrased statements:

   1. "Clark and Dodge describe self-efficacy as a reciprocal process: Confidence comes from managing one's own care, observing the results, making judgments, and drawing conclusions." (p. 5)

   2. "According to Pajares, self-efficacy beliefs provide the basis for motivation." (p. 5)

   3. "In a study of patients with HF by Stromberg et al., factors influencing self-management were categorized as inward (including the patient's personality and attitudes, disease process, and therapeutic regimen) and outward (e.g., psychosocial factors and health care professionals)." (p. 6)

9. Is the current knowledge about the research problem described? (What is known?) Current knowledge is mentioned, but after conducting a literature search and examining the results, current knowledge was judged to be incomplete and there was no synthesis of current knowledge. How did you determine that the knowledge is current? Current literature is published in past 10 years (1997-2007). Twenty-one of 23 articles met this criteria.

10. Does the literature review identify the gap(s) in the knowledge base that provides a basis for the study conducted? (What is not known?) Provide the statements made by the author that identify the gap in knowledge. "As posited by Clark, chronic disease management can produce positive outcomes; therefore, an emphasis on innovative nursing interventions that address psychologic factors and enhance self-management could potentially reduce the morbidity and mortality associated with progressive HF." (p. 1)

11. What is the focus of the present study? A mutual goal-setting intervention in participants with heart failure.

12. Is the literature review clearly organized, logically developed, and concisely written? Justify your conclusion. A literature search reveals that the literature review does not adequately cover the existing literature.

13. Does the literature review logically build a case for the study being reported? Why or why not? The literature review is not comprehensive but it is not badly written as it is woven into the discussion. It was organized, logically developed, and concisely written.

Continued

STUDY CRITICAL APPRAISAL—cont'd

14. Identify the disciplines of the authors of studies cited in this paper. Does it appear that the author searched databases outside of CINAHL for relevant studies? Both of the authors are RNs, one with a FNP-C and the other with a PhD. The authors do not appear to have searched outside CINAHL.

Performing a Literature Review

A background in reading research reports and critically appraising the literature review sections of published studies should provide assistance during a review of the literature in an area of interest. This section focuses on reviewing relevant literature to generate a picture of what is known and not known about a problem and determine whether the knowledge is ready for use in practice. For example, maybe you have noted that many hospitalized patients are elderly, and far too many of them develop pressure ulcers during their hospital stay. A brief scan using online encyclopedias such as Wikipedia or professional wikis are an excellent way to develop a basic understanding of the issue about which you are concerned. Wikis are Encyclopedias and wikis provide an introduction to the ideas, terminology and, by examining the references used, some of the landmark studies. These ideas and terminology can then be used to search the literature in greater depth. Reviewing the research literature might provide solutions for this practice problem. A substantive review of the literature requires that you be able to (1) use the library, (2) identify relevant research sources, and (3) locate these sources. Taking a little bit of time to consult with a librarian will be very useful. Some of the ways a librarian can help with the literature review are shown in Table 6–3.

Using The Library

This section provides you with information about libraries and some tips on using them. Three useful information retrieval guidelines are presented in Table 6–3. There are three major categories of libraries: public, academic, and special (Strauch, Linton, & Cohen, 1989). The **public library** serves the needs of the community in which it is located and usually contains few research reports. The **academic library** is located within an institution of higher learning. It contains numerous research reports in journals and books and provides access to many other sources on-line. Most academic libraries have an **interlibrary loan department**, which can be useful when you cannot find a particular research report. This department frequently can locate and obtain books, booklets, conference proceedings, and articles from other libraries within 1 or 2 weeks.

The **special library** contains a collection of materials on a specific topic or specialty area, such as nursing or medicine. Large hospitals, healthcare centers, and health research centers have special libraries that contain sources relevant to healthcare providers and researchers. The most comprehensive collection of national and international nursing literature is available at the Center for Nursing Scholarship in Indianapolis. Specialty libraries, such as those in hospitals, often have a librarian who will assist nurses in conducting a literature search.

Table 6–3

Librarians are information specialists. They:

- Know how to find information.
- Stock stuff in the library or have special access to information that you might find useful.
- Have all sorts of ways to help you get the information you need.
- Have unique and useful tools to find information.
- Teach ways to find information efficiently.
- Can figure out what information is good for specific kinds of purposes.
- Show you how to determine if the information you found is good for your purpose.
- Obtain information you want to use.
- Often know ways of determining how papers and reports have to be formatted and the specifics of how this is done.

They have techniques to make the access, maintenance, and creation of information easier and quicker than most people realize.

Just like not everyone who works in a hospital is a nurse or doctor, not everyone who works in a library is a librarian. If you need health care, consider consulting a healthcare provider; if you need information, consider consulting a librarian.

Guidelines for information retrieval

$ Don't spend more money than you have to; your library may already have the material you need or can get it for you.

☉ The search alone will take four times longer than you expect, even with planning help. Estimate how long you think it will take and multiply this time by four; if it takes less this expanded time, be proud of your excellent skills.

☉ If it takes more than half an hour to start getting reasonable results (not including reading the materials) start talking to friends and colleagues. Remember, librarians are colleagues who are paid to know how to find stuff and who want you to be successful.

Searching the literature has changed dramatically as the use of computers has increased. Using the library is necessary for a thorough literature review. A general Internet search can be haphazard if the searcher does not have the precise terminology. Even though many resources have been digitized and are searchable over the Internet, accessing the actual document may be expensive. There are still good-quality current books and journals that are not available in electronic form. Because the capabilities for good storage and transmission of full text has only been available for about 10 years, other needed documents, including landmark studies, may not have been digitized. Libraries have always obtained material and resources to help researchers do efficient and more effective searches, saving effort, and use of various information resources (Bernardo, 2008; Cronin, Ryan & Coughlan, 2008; Ehrlich-Jones, O'Dwyer, Stevens, & Deutsch, 2008; Hoss & Hanson, 2008; Klem & Northcutt, 2008; Lawrence, 2007; Muallem, Hough, & Schmelzer, 2008; National Library of Medicine, 2008; Schmelzer, 2008; Schnall, Rich, & Lee, 2009).

Library personnel in the reference department are familiar with the library's collections and operations and can provide assistance in using the computers to access electronic resources, as well as the myriad databases, indexes, abstracts, and reference materials in and accessible through the library. Common **library sources** for research reports include journals, books, conference proceedings, master theses, and doctoral dissertations (Strauch et al., 1989).

Identifying Relevant Research Sources

Once a problem in clinical practice is identified, the literature can be searched for studies related to this problem. Before you begin searching the literature, you should consider exactly what information you are seeking. After a brief scan of the Internet to obtain starting terminology and identify major concepts and studies, if any, an overview consultation of library resources is recommended. Using this knowledge to develop a written plan of the search strategy can save considerable time. The plan should include selecting databases to search, selecting keywords, locating relevant literature, and storing the references using reference management software. Several electronic searches, not just one, may be required to obtain the studies needed.

Selecting Databases to Search

A **bibliographical database** is a compilation of citations. A citation provides the information necessary to locate a reference. For example, the author's name, year of publication, title, journal name, volume number, issue number, and page numbers all are needed to find a journal article. A database may consist of citations relevant to a specific discipline or may be a broad collection of citations from a variety of disciplines.

Generally there are two types of bibliographic databases. There are the publishers' databases which are used by publishers to distribute their materials on-line. As the journal or book is formatted for print publication the text is made available. Searching a publisher's database is similar to using any other search engine, except you are restricted to the materials created or distributed by that publisher. You can locate materials by using words and phrases used by the various authors within these publications. Reiterative searching using synonyms is necessary and scanning the table of contents of individual issues is convenient. For example, a common publisher database is ScienceDirect *(http://www.ScienceDirect.com)*. Many libraries subscribe to publisher databases, and if you are going through your library's services many of the costs will be passed to the library, not to you.

An indexing database may be familiar to many researchers through services such as PubMed. Directed to specific audiences such as nurses or healthcare providers, or people interested in business, these are databases created after the publishers have made the materials available. A company or organization will obtain the materials from the publishers and have professional indexers read and describe the content of this material. The advantages of these types of databases are that the indexers will use standardized terms and phrases so researchers can easily find materials that are related and are on the time and money. Today, good libraries provide access to large numbers of electronic databases that supply a broad scope of the available literature nationally and internationally. Thus, library users are able to identify relevant sources quickly and also to print full-text versions of many of these sources immediately. Photocopies can be made from journals held by the library, and photocopies of articles not otherwise available often can be obtained through Interlibrary loan arrangements between your library and other libraries across the country.

It may not be necessary to go to a library to use the services you need. Authorized users can access many library services at any time and location by using the Internet. Library consultations, database searching, interlibrary loan services, full-text article downloads, and more are often available to faculty and student researchers, even those who live far from the university. The Internet can provide a link to the university library, through various digital technologies, including web pages, internet/text messaging, e-mail, and video conferencing software such as Skype.

Computers also are available for users within the library. However, each library's computerized resources differ. Written documentation usually will provide step-by-step explanations of how to use electronic resources. When you use library services for the first time, ask the library personnel for an orientation to services offered, or search for orientation material available electronically through the library's website. There are also several excellent guides available through the database vendors, the U.S. National Library of Medicine, and articles in the nursing literature that discuss the utility and same topics. Libraries subscribe to these databases because the discipline specific enhancements are invaluable to researchers. The most relevant nursing online database is CINAHL, accessible at *http://www.ebscohost.com/cinahl/*, which contains citations of nursing literature, published commonly starting in the 1980s, but some versions may have information back to the 1930s. Another database commonly used by nurse researchers is MEDLINE. The National Library of Medicine provides free access to MEDLINE through PubMed, available at *http://www.pubmed.gov*. For a variety of reasons, including the cost of receipt and storage and convenience to library users, many libraries are discontinuing subscriptions to paper versions of journals and, instead are subscribing to services that provide access to electronic versions. Libraries subscribe to vendors that, for a fee, provide software, such as OVID, EBSCOhost, Cambridge Scientific (CSA) and Gale Centgage, which can be used to access multiple bibliographical databases. Given that so many databases include different collections of full-text, libraries provide services that link between their databases to seamlessly provide the materials researchers need. This means that you can conduct a computer search on a topic, get a list of citations, identify the citations that seem useful, and select the full-text option to read the text online, print it, or save it as a computer file.

Selecting Keywords

Keywords are the major concepts or variables of a research problem or topic. These terms will be what you key in to begin a search. In most databases, phrases can be used, as well as single terms. As relevant studies are identified, they can be reviewed for other terms to be used as keywords. Alternative terms (synonyms) for concepts or variables also can be used as keywords. Most databases have a thesaurus that can be used to identify keyword search terms. Sometimes additional keywords are suggested along with the results in a preliminary search. Called Subject Headings, these words and phrases are generated from the thesaurus. Once in the database, accessing the full thesaurus separately can lead to many fruitful terms that you might not have originally considered. Truncating words may allow you to locate more citations related to that term. For example, various authors may have used intervene, intervenes, intervened, intervening, intervention, or intervenor. To capture all of these terms, a truncated term, such as interven, interven*, or interven$ (the form depends on the rule of the search engine you are using), can be used in a search. Also consider irregular plurals, such as woman becoming the plural women, as search terms. If an author is cited frequently, a search using the author's name can be performed. If the author's name is used, the term needs to be identified as an author term, not a keyword term.

Table 6-4	Written Search Record			
Database Searched	Date of Search	Search Strategy	Number of Articles Found	Percentage of Articles Relevant
CINAHL				
MEDLINE				
Academic Search Premier				
Cochrane Library				

List each search term that is used in a documented search plan. As new terms are discovered, add them to the list. For each search, record (1) the name of the database that is used, (2) the date the search is performed, (3) the exact search strategy that is used, (4) the number of articles that are found, and (5) the percentage of relevant articles that are found. Some databases can display a history of the searches attempted during the session. Capturing this list is an excellent means of quickly recording this strategy information. In the long run this saves an inordinate amount of time. You will find yourself having to go back and do additional searches based on new knowledge, and by having this record you will not have to repeat the exact same search you did earlier. You can even develop a table to record this information from multiple search strategies (Table 6–4). Save the results of each search on your computer for easy access later. Be sure to write the file name of the saved search results in the search record.

Using Reference Management Software

Reference management software can make it considerably easier to track the references that have been obtained through searches. This type of software can be used to conduct searches and store the information on all search fields for each reference obtained in a search, including the abstract. Once this is done, all of the needed citation information and the abstract are readily available electronically when the literature review is written. As you read each article, you can insert any comments into the reference file.

Reference management software has been developed to interface directly with the most commonly used word processing software. With such tools, the reference information can be organized using whatever citation style you stipulate. Citations can be inserted directly into a paper with just a keystroke or two. Some of these programs are loaded onto a specific computer and the program and information is available only through that computer. Others are Internet based and you access the program and your information that is stored at a distant location. Following are representative examples: EndNote, Refworks, and Zotero. Endnote is a commonly used software package, loaded on an individual computer (single use license). Its website along with the website with information about it is *http://www.endnote.com*. A trial version of EndNote can be downloaded from the website and used to write one or two papers. In this way, you can judge the program's effectiveness in helping track and cite references and decide whether to purchase it.

RefWorks is available through the Internet and many colleges, universities, and research institutions subscribe to the service on the behalf of their affiliates. Individual subscriptions are also available. It can be accessed at *www.refworks.com*. RefWorks does not require that you purchase software to install on your computer. Rather, it operates directly from the Internet. References can be imported directly from a bibliographical database by selecting desired items from the search, saving them in a file, and uploading them to RefWorks. As an Internet-based service, it can be put to work as an excellent aid to collaborative research.

For people who use Firefox as their browser, Zotero [zoh-TAIR-oh] is a free, easy-to-use Firefox extension that does much the same thing as EndNote and RefWorks. Although not as powerful as these other two programs, it is highly regarded. Information about it and the download link are available at *http://www.zotero.org/*.

Locating Relevant Literature

Within each bibliographic database, a search is initiated by performing a separate search of each keyword that has been identified. Search engines can be unforgiving of misspellings, so key in terms carefully, and double-check for spelling errors when results are unexpectedly sparse. Most databases allow you to indicate quickly where in the database records you wish to search for the term: in the article titles, journal names, keywords, formal subject headings, or full text of the articles. Citations usually are listed with the most recent ones first.

Most databases provide abstracts of the articles in which the term is cited, allowing you to get some sense of their content, so that you may judge whether the term is useful in relation to your selected topic. If an important reference is found, it should be saved to a file. If full text of the reference is provided, you can save a PDF or HTML version of the file.

At this point, do not attempt to examine all of the listed citations. Instead, merely note the number of citations, or "hits," that were found in the search. In some cases, the number of hits may be far too large for you to examine all of them. For example, in April 2009, a search of an on-line database (CINAHL Plus with Full Text) using the keyword *coping* yielded 19,517 hits of which 11,047 were identified as being associated with research studies. The keyword phrase *social support* yielded 7535 hits of which 6289 were research (see Figure 6–1).

After a search has been completed, save the results as a file, and record the number of citations; then perform another search using the next keyword, and so on. When you have completed this activity, you should have some sense of the extent of available literature in your area of interest. At this point, you also should have enough information to plan more complex searches.

Performing Complex Searches

A complex search combines two or more concepts or synonyms in one search. Selection of the concepts or synonyms to combine may be based on the results of previous searches. The method of performing more complex searches varies with the bibliographical database, so when a particular database is used for the first time, it is best to look for instructions and consider consulting a librarian.

In some bibliographical databases, the word *and* is used to combine terms. In some databases, AND must be in uppercase. Sometimes quotation marks must be placed around the concepts; for example, "coping and social support." In others, just typing coping and

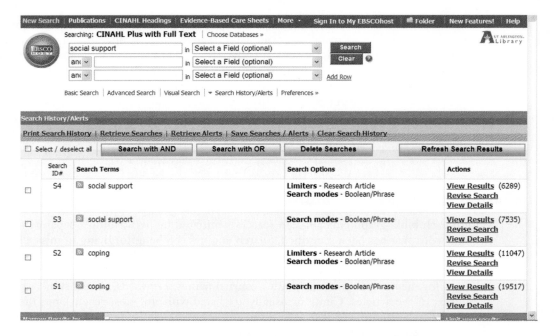

Figure 6–1. CINAHL Plus with Full Text, April 21, 2009. Search History view.

social support will find the references needed. In April 2009, combining the concepts of coping and social support yielded 1537 hits (Figure 6–2).

Searches for some topics may reveal that many hits are not useful because the selected search term includes another subject that is of no interest. For example, you may want to examine studies of coping, but not those discussing coping in relation to support. To eliminate references with the term *support*, use as your search phrase: **coping NOT support**. A number of other complex operations can be used to search databases, but the search methods described here will get you started. Instructions about how to use search options should be available in the database you are using. Some databases provide an advanced search option in which separate boxes are available for inclusion of multiple terms. For example, you might wish to include an author's last name, one or more key terms, and a journal title in a single search.

Limiting the Search

Several strategies may be used to limit a search if, after performing complex searches, you still have too many hits. The limits that can be imposed vary with the database. In CINAHL, for example, a search may be limited to English language articles. You can limit the years of a search. For example, a search might be limited to articles published in the last 10 years. Searches can be limited to find only papers that are research, are reviews, are published in consumer health journals, include abstracts, or are available in full text.

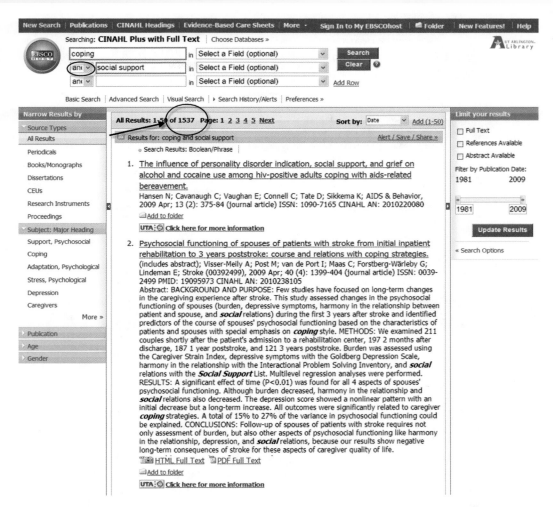

Figure 6-2. Search strategy: Coping AND Social Support (CINAHL Plus with Full Text, April 21, 2009).

When the combined search for coping and social support, described in the last section, was limited to research articles in English, there were 1300 hits. Limiting the search to research papers in English published between 2005 and 2009 yielded 499 hits (Figure 6–3).

Based on the titles, the hits that seem most relevant to a topic can be selected in Ovid software by clicking the box to the left of the reference in the list of citations and in EBSCO software by "Add to folder." Then the citations that have been selected can be either printed or saved to a file. Saving the citation to a file and then printing it with a word processing program takes considerably less paper than trying to print directly from the database. The full-text option can be selected for hits with full text available. These papers can be either printed or saved to files for printing later or reading later on the computer screen.

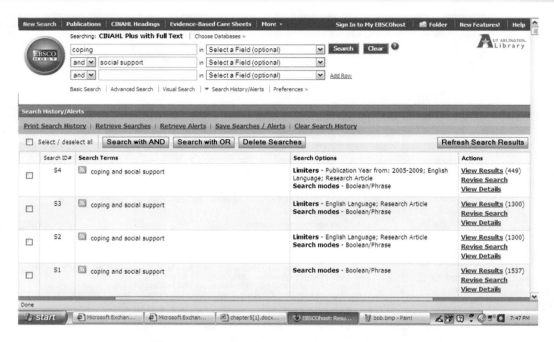

Figure 6–3. Search strategy results using Limits.

Selecting Search Fields

A **search field** is one of the various categories of information provided about an article by the bibliographical database. The fields vary with the bibliographical database. In CINAHL, With the EBSCO interface, and without selecting any specific fields, only Titles, Abstracts, and Subject headings are searched. Using the "Select a Field" drop down menus next to where you enter your keywords allows you to choose the search fields that you would like to be listed for the references you select. Common and very useful fields to use in discovering research studies include:

TX All Text
TI Title (of the article, pamphlet, chapter or book)
AU Author(s) name with the last name followed by one or more initials
AB Abstract An English-language synopsis or author abstract
Subject Heading fields (Words and phrases from the thesaurus assigned to the article to describe the contents of the article)
MW CINAHL Heading Word Word(s) that are part of the several subject heading phrase
MH Exact Subject Heading Exact word or phrase of the several subject heading thesaurus phrase
MJ Word in Major Subject Heading Word(s) that are part of the three or four subject headings describing the primary topic(s) of the article
MM Exact Major Subject Heading Exact form of one of the three or four subject headings from thesaurus that are considered the primary topics of the article

SO Publication Name Full name of journal

AF Author Affiliation The institution at which the primary author was affiliated when the article was published. This information might be useful if you wish to contact the author.

IN Instrumentation Statistical research instruments and names of clinical assessment tools used in this study.

Another good source of relevant references can be the reference lists of the articles that you retrieve through your searching. Compare the database-cited references list from articles retrieved with the list of citations obtained from your searches. This is very easy to do if you are using reference-managing software. In many cases you will find treasures that would have been missed if you had relied only on the computer search. Some of the references, which may not be journals or books listed in the databases that have been searched, may provide clues to other databases that might offer additional useful sources. These references suggest new keywords for another computer search in the databases you have been using.

Linking

Linking moves you from one website to another. In citation databases such as CINAHL, linking allows you to choose the underlined phrase full text and go directly to a full-text electronic version of an article. Sometimes it is obvious when the full text is available, but other times it may not be as obvious, even when the full text is just a few clicks away. Most libraries have programs that communicate between databases produced by different vendors, as well as many that offer individual subscriptions to which the library subscribes. These programs can identify when the library does not have the journal and fill out interlibrary loan request forms for those articles. Different libraries have different ways of letting you know this is possible, but it could be as easy as clicking on the "Click here for more information" link at the bottom of the individual citations. The time required to locate and obtain a majority of articles on a selected topic will be greatly reduced by spending just a little bit of time investigating what is available. Of course, multiple archives of full-text nursing journal articles are available, but the various archives are not always interconnected. Efforts are under way to develop linking capabilities across databases, but there still may be times when it is not as seamless as you would like.

Searching Electronic Journals

Journals are often published in both print and digital formats. A number of new nursing journals have been developed that are published only in electronic form; such a publication is referred to as an **electronic journal** or **e-journal**. Because of the high costs of publishing and distributing a printed journal, a publishing company risks losing money unless there is a very large market for the journal. As author rights issues in academic research institutions become more complicated and the trend toward institutional digital repositories increase, more and more e-journals will appear. Some of these journals are freely available over the Internet, some require free registration, and some require paid subscriptions. Most of the electronic journals are targeted to relatively small specialty audiences. These journals may have more current information on a topic than can be found in traditional journals, because articles submitted by authors are reviewed and published in electronic journals within 3 to

4 months. For articles submitted to printed journals, the time from submission to publication typically is 1 to 2 years (Fitzpatrick, 2001).

Many electronic journals have been established at universities by faculty members interested in a particular specialty area. In some cases, subscribing to the online journal may be the only way to gain access to the articles. Some electronic journals are listed in available bibliographic databases, and full-text articles from the electronic journal can be accessed through the database. However, many electronic journals are not yet in the bibliographic databases or may not be in the database you are using. Ingenta (*http://www.ingenta.com*) is a commercial website that allows the search of thousands of on-line journals from many disciplines. As of April 2009, the Directory of Open Access Journals (DOAJ, *http://www.doaj.org/*) also provides access to more than 4000 free journals containing more than 270,000 articles in all fields. Nearly 1500 of these journals are directly searchable through the DOAJ interface. The DOAJ does provide links to the remaining journals, which can then be searched individually. PubMedCentral (PMC, *http://www.pubmedcentral.nih.gov/*) is the archive of free digital biomedical and scientific journal literature. The U.S. National Institute of Health (NIH) mandates that journal articles that report the results of grant funded research be made available free to the public through this archive (NIH, n.d.). PubMed Central is getting larger daily as journal publishers open access to more articles than just those about NIH-funded projects. Although PMC can be searched separately, most databases will be able to identify these highly respected journal materials along with additional relevant materials.

Relevant articles from an electronic journal can be obtained by first locating the journal on the Internet and then scanning the titles of the published articles. Many libraries have contracts with the vendors that enable their affiliated users to have off-campus access to some of these journals and databases. Some contracts require that nonaffiliated users use the resources only within the library. Still other contracts require that all use of the resources occur in the library or other specified buildings or terminals. A list of the current electronic nursing journals is available at the following Web addresses:

- *http://www.4nursingjournals.com*
- *http://www.medbioworld.com*
- *http://highwire.stanford.edu/*

Many libraries provide lists of the electronic journals available to their affiliated users. If you are affiliated with the library, you may be able to obtain articles quite easily.

Searching the Internet

It is unlikely that studies relevant to a topic can be found by searching the Internet using general search engines; however, you may find other relevant information. One advantage of information obtained from the Internet is that it is likely to be more current than material found in books. One disadvantage is that the information is uneven in terms of accuracy. Most of the time there is no screening process for information placed on the Internet. Thus, a considerable amount of misinformation can be found, as well as some gems that might not be found elsewhere. It is important to check the source of any information obtained on the Internet so that its validity can be judged.

Although Google tends to be most familiar, a wide range of search engines are available for conducting Internet searches. Search engines vary in the following ways: (1) the approach used to search the Internet, (2) the extent of the Internet that is covered (most do not cover the entire Internet, so you may need to use more than one engine), (3) the frequency with which the search engine updates the websites that are indexed, and (4) the ease with which they are used. New search engines appear on the scene almost daily, so identifying the best search engine in this book would not be particularly useful. Currently Google Scholar *(http://scholar.google.com)* is an excellent search engine to reduce your Internet search results to those that are reasonably respected as scholarly resources. Many university libraries provide a list of other good search engines.

When a promising site is found, its location can be stored in the Web browser (using features called "favorites" or "bookmarks" in Internet Explorer, Google, or Mozilla Foxfire). Remember, however, that if a website will be used as a reference in a bibliography, the date it was visited and the address (URL [Uniform Research Locator]) it had at that time are required for proper citation.

Storing a website address on a browser simplifies return visits to check information. Additionally, many websites frequently are updated and can be regularly checked for new information. Sometimes clicking on a link (underlined or highlighted name) on one website will reveal other websites with helpful information. Following these links—**surfing the Web**—is an important part of an Internet search. Information overload is one problem that may be encountered during such a search; you may find too much information and need to be selective about what you retrieve.

Although Web browsers store a history of the websites you have visited as you move from one to another, it is wise to store their locations in the browser to avoid having to retrace the steps back through the links. Also, websites often are changed or deleted, so it is a good idea to save a particularly useful Web page as a file. Text, graphics, or both may be saved from the Web. If space on your hard drive is a problem, a memory stick will enable you to store it.

Metasearchers offer an alternative approach to searching the Internet. These programs perform a search by using multiple search engines, enabling a single search to cover more of the Web. Currently, our favorite metasearcher is Dogpile, which can be found at *http://www.dogpile.com*. Dogpile uses an innovative strategy for searching that increases the number of hits on a topic.

Systematically Recording References

The bibliographical information on a source should be recorded in a systematic manner, according to the format that will be used in the reference list. Many journals and academic institutions use the format developed by the American Psychological Association (APA, 2010). The reference lists in this book are presented using APA 6.0 format. Computerized lists of sources usually contain complete citations for references and should be filed for future use. You also can easily search a computerized database with a computer and obtain complete reference citations.

Sources that will be cited in a paper or recorded in a reference list should be cross-checked two or three times to prevent errors. Damrosch and Damrosch (1996) have identified some of the common errors that authors make when applying the APA format, and these authors provide guidelines for how to avoid such lapses in style. The sources cited in the reference list should follow the correct format for print and on-line full-text versions, as follows:

PRINT VERSION
Plawecki, H. M. (1996). Improving a manuscript's chances for acceptance. *Journal of Holistic Nursing, 14*(3).

ON-LINE FULL-TEXT VERSION
Plawecki, H. M. (1996). Improving a manuscript's chances for acceptance. *Journal of Holistic Nursing, 14*(3). DOI: 10.1177/089801019601400101.

Clarifying Evidence for Best Practices through Literature Reviews

The process of reviewing the literature in preparation for conducting a study involves careful critical appraisal of the methodology and an examination of the existing literature. Findings from each research report are clarified by the reviewer and then paraphrased. **Paraphrasing** involves expressing an author's findings clearly and concisely in the reviewer's own words. A new study is then designed to improve the methodology and strengthen the **evidence for best practices**. In recent years, it has become increasingly urgent that the literature also be reviewed to define the state of the science in a given area of practice through integrated literature reviews and meta-analyses.

Integrated Literature Reviews: State of the Science

An **integrative review of research** is conducted to identify, analyze, and synthesize the results from independent studies to determine the current knowledge (what is known and not known) in a particular area (Ganong, 1987; Hearn, Feuer, Higginson, & Sheldon, 1999; Jadad, Moher, & Klassen, 1998; Smith & Stullenbarger, 1991). For example, a group of nurses on a nursing unit may find a need for an integrated review regarding a particular patient care problem. If a review cannot be found in the literature, it may be necessary to perform one specific to the needs of the unit. The results may be used to guide the development of a protocol for the procedure or create a critical pathway tool.

The studies are selected for inclusion in the review on the basis of their quality and their relationship to a selected practice problem. Initially, therefore, the studies are read and critically appraised. Then the studies that are of the highest quality are selected, and their purposes, methods, results, and findings are compared. It may help to develop a table that includes essential information from each study so that comparisons can be made (Table 6–5) (Martin, 1997). It also may help to identify the findings that are common among the different studies and compare and contrast the outcomes of these studies. Table 6–6 was developed as an example, using the studies conducted on the prediction and prevention of pressure ulcers in adults. The next step is integrating the findings from all of the studies. The type of reasoning used during the integration of findings is synthesis. **Synthesis of sources** involves compiling the findings from all of the selected studies and analyzing and interpreting those findings. Finally, the meanings obtained from all sources are combined, or **clustered**, to specify the current state of research-based knowledge for a particular area of clinical

Table 6–5	Synthesizing Studies to Generate a Review of Literature					
Author(s) and Year	Purpose	Sample	Measurement	Treatment	Results	Findings
Allman, 1991						
Bergstrom, Braden, Laguzza, and Holman, 1987						
Berlowitz and Wilking, 1989						
Braden and Bergstrom, 1987						
Harrison, Wells, Fisher, and Prince, 1996						
Norton, 1989						
Norton, McLaren, and Exton-Smith, 1975						
Okamoto, Lamers, and Shurtleff, 1983						

Table 6–6	Comparison and Contrast Study Findings on the Prediction and Prevention of Pressure Ulcers		
Author(s) and Year	Finding 1	Finding 2	Finding 3
Allman, 1991			
Bergstrom, Braden, Laguzza, and Holman, 1987			
Berlowitz and Wilking, 1989			
Braden and Bergstrom, 1987			
Harrison, Wells, Fisher, and Prince, 1996			
Norton, 1989			
Norton, McLaren, and Exton-Smith, 1975			
Okamoto, Lamers, and Shurtleff, 1983			

practice. A number of integrated reviews of research have been written on pressure ulcer prevention.*

Expert researchers and clinicians have developed publications that summarize nursing knowledge on a variety of topics. In 1983 the first volume of the *Annual Review of Nursing Research* was published. The integrative reviews of research included in these annual publications cover relevant topics about nursing practice, nursing care delivery, nursing education, and the nursing profession. Integrative reviews also have been published in a variety of clinical and research journals. The international Cochrane Collaboration *(http://www.cochrane. org)* and the Agency for Health Care Research and Quality *(http://www.ahrq.gov)* commission

---

*See for example: Armstrong, D., & Bortz, P. (2001). An integrative review of pressure relief in surgical patients. *AORN Journal, 73*(3), 645-674.

systematic reviews on critical areas of health care. The journal *Evidence-Based Nursing* also participates in identifying clinical research for practice (Sermeus & Vanhaecht, 2000).

Meta-analyses

Meta-analyses go beyond the integrated review by performing statistical analyses using summative findings from multiple published studies. Using these strategies, it is possible to provide a global estimate of such measures as the mean number of days of hospitalization after a particular procedure or the reduction in the number of hours a patient spends in a coronary care unit resulting from a particular nursing intervention. The results from meta-analyses sometimes are referred to as benchmarking (Rudy, Lucke, Whitman, & Davidson, 2001). Meta-analyses are discussed in greater detail in Chapter 13.

Writing a Review of Literature

A well-prepared literature review documents the current knowledge on a selected topic and indicates the findings that are ready for use in practice. Often a detailed outline is developed to guide the writing of a literature review. The review of literature begins with an introduction, includes a presentation of relevant studies, and concludes with a summary of current knowledge (Burns & Grove, 2009). The headings and essential content of a literature review are briefly described as follows:

1. **Introduction.** The introduction indicates the focus or purpose of the review; describes the organization of sources; and indicates the basis for ordering the sources; for example, from least to most important or from least to most current. This section should be brief and interesting enough to capture the attention of the reader. The introduction may need to be rewritten several times in the course of developing other sections of the literature review.
2. **Data-based literature.** Data-based literature includes quality studies that are relevant for a selected evidence-based project. For each study, the purpose, sample size, design, and specific findings should be presented, with a scholarly but brief critical appraisal of the study's strengths and weaknesses. This critical appraisal should be clear and concise and include only the most relevant studies. The content from these sources is best paraphrased or summarized in your own words. If a direct quotation is used, it should be kept short to promote the flow of ideas. Long quotations often are unnecessary and interfere with the reader's train of thought.

    Ethical issues must be considered in presenting research sources (Gunter, 1981). The content from studies must be presented honestly and not distorted to support a selected evidence-based project. The weaknesses of a study need to be addressed, but it is not necessary to be highly critical of a researcher's work. The criticism should be focused on the content, be related in some way to the proposed project, and be stated as possible or plausible explanations, so that it is neutral and scholarly rather than negative and blaming. Additionally, the researcher's works that are cited in the literature review should be accurately documented.
3. **Summary.** The summary includes a concise presentation of the research knowledge about a selected topic, including what is known and not known.

KEY CONCEPTS

- The review of literature in a research report is a summary of current knowledge about a particular practice problem and includes what is known and not known about this problem.
- The literature is reviewed to summarize knowledge for use in practice or to provide a basis for conducting a study.
- Through the use of electronic databases, a large volume of references can be located quickly.
- Keywords are the major concepts or variables that must be included in a search.
- A search should be initiated by performing a separate search of each keyword that has been identified.
- Reference management software should be used to track the references obtained through the searches.
- The literature review usually begins with an introduction, includes data-based sources, and concludes with a summary of current knowledge.

REFERENCES

Allman, R. M. (1991). Pressure ulcers among bedridden hospitalized elderly. Division of Gerontology/Geriatrics, University of Alabama at Birmingham. Unpublished data compiled.

American Psychological Association. (2010). *Publication manual of the American Psychological Association* (6th ed.). Washington, DC: Author.

Barczak, C. A., Barnett, R. I., Childs, E. J., & Bosley, L. M. (1997). Fourth national pressure ulcer prevalence survey. *Advances in Wound Care*, *10*(4), 18-26.

Bergstrom, N., et al. (1994). *Treatment of pressure ulcers. Clinical Practice Guideline No. 15*. AHCPR Publication No. 95-0652. Rockville, MD: Agency for Health Care Policy and Research, Public Health Service, U.S. Department of Health and Human Services.

Bergstrom, N., Braden, B. J., Laguzza, A., & Holman, V. (1987). The Braden Scale for predicting pressure sore risk. *Nursing Research*, *36*(4), 205-210.

Berlowitz, D. R., & Wilking, S. V. (1989). Risk factors for pressure sores. A comparison of cross-sectional and cohort-derived data. *Journal of the American Geriatrics Society*, *37*(11), 1043-1050.

Bernardo, L. (2008). Finding the best evidence. Part 1: Understanding electronic databases. *JEN: Journal of Emergency Nursing*, *34*(1), 59-60.

Braden, B., & Bergstrom, N. (1987). A conceptual schema for the study of the etiology of pressure sores. *Rehabilitation Nursing*, *12*(1), 8-12.

Burns, N., & Grove, S. K. (2009). *The practice of nursing research: Conduct, critique, and utilization* (6th ed.). Philadelphia: Saunders.

Clark, F., Sanders, K., Carlson, M., Blanche, E., & Jackson, J. (2007). Synthesis of habit theory. *OTJR: Occupation, Participation & Health*, *27*(Supp 1), 7S-23S.

Cronin, P., Ryan, F., & Coughlan, M. (2008). Understanding a literature review. A step-by-step approach. *British Journal of Nursing (BJN)*, *17*(1), 38-43.

Cullum, N., Deeks, J., Sheldon, T. A., Song, F., & Fletcher, A. W. (2001). Beds, mattresses and cushions for pressure sore prevention and treatment. *The Cochrane Library (Oxford)*, *2*(20), 1-10.

Damrosch, S., & Damrosch, G. D. (1996). Methodology corner. Avoiding common mistakes in APA style: The briefest of guidelines. *Nursing Research*, *45*(6), 331-333.

Downs, F. S. (1999a). How much is enough? *Applied Nursing Research*, *12*(3), 164-165.

Downs, F. S. (1999b). How to cozy up to a research report. *Applied Nursing Research*, *12*(4), 215-216.

Ehrlich-Jones, L., O'Dwyer, L., Stevens, K., & Deutsch, A. (2008). Searching the literature for evidence. *Rehabilitation Nursing*, *33*(4), 163-169.

Fitzpatrick, J. J. (2001). Scholarly publishing: Current issues of cost and quality, fueled by the rapid expansion of electronic publishing. *Applied Nursing Research*, *14*(1), 1-2.

Ganong, L. H. (1987). Integrative reviews of nursing research. *Research in Nursing & Health*, *10*(1), 1-11.

Gunter, L. (1981). Literature review. In S. D. Krampitz & N. Pavlovich (Eds.), *Readings for nursing research* (pp. 11-16). St. Louis: Mosby.

Harrison, M. B., Wells, G., Fisher, A., & Prince, M. (1996). Practice guidelines for the prediction and prevention of pressure ulcers: Evaluating the evidence. *Applied Nursing Research*, *9*(1), 9-17.

Hearn, J., Feuer, D., Higginson, I. J., & Sheldon, T. (1999). Issues in research: Systematic reviews. *Palliative Medicine*, *13*(1), 75-80.

Hoss, B., & Hanson, D. (2008). Evaluating the evidence: Web sites. *AORN Journal, 87*(1), 124-141.

Hough, H. (2008). *Academic journals: How can you tell?* Retrieved April 20, 2009, from http://libguides.uta.edu/content.php?pid=4502.

Jadad, A. R., Moher, D., & Klassen, T. P. (1998). Guides for reading and interpreting systematic reviews. *Archives of Pediatrics and Adolescent Medicine, 152*(8), 812-817.

Klem, M., & Northcutt, T. (2008). Finding the best evidence, part 2: The basics of literature searches. *JEN: Journal of Emergency Nursing, 34*(2), 151-153.

Kottner, J., Raeder, K., Halfens, R., & Dassen, T. (2009). A systematic review of interrater reliability of pressure ulcer classification systems. *Journal of Clinical Nursing, 18*(3), 315-336.

Kübler-Ross, E. (1969). *On death and dying.* New York: Macmillan.

Lawrence, J. (2007). Techniques for searching the CINAHL database using the EBSCO interface. *AORN Journal, 85*(4), 779-791.

Lewis, M., Pearson, A., & Ward, C. (2003). Pressure ulcer prevention and treatment: Transforming research findings into consensus based clinical guidelines. *International Journal of Nursing Practice, 9*(2), 92-102.

Martin, P. A. (1997). Ask an expert: Writing a useful literature review for a quantitative research project. *Applied Nursing Research, 10*(3), 159-162.

Meyerson, K. L., & Kline, K. S. (2009). Qualitative analysis of a mutual goal-setting intervention in participants with heart failure. *Heart & Lung, 38*(1), 1-9.

Muallem, M., Hough, H., & Schmelzer, M. (2008). Searching the literature with professional databases. *Gastroenterology Nursing, 31*(5), 375-376.

Munhall, P. L. (2007). *Nursing research: A qualitative perspective* (4th ed.). Sudbury, MA: Jones & Bartlett.

National Library of Medicine. (2008, March 5). *Introduction to health services research: A self-study course.* Retrieved from http://www.nlm.nih.gov/nichsr/ihcm/index.html

National Pressure Ulcer Advisory Panel (1989). *Pressure ulcers: Incidence, economics, risk assessment. Consensus development conference statement.* West Dundee, IL: S-N Publications.

Norton, D. (1989). Calculating the risk: Reflections on the Norton Scale. *Decubitus, 2*(3), 24-31.

Norton, D., McLaren, R., & Exton-Smith, A. N. (1975). *An investigation of geriatric nursing problems in hospital.* Edinburgh: Churchill Livingstone.

Okamoto, G. A., Lamers, J. V., & Shurtleff, D. B. (1983). Skin breakdown in patients with myelomeningocele. *Archives of Physical Medicine Rehabilitation, 64*(1), 20-23.

Panel for the Prediction and Prevention of Pressure Ulcers in Adults. (1992). *Pressure ulcers in adults: Prediction and prevention. Clinical practice guidelines.* AHCPR Publication No. 92 047. Rockville, MD: Agency for Health Care Policy and Research, Public Health Service, U.S. Department of Health and Human Services.

Pinch, W. J. (1995). Synthesis: Implementing a complex process. *Nurse Educator, 20*(1), 34-40.

Pressure Ulcer Consensus Group. (2000). *Pressure ulcer prevention guidelines.* Glasgow: Author.

Rudy, E. B., Lucke, J. F., Whitman, G. R., & Davidson, L. J. (2001). Benchmarking patient outcomes. *The Journal of Nursing Scholarship, 33*(2), 185-189.

Rutledge, D. N., Donaldson, N. E., & Pravikoff, D. S. (2000). Protection of skin integrity: Progress in pressure ulcer prevention since the AHCPR 1992 guideline. *Online Journal of Clinical Innovations, 3*(5), 1-67.

Schmelzer, M. (2008). Research in practice. The importance of the literature search. *Gastroenterology Nursing, 31*(2), 151-153.

Schnall, J., & Rich, J., & Lee, A. (2009, January 20). Finding qualitative research articles. Retrieved from *http://healthlinks.Washington.edu/howto/qualitative/.*

Sermeus, W., & Vanhaecht, K. (2000). WISECARE to support evidence in practice. *Applied Nursing Research, 13*(3), 159-161.

Smith, M. C., & Stullenbarger, E. (1991). A prototype for integrative review and meta-analysis of nursing research. *Journal of Advanced Nursing, 16*(11), 1272-1283.

Stotts, N. A. (1999). Literature review. Risk of pressure ulcer development in surgical patients: A review of the literature. *Advances in wound care, 12*(3), 127-136.

Strauch, K., Linton, R., & Cohen, C. (1989). *Library research guide to nursing: Illustrated search strategy and sources.* Ann Arbor, MI: Pierian Press.

Thomas, S. A., Friedmann, E., Gottlieb, S. S., Liu, F., Morton, P. G., Chapa, D. W., Lee, H., Nahm, E. on behalf of the Sudden Cardiac Death in Heart Failure Trial Investigators (2009). Changes in pychosocial distress in outpatients with heart failure with implantable cardioverter defibrillators. *Heart & Lung, 38*(2), 109-120.

Whittemore, R. (1998). Pressure-reduction support surfaces: A review of the literature. *Journal of Wound, Ostomy, and Continence Nursing, 25*(1), 6-25.

Williams, A. (1972). A study of factors contributing to skin breakdown. *Nursing Research, 21*(3), 238-243.

7

Understanding Theory and Research Frameworks

Chapter Overview

What Is a Theory? 228
What Is a Conceptual Model? 228
Understanding the Elements of Theory 230
  Concept 230
  Defining Concepts 231
  Relational Statements 231
  Map or Model 233
Middle Range Theories 235
Practice Theories 237

Frameworks 238
Frameworks Based on Middle Range Theories 240
Frameworks for Physiological Studies 242
Frameworks Derived from Qualitative Studies 244
Frameworks Including Conceptual Nursing Models 246

Learning Outcomes

After completing this chapter, you should be able to:

1. Define theory and the elements of theory (concepts, relational statements or propositions, and model or map).
2. Describe the purpose of a study framework.
3. Describe the use of middle range and practice theories as frameworks in studies.

4. Discuss the development of theory from qualitative studies.
5. Identify study frameworks developed from conceptual nursing models.
6. Critically appraise the framework in a study.

Key Terms

Abstract, p. 228
Assumptions, p. 228
Concept, p. 230
Conceptual definition, p. 231
Conceptual model, p. 228
Concrete, p. 228
Constructs, p. 230
Existence statement, p. 231
Framework, p. 238

Implicit framework, p. 239
Map or model, p. 233
Middle range theories, p. 235
Phenomenon (phenomena), p. 228
Philosophical stance, p. 229
Philosophies, p. 229
Practice theories, p. 237

Propositions, p. 232
Relational statement, p. 231
Scientific theory, p. 242
Statements, p. 231
Substantive theory, p. 239
Tentative theory, p. 239
Theory, p. 228
Variables, p. 230

Theory is essential to research because it is the initial inspiration for developing a study. When an idea for a study emerges, researchers have a theory about what the study outcomes will be and why. This theory may not be formally stated or even written, but it is nonetheless an initial theory that stimulates ideas for a study. If a researcher tells you about the ideas of a study, you may question the use of a particular variable, or ask why particular study outcomes are expected. The explanation you receive is an expression of the researcher's theory about the study. These ideas can be developed into a framework or theoretical basis for the proposed study.

Theories have been developed in nursing to explain phenomena important to clinical practice. For example, nursing has a theory of uncertainty in illness (Mishel, 1988, 1990), a theory of health promotion behavior (Pender, Murdaugh, & Parsons, 2006), and a theory of unpleasant symptoms (Lenz, Pugh, Milligan, Gift, & Suppe, 1997). Sometimes nurses use theories developed in other disciplines, such as psychology or biology, and apply them to nursing situations. Although nurses use these theories to guide their practice, in many cases the theories have not been tested to determine whether the nursing actions proposed by the theory actually have the effects claimed. In these cases, the theory is an inspiration for the study that is developed to test its accuracy in describing the real world and its relevance for use in practice.

Sometimes nurses have read studies that included relevant theories as their frameworks. Or the theory was developed through research as was Selye's (1976) theory of stress and adaptation. Selye conducted case studies to explain the stresses that patients experience when they have changes in their health status, such as an acute appendicitis or a cancer diagnosis. Through his research, Selye found that all changes in health status are stressful to patients and their families and require adaptation. With this empirical knowledge, he developed a theory to summarize his study findings. Today, researchers might choose Selye's (1976) theory to guide them in studying patients' responses to their health problems.

As a researcher develops a plan for conducting a quantitative study, the theory on which the study is based is expressed as the framework for the study. A study framework is a brief explanation of a theory or those portions of a theory that are to be tested in a study. The study framework spells out the logic that the researcher is using in planning the study. When the study is carried out, the researcher can then answer the question, "Was this theory correct in its description of reality?" Thus, a study tests the accuracy of theoretical ideas. In explaining the study findings, the researcher will interpret those findings in relation to the theory (Burns & Grove, 2009; Smith & Liehr, 2008).

A researcher conducting a qualitative study would conduct the study, and in examining the study results would ask questions such as, "How consistent were my findings with my expectations?" or, "How consistent were my findings with the literature?" An outcome of a qualitative study is sometimes a theory that emerges from the study findings. For example, grounded theory qualitative studies are conducted to develop a theory in a selected area (Glaser & Strauss, 1967; Munhall, 2007).

An important part of critically appraising a study is to identify and evaluate the study framework. Understanding the theory on which a study is based also will help you determine whether it is appropriate to apply the study findings to your practice. To assist you in learning about theories and their use in research, this chapter describes the elements of theory, identifies types of theories, and discusses how theories provide frameworks for studies. You are also provided guidelines for critically appraising study frameworks, and these guidelines are applied to a variety of frameworks from published studies.

What Is a Theory?

Professions (such as nursing) use theories to organize their body of knowledge and establish what is known about a phenomenon. Formally, a **theory** is defined as an integrated set of defined concepts and statements that present a view of a phenomenon and can be used to describe, explain, predict, and control that phenomenon. A discussion of the description, explanation, prediction, and control of phenomenon in nursing is presented in Chapter 1.

Theories are abstract, rather than concrete. Abstract means that the theory is the expression of an idea, apart from any specific instance. An **abstract** idea focuses on more general things. **Concrete** refers to realities or actual instances—it focuses on the particular, rather than the general. For example, the word *pain* represents an abstract idea and a patient experiencing an acute, sharp, penetrating sensation in the lower right abdominal quadrate is a particular instance or concrete example of pain. This type of pain might be a particular health problem such as appendicitis.

What Is a Conceptual Model?

Conceptual model is another term that is discussed in the nursing theoretical literature. Conceptual models are similar to theories but are more abstract than theories. A **conceptual model** broadly explains phenomena of interest, expresses assumptions, and reflects a philosophical stance. A **phenomenon** (the plural form is **phenomena**) is an occurrence or a circumstance that is observed, something that impresses the observer as extraordinary, or a thing that appears to and is constructed by the mind (Johnson & Webber, 2005). Caring is a phenomenon. You provide caring as part of your nursing practice. How do you explain caring in your nursing practice? You can give a specific example of your caring for a patient, but can you make clear what caring is? Watson (1985) has developed a conceptual model of caring that expresses her philosophy of caring in nursing. Conceptual models include abstract and general concepts and relationship statements. Thus, a conceptual model can be an umbrella for a theory and studies (Fawcett & Garity, 2009). For example, Watson's theory of caring could provide philosophical ideas for the middle range theory of caring that was developed by Swanson (1991) through research.

Conceptual models also include **assumptions**, which are statements that are taken for granted or considered true, even though they have not been scientifically tested. For example, a fairly common assumption made by nurses is that "People want to assume control of their own health problems." Do you think this assumption is true? Is the assumption true for most but not all people?

Conceptual models include philosophical statements or a stance of the author(s). **Philosophies** are rational intellectual explorations of truths or principles of being, knowledge, or conduct. A **philosophical stance** is a specific philosophical view held by a person or group of people. For example, a philosophical stance might hold that there is no single reality—that reality is different for each person. What do you think?

Most disciplines have several conceptual models, each with a distinctive vocabulary. A number of conceptual models have been developed in nursing. Table 7–1 identifies just a few of these models and provides sources you might read to expand your understanding of conceptual models. For example, Roy's model (Roy & Andrews, 1999; Roy & Roberts, 1981) describes adaptation as the primary phenomenon of interest to nursing. This model identifies the elements considered essential to adaptation and describes how the elements interact to produce adaptation and thus health.

Orem (2001) considers self-care to be the phenomenon that is central to nursing. Her model explains how nurses facilitate clients to achieve self-care. Orem has also developed three theories based on her conceptual model, which provides the philosophical stance for these theories. Orem's (2001) theories are: (1) Theory of Nursing Systems, (2) Theory of Self-Care Deficit, and (3) Theory of Self-Care. A conceptual model may use the same or similar terms as those of other models but define them in different ways. For example, Roy and Orem both use the term *health* but define it in different ways. To Roy, health is determined by adaptation, and within Orem's conceptual model health is linked to levels of self-care.

Table 7–1	Conceptual Models in Nursing		
Name of the Conceptual Model	**Author**	**Focus of the Models**	**Sources of the Models**
Self-Care Deficit Theory of Nursing	Dorothy Orem	The goal is for individuals to initiate and perform self-care activities to maintain life, healthful functioning, and continual personal development.	Orem, 1995, 2001
Adaptation Model	Sister Callista Roy	The goal is adaptation; a person's adaptation level is constantly changing and is made up of focal, contextual, and residual stimuli.	Roy and Andrews, 1999; Roy and Roberts, 1981
Systems Model	Betty Neuman	This model is based on general systems theory and reflects the nature of living organisms as open systems that interact with each other and the environment.	Neuman, 1995
Theory of Caring	Jean Watson	The importance of caring in nursing is addressed in this model, which includes 10 carative factors.	Watson, 1985

Although conceptual models vary in their level of abstraction and in the breadth of phenomena they explain, they all provide an overall picture of the phenomena they address. Conceptual models, because of their level of abstraction, generally are not considered testable through research. However, the theories derived from a conceptual model can be tested, usually with the conduct of quantitative studies (Fawcett, 2005; Fawcett & Garity, 2009). The linking of conceptual nursing models to study frameworks is discussed later in this chapter.

Understanding the Elements of Theory

The first step in understanding theories is to become familiar with the elements related to theoretical ideas and their application. These elements include the concepts, definitions of concepts, relational statements, and map or model (Chinn & Kramer, 2008; Fawcett, 2005).

Concept

A concept is a term that abstractly describes and names an object, idea, or phenomenon, thus providing it with a separate identity or meaning. For example, the phenomenon *pain* introduced earlier is a concept. The concept is the basic element of a theory. Each concept in a theory needs to be defined. The meaning of the concept is conveyed in the definition developed by a theorist. The definition of a concept might be detailed and complete or might be vague and incomplete and require further development. Theories with clearly identified and defined concepts provide a stronger basis for a study framework.

Two terms closely related to concept are *construct* and *variable*. In conceptual models, concepts have very general meanings and sometimes are referred to as constructs. A construct associated with the concept of pain might be physiological responses. At a more concrete level, terms are referred to as variables and are narrow in their definition. Thus, a variable is more specific than a concept. The word *variable* implies that the term is defined so that it is measurable and suggests that numerical values of the term are able to vary ("variable") from one instance to another.

A variable related to pain might be perception of acute pain, because a specific method exists for assigning numerical values to varying amounts of acute pain. For example, the FACES Pain Scale might be used to measure *perception of acute pain* in pediatric patients (see Chapter 10 for a copy of this scale). The linkages among construct, concept, and variable are illustrated in Figure 7–1 with a clinical example.

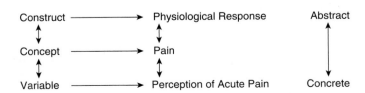

Figure 7–1. Link of theoretical elements—construct, concept, and variable.

Defining Concepts

Defining concepts allows consistency in the way the term is used. Concepts from theories have conceptual definitions that are developed by the theorist and often are clarified through research. A conceptual definition differs from the dictionary definition of a word. A **conceptual definition** is more comprehensive than a denotative (or dictionary) definition and includes associated meanings the word may have. A conceptual definition is referred to as connotative. Connotations of a term bring memories, moods, or images subtly or indirectly to mind. For example, a conceptual definition of *fireplace* might include the sense of hospitality and comfort that often are associated with fireplaces, whereas the dictionary definition is narrower and more specific: an open recess for holding a fire at the base of a chimney. Many terms commonly used in clinical nursing language have not been clearly defined. The use of these terms in theory or research requires thoughtful exploration of the connotative meanings that the terms have within nursing and a clear statement of their meaning within the particular theory or study.

A theory with clearly defined concepts provides more direction to researchers in identifying appropriate variables to examine these concepts in a study. Also the definition of a concept in a theory needs to link to the conceptual definition of the study variable and provide a basis for the operational definition of the variable. Because of the significance of conceptual definitions, it is important that you identify the researcher's conceptual definitions of study variables when you critically appraise a study. In a quantitative study, each variable in the study must be associated with a concept, a conceptual definition, and a method of measurement or operational definition. Examples of these links are presented in Table 7–2. The development of conceptual and operational definitions of variables is described in detail in Chapter 5.

Relational Statements

Statements express claims that are important to the theory. An **existence statement** declares that a given concept exists or that a given relationship between concepts occurs. For example, an existence statement might claim that a condition referred to as *stress* exists and that there is a relationship between the concept of stress and the concept of health (Selye, 1976). A **relational statement** clarifies the type of relationship that exists between or among concepts. For example, one relational statement might propose that high levels of stress are related to declining levels of health. Another more concrete relational statement might propose that smoking is related to lung damage.

Table 7–2	Links of Concepts, Variables, and Conceptual and Operational Definitions		
Concept	Variable	Conceptual Definition	Operational Definition
Pain	Perception of Acute Pain	Perception of acute pain is the patient's subjective determination of the sensations of discomfort that occur when a patient says and at the level he or she says (McCaffery, 1972).	FACES Pain Scale can be used to measure perception of acute pain in children

It is the statements of a theory that are tested through research, not the theory itself. Testing a theory involves determining the truth of each relational statement in the theory. However, a single study might test only one relational statement. As more studies examine a single relational statement, increasing evidence of the accuracy or inaccuracy of that statement is determined. Many studies are required to validate all the relational statements in a theory.

In theories, **propositions** (relational statements) can be expressed at various levels of abstraction. The statements found in conceptual models (general propositions) are at a high level of abstraction. Statements found in theories (specific propositions) are at a moderate level of abstraction (Fawcett, 2005; Johnson & Webber, 2005). Hypotheses are at a low level of abstraction and are developed to be tested in a study. Hypotheses are developed based on propositions from a theory that is the framework for the study. As statements are expressed in a less abstract way, they become narrower in scope. Statements at varying levels of abstraction that express relationships between or among the same conceptual ideas can be arranged in hierarchical form, from general to specific. This should allow the reader to see the logical links among the various levels of abstraction as shown in Table 7–3.

The abstract ideas in theories can be tested through research to verify if they hold true in the concrete reality of nursing practice. In some cases, theories are generated as a result of research. The specific instances discovered during the study are used by researchers to develop more abstract (or general) ideas about the phenomenon of interest. As discussed earlier, Selye developed his theory of stress (1976) through specific instances demonstrated in multiple studies. The specific instances discovered during a qualitative study often are used to generate theory (Munhall, 2007). Critical thinking is required to generate theory, test theory, or relate concrete realities to abstract ideas.

Table 7-3	Levels of Abstraction of Relational Statements		
Type of Relational Statement	**Common Source**	**Level of Abstraction**	**Example**
General Proposition	Conceptual Model	Very Abstract	The magnitude of the internal and external stimuli will positively influence the magnitude of the physiological response of an intact system (Roy & Roberts, 1981).
Specific Proposition	Theory	Abstract	The amount of mobility in the form of exercising positively influences the level of muscle integrity (Roy & Roberts, 1981, p. 90).
Hypothesis	Researcher formulated to test a proposition in a study	Specific to direct a study	Patients with congestive heart failure participating in a structured exercise walking program have greater muscle strength than those doing standard activities of daily living.

Map or Model

One strategy for expressing a theory or study framework is a **map or model** that graphically shows the interrelationships of the concepts and relational statements (Artinian, 1982; Fawcett, 1999; Moody, 1989; Newman, 1979). The map is sometimes referred to as a conceptual or framework map that is developed to explain the concepts contributing to or partially causing an outcome. The map should be supported by references from the literature. A conceptual map summarizes and integrates what is known about a phenomenon more succinctly and clearly than does a literary explanation, thus allowing a grasp of the "wholeness" of a phenomenon.

A conceptual map includes all of the major concepts in a theory or study framework. These concepts are linked by arrows expressing the proposed linkages between concepts. Each linkage shown by an arrow is a graphic illustration of a relational statement (proposition) of the theory. Mapping is useful in identifying gaps in the logic of the theory and reveals inconsistencies, incompleteness, and errors (Artinian, 1982).

RESEARCH EXAMPLE Study Framework

DiNapoli (2009, p. 126) conducted a study to "investigate what modifiable sociostructural variables will decrease the risk of initiating cigarette smoking before the age of 12 years among adolescent girls." DiNapoli's framework is presented as an example to promote your understanding of the following elements of a study framework: concepts, definitions of concepts, variables, and map or model. The following excerpt describes the study framework.

It was assumed in this study that the initiation of health risk behaviors, as well as its associated morbidity, is a decision made by the adolescent and that therefore a holistic view of risk and protective factors as the context for this decision must be achieved. The theoretical framework used as the context for this study, illustrated in Figure 7–2, embraces a holistic view of youth development (Brofenbrenner, 1978). The Ecological Model of Youth Development theorizes that a complex interaction between individual and contextual factors such as community, peers, family, and media influences health behavior choice. "Table 7–4 presents the variables used to examine the links between ecological levels as identified in the theoretical framework (Figure 7–2) and the dependent measure of tobacco use" (DiNapoli, 2009, pp. 127-128). Figure 7–2 is the socioecological model of health behavior that was the framework for this study. Table 7–4 includes the construct of ecological level; the concepts of youth, family, school, and community; and the variables linked to each of these framework concepts (DiNapoli, 2009).

CRITICAL APPRAISAL

DiNapoli (2009) clearly identified her study framework as the Ecological Model of Youth Development by Brofenbrenner (1978) (see Figure 7–2). The model and its description provided the context for the study. The model included the relevant concepts examined in the study, but not all concepts were examined, such as laws/norms, community economics, work setting, spiritual community, and media. It is not uncommon for researchers to study only part of the concepts and relationships in a model. The model and description clearly identify the relationships or propositions among the concepts. The concepts were linked to the study variables in a table (see Table 7–4).

Continued

CRITICAL APPRAISAL—cont'd

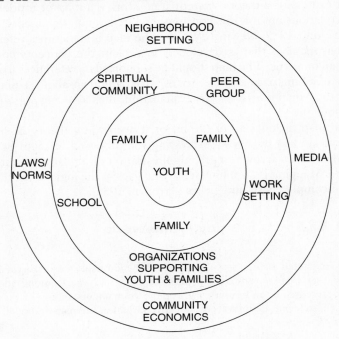

Burns & Grove: Understanding Nursing Research, 5/e

Figure 7–2. Socioecological model of health behavior. DiNapoli, P. P. (2009). Early initiation of tobacco use in adolescent girls: Key sociostructural influences. *Applied Nursing Research, 22*(2), 127.

Table 7–4 Study Variables

Ecological Level [Construct]	Variables
Youth [concept]	Emotional well-being
	Social responsibility
	Perceived risk for substance use
	Self-efficacy—school success
	Self-esteem
Family [concept]	Parenting style
	Parental values and attitudes
	Parental monitoring
	Family conflict
School [concept]	School connectedness
Community [concept]	Neighboring support
	Neighborhood monitoring

DiNapoli, P. P. (2009). Early initiation of tobacco use in adolescent girls: Key sociostructural influences. *Applied Nursing Research, 22*(2), 128.

The study findings are linked back to the framework as indicated in the following excerpt.

Although these individual-level correlates are important in terms of the characteristics of ego development, they do little to advance our understanding about the portal of risk reduction for nurses. Instead, as the theoretical framework for this current study hypothesized, the environment and interpersonal relationships play an equally important role in the decision making of adolescents that results in health behavior choice. Therefore, the level at which risk reduction should be initiated is not at the individual level but at the socio-structural level. It is important to carefully examine the context of risk reduction and direct health promotion interventions within these contexts. (DiNapoli, 2009, p. 131)

IMPLICATIONS FOR PRACTICE

DiNapoli (2009) provides specific implications for practice.

The public health message by nurses should emphasize the importance of family and community cohesion and should be followed by modeling of congruent health behaviors (e.g., caring relationships that promote emotional well-being and the availability of alternative behavior choices that promote positive ego development) to provide the risk reduction environment necessary to promote continued improvement in this preventable health problem [cigarette smoking in adolescent girls]. (DiNapoli, 2009, p. 131)

Middle Range Theories

Two types of theories are commonly used as frameworks for quantitative studies; they are middle range theories and practice or intervention theories. This section discussed middle range theories and the next section presents practice theories. Middle range theories are less abstract and narrower in scope than conceptual models. These types of theories focus on answering particular practice questions and often specify such factors as patients' health conditions, family situations, and nursing actions (Tomey & Alligood, 2006). Middle range theories tend to be more closely linked to clinical practice and research than conceptual models and thus have a greater appeal to clinicians and clinical researchers. These theories may emerge from the review of studies for the purpose of building evidence-based practice related to a particular clinical problem (Brown, 2009). Middle range theories also can be used as the framework for a study, thus contributing to the validation of the middle range theory (Liehr & Smith, 1999; Peterson & Bredow, 2004; Smith & Liehr, 2008). Table 7–5 lists some of the middle range theories currently being used as frameworks in nursing studies.

A middle range theory that has stimulated the conduct of many quantitative studies is Pender's Health Promotion Model (HPM) that was developed in 1982. The Pender HPM was last revised in 2006 and is presented in Figure 7–3. The HPM has been used as a framework in several studies that focused on defining concepts and testing relationships in this model. The HPM identifies individual characteristics and experiences that influence behavior-specific cognitions and affect to produce behavioral outcome. The individual characteristics and experiences include prior related behavior and personal biological, psychological,

Table 7-5	Middle Range Theories
Theory	**Relevant Theoretical Sources**
Acute pain	Good, 1998; Good and Moore, 1996
Acute pain management	Huth and Moore, 1998
Adaptation to chronic pain	Dunn, 2004, 2005
Adapting to diabetes mellitus	Whittemore and Roy, 2002
Adolescent vulnerability to risk behaviors	Cazzell, 2008
Bureaucratic caring	Ray, 1989
Caregiver stress	Tsai, 2003
Caring	Swanson, 1991
Chronic pain	Tsai, Tak, Moore, and Palencia, 2003
Chronic sorrow	Eakes, Burke, and Hainsworth, 1998
Culturing brokering	Jezewski, 1995
Cultural competence	Purnell, 2005
Dyspnea	Gift, 1992
Empathy	Olson and Hanchett, 1997
Entry into nursing home as a status passage	Chenitz, 1983
Generative quality of life for the elderly	Register and Herman, 2006
Health belief model	Becker, 1976
Health promotion	Pender, 1982; Pender et al., 2001, 2006
Health-related quality of life	Wilson and Cleary, 1995
Home care	Smith, Pace, Kochinda, Kleinbeck, Koehler, and Popkess-Vawter, 2002
Maternal role attainment	Mercer, 1986
Mother-infant attachment theory	Bowlby, 1969, 1973
Nursing intellectual capital	Covell, 2008
Peaceful end of life	Ruland and Moore, 1998
Peri-menopausal process	Quinn, 1991
Planned behavior	Ajzen, 1991
Postpartum depression	Beck, 1993
Recovery from schizophrenia	Noiseux and Ricard, 2008
Resilience	Polk, 1997
Self-care of elderly	Backman, 2003
Self-care management for vulnerable populations	Dorsey and Murdaugh, 2003; Jenerette, 2004
Self-efficacy	Bandura, 1982, 1989, 1997
Sensing presence and sensing space	Orticio, 2007
Social learning theory	Bandura, 1986
Socioecological model of health behavior	Brofenbrenner, 1978
Stress, appraisal, and coping	Lazarus and Folkman, 1984
Symptom management	University of California, San Francisco School of Nursing Symptom Management Group, 1994
The urine control theory	Jirovec, Jenkins, Isenberg, and Baiardi, 1999
Uncertainty in illness	Mischel, 1988, 1990
Unpleasant symptoms	Lenz, Pugh, Milligan, Gift, and Suppe, 1997

and sociocultural factors. The behavior-specific cognitions and affect include perceived benefits of action, perceived barriers to action, perceived self-efficacy, activity-related affect, interpersonal influences, and situational influences that lead to a commitment to a plan of action. The commitment to a plan for action determines the individual's health promoting behavior, which is affected by immediate competing demands.

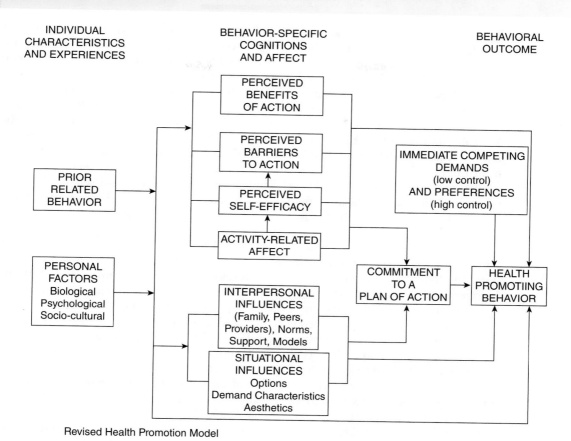

Figure 7–3. Pender Health Promotion Model. Pender, N. J., Murdaugh, C. L., & Parsons, M. A. (2006). *Health promotion in nursing practice* (5th ed.). Upper Saddle River, NJ: Pearson & Prentice Hall, 50.

Health-promoting behavior is the endpoint or action outcome in the HPM. However, health-promoting behavior is ultimately directed toward attaining positive health outcomes for the client. "Health promoting behaviors, particularly when integrated into a healthy lifestyle that pervades all aspects of living, results in improved health, enhanced functional ability, and better quality of life at all stages of development" (Pender et al., 2006, p. 57).

Health-promoting behaviors, such as balanced diet, exercise, and adequate sleep, are important to the health of individuals and society. Pender's HPM is a useful framework for future studies focused on testing interventions that might facilitate permanent, positive life-style changes in individuals and their families.

Practice Theories

Practice theories are even more specific than middle range theories. They are designed to theoretically propose specific approaches to particular nursing practice situations. Comfort

Theory (Kolcaba, 1994) is an example of a practice theory. Practice theory sometimes is referred to as prescriptive theory. Some very specific middle range theories might be considered practice theories by some researchers. One form of this level of theory is intervention theory. Such theories direct the implementation of a specific nursing intervention and provide theoretical explanations of how and why the intervention is effective in addressing a particular patient care problem. These theories are tested through programs of research to validate the effectiveness of the intervention in addressing the problem. You can find examples of these types of studies in the literature (Apóstolo & Kolcaba, 2009; Dowd, Kolcaba, Steiner, & Fashinpaur, 2007). In some cases, practice theory emerges from the guidelines that direct evidence-based practice. Now, researchers are conducting studies to examine the feasibility of implementing the evidence-based guidelines that have emerged from synthesis of findings in the research literature (Brown, 2009; Craig & Smyth, 2007). These are called translational studies, which are described in detail in Chapter 13.

An example of an intervention theory is Wellness Motivation Theory (Fleury, 1991). This theory is being implemented in a project funded by the National Institute of Nursing Research. The theory guided the development of a program titled "Motivational Intervention for Physical Activity." This program is designed to reduce disparity in health between Hispanic women and the general population, attending to cultural relevance in intervention development, implementation, and evaluation. Hispanic women have high rates of cardiovascular disease with a prevalence of overweight and obesity (71.9%) and a lack of physical activity (74%) (Perez & Fleury, 2008). The concept of motivation was used in health guides developed for Hispanic women. This health guide provided information that could lead to self-knowledge, which can be the motivating factor for planning and integrating physical activity into their daily life. Wellness Motivation Theory proposes that motivation for health behavior change leads to intention formation, intention formation leads to goal directed behavior, and goal-directed behavior leads to new positive health patterns (Fleury, 1991). The intervention project is a test of these theoretical statements.

Social support systems of the community such as the families and churches will be recruited to be involved in the project. Course content will be delivered over 12 sessions in a group format, using three teaching modes: didactic, group discussion, and "hands-on" experience. Moderate-intensity lifestyle activity will be used to promote physical activity. To determine effectiveness of their intervention, they will measure body mass index (BMI), body composition, blood pressure, walking in number of steps per day using a pedometer, and body fat distribution (Perez & Fleury, 2008). Look for the results of implementing this intervention in the research literature.

Frameworks

A **framework** is an abstract, logical structure of meaning, such as a portion of a theory, which guides the development of the study and enables the researcher to link the findings to nursing's body of knowledge. Sometimes the study framework is called the *conceptual framework* or the *theoretical framework* in a study. These terms seem to be used interchangeably in the nursing literature. Every quantitative study has a framework. This is true whether the study has a physiological, psychological, social, or cultural focus. A clearly expressed framework is one indication of a well-developed quantitative study. Perhaps the researcher expects one variable to cause another variable, such as the independent variable of aerobic exercise program causing the dependent variable of weight loss. In a well-thought-out quantitative study, the researcher explains abstractly in the framework why one variable is expected to cause the other. The idea is expressed concretely as a hypothesis to be tested through the study methodology.

In some studies the framework is derived from a well-tested theory that has been used as the framework for many quantitative studies. Many theories used as frameworks in nursing studies are from other fields and are based on theoretical works from psychology (e.g., the theory of stress and coping [Lazarus & Folkman, 1984]), physiology (e.g., The Theory of Biological Rhythms [Luce, 1970]), and sociology (e.g., The Health Belief Model [Becker, 1976]). However, over the last 10 to 15 years many middle range theories have been developed in nursing and are being used as frameworks in quantitative studies. Table 7–5 identifies several middle range theories that are being used as frameworks in nursing studies (Smith & Liehr, 2008). These published middle range theories have clearly identified concepts, definitions of concepts, and relational statements and are referred to as substantive theory.

In other quantitative studies, the framework is developed from newly proposed theory and is often called tentative theory. For example new practice theories often emerge from questions related to selected nursing problems. Additionally, new theories may arise from clinical insight suggesting that a relationship exists between or among elements important to desired nursing outcomes. These situations tend to be concrete, and they require that the researcher, using critical reasoning, express the concrete ideas in abstract language. New theories also may be developed from conceptual models or elements of existing theories not previously related.

Unfortunately, in some quantitative studies, the ideas that compose the framework remain nebulous and vaguely expressed. Although the researcher believes that the variables being studied are related in some fashion, this notion is expressed only in concrete terms. The researcher may make little attempt to explain why the variables are thought to be related. However, the rudiment of a framework is the expectation (perhaps not directly expressed) that there may be one or more important links among the study variables. Sometimes, rudimentary ideas for the framework are expressed in the introduction or literature review, in which linkages among variables found in previous studies are discussed, but then the researcher stops without fully developing the ideas as a framework. These are referred to as implicit frameworks. In most cases, a careful reader can extract an implicit framework from the text of the study. However, since the study framework is not clearly expressed, it provides limited guidance to the development and conduct of a study. Studies without frameworks limit the contribution of study findings to nursing knowledge.

The quality of a framework in a quantitative study needs to be critically appraised to determine its usefulness in directing the study and interpreting the study findings. The framework needs to be critically appraised within the context of the overall study. Thus, the following guidelines were developed to assist you in evaluating the quality of a study's framework.

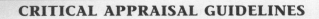

CRITICAL APPRAISAL GUIDELINES

Framework of a Study

You are encouraged to critically appraise the logical structure of a study framework using the following questions:

1. Is the study framework explicitly expressed in the study?
2. What is the name of the theory and theorist used for the framework?
3. What are the concepts in the framework? Are these concepts clearly defined?
4. Is each study variable or concept conceptually defined in the study?
5. Are the variables operational definitions consistent with its associated conceptual definitions?
6. Do the researchers clearly identify the relationship statement(s) or proposition(s) from the framework being examined by the study design?
7. Are the study findings linked back to the framework?

Critically appraising a framework of a quantitative study requires that you go beyond the framework itself to examine its linkages to other components of the study such as measurement and implementation of study variables. To answer the previous questions, first extract the concepts and conceptual definitions from the written text in the introduction, the literature review, or the discussion of the framework. Then you must judge the adequacy of the linkages of concepts to variables, the measurement of research or dependent variables, and the implementation of independent variables. You also need to determine if the study findings have been linked back to the study framework. These guidelines are used to critically appraise a framework from a middle range theory and a physiological study framework presented in the next two sections.

Frameworks Based on Middle Range Theories

Most frameworks for nursing studies are based on middle range theories. These studies test the validity of the middle range theory and also examine the parameters within which the middle range theory can be applied. Some middle range theories that were developed outside of nursing are now being used as the basis for frameworks in nursing studies. Other middle range theories were developed within nursing to explain nursing phenomena. These theories also should be tested before being applied to nursing practice.

RESEARCH EXAMPLE Framework Based on Middle Range Theory

Wilson (2005) used Pender's Health Promotion Model (Pender, Murdaugh, & Parsons, 2001), a middle range theory, as a basis for her study of *health-promoting behaviors of sheltered homeless women*. You can review Pender's HPM that was presented earlier in this chapter as Figure 7–3. Wilson (2005) implemented a descriptive study design to describe the health promoting behaviors of 137 homeless women in five shelters. The study purpose, framework, measurement methods, and key findings are presented in the following excerpt.

> The purpose of this study was to describe sociodemographic and personal characteristics, health practices, and health-promoting behaviors in a population of sheltered homeless women in a specific Midwest geographical region to increase awareness, understanding, and provide further insight into the complex area of homelessness and health.
>
> The theoretical framework for this study was based upon Pender's revised Health Promotion Model. The Health Promotion Model (HPM) provides a framework to examine influences on participation in health-promoting behaviors and provides direction for effective interventions. The HPM illustrates that each person is a multidimensional holistic individual who continually interacts with both interpersonal and physical environments and emphasizes the active role of the individual in the achievement of an improved healthy state. The 3 major constructs of the HPM (individual characteristics and experiences, behavior-specific cognition and affect, and behavioral outcomes) were used to select specific study variables as conceptualized within the model. Health-promoting behaviors, the outcome of the HPM, were examined in this population and relationships among study variables explored.
>
> Homelessness is conceptualized currently through the perspective of two levels of influences: individual and structural. Individual level issues and problems are represented by personal characteristics that contribute to vulnerability and the risk of homelessness. (Wilson, 2005, pp. 51-52)
>
> Sociodemographic and personal characteristics were measured by the Personal History Form, developed by this research ... Health-promoting behaviors were measured with the Health-Promoting Lifestyle Profile II (HPLP II). The HPLP II is used to identify patterns of health promotion lifestyles and health-promoting behaviors conceptualized as a multidimensional pattern of self-initiated actions and perceptions that serve to maintain or enhance the level of wellness. (Wilson, 2005, p. 53)
>
> Pender's HPM (Health Promotion Model) is of great value to guide health care interventions for sheltered homeless women and should be used to assess current influences and provide a framework for services directed at increasing their health. Individual characteristics and past experiences are important to assess in order to provide in-depth understanding of the individual. Immediate competing demands have direct effects on the participation of health-promoting behaviors, and, for the homeless, include issues such as availability of childcare. Additionally, basic needs (shelter, food, safety) can be viewed as competing demands as these take priority status and must be adequately addressed before health promotion needs can become a focus. (Wilson, 2005, p. 60)

CRITICAL APPRAISAL

Wilson (2005) explicitly identified the framework for her study as Pender's HPM. The framework section identified the concepts and the relationships from the HPM that were examined by the study's descriptive design. The clarity of the framework would have been enhanced by including the model of Pender's theory (see Figure 7–3). Key concepts of health-promotion behaviors, personal factors, situational factors, and competing demands were conceptually defined. The study concepts and variables were measured by the Personal History Form and the HPLP II instruments. These measurement methods were appropriate and clearly described in the study. The sample, which included subjects from five shelters for women, was of sufficient size (137 homeless women) to provide a reasonable test of Pender's HPM relationships or propositions. The study findings were clearly linked to Pender's HPM. The HPM was useful in identifying the inadequacies in health services for homeless women. The author recommended that the model be used to provide a framework for the provision of health services to homeless women.

Continued

IMPLICATIONS FOR PRACTICE

Wilson (2005) clearly identified implications for practice in her research report. The following quote identifies actions that might be taken to improve health-promotion behaviors in homeless women.

> Creation and establishment of collaborative partnerships designed to implement effective interventions and programs that will enhance the health and well-being of homeless women is of vital importance. Development of outreach services to homeless shelters as well as community sites that serve the impoverished (food banks, churches, low-income housing, community centers) is strongly warranted. Shelter-based interventions are needed that address holistic care for physical, psychological, spiritual, and social resources and not just housing, food, safety, and specific disease concerns. Interventions that support participation in health-promoting behaviors must be accessible, affordable, and appropriate to the needs and lifestyles of being homeless. Culturally appropriate interventions and programs that develop resiliency and strengthening of personal resources are needed to positively impact the health of this unique at-risk group. (Wilson, 2005, pp. 61-62)

Frameworks for Physiological Studies

The theoretical basis for physiological studies is usually derived from physiology, genetics, pathophysiology, and physics. This type of theory is called scientific theory. Scientific theory has valid and reliable methods of measuring each concept and its relational statements or propositions have been tested through research and found to be valid. Since the knowledge in these areas is well tested through research, the theoretical relationships often are referred to as laws and principles. In addition, propositions can be developed and tested using these laws and principles and then applied to nursing problems.

Developing a framework to clearly express the logic on which the study is based is helpful both to the researcher and readers of the published study. The critical appraisal of a physiological framework is no different from that of other frameworks. However, concepts and conceptual definitions in physiological frameworks may be less abstract than concepts and conceptual definitions in many psychosocial studies. Concepts in physiological studies might be such terms as cardiac output, dyspnea, wound healing, blood pressure, tissue hypoxia, metabolism, and functional status.

As the body of knowledge related to a phenomenon increases, the development of a framework to express the knowledge becomes easier. Accordingly, frameworks for quasi-experimental and experimental studies, which usually have a background of descriptive and correlational studies, generally are more easily and fully developed than frameworks for descriptive studies. Descriptive studies often examine multiple factors to understand a phenomenon not previously well studied. Theoretical work related to the phenomenon may be tentative or nonexistent. Therefore, the framework may not be as well developed.

RESEARCH EXAMPLE Critically Appraising a Physiological Framework of a Quantitative Study

Shipowick, Moore, Corbett, and Bindler (2009) conducted a quasi-experimental study to examine the effect of vitamin D on depressive symptoms of women during the winter. The study population was women with low vitamin D levels, the independent variable was vitamin D_3 supplement, and the dependent variable was depressive symptoms. A physiological framework was used to guide the development of this study and included both a framework model (Figure 7–4) and description. Shipowick et al. (2009) described their model in the following way:

> Vitamin D_3 is hydroxylated in the liver to become 25-OH vitamin D, the major circulating form of vitamin D. It is activated in the kidneys to become the hormone 1,25-OH vitamin D where it is tightly regulated. Certain organs including the brain also have the capacity to activate vitamin D (Holick & Jenkins, 2003). Both unactivated and activated vitamin D can cross the blood-brain barrier (Kiraly, Kiraly, Hawe, & Makhani, 2006). Based on these data, a biopsychological framework of vitamin D as a hormone that influences depressive symptoms served as an emerging model (Figure 7–4). Three physiological pathways between vitamin D and depressive symptoms were identified: (a) Vitamin D in the active form in the body had been shown to stimulate serotonin (Gaines, 2005), a neurotransmitter that is associated with mood elevation; (b) Vitamin D has been associated with down-regulation of glucocorticoid receptor gene activation, which is found to be up-regulated in depression; and (c) Vitamin D has also been found to be neuroprotective, shielding neurons from toxins such as glucocorticoids and other excitotoxic insults (Obradovic, Gronemeyer, Lutz, & Rein, 2006). (Shipowick et al., 222)

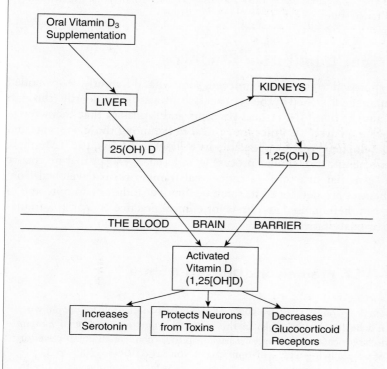

Figure 7–4. The biopsychological model of vitamin D: hormone that elevates mood. Shipowick, C. D., Moore, C. B., Corbett, C., & Bindler, R. (2009). Vitamin D and depressive symptoms in women during the winter: A pilot study. *Applied Nursing Research, 22*(3), 222.

Continued

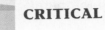

CRITICAL APPRAISAL

The framework section is a major strength of this study. Shipowick and colleagues (2009) provided a clear, concise, appropriate physiological framework for their study. The biopsychological model presented in the study provides a clear link of how vitamin D as a hormone elevates mood and decreases depressive symptoms. The study framework also provided clear conceptual definitions of the independent and dependent variables and these conceptual definitions provided a basis for operationalizing these variables in this study. The depressive symptoms were measured with the Beck Depression Inventory II and the women's vitamin D levels were determined with the serum 25-OH vitamin D levels. Both of these measurement methods are strong. The link of the study findings to the framework needed to be stronger.

IMPLICATIONS FOR NURSING PRACTICE

Shipowick et al. (2009) provided strong recommendations for future research and indicated additional research was needed before implementation in practice. However they did state the "study provided evidence to suggest that women who suffer from seasonal depressive symptoms may benefit from vitamin D_3 supplementation if serum vitamin D levels are low (<40 ng/ml). These findings are consistent with other studies that indicated that higher vitamin D levels improve sense of well-being" (Shipowick et al., 2009, p. 225). The complete study is included in Chapter 12 and a critical appraisal of the entire study is provided. We encourage you to read the study and the critical appraisal to strengthen your expertise in determining the quality of a quantitative study.

Frameworks Derived from Qualitative Studies

In qualitative studies, the approach to theorizing proceeds somewhat differently. In grounded theory research, for example, the first step in the data analysis process is to identify (through the development of substantive codes) the critical concepts and processes that characterize the phenomenon. Subsequent analysis identifies the critical links among those concepts and processes, leading to the development of a grounded theory (Glaser & Strauss, 1967; Munhall, 2007). In descriptive phenomenology, a similar process is undertaken except that no theory is developed—rather the "essential structure" (a conceptual framework) is developed from the data. Middle range theories are developed in some qualitative studies as an outcome of the study. These theories can then be used as a basis for clinical practice and/or as a framework in other qualitative or quantitative studies.

RESEARCH EXAMPLE Framework Derived from a Qualitative Study

Noiseux and Ricard (2008) conducted a grounded theory study of recovery as perceived by people with schizophrenia, family members, and health professionals. In this study, the nursing concept of human responses in situations of health/disease forms the "theoretical backdrop to or conceptual perspective for the study of the recovery process of people living with schizophrenia" (Noiseux & Ricard, 2008, p. 1150). Data for the study were obtained from people living with schizophrenia, their family members, and health professionals. There were 16 people with schizophrenia, eight women and eight men. Fifteen of the 16 participants were taking antipsychotic medication. Five family members were recruited and 20 health professionals (three psychiatrists, eight nurses, and nine educators). Data were collected through semi-structured interviews and field notes. Example questions addressed self-evaluations of their mental health; perceptions of their recovery in biopsychosocial terms; and the personal, environmental, and organizational conditions that facilitated or impeded recovery.

Noiseux and Ricard (2008) described the process of recovery using the following seven categories:

1. Experiencing schizophrenia as a "descent into hell"
   - The enormous suffering resulting from schizophrenia
   - The collapse of hopes and dreams
   - Ostracism by family and friends
2. Igniting a spark of hope
   - Despondency over a symptom-dominated existence clashes with the desire to live
3. Developing insight
   - Searching for points of reference to rebuild the sense of self
   - Discovering sources of motivation that foster the desire to live
4. Activating the instinct to fight back
   - The will to break out of an existence governed by schizophrenia symptoms
   - Perseverance in the struggle for a new life
5. Discovering keys to well-being
   - Constant search for and experimentation with new strategies
6. Maintaining a constant equilibrium between internal and external forces
   - Internal and external interactions
   - Lack of structural coherence in social and healthcare services
7. Perceiving light at the end of the tunnel
   - Recognition of indices and signs of greater well-being (pp. 1152-1153)

Using these seven categories from the descriptive analysis, a middle range theory of the recovery process was developed. The focus of the theory is not on the disease and its destructiveness, but rather provides a theoretical explanation of recovery based on the inner attributes and resources of the individual (Noiseux & Ricard, 2008).

CRITICAL APPRAISAL

The newly developed middle range theory emerging from a qualitative study does not always have the structure of theories that are tested in quantitative studies. Theoretical concepts are not yet clearly identified or defined. Theoretical statements are not yet clearly composed. Quantitative methods of measuring concepts have not yet been developed. Additional qualitative work may be required before these theoretical elements are fully developed into a theory of recovery from schizophrenia.

IMPLICATIONS FOR PRACTICE

The authors suggest that it is important

to target clinical nursing interventions at the individuals with schizophrenia so that they can identify their own keys to well-being: identify points of reference from their past that will give them a new sense of self; identify sources of motivation despite their anguish; and restore themselves to the state they were in before the disease. (Noiseux & Ricard, 2008, p. 1160)

Frameworks Including Conceptual Nursing Models

Building a body of knowledge related to a particular conceptual model requires an organized program of research. This program of research is referred to as a research tradition. A group of scholars dedicated to conducting research related to the model develop theories compatible with the model, including propositions for testing. An organized plan for testing these propositions is agreed on. Researchers conducting studies consistent with a particular research tradition often maintain a network of communication regarding their work. In some cases annual conferences focused on the model are held to share research findings, explore theoretical ideas, and maintain network contacts. Most of the conceptual models of nursing do not have well-established research traditions. However, research traditions are being developed for some of the nursing conceptual models (Fawcett, 2005; Tomey & Alligood, 2006).

RESEARCH EXAMPLE Framework Including Conceptual Nursing Model

One example of a nursing model with an emerging research tradition is the Roy Adaptation Model (RAM) (Roy & Andrews, 1999). Adaptation is the central concept in the RAM. "Adapting is the process whereby thinking and feeling people use conscious awareness and choice to create human and environmental integration" (Weinert, Cudney, & Spring, 2008, p. 364). Four major concepts are focal stimulus, contextual stimuli, coping mechanisms, and self-concept. Lévesque, Ricard, Ducharme, Duquette, and Bonin (1998) define these concepts as follows:

- Contextual stimuli: factors (internal and external) that can act on the person's perception of the focal stimulus.
- Coping mechanisms (cognator subsystem): information processing and judgment, which encompasses such activities as problem solving and decision making.
- Self-concept: the composite of beliefs and feelings that a person holds about himself or herself at a given time.

In 1999, the Boston-Based Adaptation in Nursing Research Society (BBARNS) conducted an analysis of the RAM based published research. Now (2009) they are conducting another analysis, this time combining research of the last ten years with the first analysis. These analyses are hoped to derive RAM knowledge that can be used as the theory is tested in future studies. All of the studies that are being examined have been designed to test the RAM.

Questions being asked are: (1) What has been shown in research to be accurate or valid in the propositions of the RAM? (2) What propositions have not been shown in research to be valid? (3) What measurement methods are being used to test the RAM? (4) What propositions of the theory have not yet been tested? Testing propositions of a conceptual nursing model requires including the conceptual model as well as a theory as the framework of the study.

RESEARCH EXAMPLE Framework Including Conceptual Nursing Model

Including a conceptual model as well as a theory in a framework is a relatively new idea in nursing. Therefore, few published studies have frameworks that include a conceptual model, a theory, and a conceptual map illustrating the linkage between the model and the theory. The map for such a framework must include both the conceptual model and a testable theory. Weinert and colleagues (2008) have conducted such a study in a paper entitled "Evolution of a conceptual model for adaptation to chronic illness." Their framework is shown in Figure 7–5. The purpose of the study was "to describe the evolution of 'The Women to Women Conceptual Model for Adaptation to Chronic Illness'. ... The Women to Women (WTW) is a computer-based research intervention designed to provide support and health information to middle-aged women who are chronically ill and live in rural areas of the western United States—Montana, Wyoming, North and South Dakota, Nebraska, Idaho, Oregon, and Washington" (Weinert et al., 2008, p. 365).

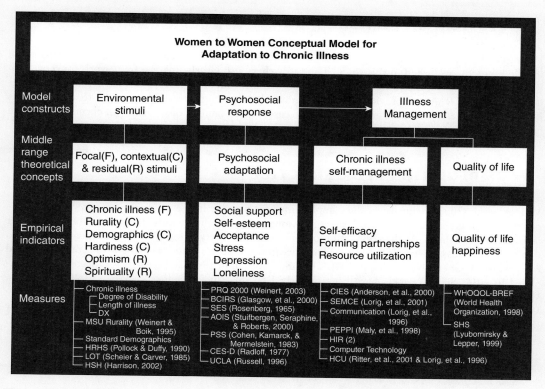

Figure 7–5. Women to women conceptual model for adaptation to chronic illness. Weinert, C., Cudney, S., & Spring, A. (2008). Evolution of a conceptual model for adaptation to chronic illness. *Journal of Nursing Scholarship, 40*(4), 366.

Continued

RESEARCH EXAMPLE—cont'd

"The study is being implemented in three phases, with the implementation of the next phase using knowledge gained from the previous phase. According to the authors "The path of the concepualization of the WTW project was traced from a single concept base to its present explanatory, multi-concept model consisting of three major adaptation model constructs (environmental stimuli, psychosocial response, and illness management) with related middle range theoretical concepts (focal, contextual, and residual stimuli, psychosocial adaptation, chronic illness self-management, and quality of life) including empirical indicators and measures for each (see Figure 7–5). The middle range theoretical concepts are useful because they are less abstract and address variables seen in particular situations that are empirically grounded and focused on practical problems and produce specific indications for practice" (Weinert et al., 2008, p. 370). The top line of the model includes the constructs from the Roy conceptual model of adaptation. The second line of the model includes the middle range theory with the selected concepts and relationships. The third line of the model includes the empirical indicators or study variables followed by their measure methods (see Figure 7–5).

CRITICAL APPRAISAL

Weinert and colleagues (2008) provided a clear link between the conceptual model of Roy (RAM) and the middle range theory tested in this study. The researchers also clearly link the framework concepts with the study variables and the variables with their measurement methods (see Figure 7–5). The studies conducted using the RAM are providing valuable knowledge that might be used by nurses to assist patients in clinical practice. The studies are providing increased understanding of women with chronic illness and how to manage their conditions using computer technology.

IMPLICATIONS FOR PRACTICE

Weinert et al. (2008) summarized their implications for practice in the following excerpt. "As the computer-based intervention is maturing, we are demonstrating its efficacy in helping rural women to better manage chronic illness. At the completion of this study, the intervention should be adequately tested so that it could be adapted for use by advanced practice nurses especially those working with people in isolated rural areas" (Weinert et al., 2008, p. 364). The studies began in 1995, and phase 3 is expected to be completed in 2010. Several papers have been published on this study (Cudney & Weinert, 2000; Cudney, Winters, Weinert, & Anderson, 2005; Hill, Schillo, & Weinert, 2004; Hill, Weinert, & Cudney, 2006; Weinert & Brandt, 1987; Weinert, Cudney & Winter, 2005). Look for more publications since 2008 by searching for the authors' names in CINAHL.

KEY CONCEPTS

- Theory is essential to research since it is the initial inspiration for developing a study and links the study findings back to the knowledge of the discipline.
- Theory is defined as an integrated set of defined concepts and statements that present a view of a phenomenon and can be used to describe, explain, predict, and control that phenomenon.

- The first step in understanding theories is to become familiar with the elements related to theoretical ideas and their application. These elements include the concepts, definitions of concepts, relational statements, and map or model.
- A conceptual model, similar to a theory but more abstract, broadly explains phenomena of interest, expresses assumptions, and reflects a philosophical stance.
- A framework is an abstract, logical structure of meaning, such as a portion of a theory, that guides the development of the study, is tested in the study, and enables the researcher to link the findings to nursing's body of knowledge.
- Every study has a framework, although some frameworks are poorly expressed or implicit.
- The framework must identify and define the concepts and the relational statements or propositions being tested and sometimes includes a model or map.
- Testing a theory involves determining the truth of each relational statement in the theory.
- Two types of theories are commonly used as frameworks for quantitative studies; they are middle range theories and practice or intervention theories.
- Middle range theories are less abstract and narrower in scope than conceptual models.
- Practice theories are even more specific than middle range theories and are designed to theoretically propose specific approaches to particular nursing practice situations.
- The theoretical basis for physiological studies is usually derived from physiology, genetics, pathophysiology, and physics and is scientific theory.
- Scientific theory has valid and reliable methods of measuring each concept, and its relational statements or propositions have been tested through research and found to be valid.
- Critically appraising a framework requires the identification and evaluation of the concepts, their definitions, and the statements linking the concepts.
- An organized program of research is important for building a body of knowledge related to the phenomena explained by a particular conceptual model.

REFERENCES

Ajzen, I. (1991). The theory of planned behavior. *Organizational Behaviour and Human Decision Processes, 50*(2), 179-211.

Apóstolo, J. L., & Kolcaba, K. (2009). The effects of guided imagery and comfort, depression, anxiety, and stress of psychiatric inpatients with depressive disorders. *Archives of Psychiatric Nursing, 23*(6), 403-411.

Artinian, B. (1982). Conceptual mapping. Development of the strategy. *Western Journal of Nursing Research, 4*(4), 379-393.

Backman, K. (2003). Middle-range theory development in nursing science: Self-care of home-dwelling elderly [Finnish]. *Holtotiede, 15*(3), 115-130.

Bandura, A. (1982). Self-efficacy mechanism in human agency. *American Psychologist, 37*(2), 122-147.

Bandura, A. (1986). *Social foundations of thought and action: A social cognitive theory.* Englewood Cliffs, NJ: Prentice-Hall.

Bandura, A. (1989). Regulation of cognitive processes through perceived self-efficacy. *Developmental Psychology, 25*(5), 729-735.

Bandura, A. (1997). *Self-efficacy: The exercise of control.* New York: W. H. Freeman.

Beck, C. T. (1993). Teetering on the edge: A substantive theory of postpartum depression. *Nursing Research, 42*(1), 42-48.

Becker, M. H. (1976). *Health belief model and personal health behavior.* Thorofare, NJ: Slack.

Bowlby, J. (1969). *Attachment and loss, vol. 1: Attachment.* London: Hogarth Press.

Bowlby, J. (1973). *Attachment and loss, vol. 2: Separation.* New York: Basic Books.

Brofenbrenner, U. (1978). *The ecology of human development: Experiments by nature and design.* Cambridge, MA: Harvard University Press.

Brown, S. J. (2009). *Evidence-based nursing: The research-practice connection.* Sudbury, MA: Jones & Bartlett.

Burns, N., & Grove, S. K. (2009). *The practice of nursing research: Appraisal, synthesis, and generation of evidence* (6th ed.). Philadelphia: Saunders.

Cazzell, M. (2008). Linking theory, evidence, and practice in assessment of adolescent inhalant use. *Journal of Addictions Nursing, 19*(1), 17-25.

Chenitz, W. C. (1983). Entry into a nursing home as status passage: A theory to guide nursing practice. *Geriatric Nursing, 4*(2), 92-97.

Chinn, P. L., & Kramer, M. K. (2008). *Integrated theory and knowledge development in nursing.* St. Louis: Mosby Elsevier.

Covell, C. L. (2008). The middle-range theory of nursing intellectual capital. *Journal of Advanced Nursing, 63*(1), 94-103.

Cudney, S., & Weinert, C. (2000). Computer-based support groups: Nursing in cyberspace. *Computers in Nursing, 18*(1), 35-43.

Cudney, S., Winters, C., Weinert, C., & Anderson, K. (2005). Social support in cyberspace: Lessons learned. *Rehabilitation Nursing, 30*(1), 25-29.

Craig, J. V., & Smyth, R. L. (2007). *The evidence-based practice manual for nurses* (2nd ed.). Edinburgh: Churchill Livingstone.

DiNapoli, P. P. (2009). Early initiation of tobacco use in adolescent girls: Key sociostructural influences. *Applied Nursing Research, 22*(2), 126-132.

Dorsey, C. J., & Murdaugh, C. L. (2003). The theory of self-care management for vulnerable populations. *Journal of Theory Construction & Testing, 7*(2), 43-49.

Dowd, T., Kolcaba, K., Steiner, R., & Fashinpaur, D. (2007). Comparison of a healing touch, coaching, and a combined intervention on comfort and stress in younger college students. *Holistic Nursing Practice, 21*(4), 194-202.

Dunn, K. S. (2004). Toward a middle-range theory of adaptation to chronic pain. *Nursing Science Quarterly, 17*(1), 78-84.

Dunn, K. S. (2005). Testing a middle-range theoretical model of adaptation to chronic pain. *Nursing Science Quarterly, 18*(2), 146-156.

Eakes, G. G., Burke, M. L., & Hainsworth, M. A. (1998). Middle-range theory of chronic sorrow. *Image-The Journal of Nursing Scholarship, 30*(2), 179-184.

Fawcett, J. (1999). *The relationship of theory and research* (3rd ed.). Philadelphia: F. A. Davis.

Fawcett, J. (2005). *Contemporary nursing knowledge: Analysis and evaluation of conceptual models and theories* (2nd ed.). Philadelphia: F. A. Davis.

Fawcett, J., & Garity, J. (2009). *Evaluating research for evidence-based nursing practice.* Philadelphia: F. A. Davis.

Fleury, J. D. (1991). Empowering potential: A theory of wellness motivation. *Nursing Research, 40*(4), 286-291.

Gaines, S. (2005). The saddest season. *Minnesota Medicine, 88*(1), 25-32.

Gift, A. G. (1992). Dyspnea. *Nursing Clinics of North America, 25*(4), 955-965.

Glaser, B. G., & Strauss, A. (1967). *The discovery of grounded theory: Strategies for qualitative research.* Chicago: Aldine.

Good, M. A. (1998). A middle range theory of acute pain management: Use in research. *Nursing Outlook, 46*(3), 120-124.

Good, M., & Moore, S. M. (1996). Clinical practice guidelines as a new source of middle range theory: Focus on acute pain. *Nursing Outlook, 44*(2), 74-79.

Hill, W., Schillo, L., & Weinert, C. (2004). Effects of a computer-based intervention on social support for chronically ill rural women. *Rehabilitation Nursing, 29*(5), 169-173.

Hill, W., Weinert, C., & Cudney, S. (2006). Influence of a computer intervention on the psychological status of chronically ill rural women: Preliminary results. *Nursing Research, 55*(1), 34-42.

Holick, M., & Jenkins, M. (2003). *The UV advantage.* New York: Ibooks Inc.

Huth, M. M., & Moore, S. M. (1998). Prescriptive theory of acute pain management in infants and children. *Journal of the Society of Pediatric Nurses, 3*(1), 23-32.

Jenerette, C. M. (2004). *Testing the theory of self-care management for vulnerable populations in a sample of adults with sickle cell disease.* Doctoral dissertation. University of South Carolina.

Jezewski, M. A. (1995). Evolution of a grounded theory: Conflict resolution through culture brokering. *Advances in Nursing Science, 17*(3), 14-30.

Jirovec, M. M., Jenkins, J., Isenberg, M., & Baiardi, J. (1999). Urine control theory derived from Roy's conceptual framework. *Nursing Science Quarterly, 12*(3), 251-255.

Johnson, B. M., & Webber, P. B. (2005). *An introduction to theory and reasoning in nursing* (2nd ed.). Philadelphia: Lippincott Williams & Wilkins.

Kiraly, S., Kiraly, M., Hawe, R., & Makhani, N. (2006). Vitamin D as a neuroactive substance: Review. *Scientific World Journal, 6*(2), 125-139.

Kolcaba, K. (1994). A theory of comfort for nursing. *Journal of Advanced Nursing, 19*(6), 1178-1184.

Lazarus, R., & Folkman, S. (1984). *Stress, appraisal, and coping.* New York: Springer.

Lenz, E. R., Pugh, C., Milligan, R. A., Gift, A. G., & Suppe, F. (1997). The middle-range theory of unpleasant symptoms: An update. *Advances in Nursing Science, 19*(3), 14-27.

Lévesque, L., Ricard, N., Ducharme, F., Duquette, A., & Bonin, J. (1998). Empirical verification of a theoretical model derived from the Roy Adaptation Model: Findings from five studies. *Nursing Science Quarterly, 11*(1), 31-39.

Lenz, E. R., Pugh, L. C., Milligan, R., Gift, A., & Suppe, F. (1997). The middle range theory of unpleasant symptoms: An update. *Advances in Nursing Science, 19*(3), 14-27.

Liehr, P., & Smith, M. J. (1999). Middle range theory: Spinning research and practice to create knowledge for the new millennium. *Advances in Nursing Science, 21*(4), 81-91.

Luce, G. (1970). *Biological rhythms in psychiatry and medicine.* Washington, DC: U.S. Public Health Service.

McCaffery, M. (1972). *Nursing management of the patient with pain.* Philadelphia: Lippincott.

Mercer, R. T. (1986). *First time motherhood: Experiences from teens to forties.* New York: Springer.

Mishel, M. H. (1988). Uncertainty in illness. *Journal of Nursing Scholarship, 20*(4), 225-232.

Mishel, M. H. (1990). Reconceptualization of the uncertainty in illness theory. *Image: Journal of Nursing Scholarship, 22*(3), 256-262.

Moody, L. E. (1989). Building a conceptual map to guide research. *Florida Nursing Review, 4*(1), 1.

Munhall, P. L. (2007). *Nursing research: A qualitative perspective* (4th ed.). Sudbury, MA: Jones & Bartlett.

Newman, M. A. (1979). *Theory development in nursing.* Philadelphia: F. A. Davis.

Neuman, B. (1995). *The Neuman systems model* (3rd ed.). Norwalk, CT: Appleton & Lange.

Noiseux, S., & Ricard, N. (2008). Recovery as perceived by people with schizophrenia, family members and health professionals: A grounded theory. *International Journal of Nursing Studies, 45*(2008), 1148-1162.

Obradovic, D., Gronemeyer, H., Lutz, V., & Rein, T. (2006). Cross-talk of vitamin D and glucocorticoids in hippocampal cells. *Journal of Neurochemistry, 96*(2), 500-509.

Olson, J., & Hanchett, E. (1997). Nurse expressed empathy, patient outcomes, and development of a middle-range theory. *Journal of Nursing Scholarship, 29*(1), 71-76.

Orem, D. E. (1995). *Nursing: Concepts of practice* (5th ed.). St. Louis: Mosby.

Orem, D. E. (2001). *Nursing: Concepts of practice* (6th ed.). St. Louis: Mosby.

Orticio, L. P. (2007). Sensing presence and sensing space: A middle range theory of nursing. *Insight: The Journal of the American Society of Ophthalmic Registered Nurses, 32*(4), 7-11.

Pender, N. J. (1982). *Health promotion in nursing practice.* Norwalk, CT: Appleton-Century-Crofts.

Pender, N. J., Murdaugh, C. L., & Parsons, M. A. (2001). *Health promotion in nursing practice* (4th ed.). Upper Saddle River, NJ: Pearson & Prentice Hall.

Pender, N. J., Murdaugh, C. L., & Parsons, M. A. (2006). *Health promotion in nursing practice* (5th ed.). Upper Saddle River, NJ: Pearson & Prentice Hall.

Perez, A., & Fleury, J. (2008). Wellness Motivation Theory in practice. *Geriatric Nursing, 30*(25), 15-20.

Peterson, S. J., & Bredow, T. S. (2004). *Middle range theories: Application to nursing research.* Philadelphia: Lippincott Williams & Wilkins.

Polk, L. V. (1997). Toward a middle-range theory of resilience. *Advances in Nursing Science, 19*(3), 1-13.

Purnell, L. (2005). The Purnell Model for cultural competence. *Journal for Multicultural Nursing & Health, 11*(2), 7-15.

Quinn, A. A. (1991). A theoretical model of the perimenopausal process. *Journal of Nurse-Midwifery, 36*(1), 25-29.

Ray, M. (1989). The theory of bureaucratic caring for nursing practice in the organizational culture. *Nursing Administration Quarterly, 13*(2), 31-42.

Register, M. E., & Herman, J. (2006). A middle range theory for generative quality of life for the elderly. *Advances in Nursing Sciences, 29*(4), 340-350.

Roy, C., & Andrews, H. A. (1999). *Roy Adaptation Model.* Norwalk, CT: Appleton & Lange.

Roy, C., & Roberts, S. L. (1981). *Theory construction in nursing: An adaptation model.* Englewood Cliffs, NJ: Prentice-Hall.

Ruland, C. M., & Moore, S. M. (1998). Theory construction based on standards of care: A proposed theory of the peaceful end of life. *Nursing Outlook, 46*(4), 169-175.

Selye, H. (1976). *The stress of life.* New York: McGraw-Hill.

Shipowick, C. D., Moore, C. B., Corbett, C., & Bindler, R. (2009). Vitamin D and depressive symptoms in women during the winter: A pilot study. *Applied Nursing Research, 22*(3), 221-225.

Smith, C. E., Pace, K., Kochinda, C., Kleinbeck, S., Koehler, J., & Popkess-Vawter, S. (2002). Caregiver effectiveness model evolution to a midrange theory of home care: A process for critique and replication. *Advances in Nursing Science, 25*(1), 50-64.

Smith, M. J., & Liehr, P. R. (2008). *Middle range theory for nursing* (2nd ed.). New York: Springer.

Swanson, K. M. (1991). Empirical development of a middle range theory of caring. *Nursing Research, 40*(3), 161-166.

Tomey, A. M., & Alligood, M. R. (2006). *Nursing theorists and their work* (6th ed.). St. Louis: Mosby.

Tsai, P. (2003). A middle-range theory of caregiver stress. *Nursing Science Quarterly, 16*(2), 137-145.

Tsai, P., Tak, S., Moore, C., & Palencia, I. (2003). Testing a theory of chronic pain. *Journal of Advanced Nursing, 43*(2), 158-169.

University of California, San Francisco School of Nursing Symptom Management Group. (1994). A model for symptom management. *Image—Journal of Nursing Scholarship, 26*(4), 272-276.

Wilson, I. B., & Cleary, P. D., (1995). Linking clinical variables and health-related quality of life: A conceptual model of patient outcomes. *Journal of American Medical Association, 273*(1), 59-65.

Watson, J. (1985). *Nursing: Human science and human care. A theory of nursing.* Norwalk, CT: Appleton & Lange.

Weinert, C., & Brandt, P. (1987). Measuring social support with the Personal Resource Questionnaire. *Western Journal of Nursing Research, 9*(4), 589-602.

Weinert, C., Cudney, S., & Spring, A. (2008). Evolution of a conceptual model for adaptation to chronic illness. *Journal of Nursing Scholarship, 40*(4), 364-372.

Weinert, C., Cudney, S., & Winter, C. (2005). Social support in cyberspace: The next generation. *Computers, Informatics, Nursing, 23*(1), 7-15.

Whittemore, R., & Roy, C. (2002). Adapting to diabetes mellitus: A theory synthesis. *Nursing Science Quarterly, 15*(4), 311-317.

Wilson, M. (2005). Health-promoting behaviors of sheltered homeless women. *Family & Community Health, 28*(1), 51-63.

8

Clarifying Quantitative Research Designs

Chapter Overview

Concepts Important to Design 253
  Causality 253
  Multicausality 254
  Probability 254
  Bias 254
  Control 255
  Manipulation 255
Designs for Descriptive and Correlational Nursing Studies 256

  Descriptive Design 256
  Correlational Design 264
Testing Causality 270
  Quasi-experimental Designs 270
  Experimental Designs 276
Defining Experimental Interventions 282
Mapping the Design 284
Role of Replication Studies in Evidence-Based Practice 285

Learning Outcomes

After completing this chapter, you should be able to:

1. Identify the designs of published studies.
2. Critically appraise the quality of designs of quantitative nursing studies.

3. Select studies sufficiently well designed to provide evidence on which practice can be based.
4. Model designs of published studies.

Key Terms

Bias, p. 254
Case study design, p. 262
Causality, p. 253
Comparative descriptive design, p. 260
Control, p. 255
Correlational design, p. 264
Descriptive correlational design, p. 264

Descriptive design, p. 256
Experimental designs, p. 276
Intervention, p. 282
Manipulation, p. 255
Model testing design, p. 268
Multicausality, p. 254
Observation, p. 255

Predictive correlational design, p. 266
Probability, p. 254
Quasi-experimental design, p. 270
Randomized clinical trial, p. 280
Replication studies, p. 285
Research design, p. 253

STUDY TOOLS

Be sure to visit http://evolve.elsevier.com/Burns/understanding for additional examples and self-tests. Also, a review of this chapter's concepts and practice exercises can be found in Chapter 8 of the Study Guide for *Understanding Nursing Research: Building an Evidence-Based Practice,* 5th edition.

A research design is a blueprint for conducting a study. The purpose of a design is to maximize control over factors that can interfere with the validity of the study findings. Just as the blueprint for a house must be individualized to the specific house being built, so must the design be made specific to a study. The control provided by the design increases the probability that the quantitative or outcomes study results will accurately reflect reality.

To critically appraise studies, you must learn how to identify the study design and evaluate threats to validity resulting from design flaws. Validity is important because studies must be well designed to contribute strong research evidence for practice (Brown, 2009). Designs that provide evidence that nursing interventions are effective in achieving desired outcomes are particularly important.

As background information necessary to identify and critically appraise designs of published studies, this chapter includes the concepts important to design, identifies some designs commonly used in nursing studies, and describes the elements of a good design. The chapter also includes content related to defining experimental interventions, mapping designs, and identifying replication studies.

Concepts Important to Design

Many terms used in discussing research design have special meanings within this context. Understanding the meanings of these concepts is critical to understanding the purpose of a specific design. Some of the major concepts used in research design for quantitative and outcomes research are causality, multicausality, probability, bias, control, manipulation, and validity.

Causality

Causality basically says that things have causes, and causes lead to effects. Not all studies examine cause and effect. Studies may describe specific variables, or examine relationships among the variables. In a critical appraisal, you must determine whether the purpose of the study is to examine causality, examine relationships among variables, or describe variables. You may be able to determine whether the purpose of a study is to examine causality by reading the purpose statement and the propositions within the framework. For example, the purpose of a causal study may be to examine the effect of a specific preoperative educational program on length of hospital stay. The proposition may state that preoperative teaching results in a decreased hospitalization period. Preoperative teaching is not the only factor affecting length of hospital stay. Other important factors include the diagnosis, type of surgery, patient's age, physical condition of the patient prior to surgery, and complications that occurred after surgery. However, from the perspective of causality, it is important to design the study so that the effect of a single cause—in this case, a preoperative education program—can be examined apart from the other factors affecting length of hospital stay.

Multicausality

Very few phenomena in nursing can be clearly linked to a single cause and a single effect. A number of interrelating variables can be involved in producing a particular effect. Thus, studies developed from a multicausal perspective will include more variables than those using a strict causal orientation. The presence of multiple causes for an effect is referred to as multicausality. For example, diagnosis, patient age, patient pre-surgical condition, and complications after surgery will be involved in causing the length of hospital stay. Because of the complexity of causal relationships, a theory is unlikely to identify every element involved in causing a particular phenomenon. However, the greater the proportion of causal factors that can be identified and examined in a single study, the clearer the understanding will be of the overall phenomenon. This greater understanding is expected to increase the ability to predict and control the effect.

Probability

Probability addresses relative rather than absolute causality. A cause may not produce a specific effect each time that particular cause occurs. Thus, researchers recognize that a particular cause *probably* will result in a specific effect. Using a probability orientation, researchers design studies to examine the probability that a given effect will occur under a defined set of circumstances. The circumstances may be variations in multiple variables.

For example, while assessing the effect of multiple variables on length of hospitalization, the researcher may choose to examine the probability of a given length of hospital stay under a variety of specific sets of circumstances. One specific set of circumstances may be that the patient had 15 minutes of preoperative teaching, underwent a specific type of surgery, was a certain age, had a particular level of health before surgery, and experienced a specific complication. The probability of a given length of hospital stay could be expected to vary as the set of circumstances vary. When examining probability, the researcher finds that hypotheses are complex, with multiple variables.

Bias

The term bias means a slant or deviation from the true or expected. Bias in a study distorts the findings from what the results would have been without the bias. Because studies are conducted to determine the real and the true, researchers place great value on identifying and removing sources of bias in their study or controlling their effects on the study findings. Quantitative designs are developed to reduce the possibility and effects of bias. Any component of a study that deviates or causes a deviation from a true measurement of the study variables contributes to distorted findings. Many factors related to research can be biased; these include attitudes or motivations of the researcher (conscious or unconscious), the components of the environment in which the study is conducted, selection of the individual subjects, composition of the sample, the groups formed, the measurement tools, the data collection process, the data, and the statistical analyses.

For example, some of the subjects for the study might be taken from a unit of the hospital in which the patients are participating in another study involving high-quality nursing care;

or one nurse, selecting patients for the study, might assign the patients who are most interested in the study to the experimental group. Each of these situations introduces bias to the study.

An important focus in critically appraising a study is to identify possible sources of bias. This requires careful examination of the researcher's report of the study methods, including strategies for obtaining subjects, implementing a study treatment, and performing measurements. However, not all biases can be identified from the published report of a study. The article may not provide sufficient detail about the methods of the study to detect all of the biases.

Control

One method of reducing bias is to increase the amount of control in the design of quantitative studies. Control means having the power to direct or manipulate factors to achieve a desired outcome. For example, in a study of preoperative teaching, subjects may be randomly selected and then randomly assigned to the experimental or control group. The researcher may control the duration of preoperative teaching sessions or intervention, the content taught, the method of teaching, and the teacher. The time that the teaching occurred in relation to surgery also may be controlled, as well as the environment in which it occurred. Measurement of the length of hospital stay may be controlled by ensuring that the number of days or hours was calculated exactly in the same way for each subject. Limiting the characteristics of subjects, such as diagnosis, age, type of surgery, and incidence of complications, is a form of control. Control is particularly important in experimental and quasi-experimental quantitative studies. The greater the researcher's control over the study situation, the more credible (or valid) the study findings. The purpose of research designs is to maximize control of elements in the study.

Manipulation

Manipulation is a form of control used most commonly in experimental or quasi-experimental research. Controlling the treatment or intervention is the most commonly used manipulation. For example, in a study of the effects of preoperative teaching, the situation might be manipulated so that one group of subjects received preoperative teaching and another did not. In a study on oral care, the frequency of care might be manipulated.

When experimental designs are used to explore causal relationships in nursing research, the nurse must be free to manipulate the variables under study. If the freedom to manipulate a variable (e.g., the type, amount, or frequency of pain control measures) is under someone else's control (e.g., a physician or the staff nurses), a bias is introduced into the study. Thus, the treatment each subject receives may differ. The researcher will then be, so to speak, comparing apples and oranges or comparing two different things. In descriptive and correlational studies, little or no effort is made to manipulate factors in the circumstances of the study. Instead, the purpose is to examine the situation as it exists. As a result of the subjective nature of observation, the possibility that bias will influence findings is greater in these types of studies.

CRITICAL APPRAISAL GUIDELINES

Study Design

When critically appraising a study, ask the following questions:

1. Is the study design descriptive, correlational, quasi-experimental, or experimental?
2. If the design is descriptive, what is the descriptive design?
3. If the design is correlational, what is the correlational design?
4. If the design is quasi-experimental or experimental, what is the quasi-experimental or experimental design?
5. If the design is quasi-experimental or experimental, which elements are controlled and what elements could have been controlled to improve the study design? What was the feasibility of controlling particular elements of the study.

Designs for Descriptive and Correlational Nursing Studies

A variety of study designs are used in nursing research; the four types most commonly used are descriptive, correlational, quasi-experimental, and experimental. Descriptive and correlational studies examine variables in natural environments and do not include treatments provided by the researcher. Quasi-experimental and experimental studies are designed to examine cause and effect. These studies are conducted to examine differences in dependent variables that are thought to be caused by independent variables (treatments). This section briefly describes the four types of designs and provides specific examples of each. More detail on specific designs is available in other sources (Burns & Grove, 2009).

The algorithm shown in Figure 8–1 may be used to determine the type of study design for a published study. The algorithm includes a series of yes or no responses to specific questions about the design. The algorithm starts with the question, "Is there a treatment?" The answer leads to the next question, with the four types of design being identified in the algorithm. Then a second algorithm provided for each type of design (descriptive, correlational, quasi-experimental, and experimental) can be used to identify the specific design used in the study.

Descriptive Design

The descriptive study is designed to gain more information about characteristics within a particular field of study. Its purpose is to provide a picture of a situation as it naturally happens. A descriptive design may be used to develop theories, identify problems with current practice, justify current practice, make judgments, or determine what other nurses in similar situations are doing. No manipulation of variables is involved in a descriptive design. In many aspects of nursing, a clearer picture of the phenomenon is needed before causality can be examined. Protection against bias is achieved through (1) conceptual and operational definitions of variables, (2) sample selection and size, (3) valid and reliable instruments, and (4) data collection procedures that partially control the environment. Descriptive studies differ in level of complexity. Some contain only two variables; others may include multiple variables.

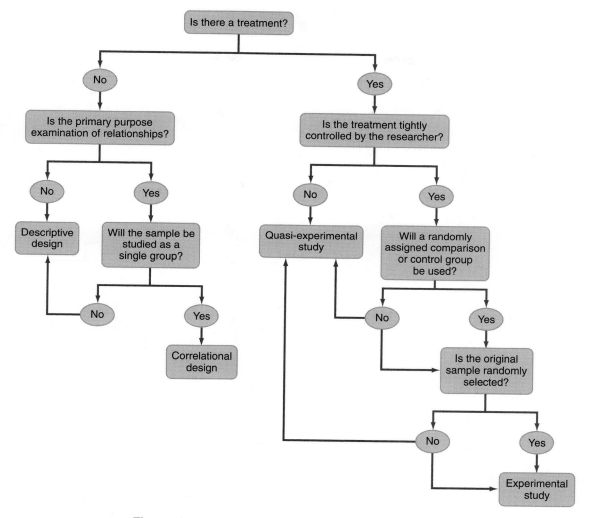

Figure 8–1. Algorithm for determining the type of study design.

Use the algorithm shown in Figure 8–2 to determine the type of descriptive design used in a published study.

Typical Descriptive Design

The most commonly used design in the category of descriptive studies is presented in Figure 8–3. The design is used to examine characteristics of a single sample. The descriptive design includes identifying a phenomenon of interest, identifying the variables within the phenomenon, developing conceptual and operational definitions of the variables, and describing the variables. The description of the variables leads to an interpretation of the theoretical meaning of the findings and the development of hypotheses.

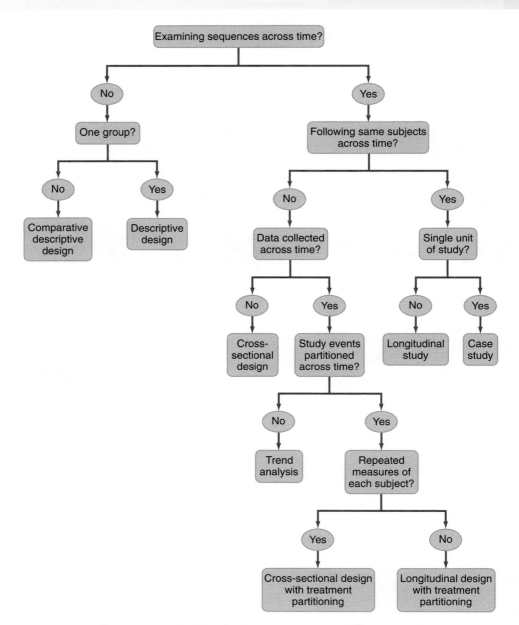

Figure 8–2. Algorithm for determining type of descriptive design.

CLARIFICATION ⟶ MEASUREMENT ⟶ DESCRIPTION ⟶ INTERPRETATION

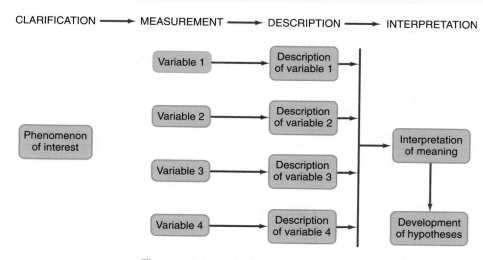

Figure 8-3. Typical descriptive design.

RESEARCH EXAMPLE

Feider, Mitchell, and Bridges (2010) published a study examining the oral care provided by RNs to orally ventilated patients. The study was published in the American Journal of Critical Care. The abstract of the study follows.

"Background Ventilator-associated pneumonia is a major threat to patients receiving mechanical ventilation in hospitals. Oral care is a nursing intervention that may help prevent ventilator-associated pneumonia.

Objectives: To describe oral care practices performed by critical care nurses for orally intubated critically ill patients and compare these practices with recommendations for oral care in the 2005 AACN Procedure Manual for Critical Care and the guidelines from the Centers for Disease Control and Prevention. Methods: A descriptive, cross-sectional design with a 31-item Web-based survey was used to describe oral care practices reported by 347 randomly selected members of the American Association of Critical-Care Nurses.

Results: Oral care was performed every 2 (50%) or 4 (42%) hours, usually with foam swabs (97%). Oral care was reported as a high priority (47%). Nurses with 7 years or more of critical care experience performed oral care more often ($P = .008$) than did less experienced nurses. Nurses with a bachelor's degree in nursing used foam swabs ($P = .001$), suctioned the mouth before the endotracheal tube ($P = .02$), and suctioned after oral care ($P < .001$) more often than other nurses. Nurses whose units had an oral care policy (72%) reported that the policy indicated using a toothbrush (63%), using toothpaste (40%), brushing with a foam swab (90%), using chlorhexidine gluconate oral rinse (49%), suctioning the oral cavity (84%), and assessing the oral cavity (73%). Oral care practices and policies differed for all those items. Conclusions: Survey results indicate that discrepancies exist between reported practices and policies. Oral care policies appear to be present, but not well used. (p. 175)

Continued

CRITICAL APPRAISAL

Study Design

1. Is the study design descriptive, correlational, quasi-experimental, or experimental?
   This is a descriptive study.

2. Did the study make comparisons?
   The researchers compared the AACCN Procedure Manual guidelines for oral care with the care provided by the nurses.

 IMPLICATIONS FOR PRACTICE

The authors found that most RNs had access to the AACCN guidelines but most did not follow the guidelines regarding the provision of oral care.

Comparative Descriptive Design

The **comparative descriptive design** (Figure 8–4) is used to describe variables and to examine differences in variables in two or more groups that occur naturally in a setting. A comparative descriptive design compares descriptive data obtained from each group and compares it in quantitative and outcomes studies. Some of the data may be measures such as marital status, job, diagnosis, age, education. The results obtained from these analyses are frequently not generalized to a population.

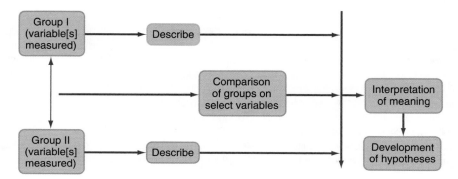

Figure 8–4. Comparative descriptive design.

RESEARCH EXAMPLE Comparative Descriptive Design

An evaluation of the hand and nasal flora of Turkish nursing students after clinical practice (Akpinar, Celebioglu, Uslu, & Uyanik, 2009).

Aim: The purpose of this study was to evaluate and compare the hand and nasal flora of nursing students before and after the clinical practice.

Background: Hospitals are places in which infective agents abound. Healthcare workers, relatives of patients, and students practicing in the hospital medium are often exposed to these infective agents. Although the role of the hand and nasal flora of healthcare workers in the development of nosocomial infections has been emphasized by earlier studies, there are a limited number of studies that investigate the hand and nasal flora of nursing students.

Design: Comparative Descriptive.

What is being compared? Infective agents on hand and nasal flora of nursing students.

Methods: This descriptive study involved 66 volunteer nursing students. Two samples of flora from both hands and nose of each student were obtained. The inoculated samples were then evaluated through routine bacteriological study methods. Chi-square and percentage calculations were used in comparisons.

Results: None of the students had methicillin-resistant *Staphylococcus aureus* or methicillin-resistant coagulase-negative *Staphylococcus* colonization in the hand samples before clinical practice, 6.1% of the students had methicillin-resistant *Staphylococcus aureus* and 4.5% had methicillin-resistant coagulase-negative *Staphylococcus* colonization after the practice. Although the differences between the rates of contamination with pathogen microorganisms in the hand and nasal flora of the student nurses before and after clinical practice were not significant, the rate of colonization after clinical practice was higher.

Conclusions: In this study, the rate of colonization after clinical practice was higher. These findings indicate that students might have been contaminated with bacteria during clinical practice.

Relevance to clinical practice: The results of this study have practical importance in clinical practice. The role of the hand and nasal flora of nursing students in the development of nosocomial infections is significant. For this reason, some precautions, such as using gloves and handwashing with special solutions when needed, should be taken to prevent nosocomial infections and protect students against associated risks. (p. 426)

CRITICAL APPRAISAL

Study Design

1. Is the study design descriptive, correlational, quasi-experimental, or experimental?
   Descriptive—this excellent descriptive study reveals some information very important to clinical practice and leads to some important questions.

2. If the design is descriptive, what is the descriptive design?
   A comparative descriptive design is used. The cultures before and after clinical practice are compared.

Continued

IMPLICATIONS FOR PRACTICE

Handwashing techniques used by nursing students (and probably other hospital staff) are not sufficient to protect the student or other patients from exposure to pathogenic organisms. Strategies used to teach effective techniques of handwashing and other measures to avoid contamination with pathogenic organisms are not adequate, at least in the hospitals used in the study. The authors suggest that it may be necessary to use precautions in addition to handwashing for protection.

Before using this information in practice, multiple studies need to be conducted in a variety of settings and a synthesis of all of the studies on the effectiveness of handwashing by nurses in healthcare facilities should be examined.

Descriptive Case Study Design

A case study design examines a single unit within the context of its real-life environment. The unit may be a person, a family, a nursing unit, or an organization. Although the number of subjects tends to be small, the number of variables in a case study usually is large. In fact, it is important to examine all variables that may have an impact on the situation being studied.

In the early twentieth century, the most common nursing study was a case study. Medical case studies were also common. Nursing case studies were published in the *American Journal of Nursing* and initiated a variety of nursing studies of patient care. As nursing research began to use more rigorous methods, the case study fell into disrepute. However, the importance of information from case studies is again being recognized. Case studies can use quantitative, qualitative, or mixed methods of data collection. It is important for the researcher to consider the multiple aspects that affect a particular case and include this essential information in the plan for data collection and analysis.

Well-designed case studies are a good source of descriptive information and can be used as evidence to support or invalidate theories. Information from a variety of sources can be collected on each concept of interest using different data collection methods. Case studies may use physiologic measures and/or valid psychosocial measures. This strategy can greatly expand the understanding of the phenomenon under study. Case studies also are useful for demonstrating the effectiveness of a therapeutic technique. In fact, the reporting of a case study can be the vehicle by which the technique is introduced to other practitioners. The case study design also has potential for revealing important findings that can generate new hypotheses for testing. Thus, the case study can lead to the design of large sample studies to examine factors identified by the case study.

The case study design depends on the circumstances of the case but usually includes an element of time. The researcher typically explores the subject's history and previous behavior patterns in detail. As the case study proceeds, the researcher may become aware of components important to the focus of the study that were not originally included in the study. Both quantitative and qualitative elements are likely to be incorporated into the case study design.

RESEARCH EXAMPLE Descriptive Case Study Design

A case study was used by Wardell, Rintala, and Tan (2008) to study the effect of healing touch with veterans experiencing chronic neuropathic pain from spinal cord injury.

Spinal cord injury often results in chronic pain syndromes that conventional pain management is unable to resolve. Healing Touch (HT) is a biofield therapy that involves using the hands to promote healing and mediate the perception of pain by affecting the energy field of the person. The practice of HT is based on the premise that the energy field has the ability to provide valuable information about the person's physical, emotional, mental, and spiritual condition and can influence the dense matter of physical form. (p. 187)

A qualitative case study approach was used to describe the experience of the patient and practitioner and to elicit information about the influence of HT on the energy field. The case study method was used because it is a complex entity operating with a number of contexts—from the physical to the ascetic (Stake, 1998). Further, the use of collective cases is an epistemological function to provide focus and understanding of a phenomenon. Pattern recognition is used to determine similarities and differences (Morse, 1994). Empirical evidence from systematic and qualitative inquiry from a series of six weekly HT sessions, including documentation from a CHTP (Certified Healing Touch Practitioner), narrative comments from interview data, and assessments for pain, were analyzed.

Two of seven cases were selected to represent cases of the experiences of the participants. These were reported as either beneficial or equivocal experience. The beneficial case demonstrates the participant finding the sessions helpful and experiencing an improved energy field pattern. The equivocal case exhibits evidence of improvement in the energy field, but this was attributed by the participant to something besides the sessions.

Data from a variety of sources were utilized in the case study process as a method of triangulation and to elucidate the qualitative findings to provide as complete a view of the energy experience as possible (Stake, 1995, 1998). This included observational recordings of the CHTPs of the energy field pretreatment and posttreatments, participant interviews, and pretest and posttest subjective measures of pain. Reliability and validity were enhanced by feedback provided during focus groups and by having the findings reviewed by a full-time CHTP with over 10 years of experience. (p. 189)

CRITICAL APPRAISAL

Study Design

1. Is the study design descriptive, correlational, quasi-experimental, or experimental?
   This is a descriptive study.

2. If the design is descriptive, what is the descriptive design?
   A case study design is used. This is a carefully planned study designed to examine areas of practice that are difficult to study.

Continued

IMPLICATIONS FOR PRACTICE

There are alternatives for pain relief when the traditional ones fail. These methods work well for some but not for others. Those without adequate pain relief should be informed of alternative approaches to pain relief (Wardell et al., 2008). The study findings will require a larger body of work before use in clinical practice.

Correlational Design

The purpose of a **correlational design** is to examine relationships between or among two or more variables in a single group in a quantitative study. This examination can occur at any of several levels: descriptive correlational, in which the researcher can seek to describe a relationship; predictive correlational, in which the researcher can predict relationships among variables; or the model testing design, in which all of the relationships proposed by a theory are tested simultaneously.

In correlational designs, a large range in the variable scores is necessary to determine the existence of a relationship. Thus, the sample should reflect the full range of scores possible on the variables being measured. Some subjects should have very high scores and others very low scores, and the scores of the rest should be distributed throughout the possible range. Because of the need for a wide variation on scores, correlational studies generally require large sample sizes. Subjects are not divided into groups, because group differences are not examined.

To determine the type of correlational design used in a published study, use the algorithm shown in Figure 8–5. More detail on specific correlational designs referred to in this algorithm is available elsewhere (Burns & Grove, 2009).

Descriptive Correlational Design

The purpose of a **descriptive correlational design** is to describe variables and examine relationships among these variables. Using this design facilitates the identification of many interrelationships in a situation (Figure 8–6). The study may examine variables in a situation that has already occurred or is currently occurring. Researchers make no attempt to control or manipulate the situation. As with descriptive studies, variables must be clearly identified and defined.

Figure 8–5. Algorithm for determining type of correlational design.

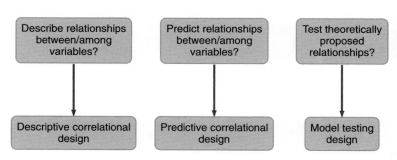

MEASUREMENT

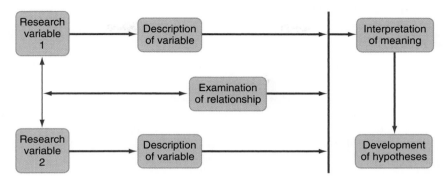

Figure 8-6. Descriptive correlational design.

 RESEARCH EXAMPLE Descriptive Correlational Design

Baker and colleagues (2008) recognized that children who suffer severe burns may face long term consequences and potentially diminished quality of life as adults. They conducted this study to determine which pencil-and-paper instrument might be a better measure of quality of life in these burn survivors. Two frequently used measures were identified, the Quality of Life Questionnaire and the SF-36 Health Survey, for comparison. Relationships between the Quality of Life Questionnaire (QLQ) and the SF-36 among young adults burned as children (Baker et al., 2008).

"Objective [purpose]: To examine the relationship between two measures that can be used to examine quality of life among pediatric burn survivors.

Design: Prospective, correlational study.

Setting: Acute and rehabilitation pediatric burn care facility.

Participants: Eighty young adult survivors of pediatric burns, who were 18-28 years of age, with burns of 30% or greater, and were at least 2 years after burns.

Interventions: Not applicable.

Main outcome measures: The SF-36 and the Quality of Life Questionnaire (QLQ) were used to assess participant's self-reported general health and long-term adjustment.

Results: Significant correlations ($p = 0.001$) were found between the total quality of life score of the QLQ and the mental component scale of the SF-36. However, no significant correlations were found between the total quality of life score of the QLQ and the SF-36 physical component scale." (p. 1163)

Continued

CRITICAL APPRAISAL

Study Design

1. Is the study design descriptive, correlational, quasi-experimental, or experimental?
   This is a correlational study.

2. If the design is correlational, what is the correlational design?
   This is a descriptive correlational design. The purpose of the study was to correlate Quality of Life Scores with SF36 scores. The SF36 gives a value for the person's mental health status and another value for their physical health status.

IMPLICATIONS FOR PRACTICE

Approximately 100,000 children are treated for burns annually, with a high percentage surviving, creating a challenge for health care professionals who need to prepare burn survivors with their psychosocial and physical well-being as adults. This study found that the SF-36 and the QLQ are measuring somewhat different aspects of psychosocial and physical adjustment. It is recommended that both tools could be useful to the burn practitioner in assessing quality of life. (Baker et al., p. 1163)

These findings are not directly useful to clinical practice unless both of the scales used in the study are being used on patients in the clinical setting. Even so, for usefulness, the two scales would need to be given to a broad base of patients so that the practitioner could judge what a specific score on the scales meant. However, effective assessment of the psychosocial and physical adjustment of burn patients is important to developing effective nursing interventions for poor adjustment.

Predictive Correlational Design

The purpose of a **predictive correlational design** is to predict the value of one variable based on values obtained for another variable(s). Prediction is one approach to examining causal relationships between variables. Because causal phenomena are being examined, the terms *dependent* and *independent* are used to describe the variables. One variable is classified as the dependent variable, and all other variables are independent variables. A predictive design (Figure 8–7) study attempts to predict the level of the dependent variable from the independent variables. The independent variables that are most effective in prediction are highly correlated with the dependent variable but not highly correlated with other independent variables used in the study. Predictive correlational designs require the development of a theory-based mathematical hypothesis proposing variables expected to effectively predict the dependent variable. Researchers then use regression analysis to test the hypothesis.

Figure 8–7. Predictive design.

Value of Intercept + Value of Independent Variable 1 + Value of Independent Variable 2 = Predicted Value of Dependent Variable

RESEARCH EXAMPLE Predictive Correlational Design

Heo et al. (2008) used a predictive correlational design to examine gender differences in and factors related to self-care behaviors among patients with heart failure.

"Background: Although self-care may reduce exacerbations of heart failure, reported rates of effective self-care in patients with heart failure are low. Modifiable factors, including psychosocial status, knowledge, and physical factors, are thought to influence heart failure self-care, but little is known about their combined impact on self-care."

Objectives: The objective of this study was to identify factors related to self-care behaviors in patients with heart failure.

Design: A cross-sectional, correlational study design was used."

"A cross-sectional design means that the researcher will divide the sample in various ways such as male and female, cardiac functional class, level of depression, etc and perform statistical correlations. The researcher is interested in which variables are most effective in predicting self-care behaviors in this population of patients. Questions the researchers asked included "Do men or women use the most self-care behaviors?" "Is the number of self-care behaviors affected by the patient's level of depression?" "Does the cardiac functional class affect the number of self-care behaviors?" The purpose of these cross-sectional analyses was to predict those patients who were most able to use self-care behaviors.

"Participants and settings: One hundred twenty-two patients (77 men and 45 women, mean age 60 ± 12 years old, 66% New York Heart Association functional class III/IV) were recruited from the outpatient clinics of an academic medical center and two community hospitals.

Methods: Data on self-care behaviors (Self-Care Heart Failure Index), depressive symptoms, perceived control, self-care confidence, knowledge, functional status, and social support were collected. Factors related to self-care were examined using hierarchical multiple regression (a statistical procedure).

Results: Mean self-care behavior scores were less than 70 indicating the majority of men and women with HF did not consistently engage in self-care behaviors. Higher self-care confidence and perceived control and better heart failure management knowledge were associated with better self-care ($r^2 = .25$, $p < .001$). Higher perceived control and better knowledge were related to better self-care behaviors in men ($r^2 = .18$, $p = .001$), while higher self-care confidence and poorer functional status were related to better self-care behaviors in women ($r^2 = .35$, $p < .001$)." (p. 1807)

CRITICAL APPRAISAL

Study Design

1. Is the study design descriptive, correlational, quasi-experimental, or experimental?
   This is a correlational study.

2. If the design is correlational, what is the correlational design?
   The design is predictive correlational. The goal of the study is to predict those patients most able to use self-care behaviors.

Continued

IMPLICATIONS FOR PRACTICE

"This study demonstrates the substantial impact of modifiable factors such as confidence in one's self-care abilities, perceived control, and knowledge on self-care behaviors. This study demonstrates that there are gender differences in factors affecting self-care, even though at baseline men and women have similar knowledge levels, physical, psychological, and behavioral status. Effective interventions focusing on modifiable factors and the unique characteristics of men and women should be provided to improve self-care behaviors in patients with heart failure." (p. 1807)

The authors point out that there are factors in the care of patients with heart failure that nursing interventions can impact. Nurses can teach self-care behaviors, facilitate the patient's use of self-care behaviors, help the patients become aware that they have control of their use of self-care behaviors, and recognize that their life will be better if they use self-care behaviors.

These findings would be strengthened by other similar studies of the same population. Nurses need to develop interventions that can be tested through research to demonstrate that their use increases self-care behaviors in this population. The interventions need to be very clearly defined so that a nurse applying that intervention in their clinical practice can anticipate an effective outcome.

Model Testing Design

Some studies are designed specifically to test the accuracy of a hypothesized causal model (middle range theory). The **model testing design** requires that all variables relevant to the model be measured. A large, heterogeneous sample is required. Investigators identify all of the paths expressing relationships between concepts and develop a conceptual map (Figure 8–8). The analysis determines whether the data are consistent with the model.

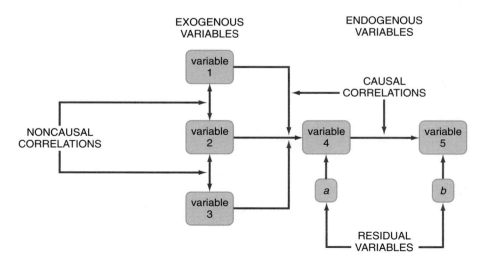

Figure 8–8. Model-testing design.

RESEARCH EXAMPLE Model Testing Design

Rempel and Fong (2005) used a model testing design to test the ability of the reasons model to predict the breastfeeding intentions of 317 first-time mothers before and after breastfeeding experience:

> The reasons model proposes that three levels of reasons for (pro) and against (con) adherence to health-related advice predict intentions: evidence-based (Level I); self-consequential (Level II); and affective, schema-related (Level III) reasons. (p. 443)

Measures included the Breastfeeding Reasons Questionnaire, Breastfeeding Intentions, and Postpartum Questionnaires. Subjects were followed from the third trimester to 12 months postpartum, with contacts at birth, 1 month, 2 months, 4 months, 6 months, 9 months, and 12 months so long as breastfeeding was continuing. Those who began breastfeeding and then stopped before the 12th month were contacted one time after discontinuation to assess actual breastfeeding duration and reasons for weaning.

Map of Model

Path analytic model: Reasons predicting breastfeeding intentions.

Findings

> "Path analyses showed that the Reasons Model was able to predict breastfeeding intentions. Level III reasons most strongly predicted prenatal and early postpartum intentions. Level II con breastfeeding reasons predicted later postpartum intentions. Breastfeeding intentions significantly predicted behavior."

The ability to predict future behavior is an important guide to nursing practice and contributes to evidence-based practice.

CRITICAL APPRAISAL

Study Design

1. Is the study design descriptive, correlational, quasi-experimental, or experimental?
   This is a correlational design.

2. If the design is correlational, what is the correlational design?
   The study uses a Model Testing Design. Using this design the researcher selects a means to measure each concept in the model, chooses a sample from a population appropriate for testing the model, gives all of the measures to each person in the sample, and then performs correlational statistical analyses designed to test models.

Continued

IMPLICATIONS FOR PRACTICE

It is important to know the reasons people give for their behavior. These reasons reflect their feelings and values. If a nurse is recommending a particular behavior, such as breastfeeding, a mother's acceptance of that recommendation must fit with her personal values and self-understanding. By understanding this, the nurse "will be in a much better position to assist individuals to make and maintain choices that will promote their own health and the health of those they love" (Rempel & Fong, 2005, p. 463).

Theoretical explanation of the pathways of cause for the preferred outcome of long-term breastfeeding is critical to the development of effective nursing interventions. The design of nursing interventions must be based on strong, well-tested theories and have strong evidence of effectiveness. Studies incorporating these principles will help to generate evidence-based guidelines for nursing practice, related in this case to the promotion of long-term breastfeeding.

Testing Causality

The experimental design is chosen to obtain a true representation of cause and effect by the most efficient means. That is, the design should provide the greatest amount of control with the least error possible. To examine cause, the researcher must eliminate all factors influencing the dependent variable other than the cause (independent variable) being studied. The effects of some factors are eliminated by controlling them (e.g., sampling criteria and highly controlled setting). Studies are designed to prevent other elements from intruding into the observation of the specific cause and effect being researched.

The essential elements of experimental research are the following:

- Random assignment of subjects to groups
- Precisely defined independent variable
- Researcher-controlled manipulation of the intervention or independent variable
- Researcher control of the experimental situation and setting, including a control or comparison group
- Clearly identified sampling criteria
- Carefully measured dependent variables
- Controlled environment for conduct of study such as laboratory setting or research unit

Quasi-experimental Designs

Use of a **quasi-experimental design** facilitates the search for knowledge and examination of causality in situations in which complete control is not possible. This type of design was developed to control as many threats to validity as possible in a situation in which some of the components of true experimental design are lacking. In experimental studies, a single group of subjects are randomly selected. Out of this group, some are randomly selected to receive the experimental treatment and the rest receive no treatment or a substitute treatment. The group that receives no treatment or a substitute treatment is referred to as a control group.

In most quasi-experimental studies, control groups are not used because of the difficulty of obtaining them. Instead, comparison groups are used. For example, the original sample

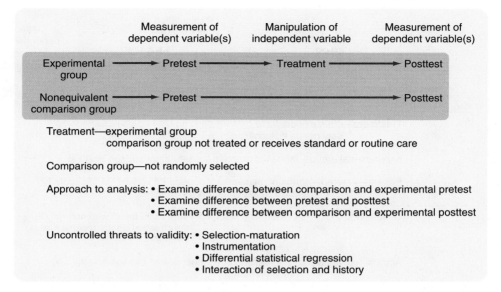

	Measurement of dependent variable(s)	Manipulation of independent variable	Measurement of dependent variable(s)
Experimental group	→ Pretest	→ Treatment	→ Posttest
Nonequivalent comparison group	→ Pretest	→	→ Posttest

Treatment—experimental group
comparison group not treated or receives standard or routine care

Comparison group—not randomly selected

Approach to analysis: • Examine difference between comparison and experimental pretest
• Examine difference between pretest and posttest
• Examine difference between comparison and experimental posttest

Uncontrolled threats to validity: • Selection-maturation
• Instrumentation
• Differential statistical regression
• Interaction of selection and history

Figure 8-9. Pretest and posttest design with a comparison group.

might be selected by a sample of convenience and then the subjects are randomly assigned to either the experimental group or comparison group. Thus, the original sample is not randomly selected but is a nonrandom sample of convenience.

In some studies, experimental and comparison subjects are selected from the same pool of potential subjects. Occasionally, with this type of design, comparison and treatment groups may evolve naturally. For example, groups may include subjects who choose a treatment as the experimental group and subjects who choose not to receive a treatment as the comparison group. These groups cannot be considered equivalent, however, because the subjects in the comparison group usually differ in important ways from those in the treatment group.

Quasi-experimental study designs vary widely. The most frequently used design in social science research is the untreated comparison group design with pretest and posttest (Figure 8–9). With this design, the researcher has a group of subjects who receive the experimental treatment (or intervention) and a comparison group of subjects who receive no treatment (or, in some cases, the standard care provided in the circumstances under study).

Another commonly used design is the posttest-only design with a comparison group (Figure 8–10). This design is used in situations in which a pretest is not possible. For example, if the researcher is examining differences in the amount of pain that a subject feels during a painful procedure, and a nursing intervention is used to reduce pain for subjects in the experimental group, it might not be possible (or meaningful) to pretest the amount of pain before the procedure. This design incorporates a number of threats to validity because of the lack of a pretest and thus is sometimes referred to as a pre-experimental design.

Use the algorithm shown in Figure 8–11 to determine the type of quasi-experimental study design used in a published study. More details about specific designs identified in this algorithm are available in other sources (Burns & Grove, 2009; Campbell & Stanley, 1963).

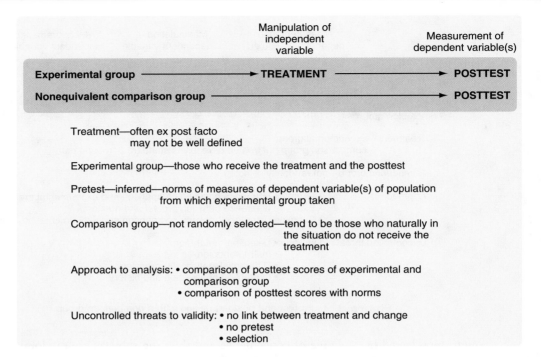

Figure 8–10. Posttest-only design with a comparison group.

RESEARCH EXAMPLE Quasi-Experimental Pretest-Posttest Design with Control Group

The following study uses a quasi-experimental design with a control group to compare the effectiveness of two treatment strategies for tuberculosis in the African country of Namibia. One group was treated using the traditional treatment strategy of having the patient travel (on foot) to the clinic to receive treatment. The other group was assigned a community nurse who traveled to the family's home to provide treatment. The nurse worked with the family as well as the patient to increase compliance with the treatment program. The two groups were then compared for degree of compliance and effectiveness. (Zvavamwe & Ehlers, 2009)

"Background: Tuberculosis (TB) remains a widespread healthcare problem in Africa, although it can be cured within 6-8 months' effective treatment. However, many patients fail to adhere to TB treatment, resulting in failure to get cured and the possible development of multi-drug resistant TB (MDR TB). A community-based TB treatment programme was started in the Omeheke region of Namibia during 2002. The efficacy of this community-based TB programme, compared to the standard hospital- and clinic-based TB treatment, was unknown.

Objectives: The major objectives were to compare TB treatment outcomes for patients who used the community-based TB with those who chose the clinic/self-administered TB treatment option; and to identify advantages and disadvantages of community-based TB care as experienced by patients who had completed their community-based TB treatment.

Design: A quasi-experimental study design was used to compare TB patients' treatment outcomes using checklists and exit interviews.

Setting: The study was conducted in the Omahekie region of Namibia.

Participants: TB patients (*n* = 332) who were hospitalized during the study period participated in the study.

Methods: Two groups of patients were selected for the study. One group received the experimental treatment, a community based TB treatment program where the nurse visited the patient at their home and the patient took their medication under the supervision of family members. The community nurse 'was used to do follow-up visits, and complete checklists, of 332 TB patients. Structured exit interviews were conducted with 101 TB patients who had completed their community-based TB treatment.' Another group of TB patients received the routine care by traveling to the clinic for care and were followed by the researchers during the study.

Results: Enhanced knowledge of TB patients improved their participation in community-based TB care. A family member was the most convenient, acceptable and accessible directly observed treatment (DOT) supervisor for 72.8% of the participants. A statistically significant difference in cure rates between community-based and the clinic/self-administered groups was found ($p = .05$) 11.78; $p \leq 0.05$; and RR = 1.35; p 0.05). The major advantages of community-based TB treatment included the ability to continue with one's daily activities during treatment and the saving of time and money. The major disadvantages included that the clinics ran out of TB drug supplies, and patients did not always have food to eat after taking their pills and they could not get sufficient rest because they had to continue doing their daily chores." (p. 302)

CRITICAL APPRAISAL

Study Design

When critically appraising a study, ask the following questions:

1. Is the study design descriptive, correlational, quasi-experimental, or experimental?
   This is a quasi-experimental study design.

2. If the design is quasi-experimental or experimental, what is the quasi-experimental or experimental design?
   The authors refer to their design as an analytic cohort prospective design. A cohort is a group of subjects that are similar in important ways. In this study there were two cohorts, one who received community care and another that received clinic care. Analytic means that the researchers plan to conduct extensive analysis on multiple variables that will be measured in both cohorts. Prospective means that the cohorts were entered in the study before treatment began.

3. If the design is quasi-experimental or experimental, which elements are controlled?
   Elements controlled:
   Clinic being attended by TB patients
   Type of treatment
   Patient education
   Precise measurement of dependent variables

Continued

CRITICAL APPRAISAL—cont'd

4. If the design is quasi-experimental or experimental, what elements could have been controlled to improve the study design?
   Follow-up on patients in both programs who did not complete treatment (would have required change in design)
   Control in clinic drug supplies throughout study.
   Development of strategy for provision of food after drug intake
   Work with family to insure specified amount of rest daily

5. If the design is quasi-experimental or experimental, what was the feasibility of controlling particular elements of the study?
   Follow-up of those patients not completing—Not feasible because of lack of researcher time in the field.
   Provision of food after drug intake—Problematic because family must provide food. Food may be scarce and family may not have enough food to provide after each dose. Family compliance may be variable.
   Specified amount of rest—There may not be enough family workers to distribute the patient's work load to other members. Compliance will be variable.

6. If the design is quasi-experimental or experimental, what was the effect of not controlling certain elements on the validity of the study findings?
   The study findings are valid for the researcher's question.
   Could have provided more information with more control. There was an assumption that the patients were unable or unwilling to be taught. The researcher found that, with teaching, the patient and family could be taught and were willing to learn. If this is the case, the researcher might include more teaching and perhaps teach both groups, thus testing only the type of care, not the compliance with teaching.

7. If the design is quasi-experimental or experimental, which elements of the design were manipulated and how they were manipulated? Manipulation usually takes place through a treatment or intervention. Sometimes more than one type of treatment or intervention is provided. In this study two treatments were provided, each repeatedly over the period of the study.
   The location of treatment—clinic versus community
   Patient and family teaching—location, amount, and content

8. If the design is quasi-experimental or experimental, how adequate was the manipulation? The term manipulation is similar to treatment or intervention. The manipulation was sufficiently adequate to statistically detect an effect. I suspect that the researcher now has ideas on how to improve the manipulation. For example, the researchers likely gained understanding in what strategies may be needed to educate the family members in the care of the person with TB.

9. What elements should have been manipulated to improve the validity of the findings? More cross patient control of the intervention. Cross patient control is to have the same degree of control in both groups. However, in a community-based intervention, this is difficult.

Overall summary of the quality of the study design. There are serious problems in the design of this study. Manipulation of the treatment in both groups to achieve equivalence of groups was poor. One would hope that a second study might be conducted to improve the amount of control in both groups, thus allowing a better test of the effectiveness of the treatment in the two groups.

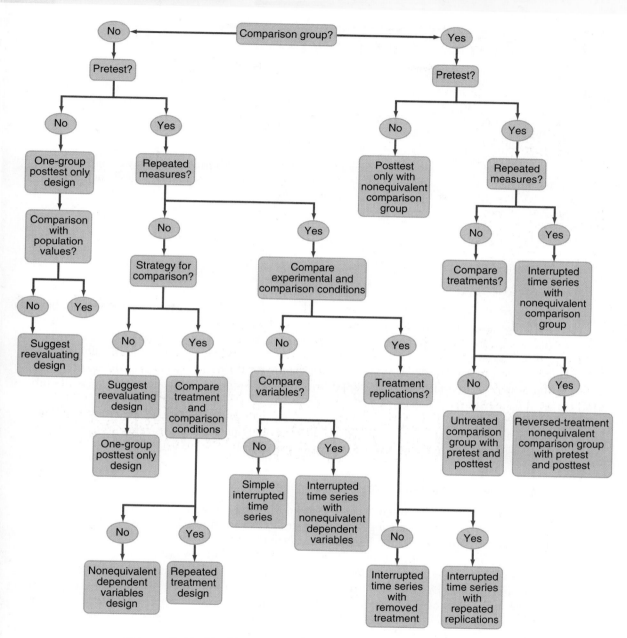

Figure 8–11. Algorithm for determining type of quasi-experimental design.

IMPLICATIONS FOR PRACTICE

TB patients on the community-based TB treatment option had better cure rates than those on clinic/self-administered TB treatment (although it cannot be inferred that the community-based treatment caused the improved cure rates, because the TB patients who did not select the community-based treatment option might have been different). The advantage experienced by patients who completed their community-based TB treatment outweighed the disadvantages. (pp. 302-303)

This information can be useful to nursing practice in caring for TB patients in many countries. For the population studied, nurses need to refine their intervention, test it again, and publish the refined intervention. This field of study would keep a group of nurse researchers actively conducting research throughout a career.

Experimental Designs

A variety of **experimental designs**, some relatively simple and others very complex, have been developed for a variety of studies focused on examining causality. In some cases, researchers may combine characteristics of more than one design to meet the needs of their study. Names of designs vary from one text to another. When reading and critically appraising a published study, determine the author's name for the design (some authors do not name the design used) and/or read the description of the design to determine the type of design used in the study.

Use the algorithm shown in Figure 8–12 to determine the type of experimental study design used in a published study. More details about specific designs referred to in Figure 8–12 are available in other texts (Burns & Grove, 2009).

Pretest-Posttest Design

The most common experimental design used in nursing studies is the pretest-posttest design with experimental and control groups. This design is shown in Figure 8–13 and is similar to the quasi-experiment design in Figure 8–9, except that the experimental study is more tightly controlled. Multiple groups (both experimental and control) can be used to great advantage in this design. For example, one control group can receive no treatment, whereas another control group receives a placebo treatment. Each one of multiple experimental groups can receive a variation of the treatment, such as a different frequency, intensity, or duration of nursing care measures. These additions greatly increase the generalizability of study findings.

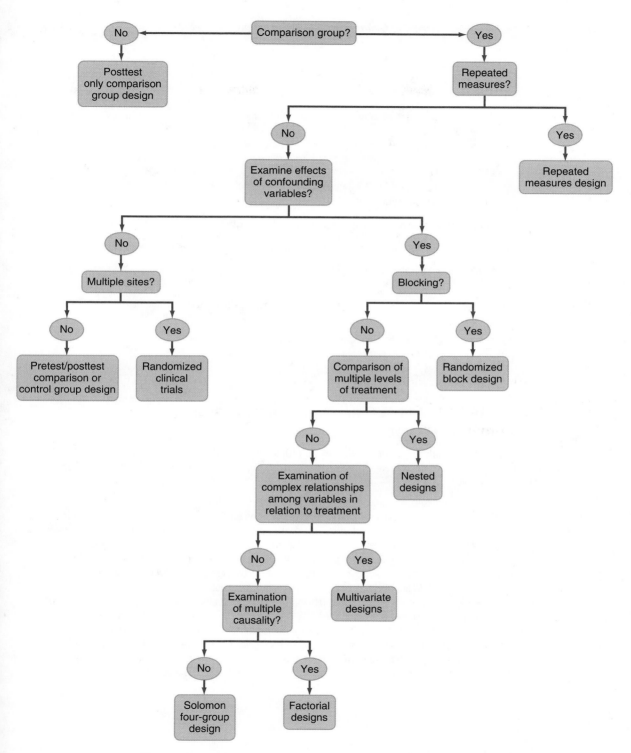

Figure 8–12. Algorithm for determining type of experimental design.

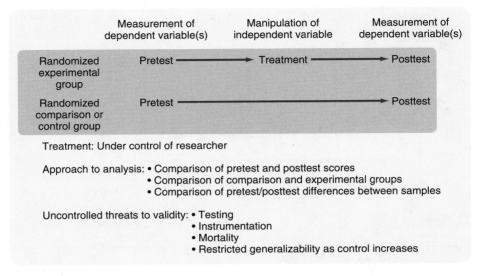

Figure 8–13. The classic experimental design: pretest-posttest control group design.

RESEARCH EXAMPLE Randomized Two-Group Experimental Design

Khare, Huber, Carpenter, Balmer, Bates, Nolen et al. (2009) conducted a study designed to reduce cardiovascular disease risk in underserved women, using the design and methods of the Illinois WISE-WOMAN Program (IWP).

"Methods: The Cooper Institute, in collaboration with the Illinois Department of Public Health and the University of Illinois at Chicago, adapted evidence-based interventions for financially disadvantaged, low literacy populations. The study used a randomized, two-group, experimental design. In total, 1021 women were recruited from the Illinois Breast and Cervical Cancer Program, which serves uninsured and underinsured women, aged 40 to 64, at or below 200% of poverty. The women were randomized to either a minimum intervention (MI) or an enhanced intervention (EI) group. Both groups received CVD risk factor screening and educational materials. Additionally, the EI group received a 12-week lifestyle intervention.

Results: Baseline comparisons show equivalent groups. IWP participants had a higher prevalence of obesity and smoking than similar national samples.

Conclusions: IWP addressed many of the cultural and implementation barriers in programs that seek to improve the health of financially disadvantaged, low literacy populations. Because of the high burden of disease, the unique study population, and the sound design, we anticipate that our future results will contribute to the translation literature, which has largely ignored significant health disparities."

CRITICAL APPRAISAL

Study Design

When critically appraising a study, ask the following questions:

1. Is the study design descriptive, correlational, quasi-experimental, or experimental?
   This was an experimental study.
   If the design is quasi-experimental or experimental, what is the design?
   The researchers refer to their study as a randomized, two-group design. Both groups received an intervention. One group received a Minimum Intervention and the other group received an Enhanced Intervention.
   If the design is quasi-experimental or experimental, which elements are controlled?
   Type of intervention
   MI—Minimum intervention
     CVD risk factor screening
     Educational materials
   EI—enhanced intervention
     CVD risk factor screening
     Educational materials
     12-Week lifestyle intervention (question, did participants have to complete the lifestyle intervention to continue in the study)

2. If the design is quasi-experimental or experimental, what elements could have been controlled to improve the study design?
   Measure changes in lifestyle and health status after treatment in both groups
   Follow-up measure of changes in lifestyle and health status after 6 months or 1 year.

3. If the design is quasi-experimental or experimental, what was the feasibility of controlling particular elements of the study? Low
   Costs of study would increase
   Loss of subjects would increase
   With loss of subjects, effect of treatment on these subjects would be lost. This would mean that the treatment would be effective only on a smaller group of the targeted population.

4. If the design is quasi-experimental or experimental, what was the effect of not controlling certain elements on the validity of the study findings?
   The findings are valid. Increasing control would broaden the range of validity.

5. If the design is quasi-experimental or experimental, which elements of the design were manipulated and how they were manipulated?
   Experimental group received 12-week lifestyle intervention while Control group did not.

6. If the design is quasi-experimental or experimental, how adequate was the manipulation?
   The manipulation was adequate to result in a statistically significant difference in the two groups

7. What elements should have been manipulated to improve the validity of the findings?
   Cannot be judged until findings are reported.

This study has a carefully planned design. One intervention builds on the other, with one treatment clearly better than the other. The careful planning provides a greater opportunity for the researchers to detect a difference in the groups if there is one.

Continued

IMPLICATIONS FOR PRACTICE

The study results were not yet reported as the text went to press. Look for them in the literature by searching for the author's names in CINAHL.

Randomized Clinical Trial

The randomized clinical trial has been used in medicine since 1945. A randomized clinical trial is a carefully designed experimental study that uses large numbers of subjects to test the effects of a treatment and compare the results with those of a control group that has not received the treatment (or that has received a traditional treatment). Until recently this design has not been used in nursing because of the extensive external funding required to conduct these studies. Subjects are drawn from a reference population, using clearly defined criteria, and then are randomly assigned to treatment or control groups. Baseline states (the state of subjects at the beginning of the study) must be comparable in all groups included in the study. The same treatment is given and is consistently applied, and outcomes are measured consistently. Care is taken to ensure that randomization procedures (procedures used to assign subjects to the experimental and control groups) are rigidly adhered to in a study. Because of the need to have large samples and generalize to a variety of clinical settings and patients, the study may be carried out simultaneously in multiple geographic locations coordinated by the primary researcher. Use of this design has the potential to greatly improve the scientific base for nursing practice (Fetter et al., 1989; Tyzenhouse, 1981). Burns and Grove (2009) have defined the criteria that must be met for a nursing study to be classified as a clinical trial.

RESEARCH EXAMPLE Randomized Clinical Trial

Sleep apnea can pose serious risks and disrupt the lives of those affected. The care provided by a physician is expensive and may be limited by the number of specialists. A plan of care that is led by nurses may be cost-effective if it is as good as the care provided by a physician. Antic and colleagues (2009) conducted a randomized clinical trial to compare a nurse-led care model to usual care provided by a physician.

Rationale: Obstructive sleep apnea (OSA) is a prevalent disease. Often limited clinical resources result in long patient waiting lists. Simpler validated methods of care are needed.

Objectives: To demonstrate that a nurse-led model of care can produce health outcomes in symptomatic moderate–severe OSA not inferior to physician-led care.

Methods: A randomized controlled multicenter non-inferiority clinical trial was performed. Of 1427 potentially eligible patients at three centers, 882 consented to the trial. Of these, 263 were excluded on the basis of clinical criteria. Of the remaining 619, 195 met home oximetry criteria for high-probability moderate-severe OSA and were randomized to 2 models of care: model A, the simplified model, using home autoadjusting positive airway pressure to set therapeutic continuous positive airway pressure (CPAP), with all care supervised by an experienced nurse; and model B, involving two laboratory polysomnograms to diagnose and treat OSA, with clinical care supervised by a sleep physician. The primary endpoint was changed in Epworth Sleepiness Scale (ESS) score after 3 months of CPAP. Other outcome measures were collected.

Measurements and Main Results: For the primary outcome change in ESS score, nurse-led management was no worse than physician-led management (4.02 vs. 4.15; difference, −0.13; 95% confidence interval: −1.52, 1.25) given a prespecified non-inferiority margin of −2 for the lower 95% confidence interval. There were also no differences between both groups in CPAP adherence at 3 months or other outcome measures. Within-trial costs were significantly less in model A. (p. 501)

Clinical trial registered with *http://www.anzctr.org.au* (ACTRN01260500006406). (Australia)

CRITICAL APPRAISAL

Study Design

When critically appraising a study, ask the following questions:
1. If the design is a clinical trial, describe the design.
   A randomized controlled multicenter non-inferiority clinical trial.
   Home oximetry criteria established for selection of all subjects.
   Patients recruited for long patient waiting lists.
   Patients randomized into control and treatment arms of the study.

Model A: All Care Supervised by an Experienced Nurse.

Use of home autoadjusting positive airway pressure to set therapeutic continuous positive airway pressure (CPAP).
   Measurement of Epworth Sleepiness Scale (ESS) before and after 3 months of treatment with CPAP.
   Measurement of cost
   Measurement of CPAP adherence at 3 months
   Other outcome measures were taken but not reported

Model B: Two Laboratory Polysomnograms to Diagnose and Treat OSA.

Clinical care supervised by a sleep physician.
   Measurement of Epworth Sleepiness Scale (ESS) before and after 3 months of treatment with CPAP.
   Measurement of CPAP adherence at 3 months
   Measurement of cost
   Other outcome measures were taken but not reported

IMPLICATIONS FOR PRACTICE

"A simplified nurse-led model of care has demonstrated non-inferior results to physician-directed care in the management of symptomatic moderate to severe OSA, while being less costly." (p. 501)

Non-inferior means that the results are no worse than those of the physician care.

Defining Experimental Interventions

In quasi-experimental and experimental studies, investigators develop an intervention that is expected to result in differences in posttest measures between the treatment and control or comparison groups. This intervention or treatment may be physiologic, psychosocial, educational, or a combination of these. The specific steps or components of the intervention need to be carefully planned, and a rationale is given for providing the intervention in a particular way. The intervention is described in detail in the published study. Labels for interventions such as "preoperative teaching" are to be avoided because they do not contribute to comprehension of the exact nature of the intervention. Readers may be easily led astray by such labels—each person has his or her own expectations of what should occur during preoperative teaching. Nursing is currently developing classifications of nursing interventions. It is hoped that these classifications will be useful to the researcher in clarifying the intervention provided. The goal of the intervention being investigated is to maximize the differences between the control and the experimental groups. Thus, it is important to choose the best intervention that can be provided under the circumstances of the study.

Although control and comparison groups traditionally have received no intervention, adherence to this expectation is not possible in many nursing studies. For example, it would be unethical not to provide preoperative teaching to a patient. Furthermore, in many studies it is possible that just spending time with a patient or having a patient participate in activities that he or she considers beneficial may in itself cause an effect. Therefore, the study often includes a control or comparison group intervention. This intervention usually is the standard care the patient would receive if a study were not being conducted. The researcher must describe in detail the standard care that the control or comparison group receives so that the study can be adequately appraised. Because the quality of this standard care is likely to vary considerably among subjects, variance in the control or comparison group is likely to be high.

CRITICAL APPRAISAL GUIDELINES

Interventions

When critically appraising the interventions in a study, ask the following questions:

1. Was the experimental intervention described in detail?
2. Was justification from the literature provided for development of the experimental intervention?
3. Was the experimental intervention the best that could be provided given current knowledge?
4. Was a protocol developed to ensure consistent or reliable implementation of the treatment with each subject throughout the study? (See Burns & Grove [2009] for a discussion of intervention protocols.)
5. Did the study report indicate who implemented the treatment? If more than one person implemented the treatment, were they trained to ensure consistency in the delivery of the treatment?

6. Was any control or comparison group intervention described? Was an intervention theory provided to explain why the intervention causes the outcomes and exactly how the intervention produced the desired effects?

Intervention research methods are presented in the textbook by Burns and Grove (2009, Chapter 13).

RESEARCH EXAMPLE Intervention—Yakson

Koreans have traditionally believed that they could relieve their sick children's pain or discomfort by gently caressing their children on the aching body part. This caressing act is called "Yakson," where "Yak" means medicine and "son" refers to hand. "A mom's hand is a Yakson" is a common idiom most Koreans have heard over the generations, and is a usual expression of the warm, loving, and caring touch of mothers who are the main caregivers of children. The work "Yakson" also implies that the hand works like medicine or treatment through love and supernatural power. The caressing action itself can be considered as the most basic and instinctive type of nursing care.

Yakson was recently studied academically, and one research study showed that Yakson is based on the concept of vital energy (i.e., Ki) released from the hand of mothers (Lee, 2003). The implementation of Yakson ... focuses on allowing an infant to receive the provider's Ki and warmth through the provider's palm, which, it was thought, could alleviate the infant's stress. During the Yakson intervention, the provider places one hand underneath the back of the infant with the other hand on the abdomen, where the internal organs are distributed most densely, as if gently wrapping the preterm infant with both hands. The assumption is that the unstable Ki of preterm infants and the stable Ki of Yakson providers communicate with each other through Yakson, which contributes to the preterm infants' comfort, alleviates of their stress, and ultimately results in a positive effect (Lee, 2003).

Im (2005) reported that Yakson increased preterm infants' (gestational age of 26 to 34 weeks) total daily intake of milk and decreased infants' heartbeat compared to the control group. In Im's study, Yakson involved administering hand resting, gentle caressing and hand resting again for 15 min a day for 15 days. Yakson was provided twice a day for 10 days by a nurse and subsequently once a day for 5 days by the preterm infants' mothers. No differences were found between experimental and control group infants in weight gain, O_2 saturation, and behavioral state (Im, 2005). Yakson also was effective in reducing the pain of term infants during heel stick procedures (Im et al., in press). A nurse provided Yakson beginning 1 minute before the heel stick through the completion of the heel stick by slowly caressing the infant's belly with one hand while placing the other hand underneath the infant's back as if wrapping the infant with two palms. The oxygen saturation levels in the Yakson group infants were maintained significantly higher than in the control group, however, there were no differences in heart rate and pain score using the Neonatal Infant Pain Scale between the Yakson group and the control group (Im et al., in press)" (p. 452).

Im, H., & Kim, E. (2009). Effect of Yakson and gentle human touch versus usual care on urine stress hormones and behaviors in preterm infants: A quasi-experimental study. *International Journal of Nursing Studies, 46*(4), 450-458.

Continued

CRITICAL APPRAISAL

Interventions

1. Was the experimental intervention described in detail?
   Yes, very careful detail.

2. Was justification from the literature provided for development of the experimental intervention?
   Yes, the relevant literature was reviewed in detail.

3. Was the experimental intervention the best that could be provided given current knowledge?
   Yes. Knowledge of this intervention is new and has been used in few studies.

4. Was a protocol developed to ensure consistent or reliable implementation of the treatment with each subject throughout the study? (See Burns & Grove [2009] for a discussion of intervention protocols.)
   Yes

5. Did the study report indicate who implemented the treatment? Yes.

6. If more than one person implemented the treatment, were they trained to ensure consistency in the delivery of the treatment? Yes, there were written directions and other nurses monitored those new to the procedure until the new user was considered competent.

7. Was any control or comparison group intervention described?
   Yes, the control or comparison group received Gentle Human Touch given by the nurses.

8. Was an intervention theory provided to explain why the intervention causes the outcomes and exactly how the intervention produced the desired effects? Yes.
   Im and Kim (2009) conducted an experimental study with a rigorous design, including a carefully implemented intervention. The study is an excellent example of experimental design.

Mapping the Design

In quasi-experimental and experimental studies, investigators can map the design to clarify the points at which measurements are taken and treatments are provided for various groups in the study. Generally, the symbol O is used for an observation or a measurement. Several measurements or observations may be indicated by this symbol. The symbol T is used for a treatment. For example, in a study with two groups, experimental and control, in which subjects received a pretest and a posttest (pretest-posttest control group design), the design can be mapped as follows:

	Pretest	Treatment	Posttest
Experimental group	O_1	T	O_2
Control or comparison group	O_1		O_2

This design map could be used for a quasi-experimental or an experimental study. In the quasi-experimental study, the control group is called the "comparison" (or "non-equivalent") group. The comparison group gets standard care and is commonly used in healthcare studies because the patients must receive care. Control group does not get care. Experimental design subjects are randomly selected and then randomly assigned to groups—typical of control group and treatment group.

If the study includes several posttests at monthly intervals, the design can be mapped as follows:

			Posttests			
	Pretest	**Treatment**	**1 mo**	**2 mo**	**3 mo**	**4 mo**
Experimental group	O_1	T	O_2	O_3	O_4	O_5
Control or comparison group	O_1		O_2	O_3	O_4	O_5

Researchers can express variations in the design map for more than two groups, by adding more rows, for repeated treatments, by placing the "T" at each place the treatment is administered, or for multiple treatments. Multiple treatments may be labeled T1, T2, T3, and so on.

Role of Replication Studies in Evidence-Based Practice

Replication studies involve reproducing or repeating a study to determine whether similar findings will be obtained (Taunton, 1989). The intent of replication is to determine whether the findings from the original study hold up despite minor changes in the research conditions. If the findings generated through replication are consistent with the original study findings, these findings are more credible and have the potential to be used in practice.

Replication is essential for knowledge development for several reasons: (1) replication establishes the credibility of the findings, (2) it extends the generalizability of the findings over a range of instances and contexts, (3) it provides support for theory development, and (4) it decreases the acceptance of erroneous results (Beck, 1994). Thus, replication studies are essential to generate evidence that can be used in practice (Brown, 2009).

Beck (1994) conducted a computerized and manual review of the nursing literature from 1983 through 1992 and found only 49 replication studies. Possibly, the number of replication studies is limited because replication is viewed by some as less scholarly or less important than original research. However, the lack of replication studies severely limits the development of a scientific knowledge base for nursing (Beck, 1994; Martin, 1995). Thus, replication of studies is an important priority for nursing because it will greatly influence the generation of nursing knowledge that can be synthesized for use in practice (Burns & Grove, 2009).

KEY CONCEPTS

- A research design is a blueprint for conducting a study that maximizes control over factors that could interfere with the validity of the findings.
- Elements central to the study design include the presence or absence of a treatment, number of groups in the sample, number and timing of measurements to be performed, method of sampling, time frame for data collection, planned comparisons, and control of extraneous variables.
- Four common types of quantitative designs are used in nursing: descriptive, correlational, quasi-experimental, and experimental.

- The three essential elements of experimental research are (1) the random assignment of subjects to groups; (2) the researcher's manipulation of the independent variable; and (3) the researcher's control of the experimental situation and setting, including a control or comparison group.
- The purpose of design is to maximize the possibility of obtaining valid answers to research questions or hypotheses. A good design provides the subjects, the setting, and the protocol within which these comparisons can be clearly examined.
- Interventions or treatments are implemented in quasi-experimental and experimental studies to determine their effect on selected dependent variables. Interventions may be physiologic, psychosocial, educational, or a combination of these.
- Critically appraising a design involves examining the study environment, sample, treatment, and measurement. Developing a map of the design can help you clarify the different elements of the design.
- Replication studies involve reproducing or repeating a study to determine whether similar findings will be obtained under similar circumstances and are essential for developing sound evidence for practice.

REFERENCES

Akpinar, R. B., Celebioglu, A., Uslu, H., & Uyanik, M. H. (2009). An evaluation of the hand and nasal flora of Turkish nursing students after clinical practice. *Journal of Clinical Nursing, 18*(3), 426-430.

Antic, N. A., Buchan, C., Esterman, A., Hensley, M., Naughton, M. T., Rowland, S., Williamson, B., Windler, S., Eckermann, S., & McEvoy, R. D. (2009). A randomized controlled trial of nurse-led care for symptomatic moderate-severe obstructive sleep apnea. *American Journal of Respiratory & Critical Care Medicine, 179*(6)I, 501-508.

Baker, C. P., Rosenberg, M., Mossberg, K. A., Holzer III, C., Blakeney, P., Robert, R., Thomas, C., & Meyer III, W. (2008). Relationships between the Quality of Life Questionnaire (QLQ) and the SF-36 among young adults burned as children. *Burns, 34*(2008), 1163-1168.

Beck, C. T. (1994). Replication strategies for nursing research. Image: *Journal of Nursing Scholarship, 26*(3), 191-194.

Brown, S. J. (2009). *Evidence-based nursing: The research-practice connection.* Sudbury, MA: Jones & Bartlett.

Burns, N., & Grove, S. K. (2009). *The practice of nursing research: Appraisal, synthesis, and generation of evidence* (6th ed.). Philadelphia: Saunders.

Campbell, D. T., & Stanley, J. C. (1963). *Experimental and quasi-experimental designs for research.* Chicago: Rand McNally.

Feider, L. L., Mitchell, P., & Bridges, E. (2010). Oral care practices for orally intubated critically ill adults. *American Journal of Critical Care, 19*(2), 175-183.

Fetter, M. S., Fink, A., Fink, B. B., Hougart, M. K., & Rushton, C. H. (1989). Randomized clinical trials: Issues for researchers. *Nursing Research, 38*(2), 117-120.

Heo, S., Moser, D. K., Lennie, T. A., Riegel, B., & Chung, M. L. (2008). Gender differences in and factors related to self-care behaviors: A cross-sectional, correlational study of patients with heart failure. *International Journal of Nursing Studies, 45*(2008) 1807-1815.

Im, H. (2005). *Effect of Yakson therapy on growth and stable state of preterm infants and on maternal attachment.* Seoul: College of Nursing, Korea University.

Im, H., & Kim, E. (2009). Effect of Yakson and Gentle Human Touch versus usual care on urine stress hormones and behaviors in preterm infants: A quasi-experimental study. *International Journal of Nursing Studies, 46*(4), 450-458.

Im, H., Kim, E., Park, E., Sung, K., & Oh, W. (2008). Pain reduction of heel stick in neonates: Yakson compared to non-nutritive sucking. *Journal of Tropical Pediatrics,* in press.

Khare, M. M., Huber, R., Carpenter, R. A., Balmer, P. W., Bates, N. J., et al. (2009). A lifestyle approach to reducing cardiovascular risk factors in underserved women: Design and methods of the Illinois WISEWOMAN Program. *Journal of Women's Health, 18*(3), 409-419.

Lee, D. (2003). *The Korean healing art of Yakson.* Seoul: Mindvision.

Martin, P. A. (1995). More replication studies needed. *Applied Nursing Research, 8*(2), 102-103.

Morse, J. M. (1994). *Critical issues in qualitative research.* Thousand Oaks, CA: Sage.

Rempel, L. A., & Fong, G. T. (2005). Why breastfeed? A longitudinal test of the Reasons Model among first-time mothers. *Psychology and Health, 20*(4), 443-466.

Stake, R. E. (1995). *The art of case study research*. Thousand Oaks, CA: Sage.

Stake, R. E. (1998). Case studies (pp. 86-109). In N. K. Denzin & Y. S. Lincoln (Eds.), *Strategies of qualitative inquiry*. Thousand Oaks, CA: Sage.

Taunton, R. L. (1989). Replication: Key to research application. *Dimensions of Critical Care Nursing, 8*(3), 156-158.

Tyzenhouse, P. S. (1981). Technical notes: The nursing clinical trial. *Western Journal of Nursing Research, 3*(1), 102-109.

Wardell, D. W., Rintala, D., & Tan, G. (2008). Study descriptions of healing touch with veterans experiencing chronic neuropathic pain from spinal cord injury. *Explore: The Journal of Science & Healing, 4*(3), 187-195.

Zvavamwe, Z., & Ehlers, V. J. (2009). Experiences of a community-based tuberculosis treatment programme in Namibia: A comparative cohort study. *International Journal of Nursing Studies, 46*(3), 302-309.

9

Examining Populations and Samples in Research

Chapter Overview

Understanding Sampling Concepts   290
  Populations and Elements   290
  Sampling or Eligibility Criteria   291
Representativeness of a Sample in Quantitative and Outcomes Research   294
  Random and Systematic Variation of Subjects' Values   294
  Acceptance and Refusal Rates in Studies   295
  Attrition and Retention Rates in Studies   296
  Random Sampling   298
  Sampling Frames   298
  Sampling Plans or Methods   298
Probability Sampling Methods   298
  Simple Random Sampling   299
  Stratified Random Sampling   301
  Cluster Sampling   302
  Systematic Sampling   303
Nonprobability Sampling Methods Used in Quantitative Research   305
  Convenience Sampling   305
  Quota Sampling   307

Sample Size in Quantitative Studies   308
  Effect Size   308
  Types of Quantitative Studies   309
  Number of Variables   310
  Measurement Sensitivity   310
  Data Analysis Techniques   310
Sampling in Qualitative Research   312
  Purposeful or Purposive Sampling   313
  Network Sampling   314
  Theoretical Sampling   316
Sample Size in Qualitative Studies   317
  Scope of the Study   318
  Nature of the Topic   318
  Quality of the Information   318
  Study Design   319
Research Settings   321
  Natural Setting   321
  Partially Controlled Setting   322
  Highly Controlled Setting   322

Learning Outcomes

After completing this chapter, you should be able to:

1. Describe sampling theory, including the concepts of population, target population, sampling criteria, sampling frame, subject or participant, sampling plan, sample, representativeness, sampling error, and systematic bias.

2. Critically appraise the sampling criteria (inclusion and exclusion criteria) used in published studies.

3. Identify the specific type of probability and nonprobability sampling methods used in published quantitative, qualitative, and outcomes studies.

4. Identify the elements of power analysis in a published quantitative study.

5. Critically appraise the sample size of published quantitative and qualitative studies.

6. Critically appraise the settings used in published quantitative, qualitative, and outcomes studies.

Key Terms

Acceptance rate, p. 295
Accessible population, p. 290
Cluster sampling, p. 302
Comparison group, p. 298
Control group, p. 298
Convenience sampling, p. 305
Effect size, p. 308
Elements, p. 291
Exclusion sampling criteria,
    p. 291
Generalization, p. 291
Heterogeneous sample, p. 291
Highly controlled setting,
    p. 322
Homogeneous sample, p. 291
Inclusion sampling criteria,
    p. 291
Intraproject sampling, p. 317
Natural (or field) setting, p. 321
Network sampling, p. 314

Nonprobability sampling,
    p. 305
Partially controlled setting,
    p. 322
Participants, p. 291
Population, p. 290
Power, p. 308
Power analysis, p. 308
Probability sampling, p. 298
Purposeful or purposive
    sampling, p. 313
Quota sampling, p. 307
Random sampling, p. 298
Random variation, p. 294
Refusal rate, p. 295
Representativeness, p. 294
Sample, p. 290
Sample attrition, p. 296
Sample retention, p. 296
Sample size, p. 308

Sampling, p. 290
Sampling or eligibility criteria,
    p. 291
Sampling frame, p. 298
Sampling plan or method,
    pp. 290, 298
Saturation of information,
    p. 317
Setting, p. 321
Simple random sampling,
    p. 299
Stratified random sampling,
    p. 301
Subjects, p. 291
Systematic sampling, p. 303
Systematic variation, p. 295
Target population, p. 290
Theoretical sampling, p. 316
Verification of information,
    p. 317

STUDY TOOLS

Be sure to visit http://evolve.elsevier.com/Burns/understanding for additional examples and self-tests. Also, a review of this chapter's concepts and practice exercises can be found in Chapter 9 of the Study Guide for *Understanding Nursing Research: Building an Evidence-Based Practice*, 5th edition.

Students often enter the field of research with preconceived notions about samples and sampling methods. Many of these notions come from exposure to television advertisements, public opinion polls, market researchers in shopping centers, and newspaper reports of research findings. A television commercial boasts that four of five doctors recommend a particular pain medication; a newscaster announces that John Jones will win the senate election by a margin of 10%; and a newspaper reports that research has shown that aggressive treatment of hypertension to maintain a blood pressure of 120/80 mm Hg or lower significantly reduces the risk for coronary artery disease and stroke.

All of these examples include a type of sampling technique. Some of the outcomes from these studies are more valid than others, because of the techniques used to obtain the samples. Thus, when critically appraising a study, you must identify the sampling method used and evaluate it for quality. The sample usually is described in the Methods section of a published research report. To judge the quality of a sample, you need an understanding of the principles of sampling theory, the types of sampling methods used in research, and the sample size.

This chapter presents the concepts of sampling theory including sampling criteria, sampling frame, and representativeness of a sample. The nonprobability and probability sampling plans or methods and sample size for quantitative and qualitative studies are detailed. The chapter concludes with a discussion of the natural, partially controlled, and highly controlled settings used for conducting research.

Understanding Sampling Concepts

Sampling involves selecting a group of people, events, behaviors, or other elements with which to conduct a study. A sampling plan, or sampling method, defines the selection process, and the sample defines the selected group of people (or elements). Samples should represent a population of people. The population might be all people who have diabetes, all patients who have had abdominal surgery, or all persons who receive care from a registered nurse. In most cases, however, it would be impossible for a researcher to study an entire population. Sampling theory was developed to determine the most effective way to acquire a sample that accurately reflects the population under study. Key concepts of sampling theory include populations, target population, sampling or eligibility criteria, accessible population, elements, representativeness, sampling frames, and sampling plans or methods. This section explains these concepts.

Populations and Elements

The population is a particular group of individuals or elements, such as people with type 2 diabetes, who are the focus of the research. The target population is the entire set of individuals or elements who meet the sampling criteria (defined in the next section), such as female, 18 years of age or older, new diagnosis of type 2 diabetes confirmed by the medical record, and not on insulin. Figure 9–1 demonstrates the link of the population, target population, and accessible population in a study. An accessible population is the portion of the target population to which the researcher has reasonable access. The accessible population might include elements within a country, state, city, hospital, nursing unit, or primary care

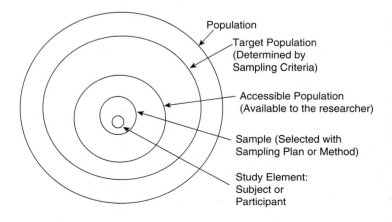

Figure 9–1. Linking population, sample, and subjects in a study.

clinic, such as the diabetics in a primary care clinic in Arlington, Texas. The researcher obtains the sample from the accessible population by using a particular sampling plan or method, such as simple random sampling. The individual units of the population and sample are called **elements**. An element can be a person, event, behavior, or any other single unit of study. When elements are persons, they are referred to as subjects or participants (see Figure 9–1). Most quantitative and outcome researchers refer to the people they study as **subjects**. Qualitative researchers refer to the individuals they study as **participants**. In quantitative and outcomes studies, researchers obtain a sample from the accessible population, and generalize findings from the sample to the accessible population and then, more abstractly, to the target population (see Figure 9–1).

Generalization extends the findings from the sample under study to the larger population. The quality of the study and the consistency of the study's findings with the findings from previous research in this area influence the extent of the generalization. If a study is of high quality with findings that are consistent with previous research, then the researchers can be confident in generalizing their findings to the target population. For example, the findings from the study of female patients with a new diagnosis of type 2 diabetes in a primary care clinic in Arlington, Texas may be generalized to the target population of adult females with type 2 diabetes managed in primary care clinics. With this information, you can decide whether it is appropriate to use this evidence in caring for the same type of patients in your practice with the goal of moving toward evidence-based practice (Brown, 2009; Cullum, Ciliska, Haynes, & Marks, 2008).

Sampling or Eligibility Criteria

Sampling criteria, also referred to as eligibility criteria, include the list of characteristics essential for eligibility or membership in the target population. For example, researchers may choose to study the effect of preoperative teaching on the outcome of length of hospital stay for adults having abdominal surgery. In this study the sampling criteria may include (1) age of at least 18 years of age or older (adults), (2) ability to speak and read English at the sixth-grade level, (3) absence of history of previous surgeries, and (4) absence of cognitive problems. The sample is selected from the accessible population that meets these sampling criteria. Sampling criteria for a study may consist of inclusion or exclusion sampling criteria, or both. **Inclusion sampling criteria** are the characteristics that the subject or element must possess to be part of the target population. In the example, the inclusion criteria are age 18 years of age or older and ability to speak and read English at the sixth-grade level. **Exclusion sampling criteria** are those characteristics that can cause a person or element to be excluded from the target population. For example, any subjects with a history of previous surgery or any cognitive problems will be excluded from the preoperative teaching study.

When the study is completed, the findings are generalized from the sample to the target population that meets the sampling criteria. The researcher may narrowly define the sampling criteria to make the sample as **homogeneous** (or similar) as possible to control for extraneous variables. Conversely, the researcher may broadly define the criteria to ensure that the study sample is **heterogeneous**, with a broad range of values or scores on the variables being studied. If the sampling or eligibility criteria are too narrow and restrictive, the researcher may have difficulty finding subjects who meet the criteria and may not be able to obtain a sufficiently large sample from the accessible population.

In discussing the generalization of findings in a published research report, investigators sometimes attempt to generalize beyond the sampling criteria. The researcher may contend that the sample was limited by the sampling criteria only for convenience in conducting the study but that the findings really apply to a larger population. Using the example preoperative teaching study, the sample may need to be limited to subjects who speak and read English because the preoperative teaching is performed in English and one of the measurement instruments requires that subjects be able to read English at the sixth-grade level. However, the researcher may believe that the findings can be generalized to non-English-speaking persons. Practicing nurses need to consider carefully the implications of using these findings with non-English-speaking populations. Perhaps such persons, because they come from another culture, do not respond to the teaching in the same way as that observed in the study population.

Generalizing to people unable to read English at the sixth-grade level also may be inappropriate. Less educated people, for example, may respond differently than other groups to the preoperative teaching. Subjects unable to read at the sixth-grade level may not be able to read or comprehend written material. They may be reluctant to ask questions when they do not understand something. Many of them may have difficulty organizing their ideas and be unable to express them to another person. They may try to conceal their lack of understanding, making it difficult to clarify misconceptions. Thus, the preoperative teaching program developed for a more educated population may be unlikely to alter the postoperative outcome or length of hospital stay of members of a poorly educated population.

For this study, the population also is limited to patients who have had no previous surgery, because such persons will have the least knowledge of the postoperative experience and how they can best care for themselves. In persons with no previous experience with surgery, pre-operative teaching could be expected to result in the greatest change in knowledge. The greater the change, the more likely it will be that the statistical procedures will detect a difference. In this hypothetical study, one group receives standard care, or the small amount of teaching the hospital routinely provides, and the other group receives the treatment. In the treatment group, the researchers can control the subjects' knowledge about how to take care of themselves after surgery by providing the information through a structured preoperative teaching program. The researchers hypothesize that the subjects will use the information to take better care of themselves after surgery, resulting in a shorter hospital stay.

However, the researchers may argue that the findings can be generalized to patients who have had previous surgeries. The effect of the preoperative teaching on patients with past surgical experience may be less than the effect on subjects without past surgical experience, because experienced patients may already know some of the information taught. However, the experienced patients also may be able to use the information to take better care of themselves after surgery and thereby shorten their hospital stay. Therefore, this may justify the researchers' claim that the findings can be generalized to patients who have had previous surgery. However, researchers need to be very cautious not to generalize beyond their sampling criteria, unless there is a sound rationale for this application on the basis of findings from previous research. The following example will assist you in identifying the inclusion and exclusion sampling criteria in a published study and determining if the criteria are appropriate for the study.

RESEARCH EXAMPLE Inclusion and Exclusion Sampling Criteria

Twiss, Waltman, Berg, Ott, Gross, and Lindsey (2009) conducted a quasi-experimental study to examine the effects of strength and weight training (ST) exercises on muscle strength, balance, and falls of breast cancer survivors (BCSs) with bone loss. The sampling or eligibility criteria for this study are presented as follows:

> Women were included if they were 35–77 years of age, had a history of stage 0 (in situ), I, or II breast cancer, a BMD [bone mineral density] T-score of –1.0 or less at any of three sites (hip, spine, forearm), were at least 6 months post breast-cancer treatment and 12 months postmenopausal, resided within 100 miles of one of four research sites (Omaha, Lincoln, Kearney, and Scottsbluff, NE), and had their physicians' permission to participate [inclusion sampling criteria]. Women were excluded if they (a) had a recurrence of breast cancer; (b) were currently taking hormone therapy, bisphosphonates, glucocorticosteroids, or other drugs affecting bone; (c) were currently engaging in ST exercises; (d) had a body mass index (BMI) of 35 or greater; (e) had serum calcium, creatinine, or thyroid stimulating hormone (if on thyroid therapy) outside normal limits; or (f) had active gastrointestinal problems or other conditions that prohibited ST exercises, risedronate, calcium, or vitamin D intake [exclusion sampling criteria]. (Twiss et al., 2009, p. 22)

CRITICAL APPRAISAL

Twiss and colleagues (2009) identified specific inclusion and exclusion sampling criteria to precisely designate the subjects in the target population. These sampling criteria probably were narrowly defined by the researchers to promote the selection of a homogeneous sample of postmenopausal BCSs with bone loss. These inclusion and exclusion sampling criteria were appropriate for the study to reduce the effect of possible extraneous variables that might impact the treatment (ST exercises) and the measurement of the dependent variables (muscle strength, balance, and falls). The last exclusion criterion identified conditions that prohibited ST exercises, conditions that made it unsafe for subjects to participate in the study. Since this is a quasi-experimental study that examined the impact of the treatment on the dependent or outcome variables, the increased controls imposed by the sampling criteria strengthened the likelihood that the study outcomes were caused by the treatment and not by extraneous variables.

IMPLICATIONS FOR PRACTICE

Twiss et al. (2009) found significant improvement in muscle strength and balance for the treatment group but no significant difference in the number of falls between the treatment and comparison groups. The researchers reported "Gains in muscle strength were 9.5% and 28.5% for hip flexion and extension, 50.0% and 19.4% for wrist flexion and extension, and 21.1% and 11.6% for knee flexion and extension. Balance improved by 39.4%. Women who exercised had fewer falls, but difference in number of falls between the two groups was not significant" (Twiss et al., 2009, p. 21). Since postmenopausal BCSs with bone loss can maintain ST exercises for 24 months and demonstrate improvement in muscle strength and balance, health professionals should encourage them to participate in ST exercises. However, additional research is needed to determine the link between ST exercises and falls and fractures this population of women experience.

Representativeness of a Sample in Quantitative and Outcomes Research

Representativeness means that the sample, the accessible population, and the target population are alike in as many ways as possible (see Figure 9–1). In quantitative and outcomes research, you need to evaluate representativeness in terms of the setting, characteristics of the subjects, and distribution of values on variables measured in the study. Persons seeking care in a particular setting may be different from those who seek care for the same problem in other settings or those who choose to use self-care to manage their problems. The setting can influence representativeness in a variety of ways. Studies conducted in private hospitals usually exclude the poor. Other settings may exclude older adults or the undereducated. People who do not have access to care are usually excluded from studies. Subjects in research centers and the care they receive are different from patients and the care they receive in community hospitals, public hospitals, veterans' hospitals, or rural hospitals. People living in rural settings may respond differently to a health situation from those who live in urban settings. Obese persons who choose to enter a program to lose weight may differ from those who do not enter such a program. Thus, gathering subjects across a variety of settings provides a more representative sample of the target population than that obtainable by limiting the study to a single setting.

A sample must be representative in terms of characteristics such as age, gender, ethnicity, income, and education, which often influence study variables. These are examples of demographic or attribute variables that might be selected by researchers for examination in their study. Researchers analyze data collected on the demographic variables to produce the sample characteristics—characteristics used to provide a picture of the sample. The sample characteristics in the preoperative teaching study, for example, may be that the mean age of the subjects is 55 years ($SD = 5.6$), a majority of the subjects are female (65%), and they have varied ethnic backgrounds (45% Caucasian, 25% African American, 23% Hispanic, and 7% Asian). The sample characteristics must be reasonably representative of the characteristics of the population. If the study includes groups, the subjects in the groups must have comparable demographic characteristics. Chapter 5 contains a more detailed discussion of demographic variables and sample characteristics.

The sample also needs to be representative relative to the variables being examined in the study. For example, if the study examines attitudes toward acquired immunodeficiency syndrome (AIDS), the sample must be representative of the distribution of attitudes toward AIDS that exist in the specified population. If a study involves blood pressures of patients in a surgical recovery room, the blood pressures of subjects must be representative of those usually noted in a surgical recovery unit.

Random and Systematic Variation of Subjects' Values

Measurement values also need to be representative. Measurement values in a study often vary randomly among subjects. **Random variation** is the expected difference in values that occurs when different subjects from the same sample are examined. The difference is random because some values will be higher and others lower than the average (mean) population value. As sample size increases, random variation decreases, improving representativeness.

Systematic variation, or systematic bias—a serious concern in sampling—is a consequence of selecting subjects whose measurement values differ in some specific way from those of the population. This difference usually is expressed as a difference in the average (or mean) values between the sample and the population. Because the subjects have something in common, their values tend to be similar to those of others in the sample but different in some way from those of the population as a whole. These values do not vary randomly around the population mean. Most of the variation from the mean is in the same direction; it is systematic. For example, the sample mean may be higher than the mean of the target population. Increasing the sample size has no effect on systematic variation. For example, if all of the subjects in a study examining some type of knowledge level have an intelligence quotient (IQ) above 120, then all of their test scores in the study are likely to be higher than those of the population mean that includes people with a wide variation in IQ scores (but with a mean IQ of 100). The IQs of the subjects will introduce a systematic bias. When systematic bias occurs in quasi-experimental or experimental studies, it can lead the researcher to think that the treatment has made a difference, when in actuality the values would have been different even without the treatment.

Acceptance and Refusal Rates in Studies

The probability of systematic variation increases when the sampling process is not random. Even in a random sample, however, systematic variation can occur when a large number of the potential subjects declines participation. As the number of subjects declining participation increases, the possibility of a systematic bias in the study becomes greater. In published studies, researchers may identify a **refusal rate**, which is the percentage of subjects who declined to participate in the study, and the subjects' reasons for not participating (Burns & Grove, 2009). You calculate the refusal rate as follows:

Refusal rate formula = number refusing ÷ number meeting sampling criteria approached × 100%

For example, if 80 potential subjects are approached to participate in the hypothetical study about the effects of preoperative teaching and 4 patients refuse, then the

$$\text{Refusal rate} = 4 \div 80 = 0.05 \times 100\% = 5\%$$

Other studies record an **acceptance rate**, which is the percentage of subjects consenting to participate in a study. You calculate the acceptance rate as follows:

Acceptance rate formula = number accepting ÷ number meeting sampling criteria approached × 100%

In the hypothetical preoperative teaching study, 4 of 80 potential subjects refused to participate—so 76 accepted. Plugging the following numbers into the stated formula gives

$$\text{Acceptance rate} = 76 \div 80 = 0.95 \times 100\% = 95\%$$

You can also calculate the acceptance and refusal rates as follows:

Acceptance rate = 100% − refusal rate, or
Refusal rate = 100% − acceptance rate

In this example, the acceptance rate was 100% − 5% (refusal rate) = 95%, which is high. In studies with a high acceptance rate and a low refusal rate, the chance for systematic variation is less, and the sample is more likely to be representative of the target population.

Attrition and Retention Rates in Studies

Systematic variation also may occur in studies with high sample attrition or mortality. Sample attrition is the withdrawal or loss of subjects from a study that can be expressed as a number of subjects withdrawing or a percentage. The percentage is the sample attrition rate and it is best if researchers include both the number of subjects withdrawing and the attrition rate. You calculate the sample attrition rate as follows:

$$\textbf{Attrition rate formula} = \textbf{Number of subjects withdrawing} \div$$
$$\textbf{Number of study subjects} \times \textbf{100\%}$$

For example, in the hypothetical study of preoperative teaching, 31 subjects—12 from the treatment group and 19 from the comparison group—withdraw, for various reasons. Loss of 31 subjects means a 41% attrition rate.

$$\text{Attrition rate} = 31 \div 76 \times 100\% = 40.795 = 41\%$$

In this example, the overall sample attrition rate was considerable (41%), and the rates differed for the two groups to which the subjects were assigned. You can also calculate the attrition rates for the groups. If the two groups were equal at the start of the study and each included 38 subjects, then the attrition rate for the treatment group was $12 \div 38 \times 100\% = 31.6 = 32\%$. The attrition for the comparison group was $19 \div 38 = 50\%$. Systematic variation is greatest when a large number of subjects withdraw from the study before data collection is completed or when a large number of subjects withdraw from one group but not the other(s) in the study. In studies involving a treatment, subjects in the comparison group who do not receive the treatment may be more likely to withdraw from the study. However, sometimes the attrition is higher for the treatment group if the intervention is complex and/or time consuming (Kerlinger & Lee, 2000). In the preoperative teaching example, there is a strong potential for systematic variation since the sample attrition rate was large (41%) and the attrition rate in the comparison group (50%) was much larger than the attrition rate in the treatment group (32%). The increased potential for systematic variation results in a sample that is less representative of the target population.

The opposite of sample attrition is the sample retention, which is the number of subjects who remain in and complete a study. You calculate the sample retention rate as follows:

$$\textbf{Sample Retention rate formula} =$$
$$\textbf{Number of subjects completing the study} \div \textbf{Number study subjects} \times \textbf{100\%}$$
$$\textbf{or}$$
$$\textbf{Sample Retention rate} = \textbf{100\%} - \textbf{Sample attrition rate}$$

In the example preoperative teaching study, 45 subjects were retained in the study that had an original sample of 76 subjects.

$$\text{Retention rate} = 45 \div 76 \times 100\% = 59.2 = 59\% \text{ or } 100\% - 41\% = 59\%$$

The higher the retention rate, the more representative the sample is of the target population and the more likely the study results are an accurate reflection of reality. Often researchers will identify either the attrition rate or the retention rate but not both. It is better to provide a rate in addition to the number of subjects withdrawing or remaining in a study. Researchers also strengthen their study by providing a rationale for the attrition of subjects from the study.

RESEARCH EXAMPLE Acceptance, Sample Retention, and Group Retention Rates

The Twiss et al. (2009) study of the effects of ST exercises on muscle strength, balance, and falls of BCSs with bone loss was introduced earlier in this chapter with the discussion of sampling criteria. It is also presented as an example here.

> A sample of 249 participants met the screening criteria and they were enrolled in the study. ... Of the 249 women, 223 completed the 24-month testing and were included in the analysis (exercise [treatment group] = 110; comparison = 113). The remaining 26 women (exercise = 14; comparison = 12) withdrew from the study before 24 months. Reasons for withdrawal included the desire for a different exercise program (*n* = 7); insufficient time (*n* = 6); intolerance to meds (*n* = 5); cancer recurrence (*n* = 5); health problems (*n* = 2); and relocation (*n* = 1). (Twiss et al., 2009, p. 22)

CRITICAL APPRAISAL

These researchers identified that 249 participants or subjects met the sampling criteria and 249 were enrolled in the study, indicating that the acceptance rate for the study was 100%. The sample retention was 223 women for a retention rate of 90% (223 ÷ 249 × 100% = 90%) and the sample attrition rate was 26 women for an attrition rate of 10% (100% − 90% = 10%). The treatment group retention was 110 women with a retention rate of 89% (110 ÷ 124 × 100% = 89%). The comparison group retention was 113 women with a retention rate of 90% (113 ÷ 125 = 90%). This study has an extremely strong acceptance rate (100%) and a very strong sample retention rate of 90% for a 24-month-long study. The retention rates for both groups were very strong and comparable (treatment group 89% and comparison group 90%). Twiss and colleagues (2009) also provided rationale for the subjects' attrition, and the reasons were varied and seemed appropriate and typical for a study lasting for 24 months. The acceptance rate, the sample and group retention rates, and the reasons for subjects' attrition indicate limited potential for systematic variation in the study sample. Thus, there is increased likelihood that the sample is representative of the target population and the results are an accurate reflection of reality. The study would have been strengthened if the researchers would have included not only the numbers but also the sample and group retention rates.

IMPLICATIONS FOR PRACTICE

The implications for practice were previously presented in the discussion of sampling criteria.

Random Sampling

From a sampling theory perspective, each person or other element in the population should have an opportunity to be selected for the sample. One method of providing this opportunity is referred to as random sampling. The purpose of random sampling is to increase the extent to which the sample is representative of the target population. However, random sampling must take place in an accessible population that is representative of the target population. It is rarely possible to obtain a random sample for clinical nursing studies because of informed consent requirements. People who volunteer to participate in a study may differ in important ways from those not willing to participate. (This chapter describes methods of achieving random samples in later sections.)

The use of the term control group is limited to those studies using random sampling methods. If researchers use nonrandom methods for sample selection, the group not receiving a treatment is a comparison group because there is an increased possibility of preexisting differences between the experimental and comparison groups. In addition, the subjects in the comparison group usually receive standard care provided for that population and the experimental group receives the treatment adding to the preexisting differences between the two groups. Often the experimental group also receives standard care to keep the groups as similar as possible.

Sampling Frames

For everyone in the accessible population to have an opportunity for selection in the sample, each person in the population must be identified. To accomplish this, the researcher must acquire a list of every member of the population, using the sampling criteria to define eligibility. This list is referred to as the sampling frame. Researchers then select subjects from the sampling frame using a sampling plan. In some studies the sampling frame cannot be identified, because it is not possible to list all members of the population. The Health Insurance Portability and Accountability Act (HIPAA) has also increased the difficulty in obtaining a sampling frame for many studies due to the requirements to protect individuals' health information.

Sampling Plans or Methods

A sampling plan or method outlines strategies used to obtain a sample for a study. Like a design, a sampling plan is not specific to a study. The plan is designed to increase representativeness and decrease systematic variation or bias. The sampling plan may use probability (random) or nonprobability (nonrandom) sampling methods. When critically appraising a study, identify the study sampling plan as either probability or nonprobability, and determine the specific method used to select a sample. The different types of probability and nonprobability sampling methods are introduced next.

Probability Sampling Methods

Probability sampling methods increase the representativeness of the sample. In probability sampling, every member (element) of the population has a probability higher than zero of

Table 9–1	Probability and Nonprobability Sampling Methods
Sampling Method	**Common Application(s)**
Probability	
Simple random sampling	Quantitative research
Stratified random sampling	Quantitative research
Cluster sampling	Quantitative research
Systematic sampling	Quantitative research
Nonprobability	
Convenience sampling	Quantitative and qualitative research
Quota sampling	Quantitative and rarely qualitative research
Purposeful or purpose sampling	Qualitative and sometimes quantitative research
Network or snowball sampling	Qualitative and sometimes quantitative research
Theoretical sampling	Qualitative research

being selected for the sample. To achieve this probability, the sample is obtained randomly. All the subsets of the population, which may differ from each other but contribute to the parameters (such as the mean and standard deviation) of the population, have a chance to be represented in the sample. The opportunity for systematic bias is less when subjects are selected randomly, although it is possible for a systematic bias to occur by chance.

Without random sampling strategies, the researcher, who has a vested interest in the study, will tend (consciously or unconsciously) to select subjects whose conditions or behaviors are consistent with the study hypotheses. The researcher may decide that person X is a better subject for the study than person Y. As another possibility, the researcher may exclude a subset of people because he or she does not agree with them, does not like them, or finds them hard to deal with. Researchers may exclude potential subjects because they are too sick, not sick enough, coping too well, not coping adequately, uncooperative, or noncompliant. By using random sampling, however, researchers leave the selection to chance, thereby increasing the validity of their studies.

There are four sampling designs that achieve probability sampling: simple random sampling, stratified random sampling, cluster sampling, and systematic sampling (Table 9–1). Probability sampling methods are used more often in quantitative research and outcomes research and are rarely used in qualitative research.

Simple Random Sampling

Simple random sampling is the most basic of the probability sampling plans. It is achieved by randomly selecting elements from the sampling frame. Researchers can accomplish random selection in a variety of ways; it is limited only by the imagination of the researcher. If the sampling frame is small, researchers can write names on slips of paper, place them in a container, mix them well, and then draw them out one at a time until they have reached the desired sample size. The most common method for randomly selecting subjects for a study is use of a computer program. The researcher can enter the sampling frame into a computer, which will then randomly select subjects until the desired sample size is achieved.

Another method for randomly selecting a study sample is use of a table of random numbers. Table 9–2 displays a section from a random numbers table. To use a table of random numbers, the researcher places a pencil or finger on the table with eyes closed. That

Table 9-2		Section from a Random Numbers Table							
06	84	10	22	56	72	25	70	69	43
07	63	10	34	66	39	54	02	33	85
03	19	63	93	72	52	13	30	44	40
77	32	69	58	25	15	55	38	19	62
20	01	94	54	66	88	43	91	34	28

number is the starting place. Then, by moving the pencil or finger up, down, right, or left, numbers are identified in order until the desired sample size is obtained. For example, you want to select 5 subjects from a population of 100 and the number 58 is initially selected as a starting point, (fourth column from the left, fourth row down), your subject numbers would be 58, 25, 15, 55, and 38. Table 9–2 is useful only when the population number is less than 100. Full tables of random numbers are available in other sources.

RESEARCH EXAMPLE Simple Random Sampling

Morea, Friend, and Bennett (2008) conducted a study to develop the Illness Self-Concept Scale (ISCS) to measure the relationship between self and illness in patients with fibromyalgia (FM). These researchers used simple random sampling in their study and described their sampling method as follows.

> Two hundred patients with FM were randomly selected from a database of 328 patients [simple random sampling method] provided by the Oregon Health & Sciences University (OHSU) and were mailed a questionnaire. All the members of the participant pool had previously been diagnosed at the OHSU Fibromyalgia Clinic using the American College of Rheumatology criteria. … Of the 200 patients selected, 173 received the questionnaire and/or were eligible to participate (12 had moved with no forwarding address, 2 were out of the country, 1 had died, and 12 reported that they no longer had fibromyalgia). Of the 173, 108 responded to the questionnaire, yielding a 62% response rated. Of the other 38%, 19 were unwilling to participate, and 46 did not respond to the questionnaire. (Morea et al., 2008, p. 566)

CRITICAL APPRAISAL

Morea and colleagues (2009) clearly indicated they used random sampling and identified the sampling frame as a list of 328 FM patients in a database provided by OHSU. These patients were consistently diagnosed with FM in the same clinic using national guidelines, ensuring a more homogeneous sample. A homogeneous sample decreases the influence of extraneous variables and increases the focus on the purpose of the study. The researchers also provided detailed rationale for the selection of 173 subjects who met sample criteria. The 62% response return rate for mailed questionnaires is very high, since the response rate to questionnaires averages 25% to 50% (Burns & Grove, 2009). In summary, the researchers used simple random sampling method, identified a complete sampling frame, had a homogenous sample of FM patients, and obtained a strong response rate to their questionnaires. These sampling activities limit the potential for systematic variation or bias and increase the likelihood that the study sample is representative of the accessible and target populations. The study would have been strengthened if the researchers had indicated how the FM patients were randomly selected from the database. The random selection was probably achieved by a computer program.

IMPLICATIONS FOR PRACTICE

Morea et al. (2008) found that the ISCS demonstrated good reliability and validity in measuring illness self-concept (ISC) in fibromyalgia patients. ISC may play a significant role in coping with fibromyalgia and the ISCS appears useful in evaluating ISC in FM and might be useful with other chronic illnesses. Future research might focus on the development of interventions to enhance ISC and promote coping with fibromyalgia and other chronic illnesses.

Stratified Random Sampling

Stratified random sampling is used in situations in which the researcher knows some of the variables in the population that are critical for achieving representativeness. Variables commonly used for stratification include age, gender, ethnicity, socioeconomic status, diagnosis, geographical region, type of institution, type of care, type of registered nurse, nursing area of specialization, and site of care. Stratification ensures that all levels of the identified variables are adequately represented in the sample. With stratification, the researcher can use a smaller sample size to achieve the same degree of representativeness relative to the stratified variable than can be derived for a large sample acquired through simple random sampling. One disadvantage is that a large population must be available from which to select subjects.

If the researcher has used stratification, he or she must define categories (strata) of the variables selected for stratification in the published report. For example, using ethnicity for stratification, the researcher may define four strata: Caucasian, African American, Hispanic, and other. The population may be 60% Caucasian, 20% African American, 15% Hispanic, and 5% other. The researcher may select a random sample for each stratum equivalent to the target population proportions of that stratum. Thus, a sample of 100 subjects would need to include approximately 60 Caucasians, 20 African Americans, 15 Hispanic, and 5 other. Alternatively, equal numbers of subjects may be randomly selected for each stratum. For example, if age is used to stratify a sample of 100 adult subjects, the researcher may obtain 25 subjects 18 to 34 years of age, 25 subjects 35 to 50 years of age, 25 subjects 51 to 66 years of age, and 25 subjects older than 66 years of age.

RESEARCH EXAMPLE Stratified Random Sampling

Willgerodt (2008, p. 395) conducted a study to test "a theoretical model examining the influence of family and peer factors on adolescent distress and risky behavior over time, using a nationally representative sample of Chinese, Filipino, and White adolescents." This study used a stratified random sample and is described as follows.

Continued

RESEARCH EXAMPLE—cont'd

Data from Wave 1 and Wave 2 of the Add Health project collected in 1994 (Wave 1) and 1995 (Wave 2; Udry, 2003) were utilized in this study. Add Health is an ecologically framed, nationally representative study of individual, family, and environmental influences on various aspects of health, including mental health and substance use. The primary sampling frame for this study included all high schools in the United States that had an 11th grade and at least 30 students in the school ($n = 26,666$). A random sample of 80 high schools was selected and stratified by region, being urban, school type, and size. The largest *feeder* school, either a middle or junior high school, for each of the 80 high schools was recruited, resulting in 80 high schools and 52 feeder schools. A random subsample of adolescents in Grades 7–12 from these schools participated in an in-home interview ($n = 12,118$), which included questions on health status, behaviors, peer networks, and family dynamics. … The sample for this study was composed of 194 Chinese, 335 Filipino, and 345 White adolescents who were randomly selected. All of the Chinese and Filipino cases with complete data were included; however, because of the large number of White cases available, a subsample of 345 cases were selected randomly, allowing the three study group sizes to remain relatively similar in size. (Willgerodt, 2008, p. 397)

CRITICAL APPRAISAL

Willgerodt (2008) obtained her subjects by randomly sampling from an existing database of a national longitudinal study of adolescent health (Add Health) (Udry, 2003). The primary study had an extremely large national random sample that was representative of Chinese, Filipino, and White youth. The random selection included both schools and adolescents within these schools from a clearly designated sampling frame. The primary study sample was stratified by region, school type, and size to ensure a national sample of adolescents was obtained who were representative of different types and sizes of schools. For her study, Willgerodt randomly selected a subsample of adolescents from the national database that was stratified by Chinese, Filipino, and White adolescents to ensure representativeness of these three ethnic groups that is consistent with the primary study sample. Thus, this study included a strong stratified randomly sampling method with a large sample size ($N = 874$), which increases the representativeness of this sample and decreases the potential for systematic error or bias.

IMPLICATIONS FOR PRACTICE

Willgerodt (2008) found for all three ethnic groups that strong family bonds significantly decreased emotional distress and risky behaviors in adolescents over time. Peer risky behaviors were found to significantly influence distress and risky behaviors among White and Filipino youth but not Chinese. These study findings increase our understanding of family and peer influences on adolescent emotional distress and risky behaviors. This knowledge could guide the development of interventions for different ethnic groups to decrease distress and risky behaviors of adolescents.

Cluster Sampling

In **cluster sampling**, a researcher develops a sampling frame that includes a list of all the states, cities, institutions, or organizations with which elements of the identified population can be linked. A randomized sample of these states, cities, institutions, or organizations can then be used in the study. In some cases, this randomized selection continues through several stages and is then referred to as multistage sampling. For example, the researcher may first randomly select states and then randomly select cities within the sampled states. Next, the researcher may randomly select hospitals within the randomly selected cities. Within the hospitals, nursing units may be randomly selected. At this level, all of the patients on the nursing unit who fit the criteria for the study may be included, or patients can be randomly selected.

Cluster sampling is used in two types of research situations. In the first such situation, the researcher considers it necessary to obtain a geographically dispersed sample but recognizes that obtaining a simple random sample will require too much travel time and expense. In the second, the researcher cannot identify the individual elements making up the population and therefore cannot develop a sampling frame. For example, a list of all people in the United States who have had open-heart surgery does not exist. Nevertheless, it often is possible to obtain lists of institutions or organizations with which the elements of interest are associated—in this example, perhaps cardiology clinics and/or university medical centers with large, well-funded cardiology departments—and then randomly select institutions from which the researcher can acquire subjects.

RESEARCH EXAMPLE Cluster Sampling

Willgerodt's (2008) study, discussed previously, included a sample obtained from a national database that was developed from the longitudinal study of adolescent health (Add Health) (Udry, 2003). This longitudinal study included both cluster sampling and stratified random sampling. The cluster sampling is evident in the identification of all high schools in the United States that had an 11th grade and at least 30 subjects in the school ($n = 26,666$) and the random selection of 80 of these high schools. The next level of the cluster sampling was to randomly select adolescents from the 80 high schools and their 52 feeder schools. Since Willgerodt sampled from this national database, her sample also included both cluster and stratified random sampling. Cluster sampling was used to ensure that a nationally representative sample of adolescents was obtained for the Add Health study and also Willgerodt's study. However, Willgerodt's (2008) study would have been strengthened by the identification of the cluster sampling method used and the rationale for using this method.

Systematic Sampling

Systematic sampling is used when an ordered list of all members of the population is available. The process involves selecting every kth individual on the list, using a starting point selected randomly. If the initial starting point is not random, the sample is nonprobability or nonrandom sample. To use this design, the researcher must know the number of elements in the population and the size of the sample desired. The population size is divided by the desired sample size, giving k, the size of the gap between elements selected from the list. For example, if the population size is $n = 1200$ and the desired sample size is $n = 100$, then $k = 12$. Thus, the researcher would include every 12th person on the list in the sample. You obtain this value by using the following formula:

$$k = \textbf{population size} \div \textbf{by the desired sample size}$$

In the example, $k = 1200$ subjects in the population ÷ 100 desired sample size = 12. Some argue that this procedure does not truly give each element of a population an opportunity to be included in the sample; it provides a random but not equal chance for inclusion (Kerlinger & Lee, 2000).

RESEARCH EXAMPLE Systematic Sampling

Rambur, McIntosh, Val Palumbo, and Reinier (2005) conducted a comparative descriptive study of job satisfaction and career retention in two groups of registered nurses (RNs) whose highest degrees were the associate degree in nursing (ADN) or the bachelor's degree in nursing (BSN). These researchers obtained their sample using systematic sampling technique:

> The study population was drawn from the roster of registered nurses by the Vermont Board of Nursing in September 2002 ($n = 7028$). For this study, advanced practice, inactive, out-of-state, foreign, and deceased nurses were excluded with a resulting population of approximately 6000. To select a sample of 3000 nurses for the study sample, the remaining list was ordered by license number and a systematic sample of every second nurse was conducted to identify the proposed sample of 3000 participants. These 3000 nurses, therefore, were a systematic sample of active RNs in Vermont in September 2002 ... Seven percent of the 3000 surveys were returned because of inaccurate postal addresses ($n = 220$) or because the nurse was deceased ($n = 2$). Of the remaining 2778 surveys, the final overall response rate was 56.7% ($n = 1574$). (Rambur et al., 2005, pp. 188-189)

CRITICAL APPRAISAL

The systematic sampling plan used by Rambur et al. (2005) has mainly strengths but also some weaknesses. The researchers made the sample more homogeneous and eliminated potential for bias by excluding advanced-practice, inactive, foreign, and deceased nurses. This resulted in a sampling frame of 6000 RNs. These researchers desired a sample size of $n = 3000$ RNs, so they systematically selected every second RN. A potential area for bias is that only 56.7%, or $n = 1574$, subjects returned their surveys and 43.3% did not. Those nurses who did not return their survey may be different in some way from those who did participate, which decreases the sample's representativeness of the target population. The return rates of surveys in studies often are low, however, and the 56.7% is above the average survey return rate of 25% to 50% (Burns & Grove, 2009). In addition, the representativeness of the sample is strengthened by the large sample size, $n = 1574$, and the use of a probability sampling method.

IMPLICATIONS FOR PRACTICE

Compared with ADN nurses, BSN nurses started their careers earlier, were employed longer, and held more positions. BSN nurses also had significantly higher job satisfaction related to autonomy and growth, job stress and physical demands, and job and organizational security. Thus, this study supports preparation of nurses with BSNs for stronger individual and social return on educational investment. Thus, hospitals need to consider this when hiring nurses because research had indicated that BSN-prepared nurses might have a more productive, satisfying, and longer career than ADN nurses.

Nonprobability Sampling Methods Used in Quantitative Research

In **nonprobability sampling**, not every element of the population has an opportunity for selection to be included in the sample. Although this approach decreases a sample's representativeness of a population, it commonly is used in nursing studies. In an analysis of studies published in six nursing journals from 1977 to 1986, only 9% used probability or random sampling (Moody, Wilson, Smyth, Schwartz, Tittle, & Van Cott, 1988). It appears that this trend continues today, because most of the nursing studies use nonprobability sampling methods. Thus, it is important to be able to discriminate among the various nonprobability sampling plans used in research.

The five nonprobability sampling plans used most frequently in nursing research are convenience sampling, quota sampling, purposive or purposeful sampling, network sampling, and theoretical sampling. Convenience and quota sampling often are used in quantitative and outcomes studies (see Table 9–1). Purposive, network, and theoretical sampling are used more frequently in qualitative research and are discussed later in this chapter.

Convenience Sampling

Convenience sampling, also called "accidental sampling," is a weak approach because it provides little opportunity to control for biases; subjects are included in the study merely because they happen to be in the right place at the right time (Burns & Grove, 2009; Kerlinger & Lee, 2000). A classroom of students, patients who attend a clinic on a specific day, subjects who attend a support group, and patients hospitalized with specific medical diagnoses or nursing problems are examples of convenience samples. The researcher simply enters available subjects into the study until the desired sample size is reached. Multiple biases may exist in the sample, some of which may be subtle and unrecognized. However, serious biases are not always present in convenience samples. According to Kerlinger and Lee (2000), a convenience sample is acceptable when it is used with reasonable knowledge and care in implementing a study.

Convenience samples are inexpensive, accessible, and usually less time consuming to obtain than other types of samples. This type of sampling provides a means to conduct studies on nursing interventions when the researchers are unable to use probability sampling. Convenience sampling method is commonly used in healthcare studies because most researchers have limited access to patients who meet study sample criteria. Probability or random sampling is not possible when the pool of potential patients is limited. Researchers often think it is best to include all patients who meet sample criteria (sample of convenience) to increase the sample size.

For some healthcare studies, the sampling frames for some populations are not available, so researchers often use a sample of convenience. Many researchers are now conducting quasi-experimental studies and clinical trials in both medicine and nursing and these types of studies frequently require the use of convenience sampling method. As a component of these study designs, subjects usually are randomly assigned to groups. This random assignment to groups, which is not a sampling method but a design strategy, does not alter the risk of biases resulting from convenience sampling but does strengthen the equivalence of the study groups. With these potential biases and the narrowly defined sampling criteria used to select subjects in most clinical trials, representativeness of the sample is a concern. To strengthen the representativeness of a sample, researchers often increase the sample size for clinical trials. Sample size is discussed later in this chapter.

RESEARCH EXAMPLE Convenience Sampling

Bay, Hagerty, and Williams (2007) used convenience sampling in their descriptive study of depression in individuals following mild-to-moderate traumatic brain injury (TBI). The researchers compared three scales to determine the best screening measure for identifying depressive symptoms in outpatients with TBI. The following excerpt describes their sampling method.

A convenience sample was recruited from five outpatient TBI programs that offered outpatient therapies for those with neurological disorders. Human investigation procedures with the injured person and their relative/significant other (R/SO) were obtained for each clinical site and written consent was obtained from the injured person and their R/SO. All centers were affiliated with large trauma hospitals in the Midwest and recruitment procedures were similar across settings. ... All persons completed the survey information in the same order, during the same testing session (unless too fatigued), and in the presence of a data collector. ... An incentive payment was offered to compensate participants for their time. ... Seventy-five persons with mild or moderate TBI participated in the study. (Bay et al., 2007, p. 4)

CRITICAL APPRAISAL

Bay's et al. (2007) used a convenience sample in conducting their study since it was the most appropriate method for the type of patients studied and had more strengths than weaknesses. The consistent recruitment of the participants and the inclusion of five TBI programs across the Midwest as settings increased the sample size and its representativeness of the target population. The sample size of 75 seems adequate considering the type of patient studied. It would have been helpful if the authors had addressed the acceptance or refusal rate for the study to determine possible sample bias. The data were collected at one session so there was no attrition noted during the study. The subjects were compensated for their time during the study, which usually increases the acceptance and retention rates for a study. Convenience sampling has a potential for bias but the consistency in subject recruitment from a variety of settings, the sample size, and the lack of sample attrition increase the sample's representativeness of the target population.

IMPLICATIONS FOR PRACTICE

Bay and colleagues (2007) found that the three depression subscales examined in their study, Neurobehavioral Functioning (NFI-D), Profile of Moods State (POMS-D), and Center for Epidemiologic Studies (CES-D), were useful in identifying depression in patients with TBI.

"Nearly 40% of this outpatient sample had significant levels of depressive symptoms. All measures were internally consistent, reliable, and highly correlated. For persons with mild-to-moderate traumatic brain injury, the CES-D was the best screening instrument because of its ease in administration, sensitivity in detecting probable major depressive disorders, its established categories of severity, and its comprehensiveness" (Bay et al., 2007, p. 2).

In summary, the researchers recommended: "Using categories of the CES-D, nurses can identify levels of depression and refer those whose score is greater than 15 to providers with special skills in TBI depression assessment and treatment" (Bay et al., 2007, p. 10).

Quota Sampling

Quota sampling uses a convenience sampling technique with an added feature—a strategy to ensure the inclusion of subject types likely to be underrepresented in the convenience sample, such as females; minority groups; and the elderly, poor, rich, and undereducated. The goal of quota sampling is to replicate the proportions of subgroups present in the target population. The technique is similar to that used in stratified random sampling. Quota sampling requires that the researcher be able to identify subgroups in the target population that are important for achieving representativeness for the problem being studied. In addition, the researcher must determine what proportion of the target population each identified subgroup represents. Quota sampling offers an improvement over convenience sampling and tends to decrease potential biases.

RESEARCH EXAMPLE Quota Sampling

McCain and colleagues (2003) used quota sampling in their quasi-experimental study of the effects of stress management on the psychoneuroimmunology outcomes in persons with human immunodeficiency virus (HIV) disease. They described their sampling method as follows:

> Quota sampling was used to achieve appropriate sample representation by gender, at a ratio of 4 males:1 female (20%). Gender subgroups were next stratified by prebaseline CD4+ cell counts [indicating the seriousness of HIV disease] to equilibrate study groups by initial CD4+ counts and, indirectly, by stage of illness ...
> Enrolled in the study were 148 individuals, 29 females (20%) and 119 males ... Study attrition was within the expected range, with 112 participants completing the intervention groups or initial waiting period (76% retention) and 102 individuals completing the 6-month follow-up visit (69% retention). The attrition rate did not differ among study groups. (McCain et al., 2003, pp. 105-106)

CRITICAL APPRAISAL

McCain and colleagues (2003) used quota sampling to ensure a gender distribution of 80% males and 20% females for their study sample (to match that in the population of all persons with HIV disease) and also equivalent CD4+ counts and stages of illness among the patients in the two study groups. The stratification by gender and CD4+ count decreased the potential for bias in the sampling method, promoted equality in the study groups, and improved the sample's representativeness of the target population. The researchers also addressed the attrition rate in terms of the total sample and the groups and indicated that this probably did not affect the study findings.

IMPLICATIONS FOR PRACTICE

McCain et al. (2003) found that a stress management intervention did improve the emotional well-being and quality-of-life scores for patients with HIV disease. Healthcare providers are encouraged to implement this stress management intervention to improve the health outcomes of patients with HIV. The researchers also recommended the testing of additional interventions that may promote the quality of life and improve the illness trajectory of patients living with HIV disease.

Sample Size in Quantitative Studies

One of the most troublesome questions that arise during the critical appraisal of a study is whether the sample size was adequate. If the study was designed to make comparisons and significant differences were found, the sample size, or number of subjects participating in the study, was adequate. Questions about the adequacy of the sample size occur only when no significance is found. Thus, when critically appraising a quantitative study in which no significance was found for at least one of the hypotheses or research questions, be sure to evaluate the adequacy of the sample size. Is there really no difference? Or was an actual difference not found because of inadequacies in the research methods, such as a small sample size?

Currently, the adequacy of the sample size in quantitative studies is evaluated using a power analysis. Power is the capacity of the study to detect differences or relationships that actually exist in the population. Expressed another way, it is the capacity to correctly reject a null hypothesis. The minimum acceptable level of power for a study is 0.8, or 80% (Cohen, 1988). This power level results in a 20% chance of a Type II error, in which the study fails to detect existing effects (differences or relationships). An increasing number of researchers are performing a power analysis before conducting their study to determine an adequate sample size. The results of this analysis usually are included in the sample section of the published study. Researchers also need to perform a power analysis to evaluate the adequacy of their sample size for all nonsignificant findings and include this in the Discussion section of their published study.

Parent and Hanley (2009) reviewed the reports of 54 randomized clinical trials published in *Applied Nursing Research*, *Heart & Lung*, and *Nursing Research* and found that sample sizes were estimated in advance in only 22% of the studies. This is of particular concern in randomized clinical trials, because they are designed to test the effect of interventions. Samples that are too small can result in studies that lack power. Polit and Sherman (1990) evaluated the sample size in 62 studies published in 1989 in *Nursing Research* and *Research in Nursing & Health*. They found that most of the studies examined had inadequate sample sizes for making comparisons between groups. The studies needed an average of 218 subjects per group to have a power level of 0.8. Therefore, in most of these studies, the risk of a Type II error—saying something is nonsignificant when it was not—was extremely high.

Other factors that influence the adequacy of sample size (because they affect power) include effect size, type of quantitative study, number of variables, sensitivity of the measurement tools, and data analysis techniques. When critically appraising the adequacy of the sample size, consider the influence of all of these factors.

Effect Size

The effect is the presence of the phenomenon examined in a study. Effect size is the extent to which the null hypothesis is false. In a study in which the researchers are comparing two populations, the null hypothesis states that the difference between the two populations is zero. However, if the null hypothesis is false, an identifiable effect is present—a difference between the two groups does exist. If the null hypothesis is false, it is false to some degree;

this is the effect size (Cohen, 1988). The statistical test tells you whether there is a difference between groups, or whether variables are significantly related. The effect size tells you the size of the difference between the groups or the *strength* of the relationship between two variables.

When the effect size is large (e.g., considerable difference between groups or very strong relationship between two variables), detecting it is easy and requires only a small sample. When the effect size is small (e.g., only a small difference between groups or a weak relationship between two variables), detecting it is more difficult and requires larger samples. The following are guidelines for categorizing the quality of the effect size:

Small effect size < 0.30

Medium effect size = 0.30 to 0.50

Large effect size > 0.50 (Burns & Grove, 2009; Cohen, 1988).

Effect size is smaller with a small sample, so effects are more difficult to detect. Increasing the sample size also increases the effect size, making it more likely that the effect will be detected and the study findings significant.

In the nursing studies examined by Polit and Sherman (1990), 52.7% of the effect sizes computed were small, with the average power being less than 0.30. That is, the probability that acceptance of the null hypothesis was correct was less than 30%, instead of the standard power of 0.8, or 80%, recommended for a study (Grove, 2007). In most cases, this flaw was the result of an insufficient sample size. Even when the effect size was moderate, the average power in the nursing studies examined was only 0.7, or 70%, with a 30% chance for error. The nursing studies reached an acceptable level of power only when the effect size was large, and 11% of these studies were underpowered. Only 15% of the studies had sufficient power for all of their analyses. When critically appraising a study, determine whether the study sample size was adequate by noting whether a power analysis was conducted and what power was achieved. Also check to see if the researchers examined the power level when findings were nonsignificant.

Types of Quantitative Studies

Descriptive studies (particularly those using survey questionnaires) and correlational studies often require very large samples. In these studies, researchers may examine multiple variables, and extraneous variables are likely to affect subject response(s) to the variables under study. Researchers often make statistical comparisons on multiple subgroups in a sample, requiring that an adequate sample be available for each subgroup being analyzed. Quasi-experimental and experimental studies use smaller samples more often than descriptive and correlational studies do. As control in the study increases, the sample size can decrease and the sample still will approximate the target population. Instruments in these studies tend to be more refined, with stronger reliability and validity. Designs that use blocking or stratification usually increase the total sample size required. Designs that use matched pairs of subjects have increased power and thus require a smaller sample (see Chapter 8).

Number of Variables

As the number of variables under study increases, the sample size needed may increase. Including variables such as age, gender, ethnicity, and education in the data analyses can increase the sample size needed to detect differences between groups. Using them only to describe the sample does not cause a problem in terms of power. A number of the studies analyzed by Polit and Sherman (1990) had sufficient sample size for the primary analyses but failed to plan for analyses involving subgroups, such as analyzing the data by age category or ethnic group. The inclusion of multiple dependent variables also increases the sample size needed.

Measurement Sensitivity

Well-developed physiological instruments measure phenomena with accuracy and precision. A thermometer, for example, measures body temperature accurately and precisely. Tools measuring psychosocial variables tend to be less precise. However, a tool that is reliable and valid measures more precisely than a tool that is less well developed. Variance tends to be higher with a less well-developed tool than with one that is well developed. For example, if you are measuring anxiety and the actual anxiety score of several subjects is 80, you may obtain measures ranging from 70 to 90 with a less well-developed tool. Much more variation from the true score occurs with new or less-developed scales than when a well-developed scale is used, which will tend to show a score closer to the actual score of 80 for each subject. As variance in instrument scores increases, the sample size needed to obtain significance increases (see Chapter 10).

Data Analysis Techniques

Data analysis techniques vary in their capability to detect differences in the data. Statisticians refer to this as the "power of the statistical analysis." An interaction also occurs between the measurement sensitivity and the power of the data analysis technique. The power of the analysis technique increases as precision in measurement increases. Larger samples are needed when the power of the planned statistical analysis is weak.

For some statistical procedures, such as the *t*-test and analysis of variance (ANOVA), equal group sizes will increase power because the effect size is maximized. The more unbalanced the group sizes are, the smaller the effect size is. Therefore in unbalanced groups, the total sample size must be larger (Kraemer & Theimann, 1987). The chi-square test is the weakest of the statistical tests and requires very large sample sizes to achieve acceptable levels of power. As the number of categories increases, the sample size needed increases. Also, if some of the categories contain small numbers of subjects, the total sample size must be increased. Chapter 11 describes the *t*-test, ANOVA, and chi-square statistical analysis techniques in more detail.

CRITICAL APPRAISAL GUIDELINES

Adequacy of the Sample in Quantitative Studies

When critically appraising the sample of quantitative studies, address the following questions:

1. Does the researcher define the target population for the study?
2. Are the sampling inclusion criteria, sampling exclusion criteria, or both clearly identified and appropriate for the study?
3. Is the sample size identified? Is a power analysis reported? Was sample size appropriate as indicated by the power analysis? If groups were included in the study, is the sample size for each group discussed?
4. Are the refusal or acceptance rates identified? Are the sample attrition or retention rates addressed? Are reasons provided for the refusal and attrition rates?
5. Is the sampling method probability or nonprobability? Identify the specific sampling method used in the study to obtain the sample.
6. Is the sampling method adequate to achieve a representative sample? Is the sample representative of the accessible and target populations?
7. Are the potential biases in the sample discussed?

RESEARCH EXAMPLE Quantitative Study Sample

Hodgins, Ouellet, Pond, Knorr, and Geldart (2008) conducted a quasi-experimental study to examine the effect of a telephone follow-up on surgical orthopedic patients' postdischarge recovery. "The sample consisted of 438 patients randomly assigned to receive routine care with or without telephone follow-up 24 to 72 hours after discharge (intervention)" (Hodgins et al., 2008, p. 218). The sample and setting are described in the following excerpt and the particular aspects of the sample have been identified in [brackets]. The sample section from Hodgins and colleagues' quantitative study is followed by a critical appraisal based on the previous guidelines and the implications for practice.

The study population consisted of adult patients admitted for either elective or emergent orthopedic surgery to a regional referral hospital in Eastern Canada [setting] between January and December 2002. The selection and inclusion criteria required that the patients be (a) English speaking, (b) able to communicate by telephone, (c) free of mental confusion, and (d) discharged to a private residence [sampling criteria]. The required sample size was estimated based on a desired power of .80, a present alpha [level of significance] = .05, 11 predictor variables, and an anticipated weak intervention effect. ... Using these criteria, we estimated that a minimum of 390 participants would be required to detect a difference in the number of postdischarge problems experienced by the intervention and control groups [power analysis]. (Power and Precision Software, Release 2.1, Biostat Software Products, Englewood, NJ) (Hodgins et al., 2008, p. 220)

The final sample consisted of 438 participants [sample size with 216 in the intervention group and 222 in the control group]. Of the 511 patients enrolled, 73 were lost to follow-up, resulting in an overall retention rate of 85.5%. Reasons for loss to follow-up included the following: unable to be contacted for the outcome interview, $n = 38$; transferred to another unit, $n = 20$; declined to participate at the time of the outcome interview, $n = 8$; death, $n = 2$; problem with data entry, $n = 1$; and unspecified, $n = 4$. A number of the recruited cases ($n = 22$) were lost before their random group assignment, which was done immediately before the telephone follow-up. (Hodgins et al., 2008, pp. 221-222)

Continued

CRITICAL APPRAISAL

Hodgins and colleagues (2008) clearly described their study population, setting, sampling criteria, and sample size that was determined with power analysis. The final sample size of 438 was strong and included 48 more subjects than the 390 subjects required by the power analysis. The retention rate of 85.5% was strong and the reasons for the attrition seemed common and not a bias for the sample based on the size of the original sample and the length of the study. The attrition of subjects was fairly comparable for the intervention group ($n = 216$) and the control group ($n = 222$). The researchers did not identify the acceptance or refusal rate that might have been a source of bias for the study.

The study would have been strengthened by the researchers clearly identifying the sampling method, which appeared to be a sample of convenience. The sample of convenience has a potential to bias the study results but adequate sample size, limited attrition, and comparable sized intervention and control groups increased the sample's representativeness of the target population (Burns & Grove, 2009; Kerlinger & Lee, 2000).

IMPLICATIONS FOR PRACTICE

Hodgins et al. (2008) found that the telephone follow-up intervention did not have a significant effect on the surgical orthopedic patients' postdischarge recovery. The limitations of the intervention included making the phone calls too early after discharge, short durations of the calls, and the limited qualifications of the nurses making the calls. In future studies, the researchers recommended the requirements of the telephone follow-up programs and the outcome measures be explicitly developed. However, the study clearly described the postdischarge experiences of surgical orthopedic patients and what nurses can do to promote their recovery. The main patient symptoms that required management in the home were pain, constipation, and swelling. Patients need to understand these symptoms and how they can manage them in their homes to promote their recovery.

Sampling in Qualitative Research

Qualitative research is conducted to gain insights and discover meaning about a particular phenomenon, situation, cultural element, or historical event (Munhall, 2007; Patton, 2002). The intent of qualitative research is an in-depth understanding of a specially selected sample and not on the generalization of the findings from a randomly selected sample to a target population, as in quantitative research. The sampling in qualitative research focuses more on experiences, events, incidents, and settings than on people (Sandelowski, 1995). Qualitative researchers often select the setting and site and then the population and phenomenon of interest (Marshall & Rossman, 2006).

The people studied in qualitative research are called participants, not subjects. Researchers attempt to select participants who are considered experts in the area of study and are willing to share rich, in-depth information about the phenomenon, situation, culture, or event being studied. For example, if the goal of the study is to describe the phenomenon of living with chronic pain, the researcher will select those individuals who are articulate and reflective, have a history of chronic pain, and are willing to share their chronic pain experience (Coyne, 1997; Munhall, 2007).

Three common sampling methods used in qualitative nursing research are purposive or purposeful sampling, network or snowball sampling, and theoretical sampling (see Table 9–1). These sampling methods enable researchers to select information-rich cases or participants who they believe will provide them the best data for their studies (Clifford, 1997). The sample selection process can have a profound effect on the quality of the research and researchers should describe this in enough depth to promote the interpretation of the findings and the replication of the study.

Purposeful or Purposive Sampling

With **purposeful sampling**, sometimes referred to as "judgmental" or "selective sampling," the researcher consciously selects certain participants, elements, events, or incidents to include in the study. Researchers may try to include typical or atypical participants or similar or varied situations. Qualitative researchers may select participants who are of various age categories, those who have different diagnoses or illness severity, or those who received an ineffective treatment rather than an effective treatment for their illness. The ultimate goal of purposeful or purposive sampling is selecting information-rich cases from which researchers can obtain in-depth information needed for their studies (Morse, 2007).

Some have criticized the purposeful sampling method because it is difficult to evaluate the accuracy or relevance of the researcher's judgment. Thus, researchers must indicate the characteristics that they desired in study participants and provide a rationale for selecting these types of individuals to obtain essential data for their study. In qualitative research, this sampling method seems to be the best way to gain insights into a new area of study or to obtain in-depth understanding of a complex experience or event.

You can combine different sampling methods with purposeful sampling such as quota purposeful sampling or purposeful random sampling. With quota purposeful sampling, researchers are able to capture major variations in a sample such as studying participants from a variety of ethnic, age, economic, or illness categories. This sampling method has some similarities to quota sampling and stratified random sampling discussed previously. Purposeful random sampling involves selecting the initial participants using purposeful sampling and then randomly selecting from that sample. "For many audiences, random sampling, even of small samples, will substantially increase the credibility of the results" (Patton, 2002, p. 240). In summary, purposeful sampling plans enable researchers to select the information-rich cases (participants, events, or situations) to gain insights and discover new meaning in their area of study (Munhall, 2007).

RESEARCH EXAMPLE Purposeful or Purposive Sampling

Pearce, Harrell, and McMurray (2008) conducted a qualitative study to explore middle-school children's understanding of physical activity. The researchers used purposeful random sampling to select the 12 children for the study.

Continued

RESEARCH EXAMPLE—cont'd

Study activities were conducted at a rural public middle school during regular school hours for 6 months … A purposeful sampling design was used to select 12 children for participation in the study. Equal age and gender cohorts were used to capture any differences in children's understanding between grades and gender. The school principal randomly selected one homeroom from the possible six to eight homerooms for each grade (sixth, seventh, and eight grades). Signed assent and consent forms were returned for 29 children (return rate 38%). Names of four children (two girls, two boys) in each grade were randomly selected from the names of all children who provided written assent and parental consent. The children's mean age was 12.5 years (range, 11-15 years), representing African-American ($n = 4$), Caucasian ($n = 6$), and Hispanic ($n = 2$) children. Each participant received a US $25 gift certificate to a local department store for each week of study participation. (Pearce et al., 2008, p. 171)

CRITICAL APPRAISAL

Pearce and colleagues (2008) clearly identified the use of a purposeful random sampling plan to select the 12 participants for their study. They also seemed to include quota sampling to ensure gender and grade levels (sixth, seventh, and eighth) were equally represented in the sample. The purposeful sampling was conducted to capture any differences or variations the children might have in their understanding of physical activity. The random selection of one homeroom by the principal and the random selection of 12 children from the 29 who assented to participate in the study added to the credibility of the study results (Patton, 2002). The study Results and Discussion sections reflected that the 12 study participants provided rich information about their understanding of physical activity.

IMPLICATIONS FOR PRACTICE

Pearce and colleagues' (2008) analysis of their study interview data reflected that the middle-school children had a very broad and concrete understanding of physical activities. They believed "if you're moving, you're doing physical activity" (Pearce et al., 2008, p. 172). Their understanding of physical activity was that it included: exercising, playing, working on the computer, and sleeping. They believed all of these activities required body movement and thus were physical activity. The children were able to easily recall activities and time duration of the activity, but had difficulty with categorizing the intensity of their activities. Thus, the middle-school children's understanding of physical activity probably does not coincide with that of most pediatric nurses and researchers. This needs to be taken into consideration when having this age of child complete questionnaires on physical activities or making recommendations to them about activities. "Thus, pediatric nurses can bridge the gap between what children know about physical activity, the activities children do, and activity measurement with interventions aimed at a better understanding of children's activity and its contribution to overall health" (Pearce et al., 2008, p. 180).

Network Sampling

Network sampling, sometimes referred to as "snowball, chain, or nominated sampling," holds promise for locating participants who would be difficult or impossible to obtain in other ways or who have not been previously identified for study (Munhall, 2007; Patton,

2002). Network sampling takes advantage of social networks and the fact that friends tend to have characteristics in common. This strategy also is particularly useful for finding subjects in socially devalued populations, such as persons who are dependent on alcohol, abuse children, commit sexual offenses, are addicted to drugs, or commit criminal acts. These persons seldom are willing to make themselves known. Other groups, such as widows, grieving siblings, or persons successful at lifestyle changes, also may be located using network sampling. Such persons typically are outside the existing healthcare system and are difficult to find. When researchers have found a few participants who meet the sampling criteria, they ask their assistance in finding others with similar characteristics.

Researchers often obtain the first few study participants through a purposeful sampling method, and expand the sample size using network sampling. This sampling method is used in quantitative studies but is more common in qualitative studies. In qualitative research, network sampling is an effective strategy for identifying subjects who can provide the greatest insight and essential information about an experience or event that is being studied (Munhall, 2007). For example if a study was being conducted to describe the lives of adolescents who are abusing substances, network sampling would enable researchers to find participants who have a prolonged history of substance abuse and were able to provide rich information about their lives in an interview (Patton, 2002).

RESEARCH EXAMPLE Network Sampling

Coté-Arsenault and Morrison-Beedy (2001) conducted a phenomenological study entitled "Women's Voices Reflecting Changed Expectations for Pregnancy after Perinatal Loss." They described the sampling plan for their study as follows:

> Following IRB [institutional review board] approval, a snowball sampling approach was used to recruit women who had experienced at least one perinatal loss and a minimum of one subsequent pregnancy. Recruitment was accomplished using various sources: personal contacts, the local perinatal loss support group, and flyers placed within the university community and local community health settings. ... The sample consisted of 21 women with diverse pregnancy and loss histories.
>
> The diversity of childbearing experiences was extensive, encompassing one woman who was currently pregnant, a woman who had given birth 14 weeks before, and women whose last birth was more than two decades prior to this study. The women had experienced from 1 to 7 losses which occurred throughout the three trimesters of pregnancy and at birth. All currently had living children. (Coté-Arsenault & Morrison-Beedy, 2001, p. 241)

CRITICAL APPRAISAL

The researchers clearly identified the networks (personal contacts, loss support group, and flyers) that were used to recruit subjects. This sampling plan successfully identified women with diverse childbearing experiences, who provided detailed data on their expectations for pregnancy after perinatal loss. Since the participants had diverse childbearing experiences, the sample size seemed to be adequate to address the purpose of the study.

Continued

IMPLICATIONS FOR PRACTICE

Coté-Arsenault and Morrison-Beedy (2001, p. 239) found that

[w]omen's stories portrayed perinatal loss as a life-altering event. Women did not feel emotionally safe in their pregnancies after loss and were afraid that those babies too would die. Despite the differences in their obstetrical and loss histories and time since loss, similarities in their responses to pregnancy far outweighed their differences. These commonalities are contained in six themes: (a) dealing with uncertainty, (b) wondering if the baby is healthy, (c) waiting to lose the baby, (d) holding back their emotions, (e) acknowledging that loss happened and that it can happen again, and (f) changing self. ... Care providers should acknowledge women's past losses, address their concerns during a current pregnancy, and recognize the potentially life-long effect perinatal loss may have on these women.

Theoretical Sampling

Theoretical sampling is used in qualitative research to develop a selected theory through the research process (Munhall, 2007). This type of sampling strategy is used most frequently with grounded theory research, since the focus of this type of research is theory development. The researcher gathers data from any person or group able to provide relevant, varied, and rich information for theory generation. The data are considered relevant and rich if they include information that generates, delimits, and saturates the theoretical codes in the study needed for theory generation (Huberman & Miles, 2002). A code is saturated if it is complete and the researcher can see how it fits in the theory. Thus, the researcher continues to seek sources and gather data until the codes are saturated, and the theory evolves from the codes and the data. Diversity in the sample is encouraged, so the theory developed covers a wide range of behaviors in varied situations and settings (Patton, 2002).

RESEARCH EXAMPLE Theoretical Sampling

Rew (2003) conducted a grounded theory study to develop a theory of self-care that was grounded in the experiences of homeless youth. The study incorporated theoretical sampling, and the sampling method was described as follows:

Theoretical sampling of homeless youths living temporarily in an urban area was used to insure a wide range of self-care experiences. Potential participants were recruited from youths seeking health and social services from a street outreach program (i.e., a clinic set up in a church basement) in central Texas. Criteria for inclusion were: (a) 16-20 years of age, (b) ability to understand and speak English, and (c) willingness to volunteer for an interview. This age group represented the majority of youths seeking services from this program. Fifteen youths (7 males, 6 females, and 2 transgendered) who were an average of 18.8 years of age volunteered to participate. Saturation (sufficient or adequate data had been collected to meet the goal of the study) was reached at the end of 12 interviews; three additional participants were recruited to verify the findings (Morse, 1998). These participants had been homeless for an average of 4.0 years. In the past year, the majority (*n* = 13) had lived in "squats," which are temporary campsites claimed by youths and other homeless persons. Demographic data and personal characteristics of these participants were summarized and pseudonyms were used to protect the identity of all participants. (Rew, 2003, p. 235)

CRITICAL APPRAISAL

Rew (2003) clearly identified the theoretical sampling method used to obtain the 15 study participants and the sampling criteria that indicated the specific individuals required for participation in the study. The participants were recruited from an urban area to ensure a wide range of self-care experiences. The researchers addressed the number of participants interviewed to reach data saturation and conducted three additional interviews to verify the findings. Researchers collected adequate data and codes were saturated to ensure the development of a grounded theory.

IMPLICATIONS FOR PRACTICE

Rew (2003) conducted a grounded theory study about the experiences of homeless youth and developed a theory of "Taking Care of Oneself in a High Risk Environment." This descriptive theory of self-care for homeless/street youth included three categories: (1) becoming aware of oneself, (2) staying alive with limited resources, and (3) handling one's own health. The study increased current understanding of the homeless experience for youth and provided a basis for further research to generate support and care for the homeless.

Sample Size in Qualitative Studies

In quantitative research, the sample size must be large enough to identify relationships among variables or to determine differences between groups. The larger the sample size and the effect size, the greater the power to detect relationships and differences in quantitative and outcomes studies. However, qualitative research focuses on the quality of information obtained from the person, situation, or event sampled, rather than on the size of the sample (Huberman & Miles, 2002; Munhall, 2007; Sandelowski, 1995).

The purpose of the study determines the sampling plan and the initial sample size. The depth of information that is obtained and needed to gain insight into a phenomenon, describe a cultural element, develop a theory, or understand a historical event determines the final number of people, sites, artifacts, or documents sampled. Morse (2007) refers to this as **intraproject sampling** or the additional sampling that is done during data collection and analysis to promote the development of quality study findings. The sample size can be too small when the data collected lack adequate depth or richness. Thus, an inadequate sample size can reduce the quality and credibility of the research findings.

The number of participants in a qualitative study is adequate when saturation and verification of information are achieved in the study area. Morse (2007) refers to these as strategies of intraproject sampling (discuss previously). **Saturation of information** occurs when additional sampling provides no new information, only redundancy of previous collected data. **Verification of information** occurs when researchers are able to further confirm hunches, relationships, or theoretical models. With grounded theory research, "sampling for verification occurs when linkages are made between categories and/or concepts in the developing analysis. In other words, as theory emerges, data collection continues" (Morse, 2007, p. 537). The theory linkages developed need to be based on data regardless of how abstract they are. Important factors that need to be considered in determining sample size are (1) scope of the study, (2) nature of the topic, (3) quality of the data, and (4) design of the study (Morse, 2000, 2007; Munhall, 2007; Patton, 2002).

Scope of the Study

If the scope of the study is broad, then researchers will need extensive data to address the study purpose, and it will take longer to reach saturation. Thus, a study with a broad scope requires more sampling of participants, events, or documents than is needed for a study with a narrow scope (Morse, 2000). For example, a qualitative study of the experience of living with chronic illness in older adulthood would require a large sample due to the broad scope of the problem. A study that has a clear focus and provides focused data collection usually has richer, more credible findings. In contrast to the study of chronic illness experiences of older adults, researchers exploring the lived experience of adults over 70 years old who have rheumatoid arthritis could obtain credible findings with a smaller sample. When critically appraising a qualitative study, determine whether the sample size was adequate for the identified scope of the study.

Nature of the Topic

If the topic of study is clear and easily discussed by the subjects, then fewer subjects are needed to obtain the essential data. If the topic is difficult to define and awkward for people to discuss, then usually more participants are needed to achieve data saturation (Morse, 2000; Munhall, 2007). For example, a phenomenological study of the experience of an adult living with a history of child sexual abuse is a very sensitive, complex topic to investigate. This type of topic probably will require increased participants and interview time to collect essential data. When critically appraising published studies, be sure to consider whether the sample size was adequate based on the complexity and sensitivity of the topic studied.

Quality of the Information

The quality of information obtained from an interview, observation, or document review influences the sample size. When the quality of the data is high, with a rich content, few participants are needed to achieve saturation of data in the area of study. Quality data are best obtained from articulate, well-informed, and communicative participants (Sandelowski, 1995). Such participants are able to share richer data in a clear and concise manner. In addition, participants who have more time to be interviewed usually provide data with greater depth and breadth. The researchers will continue sampling until saturation and verification of information is achieved to produce the best study results. Remember to consider these factors in your critical appraisal of a qualitative study:

- the quality of the information available from the participants, events, or documents
- the richness of the data collected
- the adequacy of the sample based on the findings obtained

Study Design

Some studies are designed to increase the number of interviews with each participant. When researchers conduct more interviews with a person, they probably will collect better-quality, richer data. For example, with a study design that includes an interview both before and after an event; more data are produced than with a single-interview design. Designs that involve interviewing families usually produce more data than designs with single-participant interviews. In critically appraising a qualitative study, determine the adequacy of the sample size for the chosen design (Huberman & Miles, 2002).

CRITICAL APPRAISAL GUIDELINES

Adequacy of the Sample in Qualitative Studies

When critically appraising the samples in qualitative studies, you need to address the following questions:

1. Is the sampling plan adequate to address the purpose of the study? If purposeful or purposive sampling was used, does the researcher provide a rationale for the sample selection process? If network or snowball sampling was used, does the researcher identify the networks used to obtain the sample and provide a rationale for their selection? If theoretical sampling is used, does the researcher indicate how participants are selected to promote the generation of a theory?
2. Is the sample size adequate, based on the scope of the study, nature of the topic, quality of the data, and study design?
3. Does the researcher discuss the quality of the study participants? Were the participants articulate, well informed, and willing to share information relevant to the study topic?
4. Did the sample produce saturation and verification of information in the area of the study?
5. Are the sampling criteria identified?
6. Does the researcher identify the study setting?

RESEARCH EXAMPLE Qualitative Study Sample

Turris (2009) conducted a grounded theory study to develop a theory focused on women's decisions regarding seeking treatment for symptoms of potential cardiac illness. She described her sample as follows and the particular aspects of the sample have been identified [in brackets]. The sample section from Turris' qualitative study is followed by a critical appraisal based on the previous guidelines and the implications for practice.

Sampling and procedures: At the beginning of the study, the sample was a purposive sample [sampling method] drawn from a group of women who sought ED care for the treatment of symptoms of a potential cardiac illness at one of two hospitals EDs [population, setting]. To participate in this study, individuals had to be: women, visiting either of the two EDs for treatment of the symptoms of a potential cardiac event, hemodynamically stable, 18 years of age or older, able to speak English, and competent to provide informed consent [sampling criteria]. If a woman met the inclusion criteria, permission was requested for contact

Continued

RESEARCH EXAMPLE—cont'd

several days following discharge to arrange a convenient time and location [setting] for a more formal, audiotaped interview, and she was provided with an information letter about the study.

Data analysis: Data collection and analysis were done concurrently. The accounts of 10 participants were obtained as a starting point for this project. Sampling continued to ensure that categories were "dense" and well developed; support for the relationships among the categories and the contributions of categories to the core category were explored [saturation and verification of information]. Theoretical sampling was used to collect further information [sampling method]. For example, when analysis of the data suggested age might play a role in women's decisions about treatment seeking, the accounts of younger women were actively sought [saturation and verification of information]. Upon the conclusion of the project, a total of 16 women had been interviewed [sample size]. (Turris, 2009, p. 6)

CRITICAL APPRAISAL

Turris (2009) provided extensive details of her sample and sampling plan, as set forth in the foregoing excerpt. The study population, setting, and sampling criteria were clearly identified. The focus of the purposive sampling plan was addressed, with a limited rationale for selecting this sampling plan. The rationale for the use of theoretical sampling was very clear and focused on achieving saturation and verification of study information. The sample size of 16 women seemed adequate, because saturation and verification of information was achieved. For example, when age was identified as important category in the study, accounts of younger women were sought to promote the development of the theory. The scope of the study, nature of the topic, quality of the data, and study design were addressed and seemed to support the sample size obtained. In summary, Turris (2009) provided a detailed, quality discussion of her sample and setting for her grounded theory study.

IMPLICATIONS FOR PRACTICE

Turris (2009) found that the women's decisions to seek treatment for their cardiac symptoms were influenced primarily by their roles as mothers, daughters, and wives and secondarily by their interpretation and conclusions about their symptoms. The women's decisions regarding seeking or delaying treatment were based on embodied, temporal, rational, and relational knowing. Embodied knowing is the subjective or visceral experience of the symptoms and temporal knowing is linking the symptoms to time of day such as meal time. Rational knowing comes from the media, reports, and general information women have about heart disease. Relational knowing is knowledge that comes from relationships and interactions with others that shape meaning and behavior. This study adds to the theory of treatment seeking delays and provides a greater understanding of women and their response to their cardiac symptoms. This information can be used in educating women about cardiac symptoms, encouraging them not to delay treatment, and promoting early intervention to prevent morbidity and mortality.

Research Settings

The **setting** is the site or location used to conduct a study. Three common settings for conducting nursing research are natural, partially controlled, and highly controlled. Chapter 2 initially introduced the types of settings for quantitative research. The selection of a setting in both quantitative and qualitative research is based on the purpose of the study, the accessibility of the setting or site, and the number and type of participants or subjects available in the setting. The setting needs to be clearly described in the research report with a rationale for selecting it. If the setting is partially or highly controlled, then researchers should include a discussion of how they manipulated the setting. The following sections describe the three types of research settings, with examples provided from some of the studies previously presented in this chapter.

Natural Setting

A **natural setting**, or **field setting**, is an uncontrolled, real-life situation or environment. Conducting a study in a natural setting means that the researcher does not manipulate or change the environment for the study. Descriptive and correlational quantitative studies and qualitative studies often are conducted in natural settings.

RESEARCH EXAMPLE Natural Setting

Turris (2009) conducted a grounded theory study to describe women's decisions to seek treatment for their symptoms of potential cardiac illness. She described her setting in the following excerpt:

> Setting. This project was undertaken with the approval of the university's behavioral research ethics board, as well as the relevant hospitals' ethics boards. Data were collected from two EDs in a western Canadian province, targeting one tertiary-care and one community hospital, both with more than 50,000 ED visits a year. Hospital A is a tertiary-care referral center for the province. In contrast, Hospital B is a community hospital, located in a residential suburb. Hospital B is not designated as a trauma hospital, and staff did not have the infrastructure necessary to carry out rescue angiographic procedures that might be required for the treatment of acute myocardial infarction. (Turris, 2009, p. 6)

CRITICAL APPRAISAL

Turris clearly described her study setting and provided a rational for selecting two hospital EDs. The researcher also made arrangements with the participants to conduct a more formal interview after discharge and that was probably in the participants' homes. Both of these are natural settings since no attempt was made by the researcher to manipulate the settings.

IMPLICATIONS FOR PRACTICE

Implications for practice were discussed earlier in this chapter.

Partially Controlled Setting

A **partially controlled setting** is an environment that is manipulated or modified in some way by the researcher. An increasing number of nursing studies, usually correlational, quasi-experimental, and experimental studies, are being conducted in partially controlled settings. Sometimes qualitative researchers manipulate a setting to promote the most effective environment to obtain the rich, in-depth information they need.

RESEARCH EXAMPLE Partially Controlled Setting

Pearce and colleagues (2008) used a partially controlled setting to conduct their qualitative study of middle-school children's understanding of physical activity. The interviews were conducted in group meetings with the children by grades (sixth, seventh, and eighth) in a specifically designated room in the school. The researchers described their setting in the following excerpt:

> During the meetings, children had access to Post-it notes, colored pens, and pencils, construction paper, and Play-Doh to help them express their ideas through creative expression. ... A portable SMART Board (SMART Technologies. ...) was used for free hand drawing that could be saved and directly downloaded to computer files. (Pearce et al., 2008, p. 171)

CRITICAL APPRAISAL

Pearce and colleagues (2008) clearly described their setting and how it was structured or partially controlled to promote information-rich interviews with the children. The researchers held five meetings per grade (sixth, seventh, and eighth) for a total of 15 meetings. These discussions yielded 15 transcripts, 96 pages of field notes, and 28 children's drawings.

IMPLICATIONS FOR PRACTICE

Implications for practice were discussed earlier in this chapter.

Highly Controlled Setting

A **highly controlled setting** is an artificially constructed environment developed for the sole purpose of conducting research. Laboratories, research or experimental centers, and test units in hospitals or other healthcare agencies are highly controlled settings in which experimental studies often are conducted. This type of setting reduces the influence of extraneous variables, which enables the researcher to examine accurately the effect of one variable on another. Highly controlled settings commonly are used in the conduct of experimental research.

RESEARCH EXAMPLE Highly Controlled Setting

Rasmussen and Farr (2003) conducted an experimental study of the effects of morphine and time of day on pain and beta-endorphin (BE) level in a sample of dilute brown Agouti (DBA) mice. The study was conducted in a laboratory setting, described as follows:

> The mice were housed individually in clear styrene cages in a private, controlled-access room in the laboratory animal facilities of the Comparative Medicine Department. Individual housing was used to reduce social conflict and stress, which have been shown to bring about stress-induced analgesia ... The presence of other mice in the room prevented isolation stress. Food and water were allowed ad libitum. A 12:12 light/dark cycle, with lights on at 0600, and a room temperature of 22 ± 1° C were maintained throughout the study. Experiments timed for the dark phase were performed under dim red lights. (Rasmussen & Farr, 2003, p. 107)

CRITICAL APPRAISAL

The study included the use of a highly controlled laboratory setting in terms of the housing of the mice, the light and temperature of the environment, implementation of the treatments, and the measurements of the dependent variables. Only with animals can this type of setting control be achieved in the conduct of a study. This type of highly controlled setting removes the impact of numerous extraneous variables, so that the researcher can clearly determine the effects of the independent variables on the dependent variables.

IMPLICATIONS FOR PRACTICE

Rasmussen and Farr (2003) found that morphine

> ... is used frequently to control pain, yet it also alters the endogenous BE response to acute pain. In addition, the magnitude of the increase in pain tolerance provided by morphine is not equal at all times of day. The appropriate timing of morphine administration for the treatment of acute pain should enhance the effect of the endogenous opioid system, which may decrease the need for large doses of morphine at some time points. Specifically, it may be appropriate to decrease morphine dosages during the client's active period or day to achieve this goal. (p. 113)

Because this research was conducted on animals, however, the findings cannot be generalized to humans, and additional research is needed to determine the effects of the independent variables of morphine and time of day on the dependent variables of pain and BE level in humans.

KEY CONCEPTS

- Sampling involves selecting a group of people, events, behaviors, or other elements with which to conduct a study.

- Sampling theory was developed to determine the most effective way of acquiring a sample that accurately reflects the population under study.
- Important concepts in sampling theory include population, sampling criteria, target population, accessible population, study elements, representativeness, randomization, sampling frame, and sampling plan.
- In quantitative research a sampling plan is developed to increase representativeness, decrease systematic bias, and decrease sampling error.
- The two main types of sampling plans are probability and nonprobability.
- Four sampling methods have been developed to achieve probability sampling: simple random sampling, stratified random sampling, cluster sampling, and systematic sampling.
- The five nonprobability sampling methods discussed in this chapter are convenience sampling, quota sampling, purposeful or purposive sampling, network sampling, and theoretical sampling.
- Convenience and quota sampling frequently are used in quantitative and outcomes research.
- Factors to consider in making decisions about sample size in quantitative studies include the type of study, number of variables, sensitivity of the measurement tools, data analysis techniques, and expected effect size.
- Power analysis is an effective way to determine an adequate sample size for quantitative and outcomes studies. In power analysis, effect size, level of significance (alpha = 0.05), and standard power (0.8 or 80%) are used to determine sample size for a study.
- Purposeful, network, and theoretical sampling are more commonly used in qualitative than in quantitative research.
- The number of participants in a qualitative study is adequate when saturation and verification of information is achieved in the study area.
- Important factors to consider in determining sample size for qualitative studies include: (1) scope of the study, (2) nature of the topic, (3) quality of the data collected, and (4) design of the study.
- Three common settings for conducting nursing research are natural, partially controlled, and highly controlled.

REFERENCES

Bay, E., Hagerty, B. M., & Williams, R. A. (2007). Depressive symptomatology after mild-to-moderate traumatic brain injury: A comparison of three measures. *Archives of Psychiatric Nursing, 21*(1), 2-11.

Brown, S. J. (2009). *Evidence-based nursing: The research-practice connection*. Sudbury, MA: Jones & Bartlett.

Burns, N., & Grove, S. K. (2009). *The practice of nursing research: Appraisal, synthesis, and generation of evidence* (6th ed.). Philadelphia: Saunders.

Clifford, C. (1997). *Qualitative research methodology in nursing and healthcare*. New York: Churchill Livingstone.

Cohen, J. (1988). *Statistical power analysis for the behavioral sciences* (2nd ed.). New York: Academic Press.

Coté-Arsenault, D., & Morrison-Beedy, D. (2001). Women's voices reflecting changed expectations for pregnancy after perinatal loss. *The Journal of Nursing Scholarship, 33*(3), 239-244.

Coyne, I. T. (1997). Sampling in qualitative research. Purposeful and theoretical sampling: Merging or clear boundaries. *Journal of Advanced Nursing, 26*(3), 623-630.

Cullum, N., Ciliska, D., Haynes, R. B., & Marks, S. (2008). *Evidence-based nursing: An introduction*. Oxford: Blackwell.

Grove, S. K. (2007). *Statistics for health care research: A practical workbook*. Philadelphia: Saunders.

Hodgins, M. J., Ouellet, L. L., Pond, S., Knorr, S., & Geldart, G. (2008). Effect of telephone follow-up on surgical orthopedic recovery. *Applied Nursing Research, 21*(4), 218-226.

Huberman, A. M., & Miles, M. B. (2002). *The qualitative researcher's companion*. Thousand Oaks, CA: Sage.

Kerlinger, F. N., & Lee, H. B. (2000). *Foundations of behavioral research*. New York: Harcourt Brace.

Kraemer, H. C., & Theimann, S. (1987). *How many subjects? Statistical power analysis in research*. Newbury Park, CA: Sage.

Marshall, C., & Rossman, G. B. (2006). *Designing qualitative research* (4th ed.). Thousand Oaks, CA: Sage.

McCain, N. L., Munjas, B. A., Munro, C. L., Elswick, R. K., Jr., Robins, J. L. W., Ferreira-Gonzalez, A., et al. (2003). Effects of stress management on PNI-based outcomes in persons with HIV disease. *Research in Nursing & Health, 26*(2), 102-117.

Moody, L. E., Wilson, M. E., Smyth, K., Schwartz, R., Tittle, M., & Van Cott, M. L. (1988). Analysis of a decade of nursing practice research: 1977-1986. *Nursing Research, 37*(6), 374-379.

Morea, J. M., Friend, R., & Bennett, R. M. (2008). Conceptualizing and measuring illness self-concept: A comparison with self-esteem and optimism in predicting fibromyalgia adjustment. *Research in Nursing & Health, 31*(6), 563-575.

Morse, J. M. (1998). Designing funded qualitative research. In N. K. Denzin, & Y. S. Lincoln (Eds.), *Strategies of qualitative inquiry* (pp. 56-85). Thousand Oaks, CA: Sage.

Morse, J. M. (2000). Determining sample size. *Qualitative Health Research, 10*(1), 3-5.

Morse, J. M. (2007). Strategies of intraproject sampling. In P. L. Munhall (Ed.), *Nursing research: A qualitative perspective* (4th ed., pp. 529-539). Sudbury, MA: Jones & Bartlett.

Munhall, P. L. (2007). *Nursing research: A qualitative perspective* (4th ed.). Sudbury, MA: Jones & Bartlett.

Parent, N., & Hanley, J. A. (2009). Assessing quality of reports on randomized clinical trials in nursing journals. *Canadian Journal of Cardiovascular Nursing, 19* (2), 25-31.

Patton, M. Q. (2002). *Qualitative evaluation and research methods* (3rd ed.). Thousand Oaks, CA: Sage.

Pearce, P. F., Harrell, J. S., & McMurray, R. G. (2008). Middle-school children's understanding of physical activity: "If you're moving, you're doing physical activity. *Journal of Pediatric Nursing, 23*(3), 169-182.

Polit, D. F., & Sherman, R. E. (1990). Statistical power in nursing research. *Nursing Research, 39*(6), 365-369.

Rambur, B., McIntosh, B., Val Palumbo, M., & Reinier, K. (2005). Education as a determinant of career retention and job satisfaction among registered nurses. *The Journal of Nursing Scholarship, 37*(2), 185-192.

Rasmussen, N. A., & Farr, L. A. (2003). Effects of morphine and time of day on pain and beta-endorphin. *Biological Research for Nursing, 5*(2), 105-116.

Rew, L. (2003). A theory of taking care of oneself grounded in experiences of homeless youth. *Nursing Research, 52*(4), 234-241.

Sandelowski, M. (1995). Focus on qualitative methods: Sample size in qualitative research. *Research in Nursing & Health, 18*(2), 179-183.

Turris, S. A. (2009). Women's decisions to seek treatment for the symptoms of potential cardiac illness. *Journal of Nursing Scholarship, 41*(1), 5-12.

Twiss, J. J., Waltman, N. L., Berg, K., Ott, C. D., Gross, G. J., & Lindsey, A. M. (2009). An exercise intervention for breast cancer survivors with bone loss. *Journal of Nursing Scholarship, 41*(1), 20-27.

Udry, J. R. (2003). *The National Longitudinal Study of Adolescent Health (Add Health), Waves I & II, 1994-1996; Wave III, 2001-2002 [Machine-readable data file and documentation]*. Chapel Hill, NC: Carolina Population Center, University of North Carolina at Chapel Hill.

Willgerodt, M. A. (2008). Family and peer influences on adjustment among Chinese, Filipino, and White youth. *Nursing Research, 57*(6), 395-405.

10

Clarifying Measurement and Data Collection in Quantitative Research

Chapter Overview

Concepts of Measurement Theory 328
  Directness of Measurement 328
  Levels of Measurement 329
  Measurement Error 331
  Reliability 332
  Validity 334
Accuracy, Precision, and Error of Physiological Measures 338
  Accuracy 338
  Precision 339
  Error 339

Use of Sensitivity, Specificity, and Likelihood Ratios to Determine the Quality of Diagnostic and Screening Tests 341
Measurement Strategies in Nursing 345
  Physiological Measurements 345
  Observational Measurements 348
  Interviews 350
  Questionnaires 353
  Scales 355
Process of Data Collection 361
  Data Collection Tasks 362
  Serendipity 366

Learning Outcomes

After completing this chapter, you should be able to:

1. Describe measurement theory and its relevant concepts of directness of measurement, levels of measurement, measurement error, reliability, and validity.
2. Determine the levels of measurement—nominal, ordinal, interval, and ratio—achieved by measurement methods in published studies.
3. Identify possible sources of measurement error in published studies.
4. Critically appraise the types and extent of reliability and validity of measurement methods reported in published studies.
5. Critically appraise the accuracy, precision, and error of physiological measures used in published studies.
6. Critically appraise the sensitivity, specificity, and likelihood ratios of diagnostic tests.
7. Critically appraise the measurement approaches—physiological measures, observations, interviews, questionnaires, and scales—used in published studies.
8. Critically appraise the data collection section in published studies.

Key Terms

Accuracy, p. 338
Accuracy of a screening test, p. 341
Alternate forms reliability, p. 333
Construct validity, p. 335
Content-related validity, p. 335
Data collection, p. 361
Direct measures, p. 328
Equivalence, p. 333
Error in physiological measures, p. 339
Evidence of validity from contrasting groups, p. 335

Evidence of validity from
 convergence, p. 335
Evidence of validity from
 divergence, p. 335
False negative, p. 341
False positive, p. 341
Gold standard, p. 341
Highly sensitive test, p. 342
Highly specific test, p. 342
Homogeneity, p. 334
Indirect measures, or
 indicators, p. 328
Internal consistency, p. 334
Interrater reliability, p. 333
Interval-scale measurement,
 p. 330
Interview, p. 350
Levels of measurement, p. 329
Likelihood ratios, p. 344
Likert scale, p. 357
Low sensitivity test, p. 342
Low specificity test, p. 342

Measurement, p. 327
Measurement error, p. 331
Negative likelihood ratio,
 p. 344
Nominal-scale measurement,
 p. 329
Observational measurement,
 p. 348
Ordinal-scale measurement,
 p. 330
Physiological measures,
 p. 338
Positive likelihood ratio,
 p. 344
Precision, p. 339
Questionnaire, p. 353
Random measurement error,
 p. 331
Rating scales, p. 355
Ratio-scale measurement,
 p. 330
Readability level, p. 335

Reliability, p. 332
Reliability testing, p. 333
Scale, p. 355
Sensitivity, p. 341
Serendipity, p. 366
Specificity, p. 342
Stability, p. 333
Structured interview, p. 350
Structured observational
 measurement, p. 348
Systematic measurement
 error, p. 332
Test-retest reliability, p. 333
True measure or score, p. 331
True negative, p. 341
True positive, p. 341
Unstructured interview,
 p. 350
Unstructured observations,
 p. 348
Validity, p. 334
Visual analog scale, p. 360

STUDY TOOLS

Be sure to visit http://evolve.elsevier.com/Burns/understanding for additional examples and self-tests. Also, a review of this chapter's concepts and practice exercises can be found in Chapter 10 of the Study Guide for *Understanding Nursing Research: Building an Evidence-Based Practice*, 5th edition.

Measurement is a very important part of the research process. When quality measurement methods are used in a study, it improves the accuracy or validity of study outcomes or findings. **Measurement** is the process of assigning numbers or values to individuals' health status, objects, events, or situations using a set of rules (Kaplan, 1963). For example, we measure a patient's blood pressure (BP) using a measurement method such as a stethoscope, cuff, and sphygmomanometer. Then a number or value is assigned to that patient's BP, such as 120/80. In research, variables are measured with the best possible measurement method available to produce trustworthy data that can be used in statistical analyses. Trustworthy data are essential if a study is to produce useful findings to guide nursing practice.

In critically appraising a published study, you must judge the trustworthiness or accuracy of the measurement methods used in the study. To produce trustworthy measurements, rules have been established to ensure that numbers, values, or categories will be assigned consistently from one subject (or event) to another and, eventually, if the measurement method or strategy is found to be meaningful, from one study to another. The rules of measurement established for research are similar to those used in nursing practice. For example, for pouring a liquid medication, the rule is that the specific measurement container must be placed at eye level. This ensures accuracy and precision in the dose of medication. In measuring BP, the patient should be sitting, legs uncrossed, arm relaxed on a table at heart level, cuff of accurate size placed correctly on the upper arm that is free of clothing, and stethoscope correctly placed over the brachial artery at the elbow. Following these rules ensures that the patient's BP is accurately measured and any change in BP can be attributed to a change in BP, rather than to an inadvertent change or error in the measurement technique.

Understanding the logic of measurement is important for critically appraising the adequacy of measurement methods in a nursing study. This chapter includes a discussion of important concepts of measurement theory including directness of measurement, levels of measurement, measurement error, reliability, and validity. The accuracy and precision of physiological measures and the sensitivity and specificity of diagnostic and screening tests are addressed. Some of the most common measurement methods or strategies used in nursing research are briefly described. The chapter concludes with an introduction to the essential elements of the data collection process.

Concepts of Measurement Theory

Measurement theory guides the development and use of measurement methods in research. Measurement theory was developed many years ago by mathematicians, statisticians, and other scholars and includes rules that guide how things are measured (Kaplan, 1963). These rules allow individuals to be consistent in how they perform measurements; thus, a measurement method used by one person will consistently produce similar results when used by another person. This section discusses some of the basic concepts and rules of measurement theory, including directness of measurement, levels of measurement, measurement error, reliability, and validity.

Directness of Measurement

To measure, the researcher must first identify the object, characteristic, element, event, or situation to be measured. In some cases, identifying the object to measure and determining how to measure it are quite simple, such as when the researcher measures a person's height or waist circumference. These are referred to as direct measures. **Direct measures** involve determining the value of concrete things such as height, weight, temperature, heart rate, BP, and respiration. Technology is available to measure many bodily functions and biological and chemical characteristics. The focus of measurement in these instances is on the accuracy and precision of the measurement method and process. If a patient's BP is to be accurate, it must be measured with a quality stethoscope and sphygmomanometer and must be precisely or consistently measured as discussed earlier in this chapter. Nurse researchers are also experienced in gathering direct measures of demographic variables such as age, gender, ethnic origin, diagnosis, marital status, income, and education.

However, in many cases in nursing research, the thing to be measured is not a concrete object but an abstract idea, a characteristic, or a concept such as pain, stress, caring, coping, depression, anxiety, and adherence. Researchers cannot directly measure an abstract idea, but they can capture some elements of it in their measurements, which are referred to as **indirect measures** or **indicators** of the concepts. Rarely, if ever, can a single measurement strategy measure all aspects of an abstract concept. Therefore, multiple measurement methods

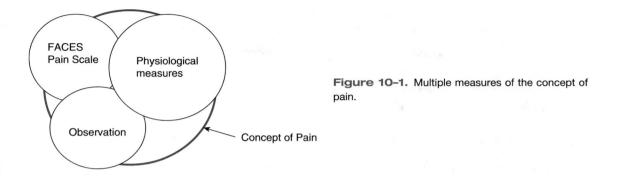

Figure 10–1. Multiple measures of the concept of pain.

or indicators are needed, and even then they cannot be expected to measure all elements of an abstract concept. For example, multiple measurement methods might be used to describe pain in a study, which decreases the measurement error and increases the understanding of pain. The measurement methods of pain might include: FACES Pain Scale; observation (rubbing and/or guarding area that hurts, facial grimacing, and crying); and physiological measures, such as pulse, respiration, and blood pressure. Figure 10–1 demonstrates multiple measures of the concept pain and demonstrates how having more measurement methods increases the understanding of the concept. The blue circle represents the concept of pain and the black circles represent the measurement methods. A larger circle is represented by physiological measures indicating these measures (pulse, blood pressure, and respirations) add more to the objective measurement of pain. Even with three different types of measurement methods being used, the entire concept of pain is not completely measured.

Levels of Measurement

Each measurement method produces data that are at different levels of measurement. The traditional levels of measurement were developed by Stevens in 1946. Stevens organized the rules for assigning numbers to objects so that a hierarchy in measurement was established. The levels of measurement, from low to high, are nominal, ordinal, interval, and ratio.

Nominal-Scale Measurement

Nominal-scale measurement is the lowest of the four measurement categories. It is used when data can be organized into categories of a defined property but the categories cannot be rank ordered. For example, you may decide to categorize potential study subjects by diagnosis. However, the category "kidney stone," for example, can't be rated higher than the category "peptic ulcer"; likewise, across categories, "ovarian cyst" is no closer to "kidney stone" than to "peptic ulcer." The categories differ in quality but not quantity. Therefore, it's not possible to say that subject A possesses more of the property being categorized than does subject B. (**RULE:** The categories must not be orderable.) Categories must be established in such a way that a datum will fit into only one of the categories. (**RULE:** The categories must be exclusive.) All of the data must fit into the established categories. (**RULE:** The categories must be exhaustive.) Data such as gender, ethnicity, marital status, and diagnoses are examples of nominal data.

Ordinal-Scale Measurement

With ordinal-scale measurement, data are assigned to categories that can be ranked. To rank data, one category is judged to be (or is ranked) higher or lower, or better or worse, than another category. Rules govern how the data are ranked. As with nominal data, the categories must be exclusive and exhaustive. With ordinal data, the quantity also can be identified (Stevens, 1946). For example, if you are measuring intensity of pain, you may identify different levels of pain. You probably will develop categories that rank these different levels of pain, such as excruciating, severe, moderate, mild, and no pain. However, in using categories of ordinal measurement, you cannot know with certainty that the intervals between the ranked categories are equal. A greater difference may exist between mild and moderate pain, for example, than between excruciating and severe pain. Therefore, ordinal data are considered to have unequal intervals.

Many scales used in nursing research are ordinal levels of measurement. For example, it's possible to rank degrees of coping, levels of mobility, ability to provide self-care, or levels of dyspnea on an ordinal scale. For dyspnea with activities of daily living (ADLs), the scale could be 0 = no shortness of breath with ADLs, 1 = minimal shortness of breaths with ADLs, 2 = moderate shortness of breath with ADLs, 3 = extreme shortness of breath with ADLs, 4 = shortness of breath so severe unable to perform ADLs without assistance. The measurement is ordinal because it's not possible to claim that equal distances exist between the rankings. A greater difference may exist between the ranks of 1 and 2 than between the ranks of 2 and 3.

Interval-Scale Measurement

Interval-scale measurement uses interval scales, which have equal numerical distances between intervals. These scales follow the rules of mutually exclusive categories, exhaustive categories, and rank ordering and are assumed to represent a continuum of values. Thus, the magnitude of the attribute can be more precisely defined. However, it is not possible to provide the absolute amount of the attribute, because the interval scale lacks a zero point. Temperature is the most commonly used example of an interval scale. The difference between the temperatures of 70° F and 80° F is 10° and is the same as the difference between the temperatures of 30° F and 40° F. Changes in temperature can be precisely measured. However, a temperature of 0° does not indicate the absence of temperature.

Ratio-Scale Measurement

Ratio-scale measurement is the highest form of measurement and meets all of the rules of other forms of measurement: mutually exclusive categories, exhaustive categories, ordered ranks, equally spaced intervals, and a continuum of values. Interval and ratio level data can be added, subtracted, multiplied, and divided because of the equal intervals and continuum of values of these data. Thus, interval and ratio data can be analyzed with statistical techniques of greater precision and strength to determine significant relationships and differences. In addition, ratio-level measures have absolute zero points (Grove, 2007; Stevens, 1946). Weight, length, and volume are commonly used as examples of ratio scales. All three have absolute zero points, at which a value of zero indicates the absence of the property being measured; zero weight means the absence of weight. Because of the absolute zero point, such statements as "Object A weighs twice as much as object B" or "Container A holds three times as much as container B" can be justified.

In critically appraising a study, you need to determine the level of measurement achieved for each measurement method. Researchers try to achieve the highest level of measurement possible for a variable because more rigorous statistical analyses can be conducted on interval and ratio level data to identify relationships and determine differences between groups (Burns & Grove, 2009).

Measurement Error

The ideal, perfect measure is referred to as the **true measure** or **score**. However, some error is always present in any measurement strategy. **Measurement error** is the difference between the true measure and what is actually measured (Burns & Grove, 2009). The amount of error in a measure varies. Thus, there may be considerable error in one measurement and very little in the next. Measurement error exists in both direct and indirect measures and can be random or systematic. With direct measures, both the object and the measurement method are visible. Direct measures, which generally are expected to be highly accurate, are subject to error. For example, a weight scale may not be accurate, a precisely calibrated thermometer may decrease in precision with use, or a tape measure may not be held at exactly the same tightness in measuring the waist of each patient. A subject in a study may be 65 years old but write illegibly on the demographic form. As a result, the age may be inaccurately entered into the study database.

With indirect measures, the element being measured cannot be seen directly. For example, you cannot see pain. You may observe behaviors or hear words that you think represent pain. But pain is a sensation that is not always clearly recognized or expressed by the person experiencing it. The measurement of pain usually is a scale but can also include observation and physiological measures as previously presented in Figure 10–1. Efforts to measure concepts such as pain usually result in measuring only part of the concept. Sometimes measures may identify some aspects of the concept but may include other elements that are not part of the concept. In Figure 10–1, the measurement methods of scale, observation, and physiological measures include things other than pain, as indicated by the parts of the circles that are outside the blue circle of the concept pain. For example, measurement methods for pain might be measuring aspects of anxiety and fear in addition to pain. However, using multiple measurement methods for examining a concept or variable in a study usually decreases the measurement error and increases the understanding of the variable being measured.

Two types of error are of concern in measurement: random error and systematic error. The difference between random and systematic error is in the direction of the error. In **random measurement error**, the difference between the measured value and the true value is without pattern or direction (random). In one measurement, the actual value obtained may be lower than the true value, whereas in the next measurement, the actual value obtained may be higher than the true value. A number of chance situations or factors can occur during the measurement process that can result in random error (Waltz, Strickland, & Lenz, 2005). For example, the person taking the measurements may not use the same procedure every time; a subject completing a paper-and-pencil scale may accidentally mark the wrong column; or the person entering the data into a computer may punch the wrong key. The purpose of measuring is to estimate the true value, usually by combining a number of values and calculating an average. Thus an average value, such as the mean, is an estimate of the true measurement. As the number of random errors increases, the precision of the estimate decreases.

Measurement error that is not random is referred to as systematic error. In **systematic measurement error**, the variation in measurement values from the calculated average is primarily in the same direction. For example, most of the variation may be higher or lower than the average that was calculated. Systematic error occurs because something else is being measured in addition to the concept. For example, a paper-and-pencil rating scale designed to measure hope may actually be measuring perceived support also. A scale used to measure subjects' weights that shows weights that are 2 pounds more than the true weights will give measures with systematic error. All of the measured weights will be high, and as a result the mean will be higher than if an accurate scale is used. Some systematic error occurs in almost any measure. Because of the importance of this type of error in a study, researchers spend considerable time and effort refining their measuring instruments to minimize systematic measurement error (Waltz et al., 2005).

In critically appraising a published study, you will not be able to judge the extent of measurement error directly. However, you may find clues to the amount of error in the published report. For example, if the researchers have described the method of measurement in great detail and provided evidence of accuracy and precision of the measurement, then the probability of error typically is reduced. If a BP cuff and sphygmomanometer are checked for accuracy, recalibrated periodically during data collection, and three readings of the blood pressure are taken and then averaged to determine a blood pressure reading for a subject, the measurement errors for blood pressure should be minimal. Measurement will also be more precise if the researcher has used a well-developed, reliable, and valid scale, like the FACES Pain Scale, instead of a newly developed scale. If a check list is developed for observation, less error occurs than if the observations for pain are unstructured. Thus, there are many steps researchers can take to decrease measurement error and increase the quality of their study findings.

Reliability

Reliability is concerned with the consistency of the measurement method. For example, if you are using a paper-and-pencil scale to measure depression, it should indicate similar depression scores each time a subject completes it within a short period of time. A scale that does not produce similar scores for a subject with repeat testing is considered unreliable (Kerlinger & Lee, 2000; Waltz et al., 2005). For example, the Center for Epidemiologic Studies Depression Scale (CES-D Scale) is a 20-item scale developed to diagnosis depression. If a subject completes this scale twice within a limited period of time, the scores should be similar, indicating the scale is reliable.

Reliability Testing

Reliability testing is a measure of the amount of random error in the measurement technique. It takes into account such characteristics as dependability, precision, stability, consistency, and reproducibility (Kerlinger & Lee, 2000; Waltz et al., 2005). Because all measurement techniques contain some random error, reliability exists in degrees and usually is expressed as a correlation coefficient (r). Cronbach's alpha coefficient is the most commonly used measure of reliability for multiple item scales (see discussion of homogeneity that follows for more details). Estimates of reliability are specific to the sample being tested. Thus, high reliability values reported for an established instrument do not guarantee that reliability will be satisfactory in another sample or with a different population. Therefore, researchers need to perform reliability testing on each instrument used in a study before performing other statistical analyses.

Reliability testing focuses on the following three aspects of reliability: stability, equivalence, and homogeneity. Stability is concerned with the consistency of repeated measures of the same attribute with the use of the same scale or instrument. It is usually referred to as test-retest reliability. This measure of reliability is generally used with physical measures, technological measures, and paper-and-pencil scales. Use of the technique requires an assumption that the factor to be measured remains the same at the two testing times and that any change in the value or score is a consequence of random error. For example, physiological measures like blood pressure equipment can be tested and then immediately retested, or the equipment can be used for a time and then retested to determine the necessary frequency of recalibration. Researchers need to include test-retest reliability results in their published studies to document the reliability of their measurement methods. For example, the CDS Depression Scale, developed in 1977 by Radloff, has been used frequently in studies over the years and has demonstrated test-retest reliability ranging from $r = 0.51$ to 0.67 in two to eight week intervals. This is very solid test-retest reliability for this scale, indicating that it is consistently measuring depression with repeat testing and recognizing that subjects' level of depression vary somewhat over time (Locke & Putnam, 2002; Sharp & Lipsky, 2002).

Reliability testing can also include equivalence, which involves the comparison of two versions of the same paper-and-pencil instrument or of two observers measuring the same event. Comparison of two observers or two judges in a study is referred to as interrater reliability. Any studies that include collecting observational data or the making of judgments by two or more data gatherers require the reporting of interrater reliability. There is no absolute value below which interrater reliability is unacceptable. However, any value below 0.80 should generate serious concern about the reliability of the data or of the data gatherer (or both). The interrater reliability value is best to be = 0.90, which means 90% reliability and 10% random error. Comparison of two paper-and-pencil instruments is referred to as alternate forms reliability, or parallel forms reliability. Alternative forms of instruments are of more concern in the development of normative knowledge testing like the Scholastic Aptitude Test (SAT) used as a college entrance requirement. The SAT has been used for decades, and there are many forms of this test with a variety of items included on each. These alternate forms of the SAT were developed to measure students' knowledge consistently and protect the integrity of the test.

Homogeneity is a type of reliability testing used primarily with paper-and-pencil instruments or scales to address the correlation of each question to the other questions within the instrument. Questions on a scale are also called items. The principle is that each item should be consistently measuring a concept like depression and so should be highly correlated with the other items. The original approach to determining homogeneity was split-half reliability. This strategy was a way of obtaining test-retest reliability without administering the test twice. Rather, the instrument items were split in odd-even or first-last halves, and a correlational procedure was performed between the two halves. Researchers have generally used the Spearman-Brown correlation formula for this procedure. One of the problems with the procedure was that although items were usually split into odd-even items, it was possible to split them in a variety of ways. Each approach to splitting the items would yield a different reliability coefficient. Therefore, the researcher could continue to split the items in various ways until a satisfactorily high coefficient was obtained.

More recently, testing the homogeneity of all the items in the instrument has been a better approach to determining reliability. Homogeneity testing examines the extent to which all the items in the instrument consistently measure the construct and is a test of internal consistency. The statistical procedures used for this process are Cronbach's alpha coefficient for interval and ratio level data. On some scales, the person responding selects between two options such as yes and no. This yields data that are dichotomous and the Kuder-Richardson formula (K-R 20) is used to estimate internal consistency. A Cronbach alpha coefficient of 1.00 indicates perfect reliability and a coefficient of 0.00 indicates no reliability. A reliability of 0.80 is usually considered a strong coefficient for a scale that has documented validity and has been used in several studies, such as the CES Depression Scale (Kerlinger & Lee, 2000; Radloff, 1977). The CES Depression Scale has strong internal consistency reliability with Cronbach's alphas ranging from 0.84 to 0.90 in field studies (Locke & Putnam, 2002; Sharp & Lipsky, 2002). For relatively new scales, a reliability of 0.70 is considered acceptable as the scale is being refined and used with a variety of samples. The stronger correlation coefficient indicates less random error and a more reliable scale. When researchers publish their studies, the results of the stability, equivalence, and/or homogeneity reliability testing done in previous research and in the present study need to be included. A measurement method must be reliable if it is to be considered a valid measure for a study variable.

Validity

The validity of an instrument is a determination of how well the instrument reflects the abstract concept being examined. Validity, like reliability, is not an all-or-nothing phenomenon; it is measured on a continuum. No instrument is completely valid. Thus, one determines the degree of validity of a measure rather than whether validity exists (Waltz et al., 2005). Validity will vary from one sample to another and one situation to another; therefore, validity testing evaluates the use of an instrument for a specific group or purpose, rather than the instrument itself. An instrument may be valid in one situation but not another. For example, the CES Depression Scale was developed to measure the depression of patients in mental health settings. Will the same scale be valid as a measure of the depression of cancer patients? You determine this by pilot testing the scale to test for validity of the instrument in a new population. In addition, the original CES Depression Scale was developed for adults, but the scale has been refined and tested with young children (4 to 6 years of age), school age children, and adolescents. Thus, different versions of this scale can be used with all ages from 4 years old to geriatric age (Sharp & Lipsky, 2002).

Currently, validity is considered a single broad method of measurement evaluation that is referred to as **construct validity** and includes content and predictive validity (Rew, Stuppy, & Becker, 1988). **Content-related validity** examines the extent to which the measurement includes all the major elements relevant to the construct being measured. This evidence is obtained from the following three sources: the literature, representatives of the relevant populations, and content experts. **Readability level** focuses on the study participants' ability to read and comprehend the content of an instrument. Readability is essential if an instrument is to be considered valid and reliable for a sample. Assessing the level of readability of an instrument is relatively simple and takes about 10 to 15 minutes. More than 30 readability formulas are available. These formulas use counts of language elements to provide an index of the probable degree of difficulty of comprehending the text. Readability formulas are now a standard part of word-processing software.

Three common types of validity presented in published studies include evidence of validity from: (1) contrasting groups, (2) convergence, and (3) divergence. You can test an instrument's **evidence of validity from contrasting groups** by identifying groups that are expected (or known) to have contrasting scores on the instrument. For example, you select samples from a group of individuals with a diagnosis of depression and a group that does not have this diagnosis. You would expect these two groups of individuals to have contrasting scores on the CES Depression Scale, adding to the construct validity of this scale.

Evidence of validity from convergence is determined when a relatively new instrument is compared with an existing instrument(s) that measures the same construct. The instruments, the new one and the existing ones, are administered to a sample concurrently. Then you evaluate results using correlational analyses. If the measures are highly positively correlated, the validity of each instrument is strengthened. For example the CES Depression Scale has shown positive correlations ranging from 0.50 to 0.80 with the Hamilton Rating Scale for depression supporting the validity of both scales (Locke & Putnam, 2002; Sharp & Lipsky, 2002).

Sometimes instruments can be located that measure a construct or concept opposite to the concept measured by the newly developed instrument. For example, if the newly developed instrument is a measure of hope, you could make a search for an instrument that measures despair. Having study participants complete both of these scales is a way to examine **evidence of validity from divergence**. Correlational procedures are performed with the measures of the two concepts. If the divergent measure (despair scale) is negatively correlated with the other instrument (hope scale), validity for each of the instruments is strengthened (Waltz et al., 2005).

The evidence of an instrument's validity from previous research and the current study needs to be included in the published report of the study. In critically appraising a study, you need to judge the validity of the measurement methods that were used. However, you cannot consider validity apart from reliability. If a measurement method does not have acceptable reliability, its validity becomes a moot issue. Unfortunately, not all published studies include information on the validity and reliability of instruments used to measure study variables.

CRITICAL APPRAISAL GUIDELINES

Directness of Measurement, Level of Measurement, Measurement Error, Reliability, and Validity

In critically appraising a published study, you need to determine the directness of measurement, level of measurement, measurement error, reliability, and validity for the different measurement methods used in a study. In most studies, the Methods section includes a discussion of measurement methods, and you can use the following guidelines to evaluate them.

1. What measurement method(s) were used to measure each study variable?
2. Was the type of measurement direct or indirect?
3. What level of measurement was achieved for each of the study variables?
4. Was reliability information provided from previous studies and for this study?
5. Was the validity of each measurement method adequately described? In some studies, researchers simply state that the measurement method has acceptable validity based on previous research. This statement provides insufficient information for you to judge the validity of an instrument.
6. Did the researchers provide adequate description of the measurement methods to judge the extent of measurement error?

RESEARCH EXAMPLE Directness of Measurement, Level of Measurement, Measurement Error, Reliability, and Validity

Whittenmore, Melkus, Wagner, Dziura, Northrup, and Grey (2009) studied the effects of a Lifestyle Change Program on the outcomes for patients with type 2 diabetes. The lifestyle program was delivered by nurse practitioners (NPs) in primary care settings. The following excerpt describes some of the measurement methods used in this study.

Outcome Measures

Data were collected at the individual (participant) and organizational (NP and site) levels at scheduled time points throughout the study. ... All data were collected by trained research assistants blinded to group assignment, with the exception of ... lipids, which were collected by experienced laboratory personnel at each site and sent to one laboratory for analysis. (Whittenmore et al., 2009, p. 5)

Efficacy data were collected on clinical outcomes of (weight loss, waist circumference, and lipid profiles); behavioral outcomes (nutrition and exercise); psychological outcomes (depressive symptoms). ... All data were collected at baseline, 3 months, and 6 months, with the exception of the laboratory data which were collected at baseline and 6 months. ... Efficacy data collection measures and times were based on the DPP [diabetes prevention program] study and modified for the short duration of this pilot study.

Weight loss was the primary outcome and was calculated as a percentage of weight loss from baseline to 6 months. ... Waist circumference and lipid profiles were secondary clinical outcomes. Waist circumference was measured by positioning a tape measure snugly midway between the upper hip bone and the uppermost border of the iliac crest. In very overweight participants, the tape was placed at the level of the umbilicus (Klein et al., 2007). Lipid profiles (LDL [low-density lipoproteins], HDL [high-density lipoproteins], total cholesterol, and total triglycerides) were determined using fasting venous blood.

Diet and exercise health-promoting behaviors were measured with the exercise and nutrition subscales of the Health-Promoting Lifestyle Profile II (eight and nine items, respectively) which has items constructed on a 4-point Likert scale and measures patterns of diet and exercise behavior (Walker, Sechrist, & Pender, 1987). This instrument has been used in diverse samples, and demonstrates adequate internal consistency (r = .70 to .90 for subscales; Jefferson, Melkus, & Spollett, 2000). The alpha coefficients for the exercise and nutrition subscales in this study were .86 and .76, respectively. …

Psychosocial data were collected on depressive symptoms, as measured by the Center for Epidemiologic Studies-Depression Scale (CES-D), a widely used scale (Radloff, 1977). The CES-D consists of 20 items that address depressed mood, guilt or worthlessness, helplessness or hopelessness, psychomotor retardation, loss of appetite, and sleep disturbance. Each item is rated on a scale of 0 to 3 in terms of frequency during the past week. The total score may range from 0 to 60, with a score of 16 or more indicating impairment. High internal consistency, acceptable test-retest reliability, and good construct validity have been demonstrated (Posner, Stewart, Marin, & Perez-Stable, 2001). The alpha coefficient was .93 for the CES-D in this sample. (Whittenmore et al., 2009, p. 6)

CRITICAL APPRAISAL

Whittenmore and colleagues (2009) measurement methods are critically appraised below using the guidelines previous introduced. The researchers had a detailed plan for data collection and the data collectors were trained and blinded to group assignment, which decrease the potential for measurement error. The variables or outcomes of weight loss, waist circumference, and lipid profiles were measured with physiological measures, which are direct measurement methods. Weight loss was calculated as a percentage, ratio level of measurement, but the researchers did not describe the precision and accuracy of the weight scales used to determine the patients' weights.

The waist circumference was measured with a tape measure, which produces ratio level data. The researchers detailed their process of measuring the participants' waists, including those who were very overweight. Their referencing indicated they used national guidelines for measuring waist circumference. Following a national measurement protocol increased the precision and accuracy of the waist measurements and decreased the potential for error.

The research assistants were trained, which strengthens the measurement process and decreases the potential for error. However, the study would have been strengthened by including the interrater reliability percentage achieved with the training of the data collectors.

The patients' lipid profiles produced ratio level data and the blood samples for these values were collected by experienced laboratory personnel at each site and sent to one laboratory for analysis. These actions increase the precision and accuracy of this measurement method and decrease the potential for measurement error.

Diet and exercise health-promoting behaviors were measured with the subscales from an established, quality Likert scale, Health-Promoting Lifestyle Profile II (Walker et al., 1987). These subscales are an indirect measure of diet and exercise and the data were analyzed as though it were interval level. The subscales had strong reliability (r = 0.70 to 0.90) when used in previous research and the reliability for the subscales in this study were strong (0.86 for diet and 0.76 for exercise). The Health-Promoting Lifestyle Profile II has been used to collect data from diverse samples, which adds to the scale validity. However, the discussion of this measurement method would have been strengthened by expanding on the scale's validity testing from previous studies.

CES-D is an indirect measure of the concept of depression and the data were analyzed as though at the interval level. The CES-D is an established scale developed in 1977 and used widely, which adds to the construct validity of the scale. The researchers also identified the focus of the 20 items of the scale, which addresses the scale's content validity. They also indicated the scale had good construct validity but

Continued

CRITICAL APPRAISAL—cont'd

provided no further specific information to support this statement. The CES-D has a history of acceptable test-retest reliability and high internal consistency. In addition, the Cronbach alpha coefficient for this sample was very strong at $r = 0.93$.

In summary, Whittenmore and colleagues (2009) appear to have selected quality measurement methods for their study. They provided the strongest information about their measurement methods for waist circumference, lipid profiles, diet, exercise, and depression. An expanded discussion of the precision and accuracy of the weight scales used to determine the participants' weights would have strengthened the measurement section of this study. In addition, the validity discussion needs to be expanded for the diet and exercise subscales and CES-D to determine the extent of measurement error.

IMPLICATIONS FOR PRACTICE

Whittenmore et al. (2009, pp. 8-9) stated "the results of this study support the feasibility of implementing a DPP by NPs in a primary care setting to adults at risk of T2D [type 2 diabetes]. ... Preliminary efficacy results of the lifestyle program indicate modest improvements with respect to clinical and behavioral outcomes. Twenty-five percent of the lifestyle participants achieved a 5% weight loss goal compared with 11% of participants in standard care." Thus, the lifestyle program has strengths and the ability to reach the targeted population of adults at risk for T2D; however further research is needed to determine the long term effects of such a program.

Accuracy, Precision, and Error of Physiological Measures

Physiological measures are measurement methods used to quantify the level of functioning of living beings (Waltz et al., 2005). The precision, accuracy, and error of physiological and biochemical measures tend not to be reported or are minimally covered in published studies. These routine physiological measures are assumed to be accurate and precise, an assumption that is not always correct. Some of the most common physiological measures used in nursing studies include BP, heart rate, weight, body mass index, and laboratory values. Sometimes researchers obtain these measures from the patient's record with no consideration given to their accuracy. For example, how many times have you heard a nurse ask a patient his or her weight, rather than weighing the patient? Thus, researchers using physiological measures need to provide evidence of their accuracy and precision and their potential for error (Burns & Grove, 2009; Gift & Soeken, 1988).

Accuracy

Accuracy is comparable to validity, in that it addresses the extent to which the instrument measures what it is supposed to in a study. For example, oxygen saturation measurements with pulse oximetry are considered comparable with the measures of oxygen saturation with arterial blood gas. Thus, pulse oximetry is an accurate measure of oxygen saturation and it has been used in studies to measure this physiological variable because it is easier, less expensive, less painful, and less invasive for research subjects. However, researchers need to document in their study the studies that have been conducted to determine the accuracy of pulse oximetry for the measurement of individuals' oxygen saturation levels.

Precision

Precision is the degree of consistency or reproducibility of measurements made with physiological instruments. Precision is comparable to reliability. The precision of most physiological instruments depends on the manufacturer and is part of quality control testing. Precision of physiological instruments over time can be maintained by following the manufacturer's instructions for care and routine testing of the instrument. Test-retest reliability is appropriate for physiological variables that have minimal fluctuations, such as the bone mineral density or weight of adults. However, test-retest reliability is inappropriate if the variables' values frequently fluctuate, such as with pulse, respirations, and BP. However, test-retest is a good measure of precision if the measurements are taken in rapid succession. For example, the national BP guidelines encourage taking three BP readings and then averaging them to get the most precise and accurate measure of BP.

Error

Sources of error in physiological measures can be grouped into the following five categories: environment, user, subject, machine, and interpretation. The environment affects both the machine and the subject. Environmental factors might include temperature, barometric pressure, and static electricity. User errors are caused by the person using the instrument and may be associated with variations by the same user, different users, or changes in supplies or procedures used to operate the equipment. Subject errors occur when the subject alters the machine or the machine alters the subject. In some cases, the machine may not be used to its full capacity. Machine error may be related to calibration or the stability of the machine. Signals transmitted from the machine are also a source of error and can result in misinterpretation (Gift & Soeken, 1988). Researchers need to report the protocols they implemented or the steps they took to prevent errors in their physiologic and biochemical measures in their published studies.

CRITICAL APPRAISAL GUIDELINES

Accuracy, Precision, and Error of Physiological Measures

When critically appraising the physiological measures in a study, consider the following questions.

1. Was the type of physiologic instrument used to measure a study variable described?
2. Was the process for obtaining, scoring, and/or recording physiological data described?
3. Were the accuracy and precision of the physiological measure addressed?
4. Did the researchers address the potential for errors with the physiological measure?

RESEARCH EXAMPLE Accuracy, Precision, and Error of Physiological Measure

Estok, Sedlak, Doheny, and Hall (2007) conducted a study to determine if menopausal women provided knowledge of their personal osteoporosis risk and knowledge about osteoporosis and prevention behaviors would increase their calcium intake and exercise. The researchers measured the women's bone mineral density (BMD) using the dual-energy X-ray absorptiometer (DXA) and used the BMD scores to determine their risk for osteoporosis. The DXA scan, the process for obtaining the BMD scores, and the meaning of the BMD scores are described in the following excerpt.

> There is low precision error and low radiation exposure in the DXA, and it can be used to measure multiple skeletal sites (Wahner & Fogelman, 1994). Measurements of bone mineral density of the AP [anterior posterior] lumbar spine (L1-L4, anterior posterior) and femur were made using the Lunar model DPX-IQ or DPX-A dual-energy X-ray absorptiometer. The DXA takes only a few minutes and can be used to predict future risk of factures in asymptomatic patients (NOF [National Osteoporosis Foundation], 2003). The results are expressed as a *T*-score and/or age-matched *Z* scores. The *T*-score is independent of age ... and is used to compare the DXA result with the mean peak bone mass of a young adult in terms of a standard deviation (*SD*). At any skeletal site, a decrease in bone mass of 1 *SD* approximately doubles the relative risk of subsequent fracture. Scores were coded using the World Health Organization [WHO] Study Group (1994) prescribed categories: 0 = normal (*T*-score above −1 *SD* in both sites); 1 = osteopenia (*T*-score between −1 and −2.5 *SD* in one or both sites); 2 = osteoporosis (*T*-score below −2.5 *SD* in one or both sites). (Estok et al., 2007, pp. 150-151)

CRITICAL APPRAISAL

Estok and colleagues (2007) provided a strong description of their physiological measurement device by discussing the accuracy, precision, and potential for error of the DXA. In addition, the scoring was described for the DXA scan with the results being standardized using WHO (1994) evidence-based guidelines for determining normal, osteopenia, and osteoporosis diagnoses. The prediction of risk for fracture was based on the NOF (2003) guidelines. In summary, the DXA is an extremely strong physiological measure that provided accurate and precise data for this study. The potential for measurement error is minimal and the scoring is nationally standardized. In addition, the DXA scan is considered a safe measurement method with low radiation exposure.

IMPLICATIONS FOR PRACTICE

Estok et al. (2007) found that the DXA results were significantly related to an increase in calcium intake by the postmenopausal women but not to the engagement in weight-bearing exercise. Evidence-based practice does designate that women over 50 years of age receive a DXA scan to determine their risk of osteopenia and osteoporosis *(www.guidelines.gov)*. Nurses need to encourage postmenopausal women to obtain their DXA scan, determine their risk for osteoporosis, and take preventative action (increase calcium intake and weight-bearing exercises). However, additional research is needed to determine effective interventions to encourage these women to increase their weight-bearing exercises.

Use of Sensitivity, Specificity, and Likelihood Ratios to Determine the Quality of Diagnostic and Screening Tests

An important part of evidence-based practice is the use of quality diagnostic and screening tests to determine the presence or absence of disease (Sackett, Straus, Richardson, Rosenberg, & Haynes, 2000). Clinicians want to know which laboratory or imaging study to order to help screen for or diagnose a disease? When the test is ordered, are the results valid or accurate? The **accuracy of a screening test** or a test used to confirm a diagnosis is evaluated in terms of its ability to correctly assess the presence or absence of a disease or condition as compared with a gold standard. The **gold standard** is the most accurate means of currently diagnosing a particular disease and serves as a basis for comparison with newly developed diagnostic or screening tests. If the test is positive, what is the probability that the disease is present? If the test is negative, what is the probability that the disease is not present? When nurse practitioners and physicians talk to their patients about the results of their tests, how sure are they that the patient does or does not have the disease? Sensitivity and specificity are the terms used to describe the accuracy of a screening or diagnostic test. You will see these terms used in studies and other healthcare literature and we want you to be aware of their definitions and usefulness for practice and research.

There are four possible outcomes of a screening test for a disease: (1) **true positive**, which is an accurate identification of the presence of a disease, (2) **false positive**, which indicates a disease is present when it is not, (3) **true negative**, which indicates accurately that a disease is not present, or (4) **false negative**, which indicates that a disease is not present when it is (Grove, 2007; Sackett et al., 2000). A 2×2 contingency table is helpful in visualizing sensitivity and specificity and these four outcomes (Table 10–1).

You can calculate sensitivity and specificity based on research findings and clinical practice outcomes to determine the most accurate diagnostic or screening tool to use in identifying the presence or absence of a disease for a population of patients. The calculations for sensitivity and specificity are provided as follows:

Sensitivity calculation = Probability of disease = $a/(a+c)$ = **True positive rate**

Specificity calculation = Probability of no disease = $d/(b+d)$ = **True negative rate**

Sensitivity is the proportion of patients with the disease who have a positive test result or true positive. The CES Depression Scale with a score of 15 or higher has 89% sensitivity

Table 10–1	Results of Sensitivity and Specificity of Diagnostic and Screening Tests		
Diagnostic Test Result	Disease Present	Disease Not Present or Absent	Total
Positive test	a (true positive)	b (false positive)	a + b
Negative test	c (false negative)	d (true negative)	c + d
Total	a + c	b + d	a + b + c + d

a = The number of people who have the disease and the test is positive (**true positive**)

b = The number of people who do not have the disease and the test is positive (**false positive**)

c = The number of people who have the disease and the test is negative (**false negative**)

d = The number of people who do not have the disease and the test is negative (**true negative**) for diagnosing depression in adults and 92% sensitivity with elderly people. The ways the researcher or clinician might refer to the test sensitivity include the following:

- A highly sensitive test is very good at identifying the diseased patient.
- If a test is highly sensitive, it has a low percentage of false negatives.
- A low sensitivity test is limited in identifying the patient with a disease.
- If a test has low sensitivity, it has a high percentage of false negatives.
- Therefore, if a sensitive test has negative results, the patient is less likely to have the disease.
- Use the acronym SnNout, which is read: High sensitivity (Sn), test is negative (N), rules the disease out (out).

Specificity is the proportion of patients without the disease who have a negative test result or true negative. The CES Depression Scale with a score of 15 or higher has 70% specificity for diagnosing depression in adults and 87% specificity with elderly people. The ways the researcher or clinician might refer to the test specificity include the following:

- A highly specific test is very good at identifying the patients without a disease.
- If a test is very specific, it has a low percentage of false positives.
- A low specificity test is limited in identifying patients without disease.
- If a test has low specificity, it has a high percentage of false positives.
- Therefore, if a specific test has positive results, the patient is more likely to have the disease.
- Use the acronym SpPin, which is read: High specificity (Sp), test is positive (P), rules the disease in (in).

CRITICAL APPRAISAL GUIDELINES

Sensitivity and Specificity of Diagnostic and Screening Texts

When critically appraising a study, you need to judge the sensitivity and specificity of the diagnostic and screening tests used in the study.

1. Was a diagnostic or screening test used in a study?
2. Are the sensitivity and specificity values provided for the diagnostic or screening test used with the study's population?

RESEARCH EXAMPLE Sensitivity and Specificity

Porter, Fleisher, Kohane, and Mandl (2003) conducted a prospective observational study to assess predictive value of parents reporting the medical history and physical signs of dehydration in their children. Their study included 132 parent-child dyads. The primary outcome was percentage of dehydration, and secondary outcomes were clinically important acidosis and hospital admission. They also compared the reports of physical signs of dehydration made by the parents and the nurse. Their study results indicated that parents' report of physical symptoms and history had a higher sensitivity (range 73% to 100%) than specificity (range 0% to 49%) for predicting dehydration of 5% or greater in their child (Table 10–2). The nurses' report of physical signs for clinically important dehydration were always more specific (33% to 93%) than the parents (17% to 82%) and usually more sensitive (10% to 100%) than the parents (0 to 91%) (Table 10–3) (Porter et al., 2003).

Table 10–2 Value of Parent-Reported History for Prediction of Clinically Important Dehydration

Historical Element (Total No. of Parents = 132)	% Sensitivity (95% CI)	% Specificity (95% CI)
Decreased oral intake	100 (75-100)	18 (8-28)
Decreased urine output	100 (75-100)	26 (15-37)
History of any vomiting during illness	100 (75-100)	3 (0-7)
History of vomiting in past 12 hours	73 (37-92)	6 (0-12)
History of any diarrhea during illness	91 (63-99)	28 (17-39)
History of diarrhea in past 12 hours	82 (50-97)	38 (26-50)
Contact with PCP by telephone (n = 131)	91 (63-99)	23 (12-34)
Contact with PCP in office (n = 131)	100 (75-100)	49 (36-62)
Previous trial of clear liquids (n = 131)	100 (75-100)	22 (12-32)

Porter, S. C., Fleisher, G. R., Kohane, I. S., & Mandl, K. D. (2003). The value of parental report for diagnosis and management of dehydration in the emergency department. *Annals of Emergency Medicine, 41*(2), 201.

Table 10–3 Diagnostic Value of Parents' and Nurses' Report of Physical Signs for Clinically Important Dehydration[*]

Physical Sign (No. of Parents/ No. of Nurses)	% Sensitivity		% Specificity	
	Parent (95% CI)	Nurse (95% CI)	Parent (95% CI)	Nurse (95% CI)
Ill appearance (71/68)	91 (63-99)	90 (60-99)	17 (7-26)	33 (21-45)
Sunken fontanelle[†] (13/11)	0 (0-84)	100 (2-100)	82 (48-98)	90 (56-100)
Sunken eyes (71/68)	64 (33-86)	70 (38-91)	37 (15-58)	59 (47-72)
Decreased tears[‡] (67/42)	91 (63-99)	100 (33-100)	25 (14-36)	33 (21-45)
Dry mouth (71/68)	64 (33-86)	100 (73-100)	42 (35-48)	49 (36-62)
Weak cry[§] (71/41)	54 (25-80)	25 (1-75)	27 (16-38)	78 (65-92)
Cool extremities (71/68)	27 (8-63)	10 (1-40)	73 (62-84)	93 (87-100)

[*]The total number of patients for this outcome equals 71. Three patients from the subset of 71 did not have nursing assessments for physical signs completed.

[†]Subset of 32 infants <9 months of age with only two cases of significant dehydration.

[‡]Parents and nurses could answer "no opportunity to observe," resulting in missing data for parents (4 patients) and nurses (26 patients).

[§]Nurses could answer "no opportunity to observe," resulting in missing data (27 patients).

Porter, S. C., Fleisher, G. R., Kohane, I. S., & Mandl, K. D. (2003). The value of parental report for diagnosis and management of dehydration in the emergency department. *Annals of Emergency Medicine, 41*(2), 202.

Continued

CRITICAL APPRAISAL

Porter and colleagues (2003) provided a quality discussion about sensitivity and specificity of predicting dehydration in young children. They detailed information in their narrative and tables about the sensitivity and specificity of nurses and parents in using certain criteria to predict dehydration in the children.

IMPLICATIONS FOR PRACTICE

In this study, the nurses' diagnostic ability to determine clinically important dehydration is the gold standard used as a basis for comparison of the parents' diagnostic ability. As expected, the nurses' were more sensitive and specific in diagnosing clinically important dehydration in children than parents, but the parents were very sensitive in reporting the child's history that was predictive of dehydration. In developing a diagnostic or screening test, researchers need to achieve the highest sensitivity and specificity possible and clinicians need to select the most sensitive and specific screening test to diagnosis diseases in their patients (Craig & Smyth, 2007; Sackett et al., 2000). However, the screening test selected for detecting a disease is dependent upon a consideration of cost as well as sensitivity and specificity.

Likelihood ratios (LRs) are additional calculations that you can perform to determine the accuracy of diagnostic or screening tests, which are based on the sensitivity and specificity results. The LRs determine the likelihood that a positive test result is a true positive and a negative test result is a true negative. The ratio of the true positive results to false positive results is known as the **positive LR** (Craig & Smyth, 2007). The positive LR is calculated as follows:

$$\text{Positive LR} = \text{Sensitivity} \div 100\% - \text{Specificity}$$

$$\text{Positive LR for Sunken Fontanelle Diagnosed by Nurse} = 100\% \div (100\% - 90\%)$$
$$= 100\% \div 10\% = 10$$

Negative LR is the ratio of true negative results to false negative results and is calculated as follows:

$$\text{Negative LR} = 100\% - \text{Sensitivity} \div \text{Specificity}$$

$$\text{Negative LR for Sunken Fontanelle Diagnosed by Nurse} = (100\% - 100\%) \div 90\%$$
$$= 0 \div 90\% = 0$$

The very high LRs that are above 10 rule in the disease or indicate that the patient has the disease. The very low LRs that are <0.1 virtually rule out the chance that the patient has the disease (Melnyk & Fineout-Overholt, 2005; Sackett et al., 2000). Understanding sensitivity, specificity, and LR increases your ability to read clinical studies and determine the most accurate diagnostic and screening tests to use in clinical practice.

Measurement Strategies in Nursing

Nursing studies examine a wide variety of phenomena and thus require an extensive array of measurement methods. Some nursing phenomena have not been examined because no one has thought of a way to measure them. This has implications for both clinical practice and research. This section describes some of the most common measurement methods used in nursing research, including physiological measurement, observational measurement, interviews, questionnaires, and scales.

Physiological Measurements

Because of measurement problems, physiological nursing research has lagged behind studies of the psychosocial dimensions of nursing practice. Some of the first physiological nursing studies examined basic care activities, such as mouth care; pressure ulcer care; the effect of preoperative teaching on postoperative recovery; and infection control related to urinary bladder catheterization, intravenous therapy, and tracheotomy care. Even at this fairly basic level, developing valid methods to measure the variables of interest was difficult and required considerable time and expense. For example, how can changes in a pressure ulcer be measured? What criteria can be used to determine the effectiveness of a mouth care regimen? Creativity and attention to detail are needed to develop effective physiological measurement strategies.

An increased need for ways to measure the outcomes of nursing care has generated more nursing studies that include physiological measures. The outcome of interest may be the outcome of all nursing care received for a particular care episode or the outcome of a particular nursing intervention. An important focus of physiological measurement is finding means to quantify changes, either directly or indirectly, that occur in physiological variables as a result of nursing care. This upsurge of interest in outcome measures has broadened the base of physiological research beyond nurse physiologists to include nurse clinicians (Brown, 2009; Craig & Smyth, 2007).

A variety of approaches for obtaining physiological measures are possible. Some measurements are relatively easy to obtain and are an extension of the measurement methods used in nursing practice, such as those used to obtain weight and BP. Other measurements are not difficult to obtain, but the method requires an imaginative approach. For example, some phenomena are traditionally only observed in clinical practice, but not measured. Some physiological measures are obtained using self-report or paper-and-pencil scales or by observation. Physiological measurements are also obtained using laboratory tests and electronic monitoring. Two studies with physiological measures are presented as examples. One study includes physiological measures obtained through self-report and the other study includes physiological measures from electronic monitoring.

RESEARCH EXAMPLE Physiological Measure Using Self-Report

Kapella, Larson, Patel, Covey, and Berry (2006) examined relationships among the physiological variables of fatigue, dyspnea, and functional status in chronic obstructive pulmonary disease (COPD) patients. These variables were measured with self-report instruments and the measurement of dyspnea is described in the following excerpt.

> Dyspnea was measured with the Chronic Respiratory Disease Questionnaire (CRQ). ... The CRQ is a disease-specific measure that was developed for use in people with COPD (Guyatt, Berman, Townsend, Pugsley, & Chambers, 1987). With the CRQ Dyspnea Scale, participants rate the dyspnea they experience during selected activities that they perform on a regular basis. It is a five-item scale with a potential range from 1 = *extremely short of breath* to 7 = *not at all short of breath*. A self-report form of the CRQ (Williams, Singh, Sewell, Guyatt, & Morgan, 2001) was used here. Cronbach's alpha for the CRQ in this study was .84. (Kapella et al., 2006)

CRITICAL APPRAISAL

The self-report CRQ Dyspnea Scale seemed to be a valid and reliable method for measuring the dyspnea experienced by patients with COPD. Kapella et al. (2006) indicated the scale was developed just for people with COPD, which adds to the validity of the scale. Sources that documented the development of the scale's validity and reliability were identified. In addition, the CRQ Dyspnea Scale was reliable in this study as indicated by the Cronbach alpha coefficient of $r = 0.84$.

IMPLICATIONS FOR PRACTICE

Kapella and colleagues (2006) found that the study participants had moderate amounts of fatigue that were situation specific and were often controlled with rest and sleep. The researchers recommend further research to increase the understanding of the symptoms of people with COPD. Using self-report measures, such as the CRQ have enabled nurses to ask research questions not previously considered, which has added to nursing's knowledge base. In addition, the scale to measure dyspnea with COPD has potential use in practice to determine the amount of dyspnea experienced by patients so the best management plan can be implemented. Thus, the insight gained could alter the nursing management of COPD patients in situations considered problematic and improve patient outcomes.

The availability of electronic monitoring equipment has greatly increased the possibilities of physiological measurement in nursing studies, particularly in critical care environments. Electronic monitoring requires placing sensors on or within the subject. The sensors measure changes in body functions such as electrical energy. For many sensors, an external stimulus is needed to trigger measurement by the sensor. Transducers convert the electrical signal. Electrical signals often include interference signals as well as the desired signal, so an amplifier may be used to decrease interference and amplify the desired signal. The electrical signal is then digitized (converted to numerical digits or values) and stored. In addition, it is immediately displayed on a monitor. The display equipment may be visual or auditory, or both. A writing recorder provides a printed version of the data. Some electronic equipment provides simultaneous recording of multiple physiological measures that are displayed on a monitor. The equipment is often linked to a computer, which allows review of data, and the computer often contains complex software for detailed analysis of the data and will provide a printed report of the analysis (Burns & Grove, 2009; DeKeyser & Pugh, 1991; Pugh & DeKeyser, 1995).

RESEARCH EXAMPLE Physiological Measures Obtained Using Electronic Monitoring

Paratz and Lipman (2006) examined the effects of manual hyperinflation (MHI) on the hemodynamics and plasma catecholamines of ventilated patients. Nurses use MHI to increase the air in the pulmonary system immediately before a ventilator is discontinued. Electronic sensors were used to measure many of the variables in this study and the measurement of the diastolic pressure, mean arterial pressure (MAP), pulmonary artery occlusion pressure (PAOP), and cardiac output (CO) are described in the following excerpt.

> Diastolic and MAP were recorded (Merlin pressure module M1006reA; Hewlett Packard) 1 minute before, during disconnection from the ventilator, at 1, 2, and 3 minutes during MHI, and at 1 and 5 minutes after MHI. The information was down-loaded to a computerized information system. PAOP was taken immediately before and after MHI at end of expiration. CO was measured by the Vigilance Cardiac Output System (Baxter Edwards Critical Care, Irwin, CA). This system employs a heated filament wrapped around a balloon flotation pulmonary artery catheter, which is positioned in the right atrium and ventricle. (Paratz & Lipman, 2006, p. 263)

CRITICAL APPRAISAL

Paratz and Lipman (2006) provided a detailed description of the electronic equipment they used to measure their study variables. This equipment appeared to have accuracy and precision in the measurement of study variables. The researchers also detailed when the measurements of variables were obtained, the recording of data, and the preparation of the data for analysis, which were done electronically to reduce the potential for error.

IMPLICATIONS FOR PRACTICE

Previous research documented that beneficial respiratory effects have been obtained from MHI; however MHI has the capacity to alter the hemodynamics of intensive care patients. Paratz and Lipman's (2006, p. 267) "study showed that there was strong indication that although the cardiac index initially decreased on application of MHI in the group of study patients, it did so by a clinically insignificant figure and the patients were able to compensate by vasoconstriction. This study gives further knowledge as to the patient selection for MHI." The findings from this study have clinical relevance for nurses working in ICU and their management of ventilator patients.

Observational Measurements

Observational measurement involves an interaction between the study participants and the observer(s) where the observer has the opportunity to watch the participant perform in a specific setting (Waltz et al., 2005). Observation can be used to collect data in qualitative research and would more likely involve unstructured observation (see Chapter 3). **Unstructured observations** involve spontaneously observing and recording what is seen. The analysis of this data may lead to a more structured observation and an observational checklist (Creswell, 2009; Marshall & Rossman, 2006; Munhall, 2007). In **structured observational measurement**, the researcher carefully defines what he or she will observe and how the observations are to be made, recorded, and coded (Waltz et al., 2005). For observations to be structured, researchers will develop a category system for organizing and sorting the behaviors or events being observed. Checklists often are used to indicate whether a behavior occurred. Rating scales allow the observer to rate the behavior or event. This provides more information for analysis than dichotomous data, which indicate only whether or not the behavior occurred.

Observation tends to be more subjective than other types of measurement and thus often is considered less credible. However, in many cases this approach is the only way to obtain important data for nursing's body of knowledge. As with any means of measurement, consistency is very important; thus, reporting interrater reliability of those doing the observations is essential.

CRITICAL APPRAISAL GUIDELINES

Observational Measurements

When critically appraising observational measures, consider the following questions:

1. Is the object of observation clearly identified and defined?
2. Are the techniques for recording observations described?
3. Is interrater reliability for the observers described?

RESEARCH EXAMPLE Observational Measurement

Liaw, Yang, Chang, Chou, and Chao (2009) conducted a study to determine the effects of a developmental supportive care (DSC) educational program provided nurses on their caregiving behaviors and the preterm infants' behaviors during bathing in a neonatal unit. These researchers provided an extensive description of their use of observational measurement to identify infant behaviors and nurse behaviors during the bathing process. The following excerpt includes part of their description of their observational measurement methods.

Nurse caregiving and infant behaviors were measured from the time that a nurse put her hands through an isolette porthole to the stage when she completed the bath and removed her hands from an incubator and left. Researchers developed two coding schemes: one was the preterm infant behavioral coding scheme for assessing preterm infant behavior responses during bath, and the other one was the nursing behavioral coding scheme for assessing nurse caregiving behavior during bath. The behaviors included in this coding scheme were only those that could be reliably recorded and observed from videotapes and with which another expert (Dr. Evelyn Thoman) agreed as being behaviors and states that could be consistently observed on video recordings. Time-triggered coding was used to measure all behaviors and states. There were four observers watching the videotapes. Two were responsible for recording infant behavior, and the other two observed nurse behavior. All behavior data were coded at 10-second intervals on a continuous basis with an electronic auditory device, and codes were typed in a Microsoft Word file. [See Table 10–4 for the infant behaviors and codes for scoring videotapes.]

Validity and Reliability

The preterm infant behaviors included in this study have been studied in other reports (Becker et al., 1999; Peters, 1998). Researchers have reported that stress behaviors, such as finger splay, leg extension, and grimace, are significantly related to ongoing caregiving procedures (Peters, 1998). ... These studies are cited as evidence to support validity of the behaviors included in this study. ... Selected nurse caregiving behaviors are based on the concepts and principles of DSC from the literature (Als, 1999; Als et al., 2003; Becker et al., 1999). Moreover, these behaviors have also been tested in other studies and could refer to behaviors that have been found to be key components of DSC. Some negative nursing behaviors, such as inappropriate position and exposure to light, which often occurred during real bathing procedures, were also included.

Interrater reliability was examined by two observers through video observations and coding. Thirty tapes were randomly selected and scored. Pearson correlation coefficients were used to calculate interrater reliability between the observers' scores. Correlation coefficients of the infant behavioral coding scheme between two observers ranged from .82 to .99, and correlation coefficients of the nursing behavior coding scheme between the other two scorers were from .91 to .98 (Liaw et al., 2009, pp. 87-89).

CRITICAL APPRAISAL

Liaw and colleagues (2009) provided an excellent description of the observations to be recorded and the process for recoding them by the observers. The coding and recoding processes were very structured to improve the validity and reliability of the observations made in the study. They provided two tables that documented the behaviors observed and the codes used when reviewing the videotapes (Table 10–4). The behaviors selected for coding were based on previous research, which strengthens the validity of the observation measures for both infant and nurse. The study included two observers coding the preterm infant behaviors from a video and they had very strong interrater reliability (0.82 to 0.99). The interrater reliability for the two observers for the nurse behaviors was also very strong, with coefficients ranging from 0.91 to 0.98. In summary, Liaw et al. (2009) provided a quality description of the highly valid and reliable observation methods used in their study.

IMPLICATIONS FOR PRACTICE

Liaw and colleagues (2009) found that the infants were less stressed and the nurses were more supportive following their DSC training. The researchers identified the following implications for practice: "Preterm infants need gentle and sensitive care to support the healthy development of their body systems, especially the brain. To significantly improve nurses' caregiving skills, they need to initially receive DSC training and to repeat the training at regular intervals—about twice a year" (Liaw et al., 2009, p. 91). The researchers also recommended that additional studies be conducted to extend the DSC type training to other nursing caregiving activities for neonates.

Continued

IMPLICATIONS FOR PRACTICE—cont'd

Table 10–4 Definitions of Infant Behaviors and Codes for Scoring Videotapes

Behavior	Code	Definition
Startle	J	A sudden movement in which the arms extend quickly outward then return toward midline: leg may flex or extend
Jerk		A sudden movement of at least a whole limb, one arm, or one leg
Tremor		A fine rhythmical movement of extremities
Extension	S	Stiff extensor positioning of extremities: salute, airplane, sitting on air, leg bracing, or other hypertonic behaviors
Arching		Movement of all limbs and trunk showing labored stretching and struggling
Squirming		Trunkal extension into an arch or head extension in prone, supine, or upright position
Finger splay	H	A sudden stiff extension of fingers and hand
Grasping		Grasping movement, with hands directed at either the baby's own face or the baby's own body, at midair, or a caregivers hands/finger/body, tubing, or bedding
Fisting		Strong hand holdings by flexing the baby's fingers and forming a fist
Grimace	G	Cry face or frown
Sucking	K	The infant sucks on one's own hands, fingers, swabs, or pacifier (although coders cannot see the baby's face, it is assumed that the baby is sucking)
Unknown	D	It is not known whether the eyes are open or closed because the coder cannot see the baby's eyes for the whole epoch
Eyes closed	C	Eyes are closed during all 10 seconds or at any time of the epoch that the baby's eyes can be seen
Eyes open	O	Eyes are open at any time during the 10 seconds
Fussing or crying	F	An intermittent fussy or sustained vocal sound of distress

Liaw, J., Yang, L., Chang, L., Chou, H., & Chao, S. (2009). Improving neonatal caregiving through a developmentally supportive care training program. *Applied Nursing Research, 22*(2), 88.

Interviews

An **interview** involves verbal communication between the researcher and the subject during which information is provided to the researcher. Although this data collection strategy is most commonly used in qualitative and descriptive studies, it also can be used in other types of quantitative studies. You can use a variety of approaches to conduct an interview, ranging from a totally **unstructured interview**, in which the content is completely controlled by the study participant, to a **structured interview**, in which the content is similar to that of a questionnaire, with the possible responses to questions carefully designed by the researcher (Creswell, 2009; Waltz et al., 2005).

Unstructured interviews, used in qualitative research to collect data, are often initiated by asking a broad question, such as "Describe for me your experience with. …" After the interview has begun, the role of the interviewer is to encourage the subject to continue talking, using techniques such as nodding the head or making sounds that indicate interest. In some cases, you may encourage the participant to elaborate further on a particular dimension of the topic of discussion (Munhall, 2007). Chapter 3 discusses unstructured interviews in qualitative research in greater detail.

During structured interviews, the researcher uses strategies to control the content of the interview. Questions the interviewer asks are designed by the researcher before the initiation of data collection, and the order of the questions is specified. In some cases the interviewer can elaborate on the meaning of the question or modify the way in which the question is asked so that the participant can understand it better. A structured interview can be used to collect quantitative data by the researcher by entering the participant's responses onto a rating scale or paper-and-pencil instrument. For example, a researcher could use a telephone interview to obtain responses to an instrument.

Because nurses frequently use interviewing techniques in nursing assessment, the dynamics of interviewing are familiar. However, using the technique for measurement in research requires greater sophistication. Interviewing is a flexible technique that allows the researcher to explore meaning in greater depth than is possible with other techniques. You can use interpersonal skills to facilitate cooperation and elicit more information. Because the response rate for interviews is higher than for questionnaires, interviewing often allows a more representative sample to be obtained. Interviewing allows collection of data from participants who are unable or unlikely to complete questionnaires, such as those who are very ill or whose ability to read, write, and express themselves is marginal.

Interviews are a form of self-report, and it must be assumed that the information provided is accurate. Because of time and costs, sample size usually is limited. Participant bias is always a threat to the validity of the findings, as is inconsistency in data collection from one subject to another (Waltz et al., 2005).

CRITICAL APPRAISAL GUIDELINES

Interviews

When critically appraising interview measurement methods in studies, you need to consider the following questions:

1. Are the interview questions relevant for the research problem and purpose and objectives, questions, or hypotheses?
2. Does the design indicate the process for conducting the interviews?
3. Do the questions tend to bias subjects' responses?

RESEARCH EXAMPLE

Interviews

Some researchers use a combination of open-ended or unstructured interview questions and structured interview questions to gather the data needed for a study. For example, Harralson (2007, p. 96) used quantitative and qualitative data collection in their mixed methods study to examine the "factors associated with delay in seeking emergency medical attention for acute ischemic symptoms in a sample of predominantly African American women." Harralson interviewed female patients who presented with symptoms of acute myocardial infarction (AMI) in a large, urban teaching hospital in the United States. The following excerpt describes the structured and unstructured interview processes used in this study.

Continued

RESEARCH EXAMPLE—cont'd

Structured Interview

The study used a structured interview to explore the variables of interest. The 45-minute interview included questions pertaining to sociodemographics, social support, general physical health, medical comorbidities, perceived and practical barriers to seeking health care, and CHD [coronary heart disease] symptoms and severity. Open-ended questions addressed the patients' experiences from symptom onset until a decision was made to seek medical attention [unstructured interview]. Open-ended questions included questions about patients' physical and emotional feelings during the experience, decision-making processes (i.e., who they told and who they sought advice from), and beliefs about what was happening to them at the onset of the symptoms of AMI [unstructured interview].

The structured interview was developed specifically for this study on the basis of a systematic review of the literature that examined concepts and factors associated with delay in seeking medical treatment. In addition, several nurses, cardiologists, and social scientists reviewed the interview.

To reduce recall bias in this study, interviews were conducted within 5 days of the acute ischemic event. This recall time frame is similar to time periods used in other studies reviewed in the background section. (Harralson, 2007, p. 98)

CRITICAL APPRAISAL

Harralson (2007) clearly indicated that the structured interview was conducted to explore the study variables. The focus of both the unstructured and structured interviews were described and seemed relevant to the study problem and purpose. The researcher based her interview questions on a review of literature and then asked several nurses, cardiologists, and social scientists to review them. These steps strengthen the content validity of the questions the researchers developed to measure the perceived and practical barriers to seeking treatment for acute ischemic symptoms by lower income, urban women. In addition, Harralson attempted to reduce recall bias by conducting the interviews within 5 days of the acute ischemic event. The structured interviews included established instruments to measure depression and social support which added strength to the data collected during the study. In summary, Harralson (2007) implemented in a reliable way both structured and unstructured interview measurement methods that had documented validity and were focused on the problem and purpose of the study.

IMPLICATIONS FOR PRACTICE

Harralson (2007) found the women on the average delayed 20.4 hours before seeking treatment for their symptoms of acute myocardial infarction (AMI). "Sixty-nine percent of the patients delayed 1 hour or more. These delays were associated with younger, African American ethnicity, poorer self-rated health, and the belief that one could not personally ever have an AMI" (Harralson, 2007, p. 96). The researcher recommended that additional education be provided to women to increase their knowledge of AMI symptoms, their personal risk factors, and the treatment of AMI. With this knowledge, women might develop a plan of action if they should experience AMI symptoms and seek treatment immediately.

Questionnaires

A **questionnaire** is a printed self-report form designed to elicit information through written or verbal responses of the subject. Questionnaires are sometimes referred to as surveys, and a study using a questionnaire may be referred to as survey research. The information obtained from questionnaires is similar to that obtained by an interview, but the questions tend to have less depth. The subject is not permitted to elaborate on responses or ask for clarification of questions, and the data collector cannot use probing strategies. However, questions are presented in a consistent manner to each subject, and opportunity for bias is less than in an interview. Questionnaires often are used in descriptive studies to gather a broad spectrum of information from subjects, such as facts about the subject or facts about persons, events, or situations known by the subject. It is also used to gather information about beliefs, attitudes, opinions, knowledge, or intentions of the subject. Like interviews, questionnaires can have various structures. Some questionnaires ask open-ended questions, which require written responses (qualitative data) from the subject. Other questionnaires ask closed-ended questions, which have only answers selected by the researcher. A modification is the use of computers to gather questionnaire data (Kerlinger & Lee, 2000).

Although you can distribute questionnaires to very large samples, either directly or through the mail or Internet, the response rate for questionnaires generally is lower than that for other forms of self-report, particularly if the questionnaires are mailed. If the response rate is lower than 50%, the representativeness of the sample is seriously in question. The response rate for mailed questionnaires usually is small (25% to 40%), so the researcher frequently is unable to obtain a representative sample, even with random sampling methods. Surveys distributed by the Internet have a greater response rate and many researchers are choosing this format if they have access to the potential subjects' e-mail addresses (Waltz et al., 2005).

Respondents commonly fail to mark responses to all of the questions, especially on long questionnaires. The incomplete nature of the data can threaten the validity of the instrument. With most questionnaires, researchers analyze data at the level of individual items, rather than adding the items together and analyzing the total scores. Responses to items usually are measured at the nominal or ordinal level.

CRITICAL APPRAISAL GUIDELINES

Questionnaires

When critically appraising a questionnaire in a published study, consider the following questions:

1. Does the questionnaire address the focus of the study outlined in the study problem and purpose and/or objective, questions, or hypotheses? Examine the description of the contents of the questionnaire in the measurement section of the study.
2. Does the study provide information on content-related validity for the questionnaire?
3. Was the questionnaire implemented consistently from one subject to another?

RESEARCH EXAMPLE Questionnaires

Kagan, Ovadia, and Kaneti (2009) conducted a study of nurses' knowledge of blood-borne pathogens (BBPs), their hand washing compliance with standard precautions (SPs), and their avoidance of therapeutic contact with BBP-infected patients. They described their questionnaire as follows:

> A structured questionnaire was built by the researchers consisting of six parts: One scale indicated sociode-mographic information; three scales indicated level of knowledge on three BBPs (HIV [human immunode-ficiency virus], HBV [hepatitis B virus], and HCV [hepatitis C virus]); one scale indicated the self-reported level of compliance with SPs; and two parts indicated understanding of SP principles and avoidance of therapeutic contact with a BBP-infected patients. One outside nursing researcher specializing in different aspects of infection control and two physicians specializing in infectious disease tested the face validity and comprehensibility of the instrument. All judges had to be in full agreement for any item to be included, and their comments were taken into account in constructing the final questionnaire. A pilot study was conducted ($n = 20$) for evaluating the data-collection process and usefulness of the questionnaire. After the pilot study, the tool was revised.
>
> Sociodemographic information was collected via 10 items addressing age, gender, family status, level of education, and academic degree, origin, profession, seniority, workplace, and job position of participant. … Knowledge related to BBPs was examined using three scales comprised of six items each for HBV, HCV, and HIV. Each scale showed perceived knowledge relating to transmission, diagnosis, symptoms, treatment, prognosis, and prevention of BBPs. … Compliance with standard precautions [SPs] was indi-cated by seven statements. … The perception of the basic principle of SP approach was indicated by the questions, "In your opinion, should every patient be treated as BBP carrier?" … Nurses' avoidance of thera-peutic contact with a BBP-infected person was measured by one question: "Does fear of possible con-tamination lead you to avoid contact with patients who are highly suspected to be infected by BBP?" (Kagan et al., 2009, pp. 15-16)

CRITICAL APPRAISAL

Kagan and colleagues (2009) clearly described the development of their questionnaire for their study. The questionnaire items addressed the study purpose which was, "To examine the relationship between nurses' knowledge of blood-borne pathogens (BBPs), their professional behavior regarding hand-washing compli-ance with standard precautions (SPs), and avoidance of therapeutic contact with BBP-infected patients" (p. 13). The researchers detailed the items on the questionnaire that were developed to measure the variables identified in the study purpose. The questionnaire items were judged for face or content validity and com-prehensibility, and the data collection process and questionnaire were pilot tested with revisions as indicated. In summary, the researchers developed a questionnaire with relevant items and documented validity.

IMPLICATIONS FOR PRACTICE

Kagan and colleagues (2009) found that the nurses' knowledge of BBPs did not increase their compliance with standard precautions. The researchers proposed that the nurses' views and attitudes might influence their compliance with hand washing more than their knowledge and they recommended this as an area for future research. The researchers also found that the nurses were avoiding therapeutic contact with the BBP-infected patients. They recommended providing educational interventions to improve the nurses' attitudes and behaviors toward patients with BBP infections.

Scales

The **scale**, a form of self-report, is a more precise means of measuring phenomena than the questionnaire. Most scales measure psychosocial variables. However, you can use scaling techniques to obtain self-reports on physiological variables such as pain, nausea, or functional capacity. The various items on most scales are summed to obtain a single score. These are referred to as summated scales. Fewer random and systematic errors occur when the total score of a scale is used (Nunnally & Bernstein, 1994). The various items in a scale increase the dimensions of the concept that are reflected in the instrument. The three types of scales described in this section that are commonly used in nursing research include rating scales, Likert scales, and visual analog scales.

Rating Scales

Rating scales are the crudest form of measure involving scaling techniques. A rating scale lists an ordered series of categories of a variable that are assumed to be based on an underlying continuum. A numerical value is assigned to each category, and the fineness of the distinctions between categories varies with the scale. Rating scales are commonly used by the general public. In conversations one can hear statements such as, "On a scale of 1 to 10, I would rank that …" Rating scales are easy to develop; however, you need to be careful to avoid end statements that are so extreme that no subject will select them. You can use a rating scale to rate the degree of cooperativeness of the patient or the value placed by the subject on nurse-patient interactions. Researchers often use this type of scale in observational measurement to guide data collection.

Some rating scales are more valid than others because they were constructed in a structured way and used in a variety of studies with different populations. For example, the Faces Pain Scale is a commonly used rating scale to assess the pain of children in clinical practice and it has proven to be valid and reliable over the years (Figure 10–2). Nurses often assess pain in adults with a numeric rating scale (NRS), presented in Figure 10–3. Using the NRS is more valid and reliable than asking a patient to rate their pain on a scale from 1 to 10.

CRITICAL APPRAISAL GUIDELINES

Rating Scales

When critically appraising a rating scale, ask the following questions.

1. Is the rating scale clearly described?
2. Are the techniques that were used to administer and score the scale provided?
3. Is information about validity and reliability of the scale described from previous studies and from this study?

0 = VERY HAPPY, NO HURT
1 = HURTS JUST A LITTLE BIT
2 = HURTS A LITTLE MORE
3 = HURTS EVEN MORE
4 = HURTS A WHOLE LOT
5 = HURTS AS MUCH AS YOU CAN IMAGINE
(Don't have to be crying to feel this much pain)

Explain to the person that each face is for a person who feels happy because he has no pain (no hurt) or sad because he has some or a lot of pain. Face 0 is very happy because he doesn't hurt at all. Face 1 hurts just a little bit. Face 2 hurts a little more. Face 3 hurts even more. Face 4 hurts a whole lot. Face 5 hurts as much as you can imagine, although you don't have to be crying to feel this bad. Ask the person to choose the face that best describes how he is feeling.

Rating scale is recommended for persons age 3 years and older.

Brief word instructions: Point to each face using the words to describe the pain intensity. Ask the child to choose face that best describes own pain and record the appropriate number.

Figure 10–2. Wong-Baker FACES Pain Rating Scale.

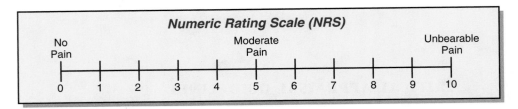

Figure 10–3. Numerical Rating Scale.

RESEARCH EXAMPLE Rating Scales

Fletcher and colleagues (2009) conducted a study of the fatigue of family caregivers of patients undergoing radiation therapy for prostate cancer. They used a numeric rating scale (NRS) to measure the fatigue of their subjects and provided the following description of their rating scale.

> Fatigue severity was measured with the 13-item Lee Fatigue Scale (LFS; Lee et al., 1991). Each item was rated on a 0 to 10 numeric rating scale (NRS), and a total score was calculated as the mean of the 13 items, with higher scores indicating greater fatigue severity. Respondents were asked to rate each item based on how they felt 'right now,' within 30 minutes of awakening (morning fatigue), and prior to going to bed (evening fatigue). The LFS has been used with healthy individuals, (Gay, Lee, & Lee, 2004; Lee et al., 1991) and patients with cancer and HIV... It was chosen for this study because it is relatively short, easy to administer, and has well established validity and reliability. The Cronbach's alpha for evening fatigue was .96 and for morning fatigue was .94 in patients undergoing evaluation for sleep disorders (Lee et al., 1999). In this sample of FCs (family caregivers) and patients, Cronbach's alphas for evening and morning fatigue at baseline were .95 and .96 respectively. (Fletcher et al., 2009, p. 129)

CRITICAL APPRAISAL

Fletcher and colleagues (2009) clearly described the LFS and how it was administered and scored when measuring fatigue severity in their study. The researchers detailed the scale's reliability for previous studies, and this study. The reported Cronbach alphas indicated that the LFS is reliable. The scale has been used in other studies with different populations, which add to the scale's validity. The researchers provided a quality discussion of the LFS that might have been strengthened by including more details on the scale's validity.

IMPLICATIONS FOR PRACTICE

Fletcher and colleagues (2009) found that the family caregivers had individual variability in their severity of fatigue, with their greatest fatigue occurring in the evenings. The researchers recommend further research to expand our understanding of these caregivers' needs and how to manage them. Based on the findings of this study, Fletcher et al. (2009, p. 125) recommended "Evaluating family caregivers for sleep disturbance, anxiety, and poor family support, as well as high levels of patient fatigue, could identify those family caregivers at highest risk for sustained fatigue trajectories." The LFS could be a useful instrument for measuring fatigue severity for both caregivers and cancer patients in clinical settings.

Likert Scale

The Likert scale is designed to determine the opinions or attitudes of study subjects. This scale contains a number of declarative statements with a scale after each statement. The Likert scale is the most commonly used of the scaling techniques. The original version of the scale included five response categories. Each response category was assigned a value, with a value of 0 or 1 given to the most negative response and a value of 4 or 5 to the most positive response (Kerlinger & Lee, 2000; Nunnally & Bernstein, 1994).

Response choices in a Likert scale most commonly address agreement, evaluation, or frequency. Agreement options may include statements such as *strongly agree, agree, uncertain, disagree,* and *strongly disagree.* Evaluation responses ask the respondent for an evaluative rating along a good/bad dimension, such as positive to negative or excellent to terrible. Frequency responses may include statements such as *never, rarely, sometimes, frequently,* and *all the time.* The terms used are versatile and are selected for their appropriateness to the stem.

Sometimes seven options are given, sometimes only four. Use of the uncertain or neutral category is controversial because it allows the subject to avoid making a clear choice of positive or negative statements. Thus sometimes only four or six options are offered, with the uncertain category omitted. This type of scale is referred to as a *forced choice version* (Nunnally & Bernstein, 1994).

A Likert scale usually consists of 10 to 20 items, each addressing an element of the concept being measured. Usually, the values obtained from each item in the instrument are summed to obtain a single score for each subject. Although the values of each item are technically ordinal-level data, the summed score is often analyzed as interval-level data. The Center for Epidemiologic Studies Depression (CES-D) Scale is a Likert scale used to assess the level of depression in patients in clinical practice and in research. Whittenmore and colleagues (2009) used the CES-D Scale in their study that was previously described. This scale has four response options, which include: *Rarely or none of the time (less than 1 day)* = 0, *Some or a little of the time (1 to 2 days)* = 1, *Occasionally or a moderate amount of time (3 to 4 days)* = 2, and *Most or all of the time (5 to 7 days)* = 3. Subjects are instructed:

> Below is a list of the ways you might have felt or behaved. Please tell me how often you have felt this way during the past week (see Figure 10–4 for a copy of the CES-D Scale). The scores on the scale can range from 0 to 60 with the higher scores indicating more depressive symptoms. A score of 16 or higher has been used extensively as the cut-off point for high depressive symptoms. The CES-D Scale was developed by Radloff in 1977 and has been used extensively over the last 30 years. The scale has strong reliability, validity, sensitivity, and specificity, which were discussed previously. (Locke & Putnam, 2002; Sharp & Lipsky, 2002)

CRITICAL APPRAISAL GUIDELINES

Likert Scales

When critically appraising a Likert scale, ask the following questions:

1. Is the Likert scale clearly described?
2. Are the techniques that were used to administer and score the scale provided?
3. Is information about validity and reliability of the scale described from previous studies and from this study?

Center for Epidemiologic Studies Depression Scale
DEPA

THESE QUESTIONS ARE ABOUT HOW YOU HAVE BEEN FEELING LATELY.
AS I READ THE FOLLOWING STATEMENTS, PLEASE TELL ME HOW OFTEN YOU FELT OR
BEHAVED THIS WAY IN THE <u>LAST WEEK</u>. [*Hand card*]. FOR EACH STATEMENT, DID YOU FEEL
THIS WAY: [Interviewer: You may help respondent focus on the whichever "style" answer is easier]

0 = **R**arely or none of the time (or less than 1 day)?

1 = **S**ome or a little of the time (or 1-2 days)?

2 = **O**ccasionally or a moderate amount of time (or 3-4 days)?

3 = **M**ost or all of the time (or 5-7 days)?

		R	S	O	M	NR
1.	I WAS BOTHERED BY THINGS THAT USUALLY DON'T BOTHER ME.	0	1	2	3	--
2.	I DID NOT FEEL LIKE EATING; MY APPETITE WAS POOR.	0	1	2	3	--
3.	I FELT THAT I COULD NOT SHAKE OFF THE BLUES EVEN WITH HELP FROM MY FAMILY AND FRIENDS.	0	1	2	3	--
4.	I FELT THAT I WAS JUST AS GOOD AS OTHER PEOPLE.	0	1	2	3	--
5.	I HAD TROUBLE KEEPING MY MIND ON WHAT I WAS DOING.	0	1	2	3	--
6.	I FELT DEPRESSED.	0	1	2	3	--
7.	I FELT THAT EVERYTHING I DID WAS AN EFFORT.	0	1	2	3	--
8.	I FELT HOPEFUL ABOUT THE FUTURE.	0	1	2	3	--
9.	I THOUGHT MY LIFE HAD BEEN A FAILURE.	0	1	2	3	--
10.	I FELT FEARFUL.	0	1	2	3	--
11.	MY SLEEP WAS RESTLESS.	0	1	2	3	--
12.	I WAS HAPPY.	0	1	2	3	--
13.	I TALKED LESS THAN USUAL.	0	1	2	3	--
14.	I FELT LONELY.	0	1	2	3	--
15.	PEOPLE WERE UNFRIENDLY.	0	1	2	3	--
16.	I ENJOYED LIFE.	0	1	2	3	--
17.	I HAD CRYING SPELLS.	0	1	2	3	--
18.	I FELT SAD.	0	1	2	3	--
19.	I FELT PEOPLE DISLIKED ME.	0	1	2	3	--
20.	I COULD NOT GET GOING.	0	1	2	3	--

Figure 10–4. Center of Epidemiological Studies-Depression Scale (CES-D).

RESEARCH EXAMPLE Likert Scale

Fletcher and colleagues (2009) also used a Likert scale to measure depression in their study of caregivers of patients undergoing radiation therapy for prostate cancer that was previously introduced. The following is a description of the Likert scale administered in their study.

> Baseline level of depression was measured with the 20-item Center for Epidemiologic Studies-Depression scale (CES-D; Radloff, 1977) [Figure 10–4]. Scores of ≥ 16 indicate the need for individuals to seek clinical evaluation for major depression. The CES-D has well established concurrent and construct validity (Carpenter et al., 1998). The Cronbach's alpha for patients with cancer was .92 (Carpenter et al., 1998). In this study, Cronbach's alphas were .84 and .83 for the FCs [family caregivers] and patients, respectively. (Fletcher et al., 2009, p. 129)

CRITICAL APPRAISAL

Fletcher and colleagues (2009) used the CES-D Scale to measure depression in their study. This Likert scale, developed in 1977 by Radloff, has been used in many healthcare studies over the last 30 years with established reliability and validity. The scale is clearly described, with methods used to complete and score the scale provided. A Cronbach's alpha value of 0.92 was reported for a previous study with cancer patients and the Cronbach alphas for this study were strong supporting the reliability of this scale.

IMPLICATIONS FOR PRACTICE

Fletcher and colleagues (2009) study findings and implications for practice were discussed previously in this chapter.

Visual Analog Scales

The **visual analog scale** (VAS) is typically used to measure strength, magnitude, or intensity of individuals' subjective feelings, sensations, or attitudes about symptoms or situations. The VAS is a line that is usually 100 mm long, with right angle "stops" at either end. You can present the line horizontally or vertically. You place bipolar anchors beyond either end of the line. These end anchors must include the entire range of sensations possible for the phenomenon being measured (e.g., all and none, best and worst, no pain and most severe pain) (Waltz et al., 2005). An example of a visual analog scale for measuring pain is in Figure 10–5.

No pain |————————————————————————————————| Pain as bad as it can possibly be

Figure 10–5. Example of a visual analog scale.

You then ask the subject to place a mark through the line to indicate the intensity of the sensation or feeling. Then, use a ruler to measure the distance between the left end of the line (on a horizontal scale) and the subject's mark. This measure is the value of the sensation. The VAS has been used to measure pain, mood, anxiety, alertness, craving for cigarettes, quality of sleep, attitudes toward environmental conditions, functional abilities, and severity of clinical symptoms (Wewers & Lowe, 1990).

The reliability of the VAS is most frequently determined by test-retest method. The correlations between the two administrations for the scale need to be moderate or strong to support the reliability of the scale (Wewers & Lowe, 1990). Because these scales are used to measure phenomena that are dynamic or erratic over time, test-retest reliability is sometimes not appropriate and the low correlation is then caused by the change in sensation versus a problem with the scale. Since the VAS contains a single item, other methods of determining reliability such as homogeneity cannot be used. The validity of the VAS is most commonly determined by correlating the VAS scores with other measures, such as rating or Likert scales, that measure the same phenomenon such as pain (Waltz et al., 2005).

CRITICAL APPRAISAL GUIDELINES

Visual Analog Scales

When critically appraising a visual analog scale, consider the following questions:

1. Is the visual analog scale included in the study report?
2. Are the techniques needed to administer and score the scale provided?
3. Is information about reliability or validity of the scale described from previous studies and/ or from this study?

Process of Data Collection

Data collection is the process of acquiring the subjects and collecting the data for the study. The actual steps of collecting the data are specific to each study and depend on the research design and measurement techniques. During the data collection period, the researcher focuses on obtaining subjects, training data collectors, collecting data in a consistent way, maintaining research controls, protecting the integrity (or validity) of the study, and solving problems that threaten to disrupt the study.

Good research reporting dictates that the researchers described the data collection process in the published study. The strategies used to approach potential subjects who meet the sampling criteria should be clear. Researchers should also specify the number and characteristics of subjects who decline to participate in the study. The approaches used to perform measurements and the time and setting for the measurements are also described. The result is a step-by-step description of exactly how, where, and in what sequence the researchers collected the data.

Many studies use data collection forms to gather data. These forms may be used to record data from the patient record or to ask the subject for such information as demographic data.

The form itself is not a measurement tool. In many cases, each item on these forms is a separate measurement. Thus, the researcher needs to report the source of information and describe the method and level of measurement of each item on the form. Figure 10–6 shows an example of a data collection form.

Data Collection Tasks

During either quantitative or qualitative research, the investigator performs five tasks during the data collection process, and these are detailed in the research report. These tasks are interrelated and run concurrently, rather than in sequence. These tasks are:

- Selecting subjects
- Collecting data in a consistent way
- Maintaining research controls as indicated in the study design
- Protecting the integrity (or validity) of the study
- Solving problems that threaten to disrupt the study

Recruiting Subjects

Subjects may be recruited only at the initiation of data collection or throughout the data collection period. The design of the study determines the method of selecting subjects. Recruiting the number of subjects originally planned is critical because data analysis and interpretation of findings depend on having an adequate sample size. The research report needs to describe the subject recruitment process.

Maintaining Consistency

The key to accurate data collection in any study is consistency. Consistency involves maintaining the data collection pattern for each collection event as it was developed in the research plan. A good plan will facilitate consistency and maintain the validity of the study. Researchers should note deviations, even if they are minor, and evaluate them for their impact on the interpretation of the findings. If a study uses data collectors, they should be trained to note deviations during the data collection process. The research report needs to reflect the data collection plan and any deviations from that plan and their effect on the study findings.

Maintaining Controls

Researchers should build research controls into the plan, to minimize the influence of intervening forces on study findings. Maintenance of these controls is essential. Many controls are not natural in a field setting, and maintaining them is not easy. In some cases the controls slip without the researcher realizing it. In addition to maintaining the controls identified in the plan, the researcher needs to continually look for previously unidentified, extraneous variables that might have an impact on the data being collected. This type of variable often is specific to a study and tends to become apparent during the data collection period. Researchers should consider the extraneous variables identified during data collection, during data analysis, and interpretation. They should also note these variables in the research report, so that future researchers can be aware of and attempt to control them.

DATA COLLECTION FORM

Subject identification number _____   Date _____

A. Age _____   B. Gender: ❏ Male   ❏ Female

C. Weight _____ pounds D. Height _____ inches

E. Surgical diagnosis _____

F. Surgery date _____   Time _____

G. Narcotics order after surgery _____
    _____

H. Narcotic administration:
    Date   Time   Type of narcotic   Dose
    1.
    2.
    3.
    4.
    5.

I. Patient instructed on Pain Scale: Date _____ Time _____
    Comments:

J. Type of treatment: ❏ TENS   ❏ Placebo-TENS   ❏ No treatment control

K. Treatment implemented: Date _____ Time _____
    Comments:

L. Dressing change: Date _____ Time _____
    Hours since surgery _____

M. Score on Visual Analogue Pain Scale _____
    Date _____   Time _____

Data collector's name _____
    Comments:

Figure 10–6. Hypothetical data collection form for Hargreaves and Lander's (1989) study, *Use of Transcutaneous Nerve Stimulation Electric for Postoperative Pain*.

Protecting Study Integrity

Maintaining consistency and controls during subject selection and data collection protects the integrity or validity of the study. In addition, the integrity of the study must be considered in a broad context. To accomplish this, the researcher needs to view the process of data collection as a whole, instead of examining single elements of data collection. Researchers need to describe how they protected the integrity of their study during data collection and any problems encountered.

CRITICAL APPRAISAL GUIDELINES

Data Collection

When critically appraising the data collection process, consider the following questions:

1. Is the recruitment and selection of study participants or subjects clearly described and appropriate?
2. Were the data collected in a consistent way?
3. Were the study controls maintain as indicated by the design? Did the design include an intervention that was consistently implemented?
4. Was the integrity of the study protected and any problems resolved?

RESEARCH EXAMPLE Data Collection

Whittenmore and colleagues (2009) developed a study to determine the effectiveness of a Diabetes Prevention Program (DPP) delivered by nurse practitioners (NPs) in primary care settings to adults who were at risk for type 2 diabetes (T2D). This study was introduced earlier and the measurement methods were described. The data collection process for this study is presented in the following excerpt.

Procedure

The NPs recruited a convenience sample of 58 adults at risk of T2D from their practices (31 treatment and 27 control group participants). The sample size for this pilot study was determined by a power analysis, recruiting 20% of what would be necessary for a clinical trial testing the intervention. ...

Intervention

Enhanced Standard Care

After informed consent was obtained and baseline data were collected, all participants (regardless of group assignment) received culturally relevant written information about diabetes prevention, a 20- to 30-minute individual session with their NP on the importance of a healthy lifestyle for the prevention of T2D, and a 45-minute individual session with a nutritionist hired for the study. ...

Lifestyle Change Program

The lifestyle change program for this pilot study was based on the protocol for the DPP (Diabetes Prevention Research Group, 1999). The goals for this program were identical to enhanced standard care, yet the approach was more intensive and based on behavioral science evidence which recognizes the difficulty inherent in diet and exercise lifestyle change. …

Outcome Measures

Data were collected at the individual (participant) and organization (NP and site) levels at scheduled time points throughout the study to evaluate the reach, implementation, and preliminary efficacy of the lifestyle program. All data were collected by trained research assistants blinded to group assignment, with exception of the GTT [Glucose Tolerance Test]. … and lipids, which were collected by experienced laboratory personnel at each site and sent to one laboratory for analysis.

Reach

Recruitment rates were documented for each NP practice. Demographic and clinical data (e.g., age, gender, socioeconomic status, ethnicity, and health history) were collected using a standard form.

Implementation

Participant measures of implementation consisted of attendance, attrition, and a satisfaction survey. The satisfaction survey was a 7-item summated scale modified from the Diabetes Treatment Satisfaction Survey (Bradley, 1994) to evaluate a DPP. … Adequate internal consistency has been reported with the original scale ($\alpha = .82$) and was demonstrated with the modified scale in this study ($\alpha = .86$).

Organizational measures of implementation consisted of NP and nutrition session documentation forms which were created with components of each session itemized. The percentage of protocol implementation was calculated by dividing the number of protocol items by the number of items completed per session. The NPs were also interviewed at 3 and 6 months to address issues of implementation. …

Data Analysis

Data were entered into databases (Microsoft Access or Excel) via an automated Teleform (Cardiff, Vista, CA) system. Mean substitution was employed for missing data of individual items on instruments (up to 15%). If more than 15% of the items were missing (rare), the subscale or scale was coded as missing data. (Whittenmore et al., 2009, pp. 4-6)

CRITICAL APPRAISAL

As can be seen in the report, Whittenmore and colleagues (2009) took very careful steps to maintain the rigor and control of their data collection by implementing a detailed plan. The recruit process, recruitment rates, selection of study participants, and informed consent process were clearly described and appropriate. The sample size was adequate for a pilot study based on a power analysis. The researchers clearly described and implemented the Lifestyle Change Program intervention to the experimental group and the standard care to both groups. The design included pre- and posttests that were scheduled and the outcome measures were collected by trained research assistants using a structured protocol. The percentage of protocol implemented was also calculated, ensuring the quality for the data collection process. The reliability of the scales used was strong but the researchers might have expanded on the description of the scales validity. The physiological measures were precise and accurate. The researchers indicated how the data were entered into the computer to promote accuracy and the actions that were taken for consistent management of missing data. In summary, Whittenmore et al. (2009) provided a detailed description of their data col-

Continued

CRITICAL APPRAISAL—cont'd

lection process that was extremely strong. Their highly structured data collection plan and process of implementation decreased the potential for error and increased the likelihood that the study findings were an accurate reflection of reality.

IMPLICATIONS FOR PRACTICE

The implications of this study's findings for practice were discussed earlier in this chapter at the end of the Concepts of Measurement Theory Section.

Solving Problems

Problems can be perceived either as a source of frustration or a challenge to researchers. The fact that the problem occurred is not as important as the success of problem resolution. Therefore, the final and perhaps most important task of the data collection period may be problem resolution. There is little in the scientific literature about the problems encountered by nurse researchers. The research reports often read as though everything went smoothly. Research journals generally do not provide sufficient space to allow description of the problems encountered, and the absence of such information may give a false impression to reviewers of research. You can obtain a more realistic picture through personal discussions with researchers about the data collection process.

Serendipity

Serendipity is the accidental discovery of something useful or valuable. During the data collection phase of studies, researchers often become aware of elements or relationships that they had not previously identified. In some published studies, therefore, the researcher has gathered data, made observations, or recorded events that were not originally planned. These newfound aspects may or may not be closely related to the planned study. Because the researcher is focused on close observation, other elements in the situation can come into clearer focus and take on new meaning. Serendipitous findings are important for the development of new insights in nursing, and they can lead to new areas of research that generate knowledge.

KEY CONCEPTS

- The purpose of measurement is to produce trustworthy evidence that can be used in examining the outcomes of research.
- The rules of measurement ensure that the assignment of values or categories is performed consistently from one subject (or event) to another and, eventually, if the measurement strategy is found to be meaningful, from one study to another.
- The levels of measurement from low to high are nominal, ordinal, interval, and ratio.

- Reliability in measurement is concerned with the consistency of the measurement technique and reliability testing focuses on equivalence, stability, and homogeneity.
- The validity of an instrument is a determination of the extent to which the instrument reflects the abstract concept being examined. Construct validity includes content-related validity and evidence of validity from examining contrasting groups, convergence, and divergence.
- Physiological measures are examined for precision, accuracy, and error in research reports.
- Diagnostic and screening tests are examined for sensitivity, specificity, and likelihood ratios.
- Common measurement approaches used in nursing research include physiological measures, observation, interviews, focus groups, questionnaires, and scales.
- The researcher performs five tasks during the process of data collection that need to be critically appraised in a research report; these include: (1) recruiting participants or subjects, (2) collecting data in a consistent way, (3) maintaining research controls according to the study design, (4) protecting the integrity (or validity) of the study, and (5) solving problems that threaten to disrupt the study.
- It is important to critically appraise the measurement methods and data collection process of a published study for threats to validity.

REFERENCES

Als, H. (1999). Reading the premature infants. In E. Golden, (Ed.), *Nurturing the premature infants: Developmental interventions in neonatal intensive care nursery* (pp. 18-85). New York: Oxford University Press.

Als, H., Gilkerson, L., Duffy, F. H., Mcanulty, G. B., Buehler, D. M., & Vandenberg, K., et al. (2003). A three-center, randomized, controlled trial of individualized developmental care for very low birth weight preterm infants: Medical neurodevelopmental, parenting and caregiving effects. *Journal of Developmental & Behavioral Pediatrics, 24*(6), 399-408.

Becker, P. T., Grunwald, P. C., & Brazy, J. E. (1999). Motor organization in very low birth weight infants during caregiving: Effects of a developmental intervention. *Developmental & Behavioral Pediatrics, 20*(5), 344-354.

Bradley, C. (1994). Diabetes treatment satisfaction questionnaire. In C. Bradley (Ed.), *Handbook of psychology and diabetes* (pp. 111-132). Melbourne, Australia: Harwood Academic Publishers.

Brown, S. J. (2009). *Evidence-based nursing: The research-practice connection.* Sudbury, MA: Jones & Bartlett.

Burns, N., & Grove, S. K. (2009). *The practice of nursing research: Appraisal, synthesis, and generation of evidence* (6th ed.). Philadelphia: Saunders.

Carpenter, J. S., Andrykowski, M. A., Wilson, J., Hall, L. A., Rayens, M. K., Sachs, B., et al. (1998). Psychometrics for two short forms of the Center for Epidemiologic Studies-Depression Scale. *Issues in Mental Health Nursing, 19*(5), 481-494.

Craig, J., & Smyth, R. (2007). *The evidence-based practice manual for nurses* (2nd ed.). Edinburgh: Churchill Livingstone Elsevier.

Creswell, J. W. (2009). *Research design: Qualitative, quantitative and mixed methods approaches* (3rd ed.). Thousand Oaks, CA: Sage.

DeKeyser, F. G., & Pugh, L. C. (1991). Approaches to physiologic measurement. In C. F. Waltz, O. L. Strickland, & E. R. Lenz (Eds.), *Measurement in nursing research* (2nd ed., pp. 387-412). Philadelphia: F. A. Davis.

Diabetes Prevention Research Group. (1999). Design and methods for a clinical trial in the prevention of type 2 diabetes. *Diabetes Care, 22*(4), 623-634.

Estok, P. J., Sedlak, C. A., Doheny, M. O., & Hall, R. (2007). Structural model for osteoporosis preventing behavior in postmenopausal women. *Nursing Research, 56*(3), 149-158.

Fletcher, B. A., Schumacher, K. L., Dodd, M., Paul, S. M., Cooper, B. A., Lee, K., et al. (2009). Trajectories of fatigue in family caregivers of patients undergoing radiation therapy for prostate cancer. *Research in Nursing & Health, 32*(2), 125-139.

Gay, C. L., Lee, K. A., & Lee, S. Y. (2004). Sleep patterns and fatigue in new mothers and fathers. *Biological Research in Nursing, 5*(4), 311-318.

Gift, A. G, & Soeken, K. L. (1988). Assessment of physiologic instruments. *Heart & Lung, 17*(2), 128-133.

Grove, S. K. (2007). *Statistics for health care research: A practical workbook.* Philadelphia: Saunders.

Guyatt, G. H., Berman, L. B., Townsend, M., Pugsley, S. O., & Chambers, L. W. (1987). A measure of quality of life for clinical trials in chronic lung disease. *Thorax, 42*(11), 773-778.

Hargreaves, A., & Lander, J. (1989). Use of transcutaneous electrical nerve stimulation for postoperative pain. *Nursing Research, 38*(3), 159-161.

Harralson, T. L. (2007). Factors influencing delay in seeking treatment for acute ischemic symptoms among lower income, urban women. *Heart & Lung, 36*(2), 96-104.

Jefferson, V. W., Melkus, G. D., & Spollett, G. R. (2000). Health promotion practices of young Black women at risk for diabetes. *Diabetes Educator, 26*(2), 295-302.

Kagan, I., Ovadia, K. L., & Kaneti, T. (2009). Perceived knowledge of blood-borne pathogens and avoidance of contact with infected patients. *Journal of Nursing Scholarship, 41*(1), 13-19.

Kapella, M. C., Larson, J. L., Patel, M. K., Covey, M. K., & Berry, J. K. (2006). Subjective fatigue, influencing variables, and consequences in chronic obstructive pulmonary disease. *Nursing Research, 55*(1), 10-17.

Kaplan, A. (1963). *The conduct of inquiry: Methodology for behavioral science.* New York: Harper & Row.

Kerlinger, F. N., & Lee, H. B. (2000). *Foundations of behavioral research* (4th ed.). Fort Worth, TX: Harcourt.

Klein, S., Allison, D. B., Heymsfield, S. B., Kelley, D. E., Leibel, R. L., Nonas, C., et al. (2007). Waist circumference and cardiometabolic risk: A consensus statement from Shaping America's Health: Association for Weight Management and Obesity Prevention; NAASO, The Obesity Society; the American Society for Nutrition and the American Diabetes Association. *Obesity, 15*(5), 1061-1067.

Lee, K. A., Hicks, G., & Nino-Murcia, G. (1991). Validity and reliability of a scale to assess fatigue. *Psychiatry Research, 36*(3), 291-298.

Lee, K. A., Portillo, C. J., & Miramontes, H. (1999). The fatigue experience for women with human immunodeficiency virus. *Journal of Obstetrics, Gynecology, and Neonatal Nursing, 28*(2), 193-200.

Liaw, J., Yang, L., Chang, L., Chou, H., & Chao, S. (2009). Improving neonatal caregiving through a developmentally supportive care training program. *Applied Nursing Research, 22*(2), 86-93.

Locke, B. Z., & Putnam, P. (2002). *Center for Epidemiologic Studies Depression Scale (CES-D Scale).* Bethesda, MD: National Institute of Mental Health, *www.nimh.nih.gov.*

Marshall, C., & Rossman, G. B. (2006). *Designing qualitative research* (4th ed.). Thousand Oaks, CA: Sage.

Melnyk, B. M., & Fineout-Overholt, E. (2005). *Evidence-based practice in nursing & healthcare: A guide to best practice.* Philadelphia: Lippincott.

Munhall, P. L. (2007). *Nursing research: A qualitative perspective* (4th ed.). Sudbury, MA: Jones & Bartlett.

National Osteoporosis Foundation (2003). *Stand up to osteoporosis. [Brochure].* Washington, DC: Author.

Nunnally, J. C., & Bernstein, I. H. (1994). *Psychometric theory* (3rd ed.). New York: McGraw-Hill.

Paratz, J., & Lipman, J. (2006). Manual hyperinflation caused norepinephrine release. *Heart & Lung, 35*(4), 262-268.

Peters, K. (1998). Bathing premature infants: Physiological and behavioral consequences. *American Journal of Critical Care, 7*(2), 90-100.

Porter, S. C., Fleisher, G. R., Kohane, I. S., & Mandl, K. D. (2003). The value of parental report for diagnosis and management of dehydration in the emergency department. *Annals of Emergency Medicine, 41*(2), 196-205.

Posner, S. F., Stewart, A. L., Marin, G., & Perez-Stable, E. J. (2001). Factor variability of the Center for Epidemiological Studies Depression Scale (CES-D) among urban Latinos. *Ethnicity & Health, 6*(2), 137-144.

Pugh, L. C., & DeKeyser, F. G. (1995). Use of physiologic variables in nursing research. *Image—Journal of Nursing Scholarship, 27*(4), 273-276.

Radloff, L. S. (1977). The CES-D scale: A self report depression scale for research in the general population. *Applied Psychological Measures, 1,* 385-394.

Rew, L., Stuppy, D., & Becker, H. (1988). Construct validity in instrument development: A vital link between nursing practice, research, and theory. *Advances in Nursing Science, 10*(4), 10-22.

Sackett, D. L., Straus, S. E., Richardson, W. S., Rosenberg, W., & Haynes, R. B. (2000). *Evidence-based medicine: How to practice and teach EBM* (2nd ed.). London: Churchill Livingstone.

Sharp, L. K., & Lipsky, M. S. (2002). Screening for depression across the lifespan: A review of measures for use in primacy care settings. *American Family Physician, 66*(6), 1001-1008.

Stevens, S. S. (1946). On the theory of scales of measurement. *Science, 103*(2684), 677-680.

Wahner, H. W., & Fogelman, I. (1994). The evaluation of osteoporosis: Dual energy X-ray absorptiometry in clinical practice. In H. W. Wahner & I. Fogleman (Eds.), *Mayo clinic proceedings* (pp. 178-195). London: Mayo Clinic.

Walker, S. N., Sechrist, K. R., & Pender, N. J. (1987). The Health-Promoting Lifestyle Profile: Development and psychometric characteristics. *Nursing Research, 36*(2), 76-81.

Waltz, C. F., Strickland, O. L., & Lenz, E. R. (2005). *Measurement in nursing and health research* (3rd ed.). New York: Springer.

Wewers, M. E., & Lowe, N. K. (1990). A critical review of visual analogue scales in the measurement of clinical phenomena. *Research in Nursing & Health, 13*(4), 227-236.

Whittenmore, R., Melkus, G., Wagner, J., Dziura, J., Northrup, V., & Grey, M. (2009). Translating the diabetes prevention program to primary care: A pilot study. *Nursing Research, 58*(1), 2-12.

Williams, J. E., Singh, S. J., Sewell, L., Guyatt, G. H., & Morgan, M. D. (2001). Development of a self-report Chronic Respiratory Questionnaire (CRQ-SR). *Thorax, 56*(12), 954-959.

World Health Organization Study Group. (1994). *Assessment of fracture risk and its application to screening for postmenopausal osteoporosis.* Geneva: World Health Organization.

11

Understanding Statistics in Research

Chapter Overview

Understanding the Data Analysis Process 372
  Preparing the Data for Analysis 372
  Describing the Sample 373
  Testing the Reliability of Measurement Methods 374
  Conducting Exploratory Analyses 374
  Conducting Confirmatory Analyses 375
  Conducting Posthoc Analyses 375
Reasoning Behind Statistics 376
  Probability Theory 376
  Decision Theory, Hypothesis Testing, and Level of Significance 377
  Inference and Generalization 378
  Normal Curve 379
  Tailedness 380
  Type I and Type II Errors 381
  Power: Controlling the Risk of a Type II Error 382
  Degrees of Freedom 383
Using Statistics to Describe 383
  Frequency Distributions 384
  Measures of Central Tendency 385
  Measures of Dispersion 387

  Understanding Descriptive Statistical Results 389
Judging Statistical Suitability 392
Using Statistics to Examine Relationships 394
  Pearson Product-Moment Correlation 394
  Factor Analysis 397
Using Statistics to Predict 398
  Regression Analysis 398
Using Statistics to Examine Causality 401
  Chi-Square Test of Independence 401
  t-Tests 404
  Analysis of Variance (ANOVA) 406
  Analysis of Covariance (ANCOVA) 408
Interpreting Statistical Outcomes 408
  Types of Results 409
  Findings 410
  Exploring the Significance of Findings 410
  Clinical Importance 410
  Conclusions 412
  Generalizing the Findings 413
  Implications for Nursing 413
  Recommendations for Further Studies 415

Learning Outcomes

After completing this chapter, you should be able to:

1. Identify the purposes of statistical analyses.
2. Describe the process of data analysis: (a) preparing the data for analysis; (b) describing the sample; (c) testing the reliability of the measurement methods; (d) conducting exploratory analysis of the data; (e) conducting confirmatory analyses guided by objectives, questions, or hypotheses; and (f) conducting posthoc analyses.
3. Differentiate probability theory from decision theory.
4. Describe the process of inferring from a sample to a population.
5. Discuss the distribution of the normal curve.
6. Compare and contrast Type I and Type II errors.

7. Identify descriptive analyses, such as frequency distributions, percentages, measures of central tendency, and measures of dispersion, conducted to describe the samples and study variables in research.

8. Describe the results obtained from the following inferential analyses: chi-square analysis, *t*-test, analysis of variance, Pearson correlation, and linear and multiple regression analyses.

9. Describe the five types of results obtained from quasi-experimental and experimental studies that are interpreted within a decision theory framework: (a) significant and predicted results, (b) nonsignificant results, (c) significant and unpredicted results, (d) mixed results, and (e) unexpected results.

10. Compare and contrast statistical significance from clinical importance of results.

11. Critically appraise statistical results, findings, conclusions, generalization of findings, nursing implications, and suggestions for further study in a study.

Key Terms

Analysis of covariance, p. 408

Analysis of variance, p. 406

Between-group variance, p. 406

Bimodal distribution, p. 385

Bivariate correlation, p. 394

Chi-square test of independence, p. 401

Clinical importance, p. 410

Coefficient of multiple determination, p. 399

Conclusions, p. 412

Confirmatory analysis, p. 375

Decision theory, p. 377

Degrees of freedom, p. 383

Dependent groups, p. 392

Descriptive statistics, p. 383

Effect size, p. 382

Empirical generalizations, p. 413

Explained variance, p. 395

Exploratory analysis, p. 374

Factor, p. 397

Factor analysis, p. 397

Findings, p. 410

Frequency distribution, p. 384

Generalization, p. 378

Grouped frequency distributions, p. 384

Implications for nursing, p. 413

Independent groups, p. 392

Inference, p. 378

Level of statistical significance, p. 377

Line of best fit, p. 398

Mean, p. 387

Measures of central tendency, p. 385

Measures of dispersion, p. 387

Median, p. 385

Mixed results, p. 409

Mode, p. 385

Multiple regression, p. 398

Negative relationship, p. 395

Nonsignificant results, p. 409

Normal curve, p. 379

One-tailed test of significance, p. 380

Outliers, p. 374

Pearson product-moment correlation, p. 394

Percentage distribution, p. 385

Positive relationship, p. 395

Posthoc analyses, p. 375

Power, p. 382

Power analysis, p. 382

Probability theory, p. 376

Range, p. 387

Recommendations for further study, p. 415

Regression analysis, p. 398

Scatterplot, p. 389

Significant and unpredicted results, p. 409

Significant results, p. 409

Standard deviation, p. 388

Standardized scores, p. 388

Symmetrical, p. 395

Total variance, p. 406

t-test, p. 404

Two-tailed test of significance, p. 380

Type I error, p. 381

Type II error, p. 381

Unexpected results, p. 410

Unexplained variance, p. 395

Ungrouped frequency distribution, p. 384

Variance, p. 387

Within-group variance, p. 406

X axis, p. 389

Y axis, p. 389

Z-score, p. 388

STUDY TOOLS

Be sure to visit http://evolve.elsevier.com/Burns/understanding for additional examples and self-tests. Also, a review of this chapter's concepts and practice exercises can be found in Chapter 11 of the Study Guide for *Understanding Nursing Research: Building an Evidence-Based Practice*, 5th edition.

The expectation that the practice of nursing be evidence-based has made it more important for clinical nurses to acquire skills in reading and evaluating the results of statistical analyses (Brown, 2009; Craig & Smyth, 2007). Nurses probably have more anxiety about data analysis and statistical results than they do about any other aspect of the research process. We hope that this chapter will dispel some of that anxiety and facilitate your critical appraisal of the results sections of studies. The statistical information in this chapter is provided from the perspective of reading, understanding, and critically appraising published quantitative studies, rather than from that of selecting statistical procedures or performing statistical analyses. To critically appraise a quantitative study, you need to be able to (1) identify the statistical procedures used; (2) judge whether these procedures were appropriate for the hypotheses, questions, or objectives of the study, and for the level of measurement of the variables; (3) comprehend the discussion of data analysis results in the study; (4) judge whether the researchers' interpretations of the results are appropriate; and (5) evaluate the clinical importance of the study's findings.

This chapter begins with a discussion of some of the more pragmatic or common aspects of quantitative data analysis procedures: the purposes of statistical analysis and the process of performing data analysis. The reasoning behind statistics is explained, and some of the more common statistical procedures used to describe variables, examine relationships, and predict and test causal hypotheses are introduced. Strategies are identified for judging the statistical suitability of study results and guidelines are provided for critically appraising the results of published studies. The chapter concludes with a discussion of the following study outcomes: findings, conclusions, generalizations, implications for nursing practice, and suggestions for further study.

Understanding the Data Analysis Process

Statistical procedures are used to examine the numerical data gathered in a study. In critically appraising a study, it may be helpful to understand the process the researcher uses to perform data analyses. The quantitative data analysis process consists of several stages: (1) preparing the data for analysis; (2) describing the sample; (3) testing the reliability of measurement methods; (4) conducting exploratory analysis of the data; (5) conducting confirmatory analysis guided by the hypotheses, questions, or objectives; and (6) conducting posthoc analysis. Although not all of these stages are equally reflected in the final published report of the study, they all contribute to the insights that can be gained from analysis of the data.

Preparing the Data for Analysis

Except in very small studies, researchers almost always use computers for data analyses. The first step of the process is entering the data into the computer. The researcher uses a systematic plan for data entry designed to reduce errors during the entry phase. After entry, the data are cleaned. This process is time intensive and tedious but essential for ensuring accuracy of the data. If the data file is small enough, every datum on the printout is cross-checked with the original datum for accuracy. Otherwise, data points are randomly checked for accuracy. All identified errors are corrected. Missing data points are identified. If the information can be obtained, the missing data are entered into the data file. If enough data are missing for certain variables, the researcher may have to determine whether the data are sufficient to perform analyses using those variables. In some cases, subjects must be excluded from an analysis because data considered essential to that analysis are missing. In examining the results of a published study, you might note that the number of subjects included in the final analyses is less than the original sample and this could be due to attrition and/or subjects with missing data being excluded from the analyses. Researchers collecting physiological data often are able to use a computer for data collection or are able to directly enter data into a computer rather than using data collection sheets, which reduce the potential for data entry errors.

Describing the Sample

Next, the researcher obtains as complete a picture of the sample as possible. First, frequencies of descriptive variables related to the sample are obtained. Estimates of central tendency (such as the mean) and dispersion (such as the standard deviation) of variables relevant to the sample are calculated. Variables relevant to the sample are called demographic variables and might include age, gender, ethnicity, education level, and health status (see Chapter 5). When a study includes more than one group (e.g., treatment group and comparison group), researchers often compare the groups in relation to the demographic variables. For example, it might be important to know whether the age distribution of the various groups was similar. This is a study strength indicating the groups are similar at the start of the study if the demographic results are similar for the groups. If the groups being compared are not equivalent in ways important to the study, the groups cannot justifiably be compared through statistical procedures. Thus the researcher must decide whether to continue the analysis process.

CRITICAL APPRAISAL GUIDELINES

Describing the Sample

When critically appraising a study, you need to examine the sample characteristics and judge the representativeness of the sample using the following questions.

1. What variables were used to describe the sample?
2. What statistical procedures were used to describe the sample?
3. Was the sample representative of the study target population?
4. If the sample is divided into groups for data analyses, was the equivalence of the groups discussed?

Testing the Reliability of Measurement Methods

After describing the sample, the researcher examines the reliability of the measurement methods used in the study. Reliability of observational or physiological measures may have been determined during the data collection phase, but will be noted again at this point. If paper-and-pencil scales were used to collect data, the Cronbach statistical procedure will be performed on the scale items to determine the alpha coefficient value (Waltz, Strickland, & Lenz, 2005). If the Cronbach alpha coefficient is unacceptably low (below 0.70), the researcher must decide whether to analyze the data collected with the instrument. A value of 0.70 is considered marginally acceptable. A Cronbach alpha coefficient value of 0.80 to 0.89 indicates that the measurement is sufficiently reliable to use in a study (see Chapter 10). The *t*-test or Pearson's Correlation statistics may be used to determine test-retest reliability (Burns & Grove, 2009).

CRITICAL APPRAISAL GUIDELINES

Testing the Reliability of Measurement Methods

When critically appraising a study, you can use the following questions to determine the reliability of the measurement methods.

1. What information was provided on the reliability of measurement methods used to gather data for the analyses?
2. What statistical procedures were used to determine the reliability of measurement methods?

Conducting Exploratory Analyses

The next step, exploratory analysis, is used to examine all of the data descriptively. This step is discussed in more detail later in the section Using Statistics to Describe. The researcher must become as familiar as possible with the nature of the data obtained on variables that will be used to answer the research questions or objectives or to test the study hypotheses. Data on each variable are examined using measures of central tendency and dispersion to determine the nature of variation in the data and identify outliers. Outliers are subjects or data points with extreme values (values that lie far from other plotted points on a graph) that seem unlike the rest of the sample. The most valuable insights from a study often come from careful examination of outliers (Tukey, 1977). In many studies, relationships among variables and differences between groups are explored using statistical procedures that also are used in confirmatory studies. However, when these procedures are used for exploratory purposes, the results are not generalized to a larger population. The results are used to give a better understanding of the data.

CRITICAL APPRAISAL GUIDELINES

Exploratory Analyses

In critically appraising a study, examine the values obtained for the study variables and ask yourself the following questions.

1. Do they appear to be representative of values you would expect to find in the population under study?
2. Is the full range of values for each variable represented in the data?
3. Did the researchers identify outliers in the sample?
4. Is it likely that data from outliers affected the results of the analyses?

Conducting Confirmatory Analyses

Researchers use **confirmatory analysis** to confirm expectations regarding data that are expressed as hypotheses, questions, or objectives. When performing confirmatory analyses, investigators generalize findings from the sample to appropriate accessible and target populations. Statistical procedures designed for the purpose of making inferences (inferential statistical procedures) are used. To justify generalization of the results of confirmatory analyses, a rigorous research methodology is needed, including a strong research design, reliable and valid measurement methods, and a large sample size.

CRITICAL APPRAISAL GUIDELINES

Confirmatory Analyses

When critically appraising a study, identify the confirmatory analyses performed.

1. What confirmatory analyses were used in the study?
2. Is the research methodology sufficiently rigorous (strong design, reliable and valid measurement methods, and adequate sample) to warrant using confirmatory analyses (Creswell, 2009)?

Conducting Posthoc Analyses

Some statistical analyses, such as chi-square analysis and analysis of variance (ANOVA), are used to test for differences among groups in studies including more than two groups. These statistical procedures indicate significant differences among groups but do not specify which groups are different. For example, a study may examine the proportion of the sample in four occupational groups of workers who are smokers to determine differences in smoking behavior among the groups. Chi-square analysis or ANOVA may show significant differences among the groups, but the researcher will not be able to determine which groups were different. In such studies, when significant differences are found, **posthoc analyses** are performed after the initial statistical analysis to identify which groups are significantly different.

CRITICAL APPRAISAL GUIDELINES

Posthoc Analyses

When critically appraising a study, address the following questions about posthoc analyses.

1. What specific posthoc analyses were done?
2. Which groups were statistically different?
3. Which groups were not statistically different?

Reasoning Behind Statistics

One reason that nurses tend to avoid statistics is that many were taught only the mathematical procedures of calculating statistical equations, with little or no explanation of the logic behind those procedures or the meaning of the results. Computation is a mechanical process usually performed by a computer, and information about the calculation procedure is not necessary to begin understanding statistical results. Here we present an approach to data analysis that will enhance your understanding of the statistical analysis process. You can then use this understanding to critically appraise data analysis techniques in the Results section of research reports.

This section presents a brief explanation of some concepts that commonly are used in statistical theory. The concepts include probability theory, decision theory, hypothesis testing, level of significance, inference, generalization, the normal curve, tailedness, Type I and Type II errors, power, and degrees of freedom. More extensive discussion of these topics can be found in other sources; we recommend our own recent textbooks (Burns & Grove, 2009; Grove, 2007).

Probability Theory

Probability theory, which is deductive, is used to explain the extent of a relationship, the probability that an event will occur in a given situation, or the probability that an event can be accurately predicted. The researcher might want to know the probability that a particular outcome will result from a nursing intervention. For example, the researcher may want to know how likely it is that urinary catheterization during hospitalization will lead to a urinary tract infection (UTI) after discharge from the hospital. The researcher also may want to know the probability that subjects in the experimental group are members of the same larger population from which the comparison group subjects were taken. Probability is expressed as a lowercase letter p, with values expressed as percentages or as a decimal value ranging from 0 to 1. For example, if the probability is 0.23, then it is expressed as $p = 0.23$. This means that there is a 23% probability that a particular outcome (such as a UTI) will occur. Probability values also can be stated as less than a specific value, such as 0.05, expressed as $p < 0.05$. (The symbol < means less than.) A study may find that the probability that the experimental group subjects were members of the same larger population as the comparison group subjects was less than or equal to 5% ($p = 0.05$). In other words, it is NOT very likely that the comparison group and the experimental group are from the same population. Put another way, you might say that there is a 5% chance that the two groups are from the same population and a 95% chance that they are not from the same population. Probability values often are stated with the results of statistical analyses. In critically appraising studies, it is useful to recognize these symbols and understand what they mean.

Decision Theory, Hypothesis Testing, and Level of Significance

Decision theory is inductive and assumes that all of the groups in a study (e.g., experimental and comparison groups) used to test a particular hypothesis are components of the same population relative to the variables under study. This expectation (or assumption) traditionally is expressed as a null hypothesis, which states that there is no difference between (or among) the groups in a study, in terms of the variables included in the hypothesis. It is up to the researcher to provide evidence for a genuine difference between the groups. For example, the researcher may hypothesize that the frequency of UTIs that occurred after discharge from the hospital in patients who were catheterized during hospitalization is no different from the frequency of such infections in those who were not catheterized. To test the assumption of no difference, a cutoff point is selected before data collection. The cutoff point, referred to as alpha (α), or the **level of statistical significance**, is the probability level at which the results of statistical analysis are judged to indicate a statistically significant difference between the groups. The level of significance selected for most nursing studies is 0.05. This means that if the level of significance found in the statistical analysis is 0.05 or less, the experimental and comparison groups are considered to be significantly different (members of different populations). In some studies, the more rigorous level of significance of 0.01 may be chosen. This may be written as $\alpha = 0.01$, particularly in tables and figures.

Decision theory requires that the cutoff point selected for a study be absolute. *Absolute* means that even if the value obtained is only a fraction above the cutoff point, the samples are considered to be from the same population, and *no* meaning can be attributed to the differences. Thus, it is inappropriate when using decision theory to state that the findings approached significance at the 0.051 level if the alpha level was set at 0.05. Using decision theory rules, this finding indicates that the groups tested are not significantly different, and the null hypothesis is accepted. On the other hand, once the level of significance has been set at 0.05 by the researcher, if the analysis reveals a significant difference of 0.001, this result is not considered more significant than the 0.05 originally proposed (Slakter, Wu, & Suzaki-Slakter, 1991). The level of significance is dichotomous, which means that the difference is either significant or not significant; there are no "degrees" of significance. However, some people, not realizing that their reasoning has shifted from decision theory to probability theory, indicate in their research report that the 0.001 result makes the findings more significant than if they had obtained only a 0.05 level of significance. The researcher may even state that the findings are highly significant, which is unacceptable from the perspective of decision theory.

From the perspective of probability theory, there is considerable difference in the risk of occurrence of a Type I error (saying something is significant when it is not) when the probability is between 0.05 and 0.001. If $p = 0.001$, the probability that the two groups are components of the same population is 1 in 1000; if $p = 0.05$, the probability that the groups belong to the same population is 5 in 100. In other words, if $p = 0.05$, then in 5 times out of 100, groups with statistical values such as those found in these statistical analyses actually are members of the same population, and the conclusion that the groups are different is erroneous.

In computer analysis, the probability value obtained from each data analysis (e.g., $p = 0.03$ or $p = 0.07$) frequently is provided on the printout and often is reported by the researcher in the published study, along with the level of significance set before data analysis was done. In summary, the probability *(p)* value reveals the risk of a Type I error. The alpha (α) value reveals whether the probability value for a particular analysis met the cutoff point for deciding whether there is a significant difference between or among groups.

CRITICAL APPRAISAL GUIDELINES

Level of Significance

When critically appraising a study level of significance, you need to ask the following questions.

1. What level of significance or α was set prior to the conduct of the study?
2. Did the findings show statistically significant differences?
3. If significant differences were found, what was the p value?
4. What was the risk of a Type I error in the study?

Inference and Generalization

An inference is a conclusion or judgment based on evidence. Statistical inferences are made cautiously and with great care. The decision theory rules used to interpret the results of statistical procedures increase the probability that inferences are accurate. A generalization is the application of information that has been acquired from a specific instance to a general situation. Generalizing requires making an inference; both require the use of inductive reasoning. An inference is made from a specific case and extended to a general truth, from a part to the whole, from the concrete to the abstract, and from the known to the unknown. In research, an inference is made from the study findings obtained from a specific sample and applied to a more general population, using the results from statistical analyses. Thus, a researcher may conclude in a research report that a significant difference was found in the number of UTIs between two samples, one in which the subjects had been catheterized during hospitalization and another in which the subjects had not. The researcher also may conclude that this difference can be expected in all patients who have been cared for in hospitals. The findings are generalized from the sample in the study to all previously hospitalized patients. Statisticians and researchers can never prove something using inference; they can never be certain that their inferences and generalizations are correct. For example, the researcher generalization of the incidence of UTIs may not have been carefully thought out; the findings may have been generalized over too broad a population. It is possible that in the more general population, there is no difference in the incidence of UTIs based on whether the patient was catheterized or not.

CRITICAL APPRAISAL GUIDELINES

Inference and Generalization

When critically appraising a study, you need to judge whether generalizations made by the researcher are justified based on the study results.

Normal Curve

The theoretical normal curve is an expression of statistical theory (Figure 11–1). A normal curve is a theoretical frequency distribution of all possible values in a population; however, no real distribution exactly fits the normal curve. The idea of the normal curve was developed by an 18-year-old mathematician, Johann Gauss, in 1795. He found that data from variables (e.g., the mean of each sample) measured repeatedly in many samples from the same population can be combined into one large sample. From this large sample, a more accurate representation can be developed of the pattern of the curve in that population than is possible with only one sample. Surprisingly, in most cases the curve is similar, regardless of the specific variables examined or the population studied.

Levels of significance and probability are based on the logic of the normal curve. The normal curve presented in Figure 11–1 shows the distribution of values for a single population. Note that 95.5% of the values are within 2 standard deviations of the mean, ranging from −2 to +2 standard deviations. (Standard deviations are defined and discussed later in the chapter under Using Statistics to Describe.) Thus, there is approximately a 95% probability that a given measured value (e.g., the mean of a group) would fall within approximately

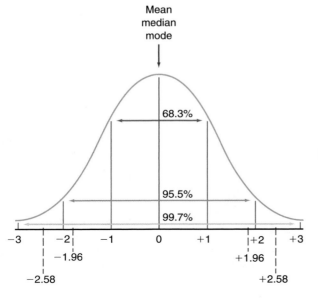

Figure 11–1. The Normal Curve.

2 standard deviations of the mean of the population, and there is a 5% probability that the value would fall in the tails of the normal curve (the extreme ends of the normal curve, below −2 (−1.96 exactly) standard deviations [2.5%] or above +2 (+1.96 exactly) standard deviations [2.5%]). If the groups being compared are from the same population (not significantly different), you would expect the value (e.g., the mean) of each group to fall within the 95% range of values on the normal curve. If the groups are from (significantly) different populations, you would expect one of the group values to be outside the 95% range of values. A statistical analysis performed to determine differences between or among groups, using a level of significance (α) set at 0.05, would test that expectation. If the statistical test demonstrates a significant difference (the value of one group does not fall within the 95% range of values), the groups are considered to belong to different populations. However, in 5% of the statistical tests, the value of one of the groups can be expected to fall outside the 95% range of values but still belong to the same population (a Type I error).

Tailedness

Nondirectional hypotheses usually assume that an extreme score (obtained because the group with the extreme score did not belong to the same population) can occur in either tail of the normal curve (Figure 11–2). The analysis of a nondirectional hypothesis is called a **two-tailed test of significance**. In a **one-tailed test of significance**, the hypothesis is directional, and extreme statistical values that occur in a single tail of the curve are of interest (see Chapter 5 for discussion of directional and nondirectional hypotheses). The hypothesis states that the extreme score is higher or lower than that for 95% of the population, indicating that the sample with the extreme score is not a member of the same population. In this case, 5% of statistical values that are considered significant will be in one tail, rather than two. Extreme statistical values occurring in the other tail of the curve are not considered significantly different. In Figure 11–3, which shows a one-tailed figure, the portion of the curve in which statistical values will be considered significant is the right tail. Developing a one-tailed hypothesis requires that the researcher have sufficient knowledge of the variables to predict

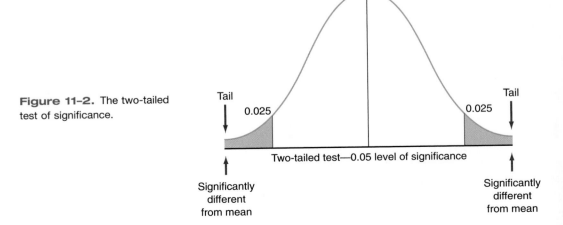

Figure 11–2. The two-tailed test of significance.

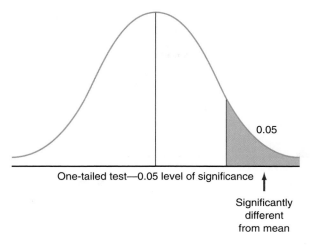

Figure 11–3. The one-tailed test of significance.

0.05

One-tailed test—0.05 level of significance

Significantly
different
from mean

whether the difference will be in the tail above the mean or in the tail below the mean. One-tailed statistical tests are uniformly more powerful than two-tailed tests, decreasing the possibility of a Type II error (saying something is not significant when it is).

CRITICAL APPRAISAL GUIDELINES

Tailedness

When critically appraising a study, you need to examine the study hypotheses and the statistical tests for tailedness.

1. Were one-tailed or two-tailed hypotheses stated in the study? One-tailed hypothesis is a directional research hypothesis that indicates the direction of the study outcome. Two-tailed hypothesis can be either a nondirectional research hypothesis or a null hypothesis.
2. If the researcher states a one-tailed hypothesis, was there sufficient knowledge on which to base a one-tailed statistical test?

Type I and Type II Errors

According to decision theory, two types of error can occur when a researcher is deciding what the result of a statistical test means: Type I and Type II. A **Type I error** occurs when the null hypothesis is rejected when it is true (e.g., when the results indicate that there is a significant difference, when, in reality, there is not). The risk of a Type I error is indicated by the level of significance. There is a greater risk of a Type I error with a 0.05 level of significance (5 chances for error in 100) than with a 0.01 level of significance (1 chance for error in 100). As the level of significance becomes more extreme, the risk of a Type I error decreases, as illustrated in Figure 11–4.

A **Type II error** occurs when the null hypothesis is regarded as true but is in fact false. For example, statistical analyses may indicate no significant differences between groups, but

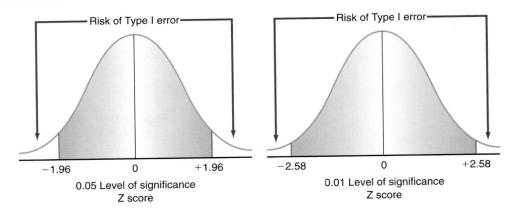

Figure 11–4. Risk of Type I error.

in reality the groups are different. There is a greater risk of a Type II error when the level of significance is 0.01 than when it is 0.05. However, Type II errors often are caused by flaws in the research methods. In nursing research, many studies are conducted with small samples and with instruments that do not precisely measure the variables under study. In many nursing situations, multiple variables interact to cause differences within populations. When only a few of the interacting variables are examined, small differences may be overlooked, which can lead to the false conclusion that there are no differences between the samples. Thus, the risk of a Type II error is high in many nursing studies.

CRITICAL APPRAISAL GUIDELINES

Type I and Type II Errors

When critically appraising a study, evaluate the risk of a Type I or Type II error.

1. What element(s) of the study could have resulted in the risk of a Type I error?
2. What element(s) of the study could have resulted in the risk of a Type II error?

Power: Controlling the Risk of a Type II Error

Power is the probability that a statistical test will detect a significant difference that exists. The risk of a Type II error can be determined using **power analysis**. Cohen (1988) has identified four parameters of a power analysis: the level of significance, sample size, power, and effect size. If three of the four are known, the fourth can be calculated using power analysis formulas. The minimum acceptable power level is 0.80. The researcher determines the sample size and the level of significance (see Chapter 9 for a detailed discussion of power analysis). **Effect size** is "the degree to which the phenomenon is present in the population, or the degree to which the null hypothesis is false" (Cohen, 1988, pp. 9-10). For example, if changes in anxiety level are measured in a group of patients before surgery, with the first measurement taken when the patients are still at home, and the second taken just before surgery, effect size will be large if a great change in anxiety occurs in the group between the two time periods. If the effect of a preoperative teaching program on the level of anxiety is measured, the effect size will be the difference in the posttest level of anxiety in the experimental group compared with that in the comparison group. If only a small change in the level of anxiety is expected, the effect size will be small. In most nursing studies, only small effect sizes can be expected. In such a study, a sample of 200 or more is needed to detect a significant difference. This small effect size occurs because nursing studies tend to use samples that are small, study designs in which threats to the validity of the design are not tightly controlled, and measurement methods that measure only large changes. The power level is required to be reported in studies that fail to reject the null hypothesis (or have nonsignificant findings). If the power level is below 0.80, you need to question the validity of nonsignificant findings.

CRITICAL APPRAISAL GUIDELINES

Power Level

When critically appraising a study's power, you need to address the following questions.

1. Were the effect size and the power level identified in the study?
2. Was a power analysis conducted to determine sample size? Was the sample size adequate for the study conducted?
3. Was the design validity strong (Burns & Grove, 2009; Creswell, 2009)? (See Chapter 8 for a discussion of design validity.)
4. Were the measurement methods in the study valid and reliable (Waltz et al., 2005)? (See Chapter 10 for a discussion of instrument reliability and validity.)

Degrees of Freedom

The concept of **degrees of freedom** *(df)* is important for calculating statistical procedures and interpreting the results using statistical tables. However, this concept is difficult to explain because of the complex mathematics involved. Degrees of freedom involve the freedom of a score value to vary given the other existing scores' values and the established sum of these scores. Degrees of freedom often are reported with statistical results.

Using Statistics to Describe

In any study in which the data are numerical, data analysis begins with **descriptive statistics** (also called *summary statistics*). For some descriptive studies, researchers limit data analyses to descriptive statistics. For other studies, researchers use descriptive statistics primarily to describe the characteristics of the sample from which the data were collected and to describe values obtained from the measurement of dependent or research variables. Descriptive statistics presented in this book include frequency distributions, measures of central tendency, measures of dispersion, and standardized scores.

Frequency Distributions

Frequency distribution usually is the first method used to organize the data for examination. There are two types of frequency distributions: ungrouped and grouped.

Ungrouped Frequency Distributions

Most studies have some categorical data that are presented in the form of an **ungrouped frequency distribution**, in which a table is developed to display all numerical values obtained for a particular variable. This approach generally is used on discrete rather than continuous data. Examples of data commonly organized in this manner are gender, ethnicity, marital status, diagnostic category of study subjects, and values obtained from the measurement of selected research and dependent variables. Table 11–1 is an example table developed for this textbook and it includes 9 different scores obtained by 50 subjects. This is an example of ungrouped frequencies since each score is represented in the table with the number of subjects receiving this score.

Grouped Frequency Distributions

Grouped frequency distributions are used when continuous variables are being examined. Many measures taken during data collection, including body temperature, vital lung capacity, weight, age, scale scores, and time, are measured using a continuous scale. Any method of grouping results in loss of information. For example, if age is grouped, a breakdown into two groups, under 65 years of age and over 65 years of age, provides less information about the data than groupings of 10-year age spans. As with levels of measurement, rules have been established to guide classification systems. There should be at least five but not more than 20 groups. The classes established must be exhaustive; each datum must fit into one of the identified classes. The classes must be exclusive; each datum must fit into only one. A common mistake occurs when the ranges contain overlaps that would allow a datum to fit into more than one class. For example, a researcher may classify age ranges as 20 to 30, 30 to 40, 40 to 50, and so on. By this definition, subjects aged 30, 40, and so on can be classified into more than one class. The range of each class must be equivalent. For example, if 10 years is the age range, each age class must include 10 years of ages. This rule is violated in some cases to allow the first and last categories to be open-ended and worded to include all scores above or below a specified point. Table 11–2 is an example of a grouped frequency distribution for income.

Table 11–1	Example of a Cumulative Frequency Table			
Score	Frequency	Percent	Cumulative Frequency *(f)*	Cumulative Percent
1	4	8	4	8
3	6	12	10	20
4	8	16	18	36
5	14	28	32	64
7	8	16	40	80
8	6	12	46	92
9	4	8	$n = 50$	100

Table 11-2	Income of Full-Time Registered Nurses ($n = 100$)	
Income	Frequency (%)
Below $40,000	5 (5%)
$40,000-49,999	20 (20%)
$50,000-59,999	35 (35%)
$60,000-70,000	25 (25%)
Above $70,000	15 (15%)

Percentage Distributions

A percentage distribution indicates the percentage of subjects in a sample whose scores fall into a specific group and the number of scores in that group. Percentage distributions are particularly useful for comparing the present data with findings from other studies that have different sample sizes. A cumulative distribution is a type of percentage distribution in which the percentages and frequencies of scores are summed, as one moves from the top of the table to the bottom. Thus, the bottom category would have a cumulative frequency equivalent to the sample size and a cumulative percentage of 100 (see Table 11–1). Frequency distributions also are displayed using tables or graphs (e.g., pie charts, bar charts, histograms, frequency polygons). Graphic displays of the frequency distribution of data from Table 11–1 are presented in Figure 11–5. You might note that in the bar and line graphs that the data distribution forms a normal curve.

Measures of Central Tendency

Measures of central tendency frequently are referred to as the midpoint in the data or as an average of the data. The measures of central tendency are the most concise statement of the nature of the data in a study. The three measures of central tendency that are commonly used in statistical analyses are the mode, median, and mean. For a data set that has a normal distribution, these values are equal (see Figure 11–1); however, they usually are different for data obtained from real samples.

Mode

The mode is the numerical value or score that occurs with greatest frequency; it does not necessarily indicate the center of the data set. The mode can be determined by examination of an ungrouped frequency distribution of the data. In Table 11–1, the mode is the score of 5, which occurred 14 times in the data set. The mode can be used to describe the typical subject or identify the most frequently occurring value on a scale item. The mode is the appropriate measure of central tendency for nominal data. A data set can have more than one mode. If two modes exist, the data set is referred to as bimodal distribution, as illustrated in Figure 11–6. A data set with more than two modes is said to be multimodal.

Median

The median is the midpoint or the score at the exact center of the ungrouped frequency distribution—the 50th percentile. The median is obtained by rank ordering the scores. If the

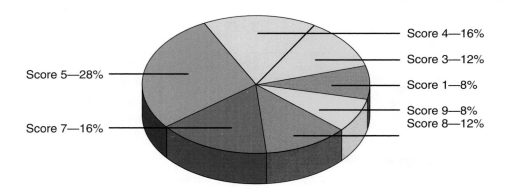

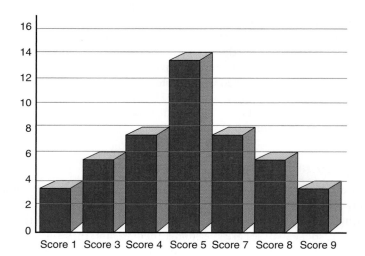

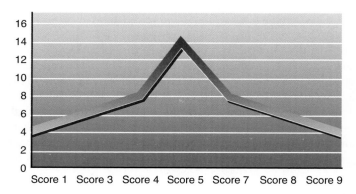

Figure 11–5. Commonly used graphic displays of frequencies distribution.

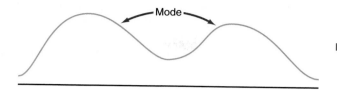

Figure 11–6. Bimodal distribution.

number of scores is uneven, exactly 50% of the scores are above the median and 50% are below it. If the number of scores is even, the median is the average of the two middle scores; thus, the median may not be one of the scores in the data set. Unlike the mean, the median is not affected by extreme scores in the data (outliers). The median is the most appropriate measure of central tendency for ordinal data. The median for the data in Table 11–1 is 5.

Mean

The most commonly used measure of central tendency is the mean. The **mean** is the sum of the scores divided by the number of scores being summed. Thus, like the median, the mean may not be a member of the data set. The mean is the appropriate measure of central tendency for interval and ratio-level data. The mean for the data in Table 11–1 is 5.28.

Measures of Dispersion

Measures of dispersion, or variability, are measures of individual differences of the members of the sample. They give some indication of how scores in a sample are dispersed or spread around the mean. These measures provide information about the data that is not available from measures of central tendency. The measures of dispersion indicate how different the scores are or the extent that individual scores deviate from one another. If the individual scores are similar, measures of variability are small, and the sample is relatively homogeneous, or similar, in terms of those scores. A heterogeneous sample has a wide variation in scores. The measures of dispersion most commonly used are range, variance, and standard deviation. Standardized scores may be used to express measures of dispersion. Scatterplots frequently are used to illustrate the dispersion in the data.

Range

The simplest measure of dispersion is the range, which is obtained by subtracting the lowest score from the highest score. The **range** for the scores in Table 11–1 is calculated as follows: $9 - 1 = 8$. The range is a difference score, which uses only the two extreme scores for the comparison. It is a very crude measure of dispersion but is sensitive to outliers. The range might also be expressed as the lowest to the highest scores. Using the data in Table 11–1, the range might also be expressed as the scores from 1 to 9.

Variance

The **variance** for scores in a study is calculated with a mathematical equation and indicates the spread or dispersion of the scores. The variance can only be calculated on data at the interval or ratio level of measurement. The numerical value obtained from the calculation depends on the measurement scale used, such as the laboratory measurement of fasting blood glucose values or the scale measurement of weights. The calculated variance value has no absolute value and can be compared only with data obtained using similar measures. Generally, however, the larger the variance value, the greater the dispersion of scores. The variance for the data in Table 11–1 is 4.94.

Standard Deviation

The **standard deviation** is the square root of the variance. Just as the mean is the average value, the standard deviation is the average difference (deviation) value. The standard deviation provides a measure of the average deviation of a value from the mean in that particular sample. It indicates the degree of error that would result if the mean alone were used to interpret the data. In the normal curve, 68% of the values will be within 1 standard deviation above or below the mean, 95% will be within 1.96 standard deviations above or below the mean, and 99% will be within 2.58 standard deviations above or below the mean (see Figure 11–1) (Grove, 2007).

The standard deviation for the data in Table 11–1 is 2.22. The mean is 5.28, so the value of a subject 1 standard deviation below the mean would be 5.28 − 2.22, or 3.06. The value of a subject 1 standard deviation above the mean would be 5.28 + 2.22, or 7.50. So approximately 68% of the sample (and perhaps the population from which it was derived) can be expected to have values in the range of 3.06 to 7.50, which is expressed as (3.06, 7.50). Extending this calculation further, the value of a subject 2 standard deviations above the mean would be 5.28 + 2.22 + 2.22 = 9.72 and the value of a subjects 2 standard deviations below the mean would be 5.28 − 2.22 − 2.22 = 0.84. Using this strategy, the entire distribution of values can be estimated (Grove, 2007). The value of a single individual can be compared with the value calculated for the total sample (e.g., mean, median, or mode). Standard deviation is an important measure, both for understanding dispersion within a distribution and interpreting the relationship of a particular value to the distribution.

Standardized Scores

Because of differences in the characteristics of various distributions, comparing a value in one distribution with a value in another is difficult. For example, perhaps you want to compare test scores from two classroom examinations. The highest possible score in one test is 100 and in the other, 70; the scores will be difficult to compare. To facilitate this comparison, a mechanism was developed to transform raw scores into **standardized scores**. Numbers that make sense only within the framework of measurements used within a specific study are transformed into numbers (standardized scores) that have a more general meaning. Transformation into standardized scores allows an easy conceptual grasp of the meaning of the score. A common standardized score is called a **Z-score**. It expresses deviations from the mean (difference scores) in terms of standard deviation units (see Figure 11–1). A score that falls above the mean will have a positive Z-score, whereas a score that falls below the mean will have a negative Z-score. The mean expressed as a Z-score is zero. The standard deviation is equal to the Z-score. Thus, a Z-score of 2 indicates that the score from which it was obtained is 2 standard deviations above the mean. A Z-score of −0.5 indicates that the score is 0.5 standard deviation below the mean.

Scatterplots

A scatterplot has two scales: horizontal and vertical. Each scale is referred to as an axis. The vertical scale is called the Y axis; the horizontal scale is the X axis. A scatterplot can be used to illustrate the dispersion of values on a variable. In this case, the X axis represents the possible values of the variable. The Y axis represents the number of times each value of the variable occurred in the sample. Scatterplots also can be used to illustrate the relationship between values on one variable and values on another. Then each axis will represent one variable. For example, if a graph is developed to illustrate the relationship between the number of days a patient has been hospitalized and the stage of the patient's decubitus ulcer, the horizontal axis represents days and the vertical axis, decubitus ulcer stage. For each unit or subject, there is a value for X and a value for Y. The point at which the values of X and Y for a single subject intersect is plotted on the graph (Figure 11–7). When the values for each subject in the sample have been plotted, the degree of relationship between the variables is revealed (Figure 11–8).

Understanding Descriptive Statistical Results

In a published study, investigators often report descriptive statistics in the text of the Results section, usually as part of the description of the sample. It also is important to report the values obtained on study variables, as well as the measures of central tendency and dispersion of each variable. In some studies, descriptive statistics may be summarized in a table. Additionally, descriptive statistics can be used to describe differences between either groups or variables. Examining differences between variables also reflects their relatedness. From a descriptive perspective of descriptive analyses, the purpose is not to test for causality, but rather to describe their differentness. Statistical procedures often used for this purpose include chi-square test and t-test.

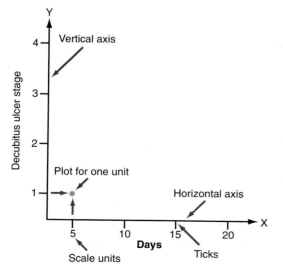

Figure 11–7. Structure of a plot.

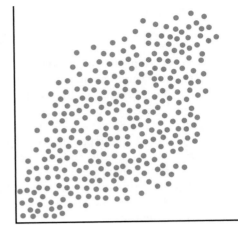

Figure 11–8. Example of a scatterplot.

RESEARCH EXAMPLE Description of the Sample

Mollaoglu and Beyazit (2009) studied the effects of a diabetic educational program on metabolic control of adults with type 2 diabetes mellitus (DM). The study included 50 subjects, with 25 patients randomly assigned to the experimental group and 25 to the control groups. The demographic variables used to describe the sample in this study included sex or gender, age, marital status, educational status, and diabetes duration. Descriptive statistics of mean, frequency, and percentage (%) were used to analyze the demographic data, and the results are presented in Table 11–3.

Table 11–3. Sociodemographic and clinical characteristics of the DM patients ($n = 50$)

Characteristics	Experimental group mean or frequency (%)	Control group mean or frequency (%)	Statistical tests t/χ^2
Sex *(n)*			
Female	16 (64.0)	13 (52.0)	χ^2: 0.73*
Male	9 (36.0)	12 (48.0)	
Age (year), mean	53.2	51.8	$t = 0.47$*
Marital status *(n)*			
Single	8 (32.0)	4 (16.0)	$\chi^2 = 2.08$*
Married	17 (68.0)	21 (84.0)	
Educational status			
No educational training	6 (24.0)	5 (20.0)	$\chi^2 = 0.11$*
Primary school	19 (76.0)	20 (80.0)	
Diabetes duration (years), M (SD)	11.14 (4.16)	12.11 (3.96)	$t = 0.83$*

*$p > 0.05$.

Adapted from Mollaoglu M., Beyazit E. (2009). Influence of diabetic education on patient metabolic control. *Applied Nursing Research, 22*(3), 186.

CRITICAL APPRAISAL

This critical appraisal is based on the questions presented earlier in this chapter for examining the description of a study sample. Mollaoglu and Beyazit (2009) developed a table that clearly presented their results from analyzing the demographic variables. The demographic variables of sex (gender), age, marital status, and educational status used to describe the sample are relevant and commonly described in most studies. The researchers also include the clinical variable of diabetes duration, which is appropriate for this study to know that the patients had Type 2 DM for many years (mean = 11.14 – 12.11 years).

The analysis techniques were appropriate for the level of measurement of the variables. Age and diabetes duration are both ratio level data and were described using means and the dispersion of diabetes duration values were described with a standard deviation. However, it would have been helpful to include the range for both variables to examine for outliers and the standard deviation for age to determine the dispersion of the subjects' ages. The other variables were either nominal (sex and marital status) or ordinal (educational status) level of measurement and were appropriately analyzed with frequencies and percentages.

The study did include two groups (experimental and control) and differences between these two groups were examined for each of the demographic and clinical variables. Differences between the experimental and control groups for age and diabetes duration, ratio level data, were appropriately analyzed with t-tests. Differences between the two groups for sex, marital status, and educational level were appropriately analyzed with chi-square tests. The groups were found to have no significant differences in demographic and clinical variables as indicated by $*p > 0.05$ at the bottom of Table 11–2. In this study, the researchers set the level of significance or $\alpha = 0.05$. Since the p values for the demographic and clinical variables were all > 0.05, this indicates no significant differences between the two groups for these variables. This is a study strength since the groups need to be as similar as possible at the start of the study so any significant differences noted at the end of the study are more likely to be due to the study intervention than to error.

IMPLICATIONS FOR PRACTICE

Mollaoglu and Beyazit (2009) implemented a structured diabetic educational program that included three sessions between the educator and the persons with diabetes. Eight weeks later the experimental group had significantly improved metabolic control as compared with the control group. Metabolic control was measured with the following dependent variables: fasting blood sugar (FBS), postprandial blood sugar (PPBS), hemoglobin A1c (HbA1c), urine glucose value, triglyceride, total cholesterol, high-density lipoprotein (HDL) cholesterol, and low-density lipoprotein (LDL) cholesterol. The researchers concluded "that the client-centered, self-care focused, home-based intervention [diabetic educational program] that is given by nurses to individuals with diabetes can help to achieve and maintain normal metabolic values" (Mollaoglu & Beyazit, 2009, p. 189). The researchers recognized the need for additional research but also encouraged nurses to use this type of educational program in caring for their patients with diabetes.

Judging Statistical Suitability

Multiple factors are involved in determining the suitability of a statistical procedure for a particular study. These include the study's (1) purpose; (2) hypotheses, questions, or objectives; (3) design; and (4) level of measurement of the variables. Determining the suitability of various statistical procedures for a particular study is not straightforward. Regrettably, there is not usually one "right" statistical procedure for a particular study.

Evaluating statistical procedures requires that you make a number of judgments about the nature of the data and what the researcher wanted to know. You need to determine (1) whether the data for analysis were treated as nominal, ordinal, or interval/ratio (see Chapter 10); (2) how many groups were in the study; and (3) whether the groups were dependent or independent. Interval/ratio levels of data are included together since the analysis techniques are the same whether the data are interval or ratio level of measurement. In **independent groups**, the selection of one subject is totally unrelated to the selection of other subjects. For example, if subjects are randomly assigned to treatment and comparison groups, the groups are independent. In **dependent groups**, subjects or observations selected for data collection are related in some way to the selection of other subjects or observations. For example, if subjects serve as their own control by using the pretest as a comparison or control group, the observations (and therefore the groups) are dependent. Also, if matched pairs of subjects are used for the comparison and treatment groups, the observations are dependent. For example, in a study of twins, one twin may be placed in the control group and the other in the treatment group. Because they are twins, they are matched on several variables.

One approach to judging the appropriateness of an analysis technique for a critical appraisal is to use an algorithm. The algorithm directs you by gradually narrowing the number of appropriate statistical procedures as you make judgments about the nature of the study and the data. An algorithm that has been helpful in judging the appropriateness of statistical procedures is presented in Figure 11–9. This algorithm identifies four factors related to the appropriateness of a statistical procedure: the research question, level of measurement of the variables, design, and type of sample. To use the algorithm in Figure 11–9, you would (1) determine whether the research question focuses on differences (I) or associations (relationships) (II), (2) determine the level of measurement (A—Nominal, B—Ordinal, or C—Interval or ratio), (3) select the design listed that most closely fits the study you are critically appraising (1, 2, or 3), and (4) determine whether the study samples are independent (a), dependent (b), or mixed (c). The lines on the algorithm are followed through each selection to identify the appropriate statistical procedure.

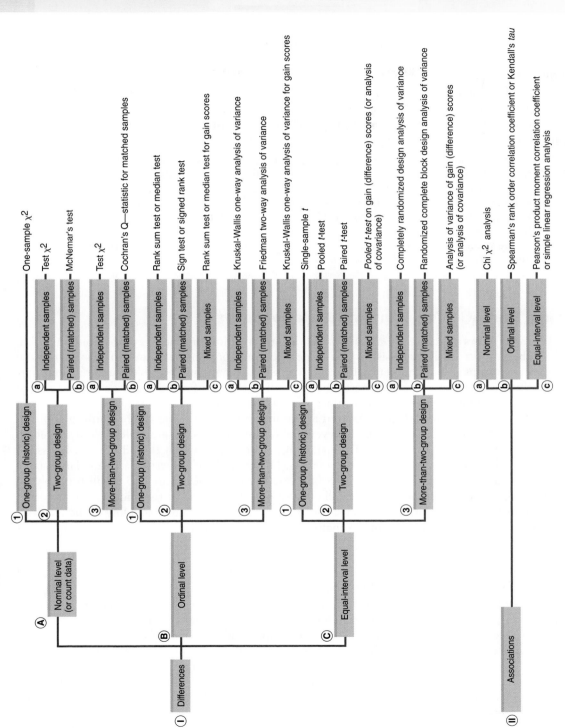

Figure 11-9. Algorithm for choosing a statistical test. From Knapp, R. B. [1985]. *Basic statistics for nurses.* Albany, NY: Delmar. Reproduced with permission.

CRITICAL APPRAISAL GUIDELINES

Statistical Suitability

When critically appraising suitability, you not only must be familiar with the statistical procedure used in the study, but also must be able to compare that procedure with others that could have been used, perhaps to greater advantage. The critical appraisals provided in the remaining part of this chapter are guided by the following questions:

1. Were the appropriate analysis techniques performed to address the study purpose or objectives, questions, or hypotheses? If so, was the focus of the analyses description, relationships, and/or differences?
2. Was the analysis technique appropriate for the level of measurement of the data (nominal, ordinal, interval, or ratio)? Use Figure 11–9 to help you determine if the appropriate analysis technique was used.
3. Were the results from the analyses clearly presented and appropriately interpreted?
4. Should additional analyses have been conducted?

Using Statistics to Examine Relationships

Investigators use correlational analyses to identify relationships between or among variables. The purpose of the analysis may be to describe relationships between variables, clarify the relationships among theoretical concepts, or assist in identifying possible causal relationships, which can then be tested by causal analyses. All of the data for the analysis need to be from a single population from which values were available on all variables to be examined in a correlational analysis. Data measured at the interval level provide the best information on the nature of the relationship. However, analysis procedures are available for most levels of measurement. Data for a correlational analysis also need to span the full range of possible values on each variable used in the analysis. For example, if values for a particular variable can range from a low of 1 to a high of 9, each of the values from 1 to 9 will probably be found in subjects in the data set. If all or most of the values are in the middle of that scoring range (4, 5, and 6) and few or none have extreme values, a full understanding of the relationship cannot be obtained from the analysis. Thus, large samples with diverse scores are desirable for correlational analyses.

Pearson Product-Moment Correlation

Pearson product-moment correlation is a parametric test used to determine relationships among variables. **Bivariate correlation** measures the extent of relationship between two variables. Data are collected from a single sample, and measures of the two variables to be examined must be available for each subject in the data set. Less commonly, data are obtained from two related subjects, such as breast cancer incidence in mothers and daughters. Correlational analysis provides two pieces of information about the data: the nature of a relationship (positive or negative) between the two variables and the magnitude (or strength) of the relationship. Scatterplots sometimes are presented to illustrate the relationship graphically (see Figure 11–8). The outcomes of correlational analyses are symmetrical, rather than asymmetrical. Symmetrical means that the analysis gives no indication of the direction of the relationship. It's not possible to establish from correlational analysis whether variable A leads to or causes variable B, or that B causes A.

Interpreting Results

The outcome of the Pearson product-moment correlation analysis is a correlation coefficient (*r*) with a value between −1 and +1. This *r* value indicates the degree of relationship between the two variables. A value of 0 indicates no relationship. A value of −1 indicates a perfect negative (inverse) correlation. In a negative relationship, a high score on one variable is correlated with a low score on the other variable. A value of +1 indicates a perfect positive relationship. In a positive relationship, a high score on one variable is correlated with a high score on the other variable. A positive correlation also exists when a low score on one variable is correlated with a low score on the other variable. The variables vary or change in the same direction, either increasing or decreasing together. As the negative or positive values of *r* approach 0, the strength of the relationship decreases (Grove, 2007). Traditionally, an *r* value of less than 0.3 or −0.3 is considered to indicate a weak relationship; a value between 0.3 and 0.5 or −0.3 and −0.5, a moderate relationship; and if the *r* value is above 0.5 or −0.5, it is considered to indicate a strong relationship (Burns & Grove, 2009). However, this interpretation of the *r* value depends to a great extent on the variables being examined and the situation in which they were measured. Therefore, interpretation requires some judgment on the part of the researcher.

When Pearson's correlation coefficient is squared (r^2), the resulting number is the percentage of variance explained by the relationship. Even when two variables are related, values of the two variables will not be a perfect match. For example, if two variables show a strong positive relationship, a high score on one variable can be expected to be associated with a high score on the other variable. However, a subject who has the highest score on one value will not necessarily have the highest score on the other variable. Thus, r^2 indicates the variance that is known by correlating two variables (Grove, 2007). There will be some variation in the relationship between values for the two variables for individual subjects. Some of the variation in values is explained by the relationship between the two variables and is called explained variance. The amount of explained variation is indicated by r^2 and is expressed as a percentage. For example, researchers may state that the relationship of the two variables anxiety and depression in their study is $r = 0.6$ and $r^2 = 0.36$ or 36%. Thus, the explained variance is 36% for the variables anxiety and depression in this study. However, part of the variation is the result of things other than the relationship and is called unexplained variance. In the example provided, 100% − 36% (explained variance) = 64% (unexplained variance). Thus, 64% of the variation in scores is a result of something other than the relationship studied—perhaps variables not examined in the study. A strong correlation has less unexplained variance than a weak correlation.

There has been a tendency to disregard weak correlations in nursing research. This approach can result in overlooking a relationship that may in fact have some meaning within nursing knowledge if the relationship is examined in the context of other variables. Three common reasons for this situation, which is similar to that of a Type II error, have been recognized. First, many nursing measurements are not powerful enough to detect fine discriminations. Some instruments may not detect extreme scores, and a relationship may be stronger than is indicated by the crude measures available. Second, correlational studies must have a wide range of scores for relationships to be detected. If the study scores are homogeneous or the sample is small, relationships that exist in the population may not show up as clearly in the sample. Third, in many cases, bivariate analysis does not provide a clear picture of the dynamics in the situation. A number of variables can be linked through weak correlations, but together they provide increased insight into situations of interest. Statistical procedures (such as regression analysis, discussed later) are available for examining the relationships among multiple variables simultaneously.

Testing the Significance of a Correlation Coefficient

Before inferring that the sample correlation coefficient applies to the population from which the sample was taken, statistical analysis must be performed to determine whether the coefficient is significantly different from zero (no correlation). With a small sample, a very high correlation coefficient can be nonsignificant. With a very large sample, the correlation coefficient can be statistically significant when the degree of association is too small to be clinically important. Therefore, in judging the significance of the coefficient, both the size of the coefficient and its statistical significance need to be considered.

RESEARCH EXAMPLE Correlation Results

Bingham and colleagues (2009) conducted a descriptive correlational study examining the relationships of obesity and cholesterol in a sample of 4013 fourth-grade children in three different countries. The purpose of this study was to describe, correlate, and compare

> two risk factors for future CVD [cardiovascular disease] in United States (U.S.), French, and Japanese children. Total serum cholesterol and two measures of overweight, including BMI [body mass index] and body fat percentage, were examined in children 9 to 10 years of age from Japan, France, and the U.S. (Whites and Blacks). (Bingham et al., 2009, p. 316)

The researchers correlated BMI with total cholesterol for males and females in the three countries and presented their results in Table 11–4.

Table 11–4. Correlation of BMI with total cholesterol

	France ($n = 570$)	Japan ($n = 1865$)	U.S. white ($n = 1226$)	U.S. black ($n = 324$)
Males				
Pearson r	0.02	0.17	0.24	0.29
p value	0.6960	0.0001	0.0001	0.0002
Females				
Pearson r	0.12	0.12	0.22	−0.14
p value	0.0494	0.0004	0.0001	0.0822

Note. Number of subjects varies slightly for each variable because of some missing data.

Bingham, M. O., Harrell, J. S., Takada, H., Washino, K., Bradley, C., Berry, D., et al. (2009). Obesity and cholesterol in Japanese, French, and U.S. children. *Journal of Pediatric Nursing, 24*(4), 318.

CRITICAL APPRAISAL

Bingham and colleagues (2009) conducted a Pearson Product Moment Correlation analysis to determine the relationships between BMI and total cholesterol for males and females from three different countries. This analysis technique was used to address the study purpose of determining the relationship between the BMI and total cholesterol. Since BMI and total cholesterol are both measured at the ratio level, this is the appropriate analysis technique for examining relationships between these two variables. The researchers clearly presented the results of the correlation of BMI with total cholesterol in table format. The table includes the group size (*n*) for each country and the *p* value for each correlation value (*r*). If the *p* values are less than $\alpha = 0.05$, then the correlations are significant. Table 11–4 includes six significant correlations and two nonsignificant correlations. The researchers noted that the numbers of subjects varied for each variable because of missing data. They might have expanded on the reasons for the missing data in the narrative of the article.

As part of the critical appraisal, you are also encouraged to interpret the results from this table. Six of the correlations or *r* values are significant, with $\alpha = 0.05$ indicating there is a statistically significant relationship between BMI and total cholesterol for the three countries. The strongest relationship was for U.S., Black males (*r* = 0.29) and the weakest relationship was for French males (*r* = 0.02) (Bingham et al., 2009). However, all the correlation values are small or <0.30 (Grove, 2007). Even the largest correlation at *r* = 0.29 only explains 8.4% of the variance between BMI and total cholesterol. This is calculated by $r^2 \times 100\% = 0.29^2 \times 100\% = 0.084 \times 100\% = 8.4\%$. The unexplained variance in this relationship is $100\% - 8.4\% = 91.6\%$. Thus, most of the correlation results in Table 11–4 are statistically significant but the clinical importance is still in question.

IMPLICATIONS FOR PRACTICE

Bingham et al. (2009, p. 320) identified the following conclusion:

> It appears that the relationship between obesity [BMI] and total cholesterol may vary by culture or ethnicity and by gender, indicating the need for more culture- and gender-specific studies in children to evaluate the relative importance of these common risk factors for developing CVD. A better understanding of the impact of culture and gender on obesity and cholesterol levels in children will help nurse clinicians as they assess children for risk factors for CVD and will provide information that may be used to develop culturally specific interventions to reduce these risk factors. It is important to monitor BMI and cholesterol in children 9-10 years old; however, additional research is needed to determine the impact of these two variables on the future development of CVD.

Factor Analysis

Factor analysis examines interrelationships among large numbers of variables and disentangles those relationships to identify clusters of variables that are most closely linked. Intellectually, you might do this by identifying categories and sorting the variables according to your judgment of the most appropriate category. Factor analysis sorts the variables into categories according to how closely related they are to the other variables. Closely related variables are grouped together into a **factor**. Several factors may be identified within a data set. Once the factors have been identified mathematically, the researcher must interpret the results by explaining why the analysis grouped the variables in a specific way. Statistical results will indicate the amount of variance in the data set that can be explained by a particular factor, and the amount of variance in the factor that can be explained by a particular variable.

Factor analysis aids in the identification of theoretical constructs; it also is used to confirm the accuracy of a theoretically developed construct. For example, a theorist may state that the concept (or construct) of "hope" consists of the following elements: (1) anticipation of the future, (2) belief that things will work out for the best, and (3) optimism. Ways can then be developed to measure these three elements, and a factor analysis can be conducted on the data to determine whether subject responses clustered into these three groupings.

Factor analysis frequently is used in the process of developing measurement instruments, particularly those related to psychological variables, such as attitudes, beliefs, values, and opinions (Burns & Grove, 2009). Thus, the measurement instrument operationalizes the theoretical construct, such as "hope." Factor analysis is used to expand the construct validity of an instrument, such as a Likert scale to measure hope. We wanted to provide you some idea of what factor analysis is when you see it in the measurement or result sections of a published study.

Using Statistics to Predict

The ability to predict future events is becoming increasingly important in today's world. People are interested in predicting who will win the football game, what the weather will be like next week, or what stocks are likely to rise in the near future. In nursing practice, as in the rest of society, the capacity to predict is crucial. For example, nurse researchers would like to be able to predict the length of a hospital stay for patients with illnesses of different severity, as well as the response of patients with a variety of characteristics to nursing interventions. Nurses also need to know what factors play an important role in a patient response to rehabilitation. Predictive analyses are based on probability theory, rather than decision theory. Prediction is one approach for examining causal relationships between or among variables.

Regression Analysis

Regression analysis is used to predict the value of one variable when the value of one or more other variables is known. The variable to be predicted in a regression analysis is referred to as the dependent variable. The dependent variable usually is measured at the interval or ratio level. The goal of the analysis is to explain as much of the variance in the dependent variable as possible. In regression analysis, variables used to predict values of the dependent variable are referred to as independent variables. If there is more than one independent variable, the analysis is referred to as **multiple regression**. In regression analysis, the symbol for the dependent variable is Y, and the symbol for the independent variable(s) is X. Scatterplots and a bivariate correlation matrix often are developed before regression analysis is performed, to examine the relationships that exist in the variables. The purpose of the regression analysis is to develop a **line of best fit** that will best reflect the values on the scatterplot. The line of best fit is often illustrated as an overlay on the scatterplot (Figure 11–10). Many types of regression analyses have been developed to analyze various types of data. One type, logistic

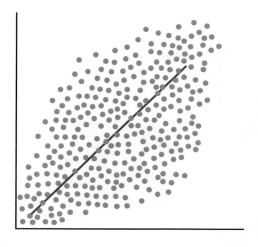

Figure 11-10. Overlay of scatterplot and best-fit line.

regression, was developed to predict values of a dependent variable measured at the ordinal level. Logistic regression is being used with increasing frequency in nursing studies (Burns & Grove, 2009).

Interpreting Results

The outcome of a regression analysis is the regression coefficient, R. When R is squared (R^2), it indicates the amount of variance in the data that is explained by the equation (Grove, 2007). When more than one independent variable is being used to predict values of the dependent variable, R^2 is sometimes referred to as the **coefficient of multiple determination**. The test statistic used to determine the significance of a regression coefficient may be t (from t-test) or F (from ANOVA). Small sample sizes decrease the possibility of obtaining statistical significance. Values for R^2 and t or F are reported with the results of a regression analysis. The calculated coefficient values may also be expressed as an equation. Many studies using regression analysis are complex, including multiple independent variables and involving more than one regression procedure. Understanding the discussion of complex results requires reading each sentence carefully for comprehension before proceeding to the next sentence.

RESEARCH EXAMPLE Regression Analysis

Cameron and colleagues (2009, p. 410) conducted their predictive correlational study for the purpose of "testing a model of patient characteristics, psychologic status, and cognitive function as predictors of self-care in persons with chronic heart failure [CHF]." The conceptual model that was tested by this study is presented in Figure 11–11. The researchers used multiple regression analysis to predict the dependent variable self-care management in CHF patients using the independent variables of age, male gender, significant comorbidity, cognitive function, depression, social situation: living with support, and self-care confidence. Cameron et al. presented their findings in Table 11–5 and included the following discussion of their table.

Continued

RESEARCH EXAMPLE—cont'd

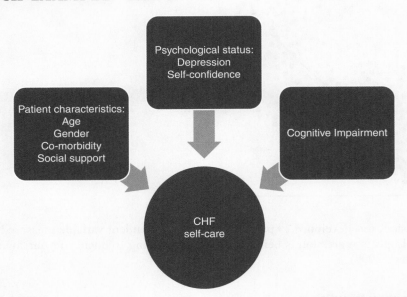

Figure 11–11. Conceptual model of factors that may influence CHF self-care. From Cameron, J., Worrall-Carter, L., Riegel, B., Lo, S. K., & Stewart, S. (2009). Testing a model of patient characteristics, psychologic status, and cognitive function as predictors of self-care in persons with chronic heart failure. *Heart & Lung, 38*(5), 411.

Table 11–5. Multiple regression analysis predicting self-care management ($n = 50$)

Predictor variables	Standardized coefficients beta	Partial R	F value	*P*	R^2
Age	0.02	0.02		0.91	
Male gender	−0.33	−0.36		0.02	
Significant comorbidity	0.33	0.33		0.03	
Cognitive function	0.25	0.25		0.09	
Depression	0.32	0.34	3.73	0.04	0.38
Social situation: living with support	−0.006	−0.007		0.97	
Self-care confidence	0.39	0.39		<0.01	

Cameron, J., Worrall-Carter, L., Riegel, B., Lo, S. K., & Stewart, S. (2009). Testing a model of patient characteristics, psychologic status, and cognitive function as predictors of self-care in persons with chronic heart failure. *Heart & Lung, 38*(5), 414.

When self-care management was regressed on the 7 independent variables, they explained 38% (*F* [7, 42] 3.73; $p = .003$) of the variance in self-care management scores [see Table 11–4]. Higher self-care confidence made the largest contribution to self-care management scores ($\beta = .39$, $p < .01$). For every point increase in self-care confidence, there was a .39 point increase in self-care management. Three other variables contributed significantly to the variance: male gender ($p < .05$), moderate-to-severe comorbidity ($p < .05$), and depressive symptoms ($p < .05$). (Cameron et al., 2009, p. 414)

CRITICAL APPRAISAL

Cameron and colleagues (2009) clearly stated their study purpose to test a model to predict self-care in patients with CHF. The model identifies the study concepts and links them to the study variables (see Figure 11–11). Multiple regression analysis is appropriate to predict a dependent variable (self-care management) using independent variables (age, male gender, significant comorbidity, cognitive function, depression, social situation, and self-care confidence). Multiple regression analysis is necessary because the study has more than one independent variable. The results of the multiple regression analysis are clearly presented in Table 11–5 and discussed in the article narrative. The study identified four independent variables, self-care confidence ($R = 0.39$), male gender ($R = -0.36$), significant comorbidity ($R = 0.33$), and depression ($R = 0.34$), to be significant predictors of the dependent variable self-care management. The results of the study are strong with these four predictor variables explaining 38% (R^2) of the variance in self-care management by CHF patients.

IMPLICATIONS FOR PRACTICE

Cameron et al. (2009, p. 416) identified the following implications for practice.

> The results of this small study add to the body of evidence that patients with heart failure overall have poor self-care maintenance and management behaviors despite the recent attention to improving this outcome. Our model of variables explained a significant amount of the variance in both self-care maintenance and management. ... Identifying patients who are least likely to engage in self-care may help in the selection of follow-up strategies required to prevent hospital readmissions and improve health outcomes. This would also allow for improved resource management, with specific groups of patients being invited to participate in CHF-MP (chronic heart failure-management program).

The researchers also provided directions for future research.

Using Statistics to Examine Causality

Causality is a way of knowing that one thing causes another. Because they can be used to understand the effects of interventions, statistical procedures that examine causality are critical to the development of nursing science. These statistics examine causality by testing for significant differences between or among groups.

Chi-Square Test of Independence

The **chi-square test of independence** determines whether two variables are independent or related; the test can be used with nominal or ordinal data. The procedure examines the frequencies of observed values and compares them with the frequencies that would be expected if the data categories were independent of each other. The procedure is not very powerful; thus, the risk of a Type II error is high (outcome of the study is nonsignificant when significant differences actually exist). Large sample sizes are needed to decrease the risk of a Type II error. Therefore, most studies using this procedure place little importance on results in which no differences are found. Researchers frequently perform multiple chi-square tests in a sample. However, results generally are presented only when a chi-square analysis shows a significant difference.

Interpreting Results

Often the first reaction to a sentence about "significant differences" by those unfamiliar with reading statistical results is panic. (The next reaction may be to skip to the next sentence—maybe that one will make more sense!) However, a sentence that looks "dense" with statistics provides a great deal of information in a small amount of space. For example, in the component "(χ^2 [1] = 18.10, p = 0.001)," the author is using chi-square (χ^2) analysis to compare two groups on a selected variable like the presence or absence of chronic illness. The author provides the degrees of freedom (df = 1), so that the reader can validate the accuracy of the results using a statistical chi-square table (see the textbook by Burns & Grove, 2009, p. 682, for a χ^2 Statistical Table). The numerical value after the first equal sign, 18.10, is the chi-square (χ^2) value obtained from calculating the chi-square equation (probably using a computer). This value has no inherent meaning other than to determine significance on a statistical table. As noted earlier, the symbol p is the abbreviation for probability. The groups were significantly different because p = 0.001, which is below the level of significance set at α = 0.05. The phrase also indicates that the probability is 0.1% (i.e., 0.001), or 1 in 1000, that these groups come from the same population. Thus, the two groups are significantly different since there is only 1 chance in 1000 the study results are an error.

If a study variable has only two categories, like presence or absence of chronic illness, the researchers know the location of the significant difference. However, the exact location of specific differences among more than two categories of variables cannot be determined from chi-square analysis alone. Chi-square analysis identifies if there is a significant difference and posthoc analyses can be used to identify the categories in which the differences lie. Posthoc analyses are statistical techniques performed in studies with more than two groups to determine which groups are significantly different. In some published studies, the researchers erroneously discuss the results as if they know where the differences are without having performed posthoc analyses. As a reader, you should view these reports with skepticism.

RESEARCH EXAMPLE Chi-Square Results

Lavoie-Tremblay and colleagues (2008) examined the influence of psychosocial work environment variables on the psychological health of new-generation nurses in Canada. The psychosocial work environment variables included effort-reward imbalance, lack of social support from colleagues and superiors, high psychological demand, low decision latitude, and elevated job strain. The nurse participants were divided into two dichotomous groups, those with high psychological distress and those with low psychological distress. The researchers conducted chi-square analysis to determine differences between the two groups of nurses for the psychosocial work environment variables and presented their findings in Table 11–6. Lavoie-Tremblay et al. noted that the two psychological distress risk groups were significantly different on three psychosocial work environment variables: (1) effort-reward balance (χ^2 [1] = 30.471, $p <$ 0.000) (2) high psychological demand (χ^2 [1] = 17.625, $p <$ 0.000), and (3) elevated job strain (χ^2 [1] = 8.96, $p <$ 0.003).

Table 11–6. Chi-square analysis of psychosocial work environment dimensions and psychological distress

Psychological distress Psychosocial work environment variables	High n	Low n	χ^2	df	p value
Effort-reward imbalance	101	79	30.471**	1	0.000
Lack of social support from colleagues and superiors	84	93	2.443	1	0.118
High psychological demand	87	71	17.625**	1	0.000
Low decision latitude	83	96	1.317	1	0.251
Elevated job strain	51	39	8.960*	1	0.003

Note. *$p \leq 0.05$; **$p \leq 0.01$.

Lavoie-Tremblay, M., Wright, D., Desforges, N., Gelinas, C., & Marchionni, C., Drevniok, U. (2008). Creating a healthy workplace for new-generation nurses. *Journal of Nursing Scholarship, 40*(3), 294.

CRITICAL APPRAISAL

Lavoie-Tremblay and colleagues (2008) clearly stated that the purpose of their study was to examine the dimensions of the psychosocial work environment that influence the psychological health of new-generation nurses. Chi-square analysis is appropriate to examine differences between the two groups of nurses that were dichotomized into high and low psychological distress. The chi-square results were clearly presented in Table 11–6 and discussed in the text of the article. Three of the psychosocial work environment variables were significantly linked to psychological distress. Since only two levels of psychological distress risk were examined, no posthoc analyses were required.

IMPLICATIONS FOR PRACTICE

Lavoie-Tremblay and colleagues (2008, p. 296) identified the following implications for practice and suggestions for further research.

As the current worldwide nursing labor shortage is expected to grow worse, retention strategies are needed that will be focused on the psychological health of new generation nurses by targeting the psychosocial work environment. Nursing managers need to revise or develop retention and workplace health-promotion strategies, tailored specifically to Nexters, to temper the effect of the nursing shortage. Research is needed on the meaning of reward at work for nursing from Generation Y. How is the effort/reward imbalance perceived? Can the way care is organized be changed to increase perceived rewards in the context of a shortage of healthcare providers and limited financial resources?

Nurse managers play a critical role in continuing to strive towards improving work environments so that new nurses do not forget the heart and soul of nursing and do remain committed to the ideals of caring that led them to the profession in the first place.

t-Tests

One of the most common analyses used to test for significant differences between two samples is the *t*-test. The *t*-test is used to examine group differences when the variables are measured at the interval or ratio level of measurement. A variety of *t*-tests have been developed for various types of samples. Frequently researchers misuse the *t*-test by using multiple *t*-tests to examine differences in various aspects of data collected in a study. This misapplication will result in an escalation of significance that increases the risk of a Type I error. The Bonferroni procedure, which controls for the escalation of significance, may be used when multiple *t*-tests must be performed on different aspects of the same data.

Interpreting Results

The result of the mathematical calculation is a *t* statistic. This statistic is compared with the *t* values in a statistical table (see Burns & Grove, 2009, p. 677). The table is used to identify the critical value of *t*. If the computed statistic is greater than or equal to the critical value, the groups are significantly different.

RESEARCH EXAMPLE *t*-Test

Mollaoglu and Beyazit (2009) conducted *t*-tests to determine differences between the experiment and control groups in their study. This study was introduced earlier in this chapter and focused on determining the effects of a structured diabetic educational program on the metabolic control of adult patients with Type 2 DM. This study was conducted using a pretest posttest design with a control group (see Chapter 8 for a model of this design). The two groups were not significantly different on the pretest, indicating the groups were similar for the dependent variables at the start of the study (Table 11–7). The experimental group received the educational program and eight weeks later the posttests were conducted. The experimental and control groups were significantly different on the posttests for all except two dependent variables (urine glucose value and HDL cholesterol). The results of the *t*-tests conducted to determine the differences on the posttests are presented in Table 11–7 and the significant results are identified with ****p* < 0.05.

CRITICAL APPRAISAL

Mollaoglu and Beyazit (2009) clearly presented the results of their *t*-test analyses for the pretests and posttests in two tables (see Tables 11–7 and 11–8). The *t*-test analysis technique was appropriate since the focus of the study was to determine differences between the experimental and control groups for selected dependent variables measured at the ratio level. It is necessary for study variables to be measured at either the interval or ratio level when using *t*-test analysis (Grove, 2007). There were significant differences between the two groups for the dependent variables FBS, PPBS, HbA1c, triglyceride, total cholesterol, and LDL cholesterol. These significant findings support the effectiveness of the diabetic educational program in improving metabolic control in diabetic patients. However, conducting multiple *t*-tests without the Bonferroni procedure raises a concern about an increased risk for a Type I error. The study would have been stronger if the data analysis had included the Bonferroni correction for multiple *t*-tests.

Table 11–7. The comparison of the E [Experimental] and C [Control] groups' preeducation metabolic control mean values

Metabolic control values	E group mean ± *SD*	C group mean ± *SD*	*t* values
FBS	178.3 ± 81.7	199.2 ± 77.6	0.92*
PPBS	263.6 ± 67.8	266.1 ± 71.0	0.12*
HbA1C	9.5 ± 1.7	9.7 ± 1.6	0.45*
Urine glucose value	248.0 ± 399.8	256.0 ± 371.4	0.07*
Triglyceride	149.0 ± 69.8	147.4 ± 49.9	0.09*
Total cholesterol	180.6 ± 38.7	190.0 ± 52.0	0.72*
HDL	44.1 ± 12.8	45.0 ± 11.9	0.25*
LDL	114.6 ± 41.8	97.9 ± 29.3	1.63*

*$p > 0.05$.

Adapted from Mollaoglu, M., & Beyazit, E. (2009). Influence of diabetic education on patient metabolic control. *Applied Nursing Research, 22*(3), 187.

Table 11–8. Distribution of E [Experimental] and C [Control] individuals' 8 weeks later metabolic control values

Metabolic control values	E group mean ± *SD*	C group mean ± *SD*	*t* values
FBS	137.1 ± 41.8	168.1 ± 62.9	2.05**
PPBS	181.0 ± 40.3	235.4 ± 62.7	3.64**
HbA1C	7.5 ± 1.3	9.6 ± 1.6	4.74**
Urine glucose value	28.8 ± 101.1	56.0 ± 125.2	0.87*
Triglyceride	145.6 ± 40.5	171.9 ± 47.6	2.10**
Total cholesterol	167.0 ± 31.9	189.7 ± 43.1	2.11**
HDL	48.4 ± 10.4	45.4 ± 13.1	0.89*
LDL	107.6 ± 36.6	87.4 ± 24.7	2.28**

*$p > 0.05$.
**$p < 0.05$.

Adapted from Mollaoglu, M., & Beyazit, E. (2009). Influence of diabetic education on patient metabolic control. *Applied Nursing Research, 22*(3), 187.

IMPLICATIONS FOR PRACTICE

The implications of the study findings for practice were discussed earlier in this chapter.

Analysis of Variance (ANOVA)

Analysis of variance (ANOVA) tests for differences between means of dependent variables. ANOVA is more flexible than other analyses, because it can be used to examine data from two or more groups. There are many types of ANOVA, some developed for analysis of data from complex experimental designs, such as those using blocking or repeated measures (Burns & Grove, 2009). Rather than focusing just on differences between means, ANOVA tests for differences in variance. One source of variance is the variance within each group, because individual scores in the group will vary from the group mean. This variance is referred to as the **within-group variance**. Another source of variation is variation of the group means around the grand mean, which is referred to as the **between-group variance**. The assumption is that if all of the samples are drawn from the same population, these two sources of variance will exhibit little difference. When these two types of variance are combined, they are referred to as the **total variance**. The test for ANOVA is always one-tailed.

Interpreting Results

The results of an ANOVA are reported as an *F* statistic. The *F* distribution table is used to determine the level of significance of the *F* statistic. (*F* statistical tables are provided in the textbook *The Practice of Nursing Research: Appraisal, Synthesis, and Generation of Evidence* by Burns and Grove, 2009, pp. 678-681.) If the *F* statistic is equal to or greater than the appropriate table value, there is a statistically significant difference between the groups. If only two groups are being examined, the location of a significant difference is clear. However, if more than two groups are under study, it is not possible to determine from the ANOVA where the significant differences lie. The researcher cannot assume that all of the groups examined are significantly different. Therefore, posthoc analyses are conducted to determine the location of the differences among groups. The frequently used posthoc tests are Bonferroni procedure, Newman-Keuls' test, Tukey's Honestly Significantly Different (HSD) test, Scheffé's test, and Dunnett's test (Burns & Grove, 2009).

RESEARCH EXAMPLE ANOVA

In a study introduced earlier in this chapter by Bingham et al. (2009), the researchers examined the relationship of obesity and cholesterol in French, Japanese, and U.S. children. They also examined differences among their four study groups (French, Japanese, U.S. White, and U.S. Black children) for the variables of height, weight, BMI, body fat percentage, and cholesterol using an ANOVA. The researchers reported their findings in Table 11–9, which included the mean and standard deviation for each variable for each of the four groups and also the ANOVA results. The ANOVA results included an *F* value and a *p* value that indicates the significance of the results. For example for the variable of height, $F = 23.3$ and $p = 0.0001$, which is a significant result since $\alpha = 0.05$. Thus, the ANOVA results demonstrate significant differences among the four groups for all variables (height, weight, BMI, body fat %, and cholesterol).

Table 11–9. BMI, body fat, and cholesterol by group

Variables	France ($n = 570$)	Japan ($n = 1865$)	U.S. white ($n = 1226$)	U.S. black ($n = 324$)	F	p
Height (cm)	137.5 ± 6.6	136.4 ± 6.4	137.3 ± 6.5	139.6 ± 7.4	23.3	0.0001
Weight (kg)	32.3 ± 6.3	32.5 ± 6.6	35.3 ± 9.1	37.9 ± 10.3	71.8	0.0001
BMI (kg/m²)	17.0 ± 2.4	17.3 ± 2.6	18.6 ± 3.6	19.2 ± 3.9	78.6	0.0001
Body fat (%)	17.7 ± 6.8	18.8 ± 5.9	23.1 ± 10.3	22.1 ± 11.4	84.6	0.0001
Cholesterol (mmol/L)	4.73 ± 0.89	4.38 ± 0.66	4.25 ± 0.75	4.47 ± 0.82	54.7	0.001
Cholesterol conversion (mg/dl)	183.0 ± 34.6	169.4 ± 25.5	164.3 ± 29.1	172.7 ± 31.9		

Note. Number of subjects varies slightly for each variable because of some missing data.
Bingham, M. O., Harrell, J. S., Takada, H., Washino, K., Bradley, C., Berry, D. et al. (2009). Obesity and cholesterol in Japanese, French, and U.S. children. *Journal of Pediatric Nursing, 24*(4), 317.

CRITICAL APPRAISAL

Bingham and colleagues (2009) conducted their study for the purpose of determining differences among four groups of children (French, Japanese, U.S. Black, and U.S. White) on the variables of height, weight, BMI, body fat percentage, and total cholesterol. These study variables were measured at the ratio level of measurement. ANOVA is the appropriate analysis technique to use with two or more study groups and for variables measured at least at the interval level of measurement. These researchers clearly presented their ANOVA results in table format and discussed these results in the result section of their article.

> The U.S. Black children were the tallest, followed by French, U.S. White, and Japanese participants, with minimal differences in height between the French and U.S. White children. Weight was highest in the U.S. Black children and lowest in French children. BMI was highest in U.S. Black children, followed by U.S. White, Japanese, and French children. Body fat percentage was highest in U.S. White children and lowest in French children. Findings were quite different for total cholesterol, which was highest in French children and lowest in U.S. White children. (Bingham et al., 2009, p. 317)

The researchers did not discuss conducting a posthoc analysis technique to determine exactly where the differences were among the four groups (French, Japanese, U.S. Black, and U.S. White children) for the study variables. This study would have been strengthened by a discussion of posthoc analysis to determine exactly where the differences occurred among the four groups for the study variables. You must question any of the discussions of specific group differences without the posthoc analyses.

IMPLICATIONS FOR PRACTICE

Bingham et al. (2009) noted the following findings from their study.

> Japanese and French children were significantly leaner than U.S. Children (Black and White), with U.S. Black children having the highest BMI (19.2) and U.S. White children the highest body fat percentage

Continued

IMPLICATIONS FOR PRACTICE—cont'd

(23.1%)… The noted increase in childhood obesity in the United States has been described as resulting from a combination of factors including biological, social, and environmental that may vary and interact differently by country, culture, and race/ethnicity. … The results of our comparison reinforce the need for standards to assess obesity using the same methods of measurement. This uniformity would enable researchers and clinicians to better document and understand differences between countries or ethnic groups and provide more consistency to assess change over time. (Bingham et al., 2009, pp. 318-319)

These researchers recommended the BMI as the best measure of overweight children, but acknowledged that the cut off point for risk of or actual clinical complications is still unclear. They recommended additional studies of children in the United States and other countries to determine the link of obesity and total cholesterol with CVD.

Analysis of Covariance (ANCOVA)

Analysis of covariance (ANCOVA) allows the researcher to examine the effect of a treatment apart from the effect of one or more potentially confounding variables (see Chapter 5 for a discussion of confounding variables). Potentially confounding variables that commonly are of concern include pretest scores, age, education, social class, and anxiety level. These variables would be confounding if they were not measured and if their effects on study variables were not statistically removed by performing regression analysis before performing ANOVA. This strategy removes the effect of differences among groups that is due to a confounding variable. Once this effect is removed, the effect of the treatment can be examined more precisely. This technique sometimes is used as a method of statistical control when it is not possible to design the study so that potentially confounding variables are controlled. However, control through careful planning of the design is more effective than statistical control.

ANCOVA may be used in pretest-posttest designs in which differences occur in groups on the pretest. For example, people who achieve low scores on a pretest tend to have lower scores on the posttest than those whose pretest scores were higher, even if the treatment had a significant effect on posttest scores. Conversely, if a person achieves a high pretest score, it is doubtful that the posttest will indicate a strong change as a result of the treatment. ANCOVA maximizes the capacity to detect differences in such cases. This information was provided so you might understand why ANCOVA analysis is conducted and to determine the confounding variables in the study.

Interpreting Statistical Outcomes

To be useful, the evidence from data analysis must be carefully examined, organized, and given meaning. Evaluating the entire research process, organizing the meaning of the results, and forecasting the usefulness of the findings, all of which are involved in interpretation, require high-level intellectual processes. In this segment of a study, the researcher translates the results of analysis into findings and then interprets them by attaching meaning to the findings.

Within the process of interpretation are several intellectual activities that can be isolated and explored, including examining evidence, forming conclusions, considering implications, exploring the significance of the findings, generalizing the findings, and suggesting further studies. This information usually is included in the final section of published studies, which often is entitled Discussion.

Types of Results

Interpretation of results from quasi-experimental and experimental studies traditionally is based on decision theory, with five possible results: (1) significant results that agree with those predicted by the researcher, (2) nonsignificant results, (3) significant results that are opposite those predicted by the researcher, (4) mixed results, and (5) unexpected results (Kerlinger & Lee, 2000). In critically appraising a study, you must identify which types of results were presented in the study.

Significant and Predicted Results

Significant results agree with those predicted by the researcher and support the logical links developed by the researcher among the framework, questions, variables, and measurement tools. In examining the results, however, you must consider the possibility of alternative explanations for the positive findings. What other elements could possibly have led to the significant results?

Nonsignificant Results

Nonsignificant (or inconclusive) results, often referred to as "negative" results, may be a true reflection of reality. In that case, the reasoning of the researcher or the theory used by the researcher to develop the hypothesis is in error. If it is, the negative findings are an important addition to the body of knowledge. But the results also may stem from a Type II error resulting from inappropriate methodology, a biased sample, a small sample, problems with internal design validity, inadequate measurement, weak statistical measures, or faulty analysis. In such instances, the reported results could introduce faulty information into the body of knowledge (Angell, 1989). Negative results do not mean that no relationships exist among the variables. Negative results indicate only that the study failed to find any. Nonsignificant results provide no evidence of either the truth or the falsity of the hypothesis.

Significant and Unpredicted Results

Significant and unpredicted results are the opposite of those predicted by the researcher and indicate that flaws are present in the logic of both the researcher and the theory being tested. If the results are valid, however, they constitute an important addition to the body of knowledge. For example, a researcher may propose that social support and ego strength are positively correlated. If the relevant study shows instead that high social support is correlated with low ego strength, the result is the opposite of that predicted.

Mixed Results

Mixed results probably are the most common outcome of studies. In this case, one variable may uphold predicted characteristics whereas another does not; or two dependent measures of the same variable may show opposite results. These differences may be caused by methodology problems, such as differing reliability or sensitivity of two methods of measuring variables. The mixed results also may indicate that existing theory should be modified.

Unexpected Results

Unexpected results usually are relationships found between variables that were not hypothesized and not predicted from the framework being used. Most researchers examine as many elements of data as possible, in addition to those directed by the questions. These findings can be useful in the modification of existing theory and the development of both new theories and later studies. In addition, unexpected or serendipitous results are important evidence for developing the implications of the study. However, serendipitous results must be interpreted carefully, because the study was not designed to examine these results.

Findings

Results in a study are translated and interpreted to become study findings, which are a consequence of evaluating evidence from a study. Although much of the process of developing findings from results occurs in the mind of the researcher, evidence of these thought processes can be found in published research reports.

Exploring the Significance of Findings

The significance of a study is associated with its importance in contributing to nursing's body of knowledge. Significance is not a dichotomous characteristic because studies contribute in varying degrees to the body of knowledge. Significance may be associated with the amount of variance explained, the degree of control in the study design to eliminate unexplained variance, or the ability to detect statistically significant differences. To the extent possible at the time the study is reported, the researcher is expected to clarify the significance.

A few studies, referred to as "landmark studies," become important reference points in the discipline (Johnson, 1972; Passos & Brand, 1966; Van Aernam & Lindeman, 1971; Williams, 1972). The true importance of a particular study may not become apparent for years after publication. Certain characteristics, however, are associated with the significance of studies: Significant studies make an important difference in people's lives; it is possible to generalize the findings far beyond the study sample so that the findings have the potential of affecting large numbers of people. The implications of significant studies go beyond concrete facts to abstractions and lead to the generation of theory or revisions of existing theory. A very significant study has implications for one or more disciplines in addition to nursing. The study is accepted by others in the discipline and frequently is referenced in the literature. Over a period of time, the significance of a study is measured by the number of other studies it generates.

Clinical Importance

The strongest findings of a study are those that have both statistical significance and clinical importance. Clinical importance is related to the practical relevance of the findings. There is no common agreement in nursing about how to evaluate the clinical importance of a finding. The effect size, however, can be used to determine clinical importance. For example, one group of patients may have a body temperature 0.1° F higher than that of another group. Data analysis may indicate that the two groups are statistically significantly different, but the findings have no clinical importance. The difference is not sufficiently important to warrant changing patient care. In many studies, however, it is difficult to judge how much change would constitute clinical importance. In studies testing the effectiveness of a treatment, clinical importance may be demonstrated by the proportion of subjects who showed improvement or the extent to which subjects returned to normal functioning. But how much improvement must subjects demonstrate for the findings to be considered clinically important? Questions also arise regarding who should judge clinical importance: the patients and their families, the clinician, the researcher, or society at large? At this point in the development of nursing knowledge, clinical importance or relevance is ultimately a value judgment (LeFort, 1993).

CRITICAL APPRAISAL GUIDELINES

Findings and Significance of Findings

When critically appraising a study, be sure to address the following questions.

1. What are the study findings? Did the study include significant and nonsignificant findings?
2. Were the findings appropriate based on the statistical results?
3. Were the study findings linked to previous research findings?
4. Were the findings clinically important?

RESEARCH EXAMPLE Findings and Significance of Findings

The findings from the Cameron et al. (2009) study, introduced earlier in this chapter, are presented as an example. The focus of this study was to test a model of the factors that may influence the self-care of patients with CHF. The model, presented in Figure 11–11, was tested with regression analysis and the results were presented in Table 11–5. Some of the key study findings are presented in the following excerpt.

In the current study the hypothesized model of 7 variables explained a significant amount of the variance in self-care maintenance and management. ... The correlation between gender and self-care management was surprising, albeit consistent with the results of other investigators. ... Our results also lend support that depression is associated with poor self-care, which may be linked to the interplay between self-efficacy and depression. ... We hypothesized that cognitive function would have a meaningful influence on self-care. It was therefore surprising to find that impaired cognitive function contributed to the model but individually did not significantly correlate with self-care maintenance or management. ... Failure to support this hypothesis could be due to the manner in which cognition was measured. ... Overall, self-care was low in this sample, which may reflect the newness of the diagnosis. Only half of the patients followed self-care maintenance instructions, such as daily weighing; most did not understand the significance of their symptoms. Despite being able to evaluate their symptoms, they were not proactive in implementing any self-care actions. (Cameron et al., 2009, pp. 414-416)

Continued

CRITICAL APPRAISAL

Cameron and colleagues (2009) discussed both their significant and nonsignificant findings, which were consistent with their study results. The findings were also linked with the findings of previous research and possible reasons were provided for nonsignificant findings. The regression analysis significantly predicted 38% of the variance of self-care management in patients with CHF. The findings are also clinically important because of the increased ability to predict self-care management in this population.

IMPLICATIONS FOR PRACTICE

The implications for practice were discussed earlier in this chapter.

Conclusions

Conclusions are a synthesis of the findings. In forming conclusions, the researcher uses logical reasoning, creates a meaningful whole from pieces of information obtained through data analysis and findings from previous studies, remains receptive to subtle clues in the data, and considers alternative explanations of the data. One of the risks in developing conclusions is going beyond the data, or forming conclusions that are not warranted by the data. This occurs more frequently in published studies than one would like to believe.

CRITICAL APPRAISAL GUIDELINES

Conclusions

When critically appraising study conclusions, you need to address the following questions.

1. What were the conclusions?
2. Were the conclusions appropriate based on the study results and findings?

RESEARCH EXAMPLE Conclusions

In their study of the self-care activities of CHF patients, Cameron and colleagues (2009) formed the following conclusions based on their study results and findings.

> This suggests that patient education alone does not improve self-care practice. Our results lend further evidence to the growing body of knowledge surrounding the number of nonmodifiable factors that influence self-care practices. These factors must be considered when developing appropriate follow-up strategies and education programs for patients with CHF. ... Patients with CHF are encouraged to become active participants in their care, which requires them to be able to interpret the importance of symptom changes, implement appropriate remedies, and evaluate their effectiveness. To compound the self-care decision-making process, patients with CHF are elderly, have concomitant comorbid illnesses, and often have changes in cognition, which may influence their capacity to become effective self-care managers. (Cameron et al., 2009, p. 416)

CRITICAL APPRAISAL

Cameron et al. (2009) provide specific conclusions for their study at the end of their research report and clearly labeled the section Conclusions. The conclusions were consistent with their study results and findings. The researchers also build on their conclusions with recommendations for further research, which are presented later in this section.

Generalizing the Findings

Generalization extends the implications of the findings from the sample studied to a larger population. For example, if the study was conducted on CHF patients, it may be possible to generalize the findings to persons with other chronic illnesses or to healthy people. Cameron and colleagues (2009) were very cautious in making generalizations related to their study findings. They indicated that their study was small ($n = 50$) and provided significant findings of some of the variables that influence self-care of patients with CHF. Thus, they generalized only to the target population of this study, which included patients with CHF.

How far can generalizations be made? From a very narrow perspective, it is not feasible to generalize from the sample on which the study was conducted; any other sample is likely to be different in some way. Researchers with a conservative view consider generalization particularly risky if the sample was not randomly selected. According to Kerlinger and Lee (2000), unless special precautions are taken and efforts made, the research results frequently are not representative and therefore are not generalizable. Most nurse researchers are not this conservative in making generalizations.

Empirical generalizations are based on accumulated evidence from many studies and are important for the verification of theoretical statements or the development of new theory. Empirical generalizations constitute the base of a science and contribute to scientific conceptualization. Nursing has few empirical generalizations at this time.

CRITICAL APPRAISAL GUIDELINES

Generalizing the Findings

When critically appraising a study, be sure to consider generalization of the findings by asking the following questions.

1. To what population(s) did the researchers generalize the study findings?
2. Were the generalizations appropriate?

Implications for Nursing

Implications for nursing are the meanings of conclusions from scientific research for the body of nursing knowledge, theory, and nursing practice. Implications are based on but are more specific than conclusions, and they provide specific suggestions for implementing the findings in nursing. For example, a researcher may suggest how nursing practice should be modified. If a study indicates that a specific solution is effective in decreasing pressure ulcers in hospitalized elderly patients, the implications will state how the care of elderly patients needs to be modified to prevent pressure ulcers. Interventions with extensive research support provide the basis for developing evidence-based guidelines (see Chapter 13).

CRITICAL APPRAISAL GUIDELINES

Implications for Nursing

When critically appraising a study, you might address the following questions related to the implications for nursing identified by the researchers.

1. What implications for nursing knowledge, theory, and practice were identified?
2. Were the implications for nursing practice appropriate based on the study findings and conclusions?
3. Were there additional implications for nursing knowledge, theory, and practice that were not considered by the researchers?

RESEARCH EXAMPLE Implications for Nursing

Cameron et al. (2009, p. 416) identified the following implications for practice.

> The results of this small study add to the body of evidence that patients with heart failure overall have poor self-care maintenance and management behaviors despite the recent attention to improving this outcome. Our model of variables explained a significant amount of the variance in both self-care maintenance and management. ... Identifying patients who are least likely to engage in self-care may help in the selection of follow-up strategies required to prevent hospital readmissions and improve health outcomes. This would also allow for improved resource management, with specific groups of patients being invited to participate in CHF-MP (chronic heart failure-management program].

CRITICAL APPRAISAL

Cameron and colleagues (2009) provided a separate section at the end of their article that included the heading Implications for Research and Practice. They clearly presented their implications for nursing practice that seem appropriate based on the study findings and conclusions. The authors stressed the need for additional research in the area of self-care management by CHF patients. Thus, we would support the recommendation for additional research before expanding on the implications for nursing practice.

Recommendations for Further Studies

In every study, the researcher gains knowledge and experience that can be used to design a better study next time. Therefore, the researcher often will make suggestions for future studies that emerge logically from the present study. **Recommendations for further study** may include replications or repeating the design with a different or larger sample, using different measurement methods, or testing a new treatment. Recommendations also may include the formation of hypotheses to further test the framework in use. This section provides other researchers with ideas for future studies needed to develop the knowledge needed for evidence-based practice (Brown, 2009; Craig & Smyth, 2007; Cullum, Ciliska, Haynes, & Marks, 2008).

CRITICAL APPRAISAL GUIDELINES

Recommendations for Further Studies

When critically appraising a study, you need to address the following questions related to recommendations for further research.

1. Did the researchers make recommendations for further studies?
2. Were these recommendations based on the study results, findings, limitations, and conclusions?

RESEARCH EXAMPLE Recommendations for Further Studies

Cameron and colleagues (2009, p. 416) made the following recommendations for future research:

> Future studies investigating the correlation between self-care and cognitive function should be conducted in a larger sample with more sensitive screening tools for identifying mild cognitive impairments affecting frontal and temporal lobes of the brain. ... Further research is recommended to investigate the interplay between nonmodifiable factors and the application of CHF-management strategies selectively directed to those in greatest need for improvements in self-care, such as those who are depressed, cognitively impaired, young, or female, and those with few comorbidities and less confidence in their ability to perform self-care.

CRITICAL APPRAISAL

Cameron and colleagues (2009) provided clearly stated recommendations for further research. These recommendations address the questions or concerns that the researchers identified in their discussion of their findings, such as the measurement of cognitive function in this population. These recommendations also addressed some of the limitations noted by the researchers, which were small sample size with limited numbers of women included as subjects. Thus, these recommendations seem to be based on the study results, findings, limitations, and conclusions.

KEY CONCEPTS

- In critically appraising a quantitative study, you need to (1) identify the statistical procedures used; (2) judge whether these statistical procedures were appropriate for the hypotheses, questions, or objectives of the study and the data available for analysis; (3) comprehend the discussion of data analysis results; (4) judge whether the author interpretation of the results is appropriate; and (5) evaluate the clinical significance of the findings.
- Quantitative data analysis has several stages: (1) preparing the data for analysis; (2) describing the sample; (3) testing the reliability of measurement methods; (4) conducting exploratory analysis of the data; (5) conducting confirmatory analyses guided by the hypotheses, questions, or objectives; and (6) conducting posthoc analyses.
- Understanding the concepts of statistical theory will assist you in critically appraising quantitative studies.
- Probability theory, which is deductive, is used to explain a relationship, the probability of an event occurring in a given situation, or the probability of accurately predicting an event.
- Decision theory, which is inductive, assumes that all of the groups in a study (such as experimental and comparison or control groups) used to test a particular hypothesis are components of the same population in relation to the variables under study.
- A Type I error occurs when the null hypothesis is rejected when it is true. Thus, the researchers conclude that significant results exist in a study, when in reality they do not. The risk of a Type I error is indicated by the level of significance or α.
- A Type II error occurs when the null hypothesis is accepted when it is false. Thus, the researchers conclude the study results are nonsignificant when in actuality the results are significant. Type II errors often are a consequence of flaws in the research methods. The risk of a Type II error can be determined using power analysis.
- Summary statistics include frequency distributions, percentages, measures of central tendency, and measures of dispersion.
- Statistical analyses conducted to examine relationships included in this book are Pearson Product-Moment Correlation and factor analysis.
- Regression analysis is conducted to predict the value of one dependent variable using one or more independent variables.
- Statistical analyses conducted to examine causality included in this text are chi-square, *t*-test, analysis of variance, and analysis of covariance.
- Interpretation of results from quasi-experimental and experimental studies traditionally is based on decision theory, with five possible results: (1) significant results that agree with those predicted by the researcher, (2) nonsignificant results, (3) significant results that are opposite those predicted by the researcher, (4) mixed results, and (5) unexpected results.
- In the Discussion section of a study report, researchers examine evidence from the study results, form findings and conclusions, explore the significance of the findings and conclusions, determine the ability to generalize the findings, consider implications for nursing, and make recommendations for further studies.
- In critically appraising a study, you will need to evaluate the appropriateness and completeness of the researchers' results and discussion sections.

REFERENCES

Angell, M. (1989). Negative studies. *The New England Journal of Medicine, 321*(7), 464-466.

Bingham, M. O., Harrell, J. S., Takada, H., Washino, K., Bradley, C., Berry, D., et al. (2009). Obesity and cholesterol in Japanese, French, and U.S. children. *Journal of Pediatric Nursing, 24*(4), 314-322.

Brown, S. J. (2009). *Evidence-based nursing: The research-practice connection*. Sudbury, MA: Jones & Bartlett.

Burns, N., & Grove, S. K. (2009). *The practice of nursing research: Appraisal, synthesis, and generation of evidence* (6th ed.). Philadelphia: Saunders.

Cameron, J., Worrall-Carter, L., Riegel, B., Lo, S. K., & Stewart, S. (2009). Testing a model of patient characteristics, psychologic status, and cognitive function as predictors of self-care in persons with chronic heart failure. *Heart & Lung, 38*(5), 410-418.

Cohen, J. (1988). *Statistical power analysis for the behavioral sciences* (2nd ed.). New York: Academic Press.

Craig, J. V., & Smyth, R. L. (2007). *The evidence-based practice manual for nurses* (2nd ed.). Edinburgh: Churchill Livingstone.

Creswell, J. W. (2009). *Research design: Qualitative, quantitative and mixed methods approaches* (3rd ed.). Thousand Oaks, CA: Sage.

Cullum, N., Ciliska, D., Haynes, R. B., & Marks, S. (2008). *Evidence-based nursing: An introduction*. Oxford, UK: Blackwell Publishing.

Grove, S. K. (2007). *Statistics for health care research: A practical workbook*. St. Louis: Saunders Elsevier.

Johnson, J. E. (1972). Effects of structuring patients' expectations on their reactions to threatening events. *Nursing Research, 21*(6), 499-504.

Kerlinger, F. N., & Lee, H. B. (2000). *Foundations of behavioral research* (4th ed.). Fort Worth, TX: Harcourt College Publishers.

Knapp, R. B. (1985). *Basic statistics for nurses*. Albany, NY: Delmar.

Lavoie-Tremblay, M., Wright, D., Desforges, N., Gelinas, C., Marchionni, C., & Drevniok, U. (2008). Creating a healthy workplace for new-generation nurses. *Journal of Nursing Scholarship, 40*(3), 290-297.

LeFort, S. M. (1993). The statistical versus clinical significance debate. *Image—The Journal of Nursing Scholarship, 25*(1), 57-62.

Mollaoglu, M., & Beyazit, E. (2009). Influence of diabetic education on patient metabolic control. *Applied Nursing Research, 22*(3), 183-190.

Passos, J. Y., & Brand, L. M. (1966). Effects of agents used for oral hygiene. *Nursing Research, 15*(3), 196-202.

Slakter, M. H., Wu, Y. B., & Suzaki-Slakter, N. S. (1991). *, **, and ***: Statistical nonsense at the 0.00000 level. *Nursing Research, 40*(4), 248-249.

Tukey, J. W. (1977). *Exploratory data analysis*. Reading, MA: Addison-Wesley.

Van Aernam, B., & Lindeman, C. A. (1971). Nursing intervention with the presurgical patient: The effects of structured and unstructured preoperative teaching. *Nursing Research, 20*(4), 319-332.

Waltz, C. F., Strickland, O. L., & Lenz, E. R. (2005). *Measurement in nursing and health research* (3rd ed.). New York: Springer.

Williams, A. (1972). A study of factors contributing to skin breakdown. *Nursing Research, 21*(3), 238-243.

12

Critical Appraisal of Quantitative and Qualitative Research for Nursing Practice

Chapter Overview

Examining the Elements of an Intellectual
  Critical Appraisal of Quantitative and
  Qualitative Studies   419
Roles of Nurses in Conducting Intellectual
  Critical Appraisals of Studies   421
Understanding the Quantitative Research
  Critical Appraisal Process   422

Phase 1: Comprehension   422
Phases 2 and 3: Comparison and Analysis   425
Phase 4: Evaluation   427
Critical Appraisal of a Quantitative Study   428
Understanding the Qualitative Research
  Critical Appraisal Process   442

Learning Outcomes

After completing this chapter, you should be able to:

1. Describe the roles of nurses in critically appraising studies to determine the credibility of the findings.
2. Describe the four phases of critical appraisal for a quantitative study: Comprehension or identification of the steps of the research process, comparison and analysis resulting in description of study strengths and weaknesses,

and evaluation of the quality and credibility of the study findings.
3. Conduct a critical appraisal of a quantitative research report.
4. Describe the guidelines for conducting critical appraisals of qualitative studies.
5. Conduct a critical appraisal of a qualitative research report.

Key Terms

Analysis phase, p. 425
Comparison phase, p. 425
Comprehension phase,
  p. 422
Critical appraisal, p. 419

Critical appraisal of
  quantitative studies,
  p. 419
Critical appraisal of
  qualitative studies, p. 442

Evaluation phase, p. 427
Intellectual critical appraisal
  of a study, p. 419

STUDY TOOLS

Go to your Companion CD for interactive review questions related to this chapter. Also, be sure to visit *http://evolve.elsevier.com/Burns/understanding* for additional review questions, critical appraisal activities, and more. For additional content review of the processes for critically appraising quantitative and qualitative studies, go to Chapter 12 of the *Study Guide for Understanding Nursing Research*, 5th edition.

The nursing profession continually strives for evidence-based practice, which includes critically appraising studies, synthesizing the findings, and applying the scientific evidence in practice (Brown, 2009; Craig & Smyth, 2007; Melnyk & Fineout-Overholt, 2005). Thus, critically appraising studies is an essential step toward basing your practice on empirical evidence. The term **critical appraisal** or critique is an examination of the quality or credibility of a study. Critique is often associated with criticize; a term that is frequently viewed as negative. In the arts and sciences, however, critique is associated with critical thinking and evaluation—tasks requiring carefully developed intellectual skills. This type of critical appraisal or critique is referred to as an intellectual critical appraisal. An intellectual critical appraisal is directed at the element that is created, rather than at the creator, and involves the evaluation of the quality of that element. For example, it is possible to conduct an intellectual critical appraisal of a work of art, an essay, or a study.

The idea of the intellectual critical appraisal was introduced early in this book and has been woven throughout the chapters. As each step of the research process was introduced, guidelines were provided to direct the critical appraisal of that step in a research report. This chapter summarizes and builds on previous critical appraisal content and provides direction for conducting critical appraisals of both quantitative and qualitative studies. Thus, Chapter 12 focuses on critically appraising individual studies to evaluate the quality and credibility of the study and its findings. The background provided by this chapter serves as a foundation for the critical appraisal of research syntheses. There are different types of research syntheses, such as systematic reviews, meta-analyses, integrative reviews, metasummaries, and metasyntheses, and these are discussed in Chapter 13.

The elements of intellectual critical appraisal of quantitative and qualitative studies used by nurses are described to assist you in determining the quality of the findings generated by individual studies. The steps for **critical appraisal of quantitative studies** (comprehension, comparison, analysis, and evaluation) are presented in detail. An example critical appraisal of a published quantitative study is provided. The chapter concludes with the critical appraisal process for qualitative studies and an example critical appraisal of a qualitative study.

Examining the Elements of an Intellectual Critical Appraisal of Quantitative and Qualitative Studies

An **intellectual critical appraisal of a study** involves a careful, complete examination of that study to judge its strengths, weaknesses, meaning, credibility, and significance for practice. A high-quality study focuses on a significant problem, demonstrates sound methodology, produces credible findings, and provides a basis for additional studies (Brown, 2009; Burns & Grove, 2009). Ultimately, the findings from several quality studies can be synthesized to provide empirical evidence for use in practice (Craig & Smyth, 2007; Stevens, 2005; Whittemore, 2005).

CRITICAL APPRAISAL GUIDELINES

Intellectual Critical Appraisal of a Study

When conducting an intellectual critical appraisal of a study, you must address these questions. Answering these questions requires careful examination of the problem, purpose, literature review, framework, methods, results, and findings of the study.

1. Was the research problem significant? Will the study problem and purpose generate or refine knowledge for nursing practice?
2. What are the major strengths of the study?
3. What are the major weaknesses of the study?
4. Did the researchers use sound methodology?
5. Do the findings from the study accurately reflect reality? Are the findings credible?
6. Are the findings consistent with those from previous studies?
7. Can the study be replicated by other researchers?
8. What are the implications of the findings for nursing practice?

An intellectual critical appraisal of a study involves the application of some basic guidelines to assist you in answering the preceding questions. These guidelines, presented in Table 12–1, stress the importance of critiquing the entire study and clearly, concisely, and objectively identifying the study's strengths and weaknesses. All studies have weaknesses or flaws; if every flawed study were discarded, no scientific evidence would be available for use in

Table 12–1	Steps for Conducting Intellectual Critical Appraisal of Quantitative and Qualitative Studies

Read and critically appraise the entire study. A research critical appraisal involves examining the quality of all steps of the research process.

Examine the organization and presentation of the research report. A well-prepared report is complete, concise, clearly presented, and logically organized. It does not include excessive jargon that is difficult for students and practicing nurses to read. The references need to be complete and presented in a consistent format.

Examine the significance of the problem studied for nursing practice. The focus of nursing studies needs to be on significant practice problems if a sound knowledge base is to be developed for the profession.

Indicate the type of study and identify the steps or elements of the study. This might be done as an initial critical appraisal of a study by a nursing student. This indicates your knowledge of the different types of quantitative and qualitative studies and the steps or elements included in these studies.

Identify the strengths and weaknesses of a study. All studies have strengths and weaknesses, so attention must be given to all aspects of the study.

Be objective and realistic in identifying the study's strengths and weaknesses. Be balanced in your critical appraisal of a study. Try not to be overly critical in identifying a study's weaknesses or overly flattering in identifying the strengths.

Provide specific examples of the strengths and weaknesses of a study. Examples provide evidence for your critical appraisal of the strengths and weaknesses of a study.

Provide a rationale for your critical appraisal. Include justifications for your critical appraisal, and document your ideas with sources from the current literature. This strengthens the quality of your critical appraisal and documents the use of critical thinking skills.

Evaluate the quality of the study. Describe the credibility of the findings, consistency of the findings with those from other studies, and the quality of the study conclusions.

Discuss the usefulness of the findings for practice. The findings from the study need to be linked to the findings of previous studies and examined for use in clinical practice.

practice. In fact, science itself is flawed. Science does not completely or perfectly describe, explain, predict, or control reality. However, improved understanding and increased ability to predict and control phenomena depend on recognizing the flaws in studies and science. Additional studies can then be planned to minimize the weaknesses of earlier studies. You also need to recognize a study's strengths to determine the quality of a study and the credibility of its findings. Adding together the strong points from multiple studies slowly builds a solid base of evidence for practice.

Two nursing research journals, *Scholarly Inquiry for Nursing Practice: An International Journal* and *Western Journal of Nursing Research* include commentaries (partial critical appraisals) after some of the published research reports. In these journals, authors receive critical appraisals of their work and have an opportunity to respond to these reviews. Published critical appraisals usually increase the reader's understanding of the study and ability to critically appraise other studies. A less formal critical appraisal of a published study might appear as a letter to the editor. Readers have the opportunity to comment on the strengths and weaknesses of published studies by writing to the editors of journals.

Roles of Nurses in Conducting Intellectual Critical Appraisals of Studies

Scientists in every field, including nursing, critically appraise research to broaden their understanding, determine evidence for use in practice, and provide a background for developing new studies. All nurses, including students, practicing nurses, educators, administrators, and researchers, need a background in critically appraising studies. Basic knowledge of the research process and the critical appraisal process often is provided early in professional nursing education at the baccalaureate level. More advanced critical appraisal skills are taught at the master's and doctorate levels, with critical appraisal skills increasing as knowledge of the research process increases.

As a student or practicing nurse, you are encouraged to critically appraise published studies on relevant clinical topics, to increase your understanding of the research process, promote your interest in reading research articles, and improve your ability to determine how the accumulated empirical evidence can be used in practice. Critical appraisals of studies by practicing nurses are essential for expanding understanding and making changes in practice. Nurses in practice need to constantly update their nursing interventions in response to current research knowledge. Critical appraisal is an essential component of providing evidence-based practice. In addition, accrediting agencies for healthcare facilities require that policy and procedure manuals used to direct care be based on research.

Educators critically appraise studies to update their knowledge of research findings. This knowledge provides a basis for developing and refining content taught in classroom and clinical settings. Instructors and textbooks often identify the nursing interventions that were tested through research. Many educators who conduct studies critically appraise research as a basis for planning and implementing their own studies. Researchers often focus on one problem area and update their knowledge base by critically appraising new studies in this area. The outcome of the critical appraisal influences the selection of research problems, identification of frameworks, development of methodologies, and interpretation of findings in future studies.

Understanding the Quantitative Research Critical Appraisal Process

The critical appraisal process for quantitative studies includes four phases: comprehension, comparison, analysis, and evaluation (Burns & Grove, 2009). These phases initially occur in sequence and presume accomplishment of the preceding steps. However, after you gain experience in the critical appraisal process, you will be able to perform several of these phases simultaneously. Conducting a critical appraisal is a complex mental process that is stimulated by raising questions. Thus relevant questions are provided for each phase of the critical appraisal process. The comprehension phase involves identification of the steps of the research process and is covered separately because students who are new to critically appraising studies need to start with this phase. The comparison and analysis phases are presented together because they often occur simultaneously in the mind of the person conducting the critical appraisal as they describe the strengths and weaknesses of a study. Evaluation is covered separately because it requires increased expertise and builds on the knowledge generated from the comprehension, comparison, and analyses phases of the critical appraisal process. Each of these critical appraisal phases involves examination of the steps of the quantitative research process and identification of the strengths and weaknesses of these steps.

Phase 1: Comprehension

The comprehension phase is the first step in the critical appraisal process for quantitative studies. This critical appraisal phase involves understanding the terms and concepts in the report and identifying the steps of the research process, such as the problem, purpose, framework, design, sample, measurement methods, data collection and analysis, and findings. It is also necessary to grasp the nature, significance, and meaning of these steps in a research report.

The first steps of the Comprehension Phase include reviewing the abstract, reading the entire study, and examining the references (see Table 12-1). Next, the presentation of the study is evaluated using the following questions: Was the writing style clear and concise? Were relevant terms clearly defined? Were the following major sections of the research report clearly identified?

1. Introduction section with the problem, purpose, literature review, framework, study variables, and objectives, questions, or hypotheses.
2. Methods section with the design, sample, measurement methods, and data collection.
3. Results section with data analysis and specific results.
4. Discussion section with the findings, conclusions, limitation, generalizations, implications for practice, and suggestions for future research (Burns & Grove, 2009; Creswell, 2009).

You are encouraged to underline terms you do not understand and look them up in the glossary at the back of this book. Next, it may help to read the article a second time and highlight and label each step of the research process.

CRITICAL APPRAISAL GUIDELINES

Comprehension Phase Including Identification of the Steps of the Research Process

To write a critical appraisal that demonstrates comprehension of the study steps, concisely identify each step of the research process, and briefly respond to the following questions. Do not answer the questions with a yes or no; rather, provide a rationale or include examples or content from the study to address the questions.

1. Did the abstract include key elements of purpose, design, sample, selected results, and conclusions?
2. What is the study problem?
3. What is the study purpose?
4. Does the literature review include current, relevant previous studies and theories?
5. Is a particular theory or model identified as a framework for the study? Is a map or model of the framework provided for clarity?
6. Are research objectives, questions, or hypotheses used to direct the conduct of the study? Identify these.
7. Are the major variables (independent and dependent variables or research variables) identified and defined (conceptually and operationally)? Identify and define these variables.
8. What attribute or demographic variables are examined in the study?
9. What design was used to conduct the study?
   a. Does the study include a treatment or intervention? If so, identify the intervention.
   b. If the study has more than one group, how were the subjects assigned to groups?
10. Are the following elements of the sample described?
   a. Identify inclusion and exclusion sample criteria.
   b. Identify the sampling method.
   c. Discuss the sample size, power analysis, acceptance rate, and attrition rate.
11. Was institutional review board approval obtained from the university and/or agency in which the study was conducted? Was informed consent obtained from the subjects?
12. What was the study setting?
13. Are the measurement methods described? Identify the name of each measurement method, the author, the type of measurement method, level of measurement achieved, and reliability and validity of the scales used or the precision and accuracy of physiological measures. Complete the following table with information about the measurement methods in the study. An example table is provided on the following page to assist you.
14. How were study procedures implemented and data collected during the study?
15. What statistical analyses are included in the research report?
   a. Identify the analysis techniques used to describe the sample.
   b. Complete the following table with the analysis techniques conducted in the study: (1) identify the focus (description, relationships, or differences) of each analysis technique; (2) list the statistical procedures; (3) list the statistics; (4) identify specific results; and (5) provide a specific probability values (*p*). An example table is provided on the following page to assist you.

Continued

CRITICAL APPRAISAL GUIDELINES—cont'd

Measurement Methods Table

Name of Measurement Method	Author	Type of Measurement Method	Level of Measurement	Reliability or Precision	Validity or Accuracy
Beck Depression Inventory	Beck	Likert Scale	Interval/Ratio	Cronbach alphas of 0.82-0.92 from previous studies and 0.84 for this study. Reading level at 6th grade.	Construct validity: Content validity from concept analysis, literature review, and reviews of experts. Convergent validity with Zung Depression Scale. Prediction validity of patients' future depression episodes. Successive use validity with previous studies and this study.
Omron Blood Pressure (BP) Equipment	Health Care Equipment Agency	Physiologic measurement method	Interval/Ratio	Test-retest values of BPs in previous studies. BP equipment new and recalibrated every 50 BP readings in this study. Average 3 BP readings to determine BP.	Documented accuracy of systolic and diastolic BPs to 1 mm mercury by company developing Omron BP cuff. Designated protocol for taking BP. Average 3 BP readings to determine BP.

Data Analysis Table

Purpose of Analysis	Analysis Technique	Statistic	Results	Probability (p)
Description of subjects' age	Mean, Standard deviation, and Range	X SD range	65.34 6.71 18-88	
Difference between males and females on blood pressure	t-test	t	2.75	$p = 0.01$
Difference between treatment group and the comparison group on weight lost	Analysis of Variance	F	4.88	$p = 0.03$
Relationships between depression and anxiety	Pearson Product Moment Correlation	R	0.48	$p = 0.02$

16. What is the researcher's interpretation of the findings?
17. What limitations of the study are identified by the researchers?
18. What conclusions did the researchers identify based on this study and previous research?
19. Describe how the researcher generalized the findings?
20. What implications do the findings have for nursing practice?
21. What suggestions are made for further studies?

Phases 2 and 3: Comparison and Analysis

Critical appraisal phases 2 and 3 (comparison and analysis) are frequently done simultaneously when critically appraising a study. The comparison phase requires knowledge of what each step of the research process should be like, and then the ideal is compared with the real. During the comparison phase, you must examine the extent to which the researcher followed the rules for an ideal study. Examine the steps of the study, such as the problem, purpose, framework, methodology, and results, based on the content presented in Chapters 4 to 11 of this book. Did the researchers rigorously develop and implement the study? What are the strengths of the study? What are the weaknesses of the study?

The analysis phase involves a critical appraisal of the logical links connecting one study element with another. For example, the presentation of the problem must provide a background and direction for the statement of the purpose. In addition, the overall logical development of the study must be examined. The variables identified in the study purpose should be consistent with the variables identified in the research objectives, questions, or hypotheses. These variables must be conceptually defined in light of the study framework. The conceptual definitions need to provide the basis for the operational definitions of the study variables. The study design needs to be appropriate for the investigation of the purpose of the study and for the specific objectives, questions, or hypotheses. The instruments used in the study need to adequately measure the variables. The sample selected should be representative of the population identified in the problem and purpose. Analysis techniques provide results that address the purpose and the specific objectives, questions, or hypotheses. To determine the current knowledge of the study problem, the findings from a study need to be linked to the framework and the findings from previous research. These findings are synthesized in the conclusions so that they can be generalized to individuals other than the study subjects. Depending on the quality of the findings, the researcher indicates the use of the findings in nursing practice. All steps of the research process provide a basis for the identification of future research projects. The steps of the research process need to be precisely developed and strongly linked to each other to conduct a quality study.

Guidelines for Comparison and Analysis of a Quantitative Research Report

To conduct the comparison and analysis steps, review the chapters in this text, as well as other references describing the steps of the research process (Brown, 2009; Burns & Grove, 2009; Craig & Smyth, 2007; Creswell, 2009; Munro, 2005; Robinson, 2001; Santacroce, Maccarelli, & Grey, 2004). Then compare the steps in the study you are critically appraising with the criteria established for each step in this textbook or other sources (Phase 2, Comparison). Next analyze the logical links among the steps of the study (Phase 3, Analysis). The guidelines in this section should assist you in implementing the phases of comparison and analysis for each step of the research process. Questions relevant to analysis are identified; all other questions direct the comparison of the steps of the study with the ideal. Use these questions to determine how rigorously the steps of the research process were implemented in published studies. Indicate the strengths and weaknesses for the different steps of the research process. When identifying study strengths or weaknesses, provide examples from the study and state a rationale, along with documentation to support your conclusions. In addition, identify the strengths in the logical way the steps of the study are linked together or any breaks or weaknesses in the links of a study's steps.

CRITICAL APPRAISAL GUIDELINES: QUANTITATIVE STUDY

Comparison and Analysis Resulting in a Description of Study Strengths and Weaknesses

The written critical appraisal should be a narrative summary of the strengths and weaknesses that you note in the study. Use the following guidelines to examine the significance of the problem, fit of the framework, rigor of the methodology, and quality and relevance of the findings in published studies.

1. Research problem and purpose
   a. Is the problem clinically significant and relevant to nursing?
   b. Does the purpose narrow and clarify the focus or aim of the study?
2. Literature review: Does the literature review provide a rationale and direction for the study? (Analysis)
   a. Study framework: Is the framework presented with clarity and linked to the study purpose, variables, and findings? (Analysis)
3. Research objectives, questions, or hypotheses: Are the objectives, questions, or hypotheses logically linked to the study purpose, framework, design, and results? (Analysis)
4. Variables
   a. Do the variables reflect the concepts identified in the framework? (Analysis)
   b. Are the variables clearly defined (conceptually and operationally) based on previous research and/or theories?
5. Design
   a. Does the design provide a means to examine all of the objectives, questions, or hypotheses and the study purpose? (Analysis)
   b. What are the strengths and weaknesses of the design?
   c. If the study had a treatment, is it consistently implemented? Who is blinded to the treatment, subjects, data collectors, researchers? Being blinded to the treatment decreases potential for bias (Brown, 2002; Santacroce et al., 2004).
   d. If the study has treatment and comparison groups, are these groups equivalent?
6. Sample, population, and setting
   a. What are the potential biases in the sampling method?
   b. Is the sample size sufficient to avoid a Type II error? Was the sample size determined by a power analysis? Was the attrition rate high?
   c. Are the rights of human subjects protected? Are the HIPAA privacy regulations followed in conducting the study? (Olsen, 2003)
   d. Is the setting used in the study typical of clinical settings?
7. Measurements
   a. Are the measurement methods clearly described? (Roberts & Stone, 2003)
   b. Respond to the following questions that are relevant to the measurement approaches used in the study.
   c. Scales and questionnaires
      (1) Are techniques to administer, complete, and score the instruments provided?
      (2) Are the reliability and validity of the instruments described?
      (3) If the instrument was developed for the study, is the instrument development process described?

    d. Observation

       (1) Are the techniques for recording observations described?

       (2) Is interrater reliability described?

    e. Physiological measures

       (1) Are the accuracy, precision, and error of the physiological instruments discussed?

       (2) Are the methods for recording data from the physiological measures clearly described?

8. Data collection

    a. Is the training of data collectors clearly described and adequate?

    b. Is the data collection process conducted in a consistent manner?

    c. Are the data collection methods ethical?

9. Data analyses

    a. Do data analyses address each objective, question, or hypothesis?

    b. Are data analysis procedures appropriate to the type of data collected? (Duffy, 1988)

    c. Are tables and figures used to synthesize and emphasize certain findings? (Burns & Grove, 2009)

    d. If the results were nonsignificant, was the sample size sufficient to detect significant differences? Was a power analysis conducted to examine nonsignificant findings?

10. Interpretation of findings

    a. Are significant and nonsignificant findings explained?

    b. Were the statistically significant findings also examined for clinical significance?

    c. Did the researchers identify important study limitations?

    d. Are the conclusions based on statistically and clinically significant results? (Analysis)

    e. Is the generalization of the study findings appropriate based on the findings of this study and previous research? (Analysis)

    f. Are the implications for practice consistent with study conclusions? (Analysis)

    g. Are relevant ideas provided for future research?

Phase 4: Evaluation

During the evaluation phase of a research critical appraisal, the meaning and significance of the study findings are examined. The evaluation becomes a summary of the study's quality that builds on conclusions reached during the first three phases (comprehension, comparison, and analysis) of the critical appraisal. This level of critical appraisal may or may not be conducted by a nursing student in a baccalaureate degree program. The guidelines for the evaluation phase are provided for those students who want to perform a more comprehensive critical appraisal to determine the quality and credibility of the study and its findings.

Guidelines for Evaluation of a Quantitative Research Report

The evaluation phase involves reexamining the findings, conclusions, limitations, implications for nursing, and suggestions for further study, which usually are presented in the Discussion section of a research report. All nurses should be able to determine the value of research findings in the development of nursing knowledge and for use in practice. The evaluation phase involves developing a summary of the study's quality and credibility. This summary is a narrative that usually is the last one or two paragraphs of a critical appraisal.

CRITICAL APPRAISAL GUIDELINES: QUANTITATIVE STUDY

Evaluation of Quality and Credibility of Study Findings

Using the following questions as a guide, summarize the quality of the study, the credibility of the findings, and the usefulness of the findings for nursing practice and to direct future studies.

1. Are the findings valid or an accurate reflection of reality? Do you have confidence in the findings?
2. What do the findings add to the current body of knowledge? For example, do the findings support the study framework and are they consistent with previous studies?
3. Can the findings from the study be generalized from the study sample to the population?
4. Do the findings have potential for use in nursing practice?

Critical Appraisal of a Quantitative Study

A critical appraisal was conducted of the quasi-experimental study by Shipowick, Moore, Corbett, and Bindler (2009) and presented as an example in this chapter. The research report titled, *Vitamin D and Depressive Symptoms in Women During the Winter: A Pilot Study*, is included in this section. This study examines the effects of a vitamin D_3 supplement on depressive symptoms in women with low vitamin D levels. This study is followed by the four phases for critically appraising a quantitative study: comprehension, comparison, analysis, and evaluation.

Nursing students and RNs usually conduct critical appraisals that are focused on comprehension, which includes identifying the steps of the research process in a study. The comprehension critical appraisal may be written in outline format, with headings identifying the steps of the research process. A more in-depth critical appraisal includes not only the comprehension step but also the comparison, analysis, and evaluation phases. We encourage you to read the Shipowick et al. (2009) study and conduct a comprehension critical appraisal using the guidelines presented at the beginning of this chapter. Compare your ideas with the critical appraisal presented in this chapter.

RESEARCH EXAMPLE Quantitative Study
Vitamin D and Depressive Symptoms in Women During the Winter: A Pilot Study

Clarissa Drymon Shipowick, BSW, RNC, C. Barton Moore, MD, Cynthia Corbett, PhD, RN, and Ruth Bindler, PhD, RNC

ELSEVIER

Available online at www.sciencedirect.com

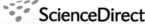

ScienceDirect

Applied Nursing Research 22 (2009) 221–225

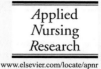

Applied Nursing Research

www.elsevier.com/locate/apnr

Vitamin D and depressive symptoms in women during the winter: A pilot study

Clarissa Drymon Shipowick, BSW, RNC[a],*, C. Barton Moore, MD[b],
Cynthia Corbett, PhD, RN[c], Ruth Bindler, PhD, RNC[c]

[a]*Washington State University, Richland, WA 99352, USA*
[b]*Blue Mountain Medical Group, Walla Walla, WA 99362, USA*
[c]*College of Nursing, Washington State University, Spokane, WA 99224, USA*

Received 15 June 2007; revised 27 July 2007; accepted 9 August 2007

Abstract

Background: Research indicates that vitamin D supplementation may decrease depressive symptoms during the winter months.
Method: In this study, nine women with serum vitamin D levels <40 ng/ml were administered the Beck Depression Inventory (BDI)-II. After vitamin D_3 supplementation, six of these women completed the BDI-II and had their serum vitamin D levels reassessed.
Results: Vitamin D supplementation was associated not only with an increase in the serum D levels by an average of 27 ng/ml but also with a decline in the BDI-II scores of an average of 10 points.
Discussion: This study suggests that supplemental vitamin D_3 reduces depressive symptoms.
© 2009 Elsevier Inc. All rights reserved.

1. Vitamin D and depressive symptoms in women during the winter

It has been hypothesized that low vitamin D levels in the winter account for exacerbation of melancholia (Vasquez, Manso, & Cannell, 2004). Vitamin D can be obtained through food consumption or synthesized by the body from sun exposure. For people living in northern climates (above 37° latitude), the oblique angle of the sun's rays during the autumn and winter precludes vitamin D synthesis, and vitamin D deficiency or insufficiency is common (Rucker, Allen, Fick, & Hanley, 2002).

In the United States, laboratories use a different version of the metric system (nanograms per milliliter) to measure 25-OH serum vitamin D levels, whereas the International System of Units is used worldwide (nanomoles per liter). The following 25-OH serum vitamin D levels are used as criteria for this study. Vitamin D deficiency is defined as serum levels <20 ng/ml or <50 nmol/L. The prefix *nano* is one billionth of a unit of measurement (Pickett, 2000). Vitamin D insufficiency is defined as serum vitamin D levels >20 but <40 ng/ml or >50 but <100 nmol/L. Optimal vitamin D levels are defined as between 40 and 65 ng/ml or between 100 and 160 nmol/L (Vasquez et al., 2004). Toxic levels do not occur until circulating levels are greater than 125 ng/ml or 312 nmol/L (Holick & Jenkins, 2003).

Research shows that women are more susceptible to depression than men (Kornstein & Sloan, 2003). Women under 40 years of age are four times more likely to have seasonal affective disorder than men (Gaines, 2005). According to the World Health Organization (WHO), by 2020, depression will be the leading cause of disability worldwide (WHO, 2000).

Studies indicate that vitamin D deficiency is associated with increased depressive symptoms (Armstrong et al., 2006; Jorde, Waterloo, Haug, & Svartberg, 2005). Thus, vitamin D supplementation may provide a natural, inexpensive, and accessible remedy for seasonal mood fluctuations and an adjunct for individuals with depressive symptoms.

2. Purpose of the study

The following research questions guided the study: (a) Is there a significant relationship between serum vitamin D

* Corresponding author. Tel.: +1 509 522 2747.
E-mail address: cshipowick@charter.net (C.D. Shipowick).

0897-1897/$ – see front matter © 2009 Elsevier Inc. All rights reserved.
doi:10.1016/j.apnr.2007.08.001

Continued

RESEARCH EXAMPLE—cont'd

222   *C.D. Shipowick et al. / Applied Nursing Research 22 (2009) 221–225*

levels and depressive symptoms? and (b) Do depressive symptoms in women with low serum vitamin D levels improve 8 weeks after initiation of vitamin D₃ supplementation (5,000 IU daily) during the fall and winter?

3. Conceptual model

Vitamin D₃ is hydoxylated in the liver to become 25-OH vitamin D, the major circulating form of vitamin D. It is activated in the kidneys to become the hormone 1,25-OH vitamin D where it is tightly regulated. Certain organs including the brain also have the capacity to activate vitamin D (Holick & Jenkins, 2003). Both unactivated and activated vitamin D can cross the blood–brain barrier (Kiraly, Kiraly, Hawe, & Makhani, 2006). Based on these data, a biopsychological framework of vitamin D as a hormone that influences depressive symptoms served as an emerging model (Fig. 1). Three physiologic pathways between vitamin D and depressive symptoms were identified: (a) Vitamin D in its active form in the body has been shown to stimulate serotonin (Gaines, 2005), a neurotransmitter that is associated with mood elevation; (b) Vitamin D has been

associated with down-regulation of glucocorticoid receptor gene activation, which is found to be up-regulated in depression; and (c) Vitamin D has also been found to be neuroprotective, shielding neurons from toxins such as glucocorticoids and other excitotoxic insults (Obradovic, Gronemeyer, Lutz, & Rein, 2006).

4. Literature review

In a descriptive study of patients with fibromyalgia ($N = 75$; 70 females and 5 males) at a clinic in Belfast, Ireland, during the winter season, 10% were found to be vitamin D deficient, 42% had levels that were labeled inadequate, and only 23% had levels considered to be adequate (Armstrong et al., 2006). The Hospital Anxiety and Depression Scale (HADS), a tool used to measure mood disorders, was completed by these patients. Using a Kruskal–Wallis analysis of variance (ANOVA), a statistically significant difference ($p \le .05$) between the HADS scores of the group with the lowest vitamin D levels and the other two groups was found, suggesting a link between anxious and depressive symptoms and vitamin D deficiency.

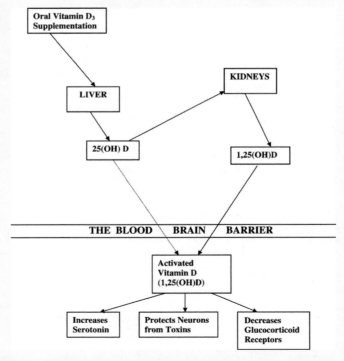

Fig. 1. The biopsychological model of vitamin D: hormone that elevates mood. From *The UV Advantage* (Fig. 1.3: New understanding of how vitamin D benefits health), by M. Holick & M. Jenkins, 2003, New York, NY: Ibooks Inc. Adapted with permission.

CHAPTER 12 *Critical Appraisal of Quantitative and Qualitative Research for Nursing Practice* **431**

C.D. Shipowick et al. / Applied Nursing Research 22 (2009) 221–225 223

Table 1
Paired samples statistics and tests (n = 6)

Paired samples	M	Difference in means	SD	Average SD	t	p
BDI-II (1)	31.8333	10.66667	4.79236	7.7616	3.366	.020
BDI-II (2)	21.1667		11.07098			
25-OH-D (1)	21.8333	−26.33333	8.32867	15.68014	−4.114	.009
25-OH-D (2)	48.1667		20.01416			

In an Australian study during the summer, serum vitamin D levels were collected from patients with unipolar and bipolar depression (N = 17). Only 3 of the 17 participants had adequate vitamin D levels. The mean serum vitamin D level among the general population in the same geographic area was found to be 34 nmol/L higher. This study suggests that a higher proportion of depressed patients are vitamin D deficient (Berk et al., 2007).

The Tromso study, conducted in northern Norway, measured serum calcium and parathyroid hormone levels in 7,950 participants. Subsequently, a secondary analysis of 21 participants who had been experiencing secondary hyperparathyroidism without renal failure was conducted. The 21 participants with altered calcium metabolism demonstrated neuropsychological problems. A relationship between serum vitamin D levels and depressive symptoms was also documented. Using ANOVA, there was a statistically significant association between serum vitamin D levels and the Beck Depression Inventory (BDI) scores, indicating that a low serum level was indicative of high depressive symptoms. This association did not appear to be the result of covariation with any other variables. Low serum vitamin D levels correlated with higher BDI scores, identifying a negative correlation between vitamin D levels and depressive symptoms (Jorde et al., 2005).

5. Methods and procedure

Following university institutional review board approval and the approval of the clinical agency where the study was carried out, a quasi-experimental pretest–posttest design was implemented with female participants acting as their own pre–post control. Female patients (N = 9) being treated at a medical clinic in southeastern Washington for vitamin D deficiency or insufficiency voluntarily participated in this study. Initial evaluations took place between January and March. During these months, vitamin D stores are typically low and the impact of vitamin D supplementation should be most visible in participants. The following were excluded from the study: (a) those with mental impairments such as dementia or language barriers that may have inhibited answering written questions; (b) women who were using or planned to use tanning beds or other phototherapy; (c) women who planned on traveling to sunnier, more tropical areas (e.g., Mexico, Hawaii, Arizona) during the winter; and (d) women taking or planning to take antidepressants.

Per usual medical care at the clinic, participants had who blood tests that indicated serum vitamin D levels below 40 ng/ml

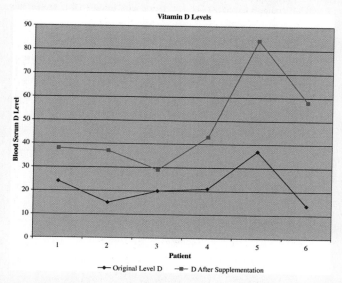

Fig. 2. Comparing vitamin D levels before and after supplementation. This graph shows that vitamin D₃ supplementation is associated with an increase in serum 25-OH vitamin D levels by an average of 27 ng/ml after 8 weeks.

Continued

RESEARCH EXAMPLE—cont'd

224   *C.D. Shipowick et al. / Applied Nursing Research 22 (2009) 221–225*

were advised to initiate vitamin D_3 supplementation (5,000 IU) by their physician. Before vitamin D_3 supplementation, women were informed of the research opportunity. Women agreeing to participate completed the BDI-II survey prior to initiating vitamin D_3 supplementation. The BDI-II is a commonly used depression screening tool with demonstrated reliability and validity. The following criteria are used universally in the scoring of the BDI-II and for this study. Potential scores range from 0 to 63 with normal (0–13), mild depression (14–19), moderate depression (20–28), and severe depression (29–63) as designated. After the 8 weeks of D_3 supplementation, participants returned to the clinic to have their vitamin D level rechecked per usual clinic protocol and once again completed the BDI-II survey. Participants gave permission for their medical records to be accessed to document serum vitamin D levels for the study. Of the nine participants, six provided BDI-II and serum vitamin D levels 8 weeks after vitamin D_3 supplementation.

6. Data analysis and results

SPSS 14.0 was used to perform statistical analysis. The participants who did not complete the postsupplement measurements were not included in the correlational and inferential analyses. Cronbach's alpha for the BDI-II was .81 at baseline and .95 at follow-up.

Six participants completed the study. This subsample had a mean age of 42.2 years ($SD = 13.17$, range = 23–55). Their

baseline and follow-up mean serum vitamin D levels were 21.8 ($SD = 8.33$, range = 14–37) and 48.2 ($SD = 20.01$, range = 29–84), respectively ($t = -4.11$, $p = .009$). The baseline and follow-up mean BDI-II scores were 31.8 ($SD = 4.79$, range = 26–40) and 21.2 ($SD = 11.07$, range = 8–37), respectively ($t = 3.37$, $p = .02$; Table 1). Normal serum vitamin D levels (>40 ng/ml) were achieved after supplementation for three participants (Fig. 2). These same three participants had BDI-II scores of 14 or below after supplementation (Fig. 3).

7. Discussion

Following supplementation, serum vitamin D levels increased in all participants with an average increase of 27 ng/ml. At the prescribed intake of 5,000 IU daily, a significant reduction in depressive symptoms was realized after supplementation. Further, among the three women with a postsupplementation serum vitamin D level greater than 40, all had BDI-II scores of 14 or less, suggestive of normal mood with minimal depressive symptoms.

The Armstrong study statistically associated depressive and anxious symptoms with low serum vitamin D levels. The Berk study found low vitamin D levels prevalent in patients diagnosed with unipolar or bipolar depression, and the Tromso study associated low vitamin D levels with higher scores on the BDI, indicative of depressive symptoms. The current study associated higher vitamin D levels with lower BDI-II scores, indicating less depressive

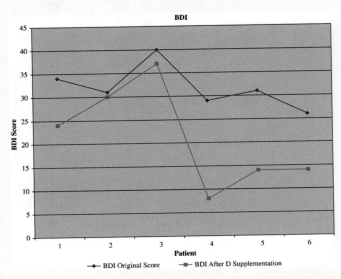

Fig. 3. Comparing BDI-II scores before and after supplementation. This graph shows that vitamin D supplementation is associated with a decline (improved mood: a negative correlation) in BDI-II scores of an average of about 10 points.

symptoms with more optimal vitamin D levels. Further research with a larger sample size and stronger design is warranted to continue to investigate the clinical utility of vitamin D_3 supplementation.

8. Limitations and conclusions

Replication of this study with a larger, adequately powered sample is needed to provide a more definitive understanding of the relationship between vitamin D supplementation and seasonal depressive symptoms. Additionally, further research to determine factors related to vitamin D_3 dosing is needed. The reasons for three of the women not achieving serum vitamin D_3 levels above 40 ng/ml are unclear. It may be that these women were not consistently taking vitamin D_3, that they required longer than 8 weeks of supplementation to achieve optimal vitamin D levels, or that a higher vitamin D_3 dose was needed to achieve optimal vitamin D levels. More frequent analyses of serum vitamin D levels and measuring adherence to supplementation are warranted in future studies. Future studies should be conducted with a randomized and blinded design to account for placebo effect.

In summary, this pilot study provides evidence to suggest that women who suffer from seasonal depressive symptoms may benefit from vitamin D_3 supplementation if serum vitamin D levels are low (<40 ng/ml). These findings are consistent with other studies that indicate that higher vitamin D levels improve sense of well-being (Armstrong et al., 2006; Berk et al., 2007; Jorde et al., 2005).

Acknowledgments

We are grateful to Robert Bendall for his statistical expertise and to Mary DeRose for her work behind the scenes and her troubleshooting expertise.

References

Armstrong, D. J., et al. (2006). Vitamin D deficiency is associated with anxiety and depression in fibromyalgia. *Clinical Rheumatology, 26*(4), 348–355.

Berk, M., et al. (2007). Vitamin D deficiency may play a role in depression. *Medical Hypotheses, 4*(1), 1–4.

Gaines, S. (2005). The saddest season. *Minnesota Medicine, 88*, 25–32.

Holick, M., & Jenkins, M. (2003). *The UV advantage.* New York, NY: Ibooks Inc.

Jorde, R., Waterloo, K., Saleh, F., Haug, E., & Svartberg, J. (2005). The Tromso study. *Journal of Neurology, 10*, 27–32.

Kiraly, S., Kiraly, M., Hawe, R., & Makhani, N. (2006, January). Vitamin D as a neuroactive substance: Review. *Scientific World Journal, 6*, 125–139.

Kornstein, S., & Sloan, D. (2003). Gender differences in depression and response to antidepressant treatment. *Psychiatric Clinics North America, 26*, 581–594.

Obradovic, D., Gronemeyer, H., Lutz, B., & Rein, T. (2006). Cross-talk of vitamin D and glucocorticoids in hippocampal cells. *Journal of Neurochemistry, 96*, 500–509.

Pickett J, (Ed.) (2000). *The American heritage dictionary of the English language.* 4th ed. Boston: Houghton Mifflin Company, p. 1167.

Rucker, D., Allen, J., Fick, G., & Hanley, D. (2002). Vitamin D insufficiency in a population of healthy western Canadians. *Canadian Medical Association Journal, 166*, 1517–1524.

Vasquez, A., Manso G., & Cannell, J. (2004). The clinical importance of vitamin D: A paradigm shift with implications for all healthcare providers. *Alternative Therapies in Health and Medicine, 10*, 28–36.

World Health Organization. (2000). Setting the WHO agenda for mental health. *Bulletin of the World Health Organization*, (Vol. 78, p. 500).

COMPREHENSION CRITICAL APPRAISAL

1. *Abstract:* The study abstract included the problem, sample of women with serum vitamin D levels <40 ng/ml, sample size of 9 with 6 completing the study, treatment of vitamin D_3 supplementation, dependent variable of depressive symptoms measured with the Beck Depression Inventory II (BDI-II), key results, and conclusions. The study purpose and design were not included in the abstract.

2. *Problem:* "Research shows that women are more susceptible to depression than men (Sloan & Kornstein, 2003). Women under 40 years of age are four times more likely to have seasonal affective disorder than men (Gaines, 2005). According to the World Health Organization (WHO), by 2020, depression will be the leading cause of disability worldwide (WHO, 2000). Studies indicate that vitamin D deficiency is associated with increased depressive symptoms (Armstrong, Meenagh, Bickle, Lee, Curran, Finch, 2007; Jorde, Waterloo, Salech, Haug, & Svartberg, 2006). Thus, vitamin D supplementation may provide a natural, inexpensive, and accessible remedy for seasonal mood fluctuations and an adjunct for individuals with depressive symptoms" (Shipowick et al., 2009, p. 429).

Continued

RESEARCH EXAMPLE—cont'd

3. *Purpose:* The purpose is not clearly stated in the study but it is evident from the title and problem that the purpose of this quasi-experimental study was to examine the effect of vitamin D_3 supplementation on depressive symptoms of women during the winter months.

4. *Literature review:* A minimal review of literature is presented in the article. Shipowick et al. (2009) identified three studies that linked vitamin D to depression. Armstrong et al. (2007) found that patients with the lowest vitamin D levels had the highest anxiety and depression scores. This suggested a link between anxious and depressive symptoms and vitamin D deficiency. Berk et al. (2007) found that a higher proportion of depressed patients were vitamin D deficient, supporting the link between depression and vitamin D level. Jorde et al. (2006) found a "statistically significant association between serum vitamin D levels and the Beck Depression Inventory (BDI) scores, indicating that a low serum level was indicative of high depressive symptoms" (p. 431).

5. *Framework:* A biopsychological model (see Figure 12–1) is clearly presented as the framework for this study. Shipowick et al. (2009) described their model in the following way. "Vitamin D_3 is hydroxylated in the liver to become 25-OH vitamin D, the major circulating form of vitamin D. It is activated in the kidneys to become the hormone 1,125-OH vitamin D where it is tightly regulated. Certain organs including the brain also have the capacity to activate vitamin D (Holick & Jenkins, 2003). Both unactivated and activated vitamin D can cross the blood-brain barrier (Kiraly, Kiraly, Hawe, & Makhani, 2006). Based on these data, a biopsychological framework of vitamin D as a hormone that includes depressive symptoms served as an emerging model (Figure 12–1, p. 435). Three physiological pathways between vitamin D and depressive symptoms were identified: (a) Vitamin D in the active form in the body had been shown to stimulate serotonin (Gaines, 2005), a neurotransmitter that is associated with mood elevation; (b) Vitamin D has been associated with down-regulation of glucocorticoid receptor gene activation, which is found to be un-regulated in depression; and (c) Vitamin D has also been found to be neuroprotective, shielding neurons from toxins such as glucocorticoids and other excitotoxic insults (Obradovic, Gronemeyer, Lutz, & Rein, 2006)" (p. 430).

6. *Research Questions and Hypothesis*: "The following research questions guided the study: (a) Is there a significant relationships between serum vitamin D levels and depressive symptoms? and (b) Do depressive symptoms in women with low serum vitamin D levels improve 8 weeks after initiation of vitamin D_3 supplementation (5,000 IU daily) during the fall and winter?" (pp. 429–430).

7. *Variables:* Shipowick et al. (2009) clearly presented the conceptual and operational definitions for the independent and dependent variables. The conceptual and operational definitions for vitamin D supplementation and depressive symptoms are provided in the following.

Independent Variable: Vitamin D_3 Supplementation

Conceptual Definition

Vitamin D_3 improves depressive symptoms through three physiological pathways: (a) its active form in the body stimulates serotonin, a neurotransmitter associated with mood elevations; (b) it is associated with down-regulation of glucocorticoid receptor gene activation, which is up-regulated in depression; and (c) it is neuroprotective, shielding neurons from toxins such as glucocorticoids and other excitotoxic insults.

Operational Definition

The treatment of vitamin D_3 supplementation was implemented by providing the subjects with 5000 IU of vitamin D_3 daily for 8 weeks.

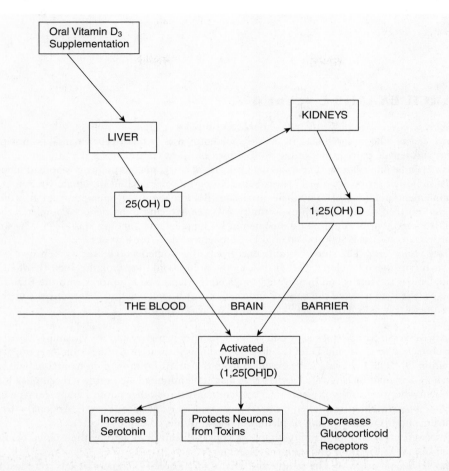

Figure 12–1. The biopsychological model of vitamin D: hormone that elevates mood. From The UV Advantage Fig. 1.3: Holick, M., & Jenkins, M. (2003). *New understanding of how vitamin D benefits health.* New York: Ibooks Inc. Adapted with permission. Shipowick, C. D., Moore, C. B., Corbett, C., & Bindler, R. (2009). Vitamin D and depressive symptoms in women during the winter: A pilot study. *Applied Nursing Research, 22*(3), 222.

Dependent Variable: Depressive Symptoms

Conceptual Definition

Depressive symptoms are influenced by levels of serotonin, actions of glucocorticoid receptors, and neurons exposed to toxins.

Operational Definition

Depressive symptoms were measured with the Beck Depression Inventory II (BDI-II) Likert scale.

Continued

RESEARCH EXAMPLE—cont'd

8. *Attribute variables:* The only attribute variable identified was age.
9. *Research design:* The research design was clearly identified as "a quasi-experimental pretest-posttest design with female participants acting as their own pre-post control" (p. 431).
    a. *Treatment or Intervention:* "Per usual medical care at the clinic, participants who had blood tests that indicated serum vitamin D levels below 40 ng/ml were advised to initiate vitamin D_3 supplementation (5000 IU) by their physicians. Before vitamin D_3 supplementation, women were informed of the research opportunity. Women agreeing to participate completed the BDI-II survey prior to initiating the vitamin D_3 supplementation" (pp. 431–432). The women participants took the 5000 IU vitamin D_3 supplement daily for 8 weeks.
    b. *Group Assignment:* The study has only one group of 9 women who served as their own control. This means they completed BDI-II scale as the pretest and then took the 5000 IU of vitamin D_3 supplement treatment and then were posttested for depressed symptoms with the BDI-II. Thus, the pretest is considered the control and the posttest is conducted to determine the effect of the treatment (Burns & Grove, 2009).
10. Sample
    a. *Sample criteria:* Sample inclusion criteria were females being treated for vitamin D deficiency or insufficiency with vitamin D level below 40 ng/ml as measured by the serum level of 25-OH vitamin D. "The following were excluded from the study: (a) those with mental impairments such as dementia or language barriers that may have inhibited answering written questions; (b) women who were using or planned to use tanning beds or other phototherapy; (c) women who planned on traveling to sunnier, more tropical areas (e.g., Mexico, Hawaii, Arizona) during the winter; and (d) women taking or planning to take antidepressants" (p. 431).
    b. *Sampling method:* Nonprobability sample of convenience is indicated by the women being asked to take part in the study and then they voluntarily participated.
    c. *Sample size and attrition:* The sample size was $N = 9$. Three (33%) participants were lost from the study and 6 (67%) completed. This study included no mention of power analysis or acceptance rate for study participation.
11. *Institutional review board and type of consent:* "Following university institutional review board approval and the approval of the clinical agency where the study was carried out … Before vitamin D_3 supplementation, women were informed of the research opportunity. Women agreeing to participate completed the BDI-II. …" (p. 431).
12. Study setting: The setting was a medical clinic in southeastern Washington. The women took the vitamin D_3 supplements daily in their homes.
13. Measurement methods: The study only included one dependent variable that was measured with one measurement method, the BDI-II Likert scale. However, the sample inclusion criteria required that the women have a serum 25-OH vitamin D level. Therefore both of the measurement methods are included in the following table.

Name of Measurement Method	Author	Type of Measurement Method	Level of Measurement	Reliability or Precision	Validity or Accuracy
Beck Depression Inventory II (BDI-II)	Beck	Likert Scale	Interval	BDI-II commonly used depression screening tool with demonstrated reliability. For this study, the BDI-II had Cronbach alphas of 0.81 at baseline and 0.95 at follow-up.	BDI-II had demonstrated validity in previous studies and was used in Jorde et al. (2005) study cited in the review of literature. Successive use validity since scale is used in previous studies and the current study.
25-OH vitamin D level	Unknown	Physiologic measurement method: Laboratory test of serum vitamin D level	Ratio	Precision of lab test not addressed in the study. No discussion of the collection and analysis of the serum for the vitamin D levels. Serum collection was done in same clinic for pre- and posttests.	Vitamin D is hydroxylated in the liver to become 25-OH vitamin D, the major circulating form of vitamin D. Thus, 25-OH vitamin D is the most accurate measure of vitamin D in the body to identify deficiencies.

14. *Data collection procedures:* The women were screened for their 25-OH vitamin D level in January to March. If the vitamin D level was <40 ng/ml, the women were informed of the study and asked to participate. Those volunteering to participate in the study then were asked to complete the BDI-II and then started on the 5000 IU of vitamin D_3 every day for 8 weeks. At the end of the 8th week, the women again were asked to complete the BDI-II to document their depression symptoms. The 25-OH vitamin D level was also determined. Those involved in treatment implementation and data collection were not identified. The training of individuals for data collection and implementation of the treatment was not described.

15. *Statistical analyses:* The Statistical Package for the Social Sciences (SPSS) 14.0 was used to perform the statistical analyses. Only the 6 participants completing the study were included in the analyses. The analyses conducted are summarized in the following table.

Continued

RESEARCH EXAMPLE—cont'd

Purpose of Analysis	Analysis Technique	Statistic	Results	Probability (p)
Description of subjects' age	Mean, Standard deviation, and Range	X SD $range$	42.2 13.17 23-55	
Description of Depression Symptoms measured with the BDI-II	Mean Standard deviations Differences in means Line Graph	$\bar{X}$ SD Average SD Mean Difference	Pretest Posttest 31.8333 21.1667 4.79236 7.7616 10.66667 Figure 12-3	
Description of 25-OH vitamin D levels	Mean Standard deviations Differences in means Line Graph	$\bar{X}$ SD Average SD Mean Difference	Pretest Posttest 21.8333 48.1667 8.32867 15.68014 −26.33333 Figure 12–2	
Difference between the pretest and the posttest on depressive symptoms	Dependent or paired t-test	t	3.366	$p = 0.020$
Difference between the pretest and posttest for 25-OH vitamin D level	Dependent or paired t-test	t	−4.114	$p = 0.009$

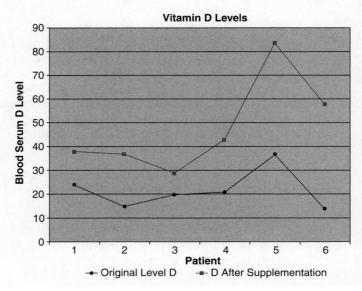

Figure 12–2. Comparing vitamin D levels before and after supplementation. This graph shows that vitamin D_3 supplementation is associated with an increase in serum 25-OH vitamin D levels by an average of 27 ng/ml after 8 weeks. Shipowick, C. D., Moore, C. B., Corbett, C., & Bindler, R. (2009). Vitamin D and depressive symptoms in women during the winter: A pilot study. *Applied Nursing Research, 22*(3), 223.

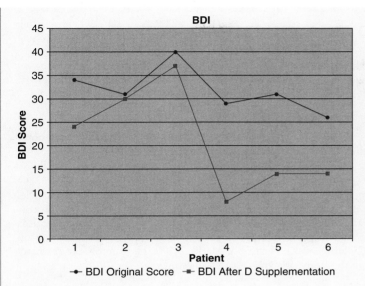

Figure 12–3. Comparing BDI-II scores before and after supplementation. This graph shows that vitamin D supplementation is associated with a decline (improved mood: a negative correlations) in BDI-II scores of an average of 10 points. Shipowick, C. D., Moore, C. B., Corbett, C., & Bindler, R. (2009). Vitamin D and depressive symptoms in women during the winter: A pilot study. *Applied Nursing Research, 22*(3), 224.

16. *Interpretation of findings:* "Following supplementation, serum vitamin D levels increased in all participants with an average increase of 27 ng/ml. At the prescribed intake of 5000 IU daily, a significant reduction in depressive symptoms was realized after supplementation. Further, among the three women with a postsupplementation serum vitamin D level greater than 40, all had BDI-II scores of 14 or less, suggestive of normal mood with minimal depressive symptoms" (p. 432).

17. *Limitations of the study:* The small sample size was identified as a limitation. The reasons for three of the women not achieving serum vitamin D_3 levels above 40 ng/ml were unclear. Maybe they were not taking the vitamin D_3 consistently or needed longer than 8 weeks to achieve optimal vitamin D levels of 40 to 65 ng/ml. The design was identified as a limitation and Shipowick et al. (2009) recommended the use of stronger designs in future studies.

18. *Conclusions:* "In summary, this pilot study provides evidence to suggest that women who suffer from seasonal depressive symptoms may benefit from vitamin D_3 supplementation if serum vitamin D levels are low (<40 ng/ml). These findings are consistent with other studies that indicate that higher vitamin D levels improve sense of well-being (Armstrong et al., 2007; Berk et al., 2007; Jorde et al., 2006)" (p. 433).

19. *Implications for nursing:* The researchers provide no specific implications for nursing practice.

20. *Suggestions for further research:* "Further research with a larger sample size and stronger design is warranted to continue to investigate the clinical utility of vitamin D_3 supplementation. ... Replication of this study with a larger, adequately powered sample is needed to provide a more definitive understanding of the relationship between vitamin D supplementation and seasonal depressive symptoms. Additionally, further research to determine factors related to vitamin D_3 dosing is needed. ... More frequent analyses of serum vitamin D levels and measuring adherence to supplementation are warranted in future studies. Future studies should be conducted with a randomized and blinded design to account for placebo effect" (p. 433).

Continued

COMPARISON AND ANALYSIS CRITICAL APPRAISAL

This section discusses the strengths and weaknesses of the steps of the research process and the logical links among these steps. The abstract, problem, purpose, literature review, framework, methodology, results, and discussion elements of the article are critically appraised.

Abstract

The abstract is very brief and includes the study problem, sample size, significant results, and conclusions. The abstract would have been strengthened by including the study purpose and design.

Problem and Purpose

The research problem is clearly identified in the abstract and in the first few paragraphs of the article. This is a significant clinical problem that could be detected, managed, and monitored by nurses in collaboration with physicians. Vitamin D insufficiency is a very common problem in health care today, as is depression. Additional research is needed to determine the impact of vitamin D supplementation on depression symptoms (Brown, 2009; Cullum, Ciliska, Haynes, & Marks, 2008). The purpose is not clearly stated in the study, but is inferred from the study title and research questions.

Literature Review

The literature review is brief, including only three studies, and would have been strengthened by the addition of more quasi-experimental studies focused on the impact of vitamin D supplementation on mood. However, the three studies cited do provide a basis for conducting this study. A final summary of what is known and not known about the problem studied would have added clarity to the literature review (Burns & Grove, 2009).

Framework

The framework section is a major strength of this study. Shipowick and colleagues (2009) provided a clear, concise, appropriate physiological framework for their study. The biopsychological model presented in the study provides a clear link of how vitamin D as a hormone elevates mood and decreases depressive symptoms. The study framework also provided clear conceptual definitions of the independent and dependent variables, and these conceptual definitions provided a basis for operationalizing these variables in this study (Burns & Grove, 2009).

Methods

The study design is a single group pretest and posttest, with subjects serving as their own control. This is a weak design because there is only a treatment group and no comparison group to determine if the treatment is effective or if the change from pre- to posttest is caused by extraneous variables (Burns & Grove, 2009; Creswell, 2009). However, the design does provide a means to examine the two research questions. The sample size was small, with $N = 9$, and no power analysis was conducted to determine an adequate sample size for the study. In addition, the study has a high 33% attrition, with 3 subjects dropping out of the study before the 8 weeks of the treatment are completed (Grove, 2007). No rationale is provided for why the subjects did not complete the study. However, the study results were significant, indicating the sample was adequately powered and no Type II error occurred (Burns & Grove, 2009).

The sampling method was one of convenience and there is greater potential for sampling error with a nonprobability sample than a random sample. However, the researchers provide very strong sample inclusion and exclusion criteria that limit the potential effects of extraneous variables and improve the representativeness of the sample. Only the age of the participants are described, and it might have been helpful to include the ethnicity and history of depression. The study was ethical, because it was approved for conduct by the institutional review boards of the university and clinic and informed consent was obtained from the study participants (Creswell, 2009).

The study included a strong treatment of vitamin D_3 supplementation of 5000 IU daily for 8 weeks. The researchers needed to provide more detail, however, about how the treatment was implemented. If the treatment was implemented by more than one person, the training to promote consistency in the treatment needs to be addressed (Santacroce et al., 2004).

The BDI-II is a strong measurement strategy for depression and has been used in many other studies over the years. In addition, the Cronbach alphas were strong and supported the reliability of this scale in this study. However, the measurement section would have been strengthened by a more detailed discussion of the reliability and validity of the BDI-II based on previous research (Roberts & Stone, 2003; Robinson, 2001). The researchers discussed the scoring for the BDI-II and indicated that the scores could range from 0 to 63. They also indicated the meaning for the different scores with normal being scores from 0 to 13, mild depression included scores from 14 to 19, moderate depression included scores from 20 to 28, and severe depression included scores from 29 to 63.

The 25-OH vitamin D level is the strongest measurement of vitamin D levels in the body and is the most effective way to identify women with insufficient vitamin D levels. Additional discussion was needed, however, of the precision and accuracy of this laboratory test in the study (DeKeyser & Pugh, 1990). Shipowick et al. (2009) did not indicate who collected the data. If more than one person collected data, the reliability or consistency of the data collection process needs to be addressed (Burns & Grove, 2009; Santacroce et al., 2004).

Results

The statistical techniques used to analyze data from the BDI-II and the 25-OH vitamin D levels were clearly identified and appropriate. The analysis techniques (descriptive and inferential) are appropriate for the level of measurement of the variables (Grove, 2007; Munro, 2005). The results are clearly and concisely presented in narrative form, table, and graphs to facilitate understanding. The sample size was small but adequate to detect significant differences between the pre- and posttests for depression symptoms and the vitamin D levels. This section would have been strengthened by linking the results to the two research questions.

Discussion

The findings were as expected, and the statistical and clinical significance of the findings are clearly addressed (Burns & Grove, 2009). The findings were supportive of the study framework and consistent with previous research, and this was documented in the article. The conclusions were clearly expressed and appropriate based on the study results and findings. The researchers identified the study limitations and provided specific, appropriate ideas for future studies to overcome the limitations of this study. The researchers did not make recommendations for nursing practice but focused on the need for additional research before making changes in practice.

EVALUATION CRITICAL APPRAISAL

This study examines significant clinical problems (seasonal depression and vitamin D deficiencies in women) and examines the effectiveness of vitamin D_3 supplementation for these problems. This study has many strengths and some weaknesses, which leads one to conclude that the findings are credible and an

Continued

EVALUATION CRITICAL APPRAISAL—cont'd

accurate reflection of reality. The findings, women who suffer from seasonal depressive symptoms may benefit from vitamin D_3 supplementation if their vitamin D levels are low, are supportive of the study framework (see Figure 12–1). In addition, these findings are consistent with those of previous researchers (Armstrong et al., 2007; Berk et al., 2007; Jorde et al., 2006).

The findings of the Shipowick et al. (2009) study increase our understanding of the link between vitamin D and depressive symptoms in women and provide direction for future studies. Vitamin D_3 has a potential to be an effective treatment for seasonal depression in women with low vitamin D levels. Because of the small sample size and the limitations of the study design, however, the researchers do not recommend generalizing these findings from the sample to the population. Shipowick and colleagues provide excellent, detailed directions for future studies. They do not recommend using the findings in practice at this time. Clinically, patients are currently being tested for deficiencies in vitamin D levels and treated with 5000 IU of vitamin D_3. Even though research is still inadequate to recommend treatment of depressive symptoms with vitamin D, this is an important area for further research.

Understanding the Qualitative Research Critical Appraisal Process

Nurses in every phase and field of practice need experience in critically appraising both qualitative and quantitative studies. Although qualitative studies require a different approach to critical appraisal than used when appraising a quantitative study (Sandelowski, 2008), appraisal in both cases has a common purpose—determining the rigor with which the methods were applied. Critical appraisal of qualitative studies focuses on how the integrity of the design and methods will affect the credibility and meaningfulness of the findings and their usefulness in clinical practice (Pickler, 2007). Burns (1989) first described the standards for rigorous qualitative research 20 years ago. Since that time, other criteria have been published (Cesario, Morin, & Santa-Donato, 2002; Clissett, 2008; Fossey, Harvey, McDermott, & Davidson, 2002; Morse, 1991; Pickler, 2007) and have been the source of considerable debate (Barbour & Barbour, 2003; Cohen & Crabtree, 2008; Nelson, 2008; Stige, Malterud, & Midtgarden, 2009; Whittemore, Chase, & Mandle, 2001).

Two nurse researchers who shaped the ongoing dialogue on qualitative research are Dr. Margarete Sandelowski from the University of North Carolina at Chapel Hill and Dr. Julie Barroso from Duke University School of Nursing. They obtained two grants for the study of *Analytic Techniques for Qualitative Metasynthesis* from the National Institute of Nursing Research/National Institutes of Health (R01 NR004907). They developed their analysis techniques by examining all the qualitative studies conducted with women living with HIV infection. As they read the 114 reports of these studies, they realized they needed a consistent method of deconstructing and appraising the reports. Their critical appraisal method was first published as an article (Sandelowski & Barroso, 2002) and was included in the book that resulted from their studies, *Handbook for Synthesizing Qualitative Research* (Sandelowski & Barroso, 2007). Their methods of critically appraising qualitative studies are adapted for this text.

CRITICAL APPRAISAL GUIDELINES: QUALITATIVE STUDIES

Problem Statement

1. Identify the clinical problem and research problem that led to the study. What was not known about the clinical problem that, if it were known, nurses could use the information to make a difference? This gap in knowledge is the research problem.
2. How did the author establish the significance of the study? In other words, why should the reader care about this study? Look for statements about human suffering, costs of treatment, or the number of people affected by the clinical problem.

Purpose and Research Questions

1. Identify the purpose of the study. An author may clearly state the purpose of the study or may describe the purpose as the study goals, objectives, or aims.
2. List research questions that the study was designed to answer. If the author does not explicitly provide the questions, attempt to infer the questions from the answers. What information did the author include as findings?
3. Were the purpose and research questions related to the problem?
4. Were qualitative methods appropriate to answer the research questions?

Literature Review

In some research articles, the literature review will be identified clearly as a Review of the Literature. Some authors may incorporate the review into a section titled Background and Significance.

1. Did the author cite quantitative and qualitative studies relevant to the focus of the study? What other types of literature did the author include?
2. Are the references current? For qualitative studies, the author may have included studies older than the 5-year limit typically used for quantitative studies. Findings of older qualitative studies may be relevant to a qualitative study.
3. Identify the disciplines of the authors of studies cited in this paper. Does it appear that the author searched databases outside of CINAHL for relevant studies?
4. Did the author evaluate or indicate the weaknesses of the available studies?
5. The literature review should be a synthesis of what is known and not known.
   An author may have been unable to include all the studies and literature relevant to the study because of the page limitations of the journal. Did the literature review include adequate information to build a logical argument? Another way to ask the question is, Did the author provide enough evidence to support the verdict that the study was needed?

Frame of Reference

Qualitative studies emerge from a variety of philosophical or theoretical perspectives. For example, some qualitative researchers ascribe to a philosophical perspective such as phenomenology. The methods used by qualitative researchers are determined by the philosophical foundation of their work. Some researchers may not specify a philosophy but

Continued

CRITICAL APPRAISAL GUIDELINES—cont'd

identify a theory that provides a context for the study, such as a theory of coping or a theory of symptoms.

1. Did the author identify a specific perspective from which the study was developed? If so, what was it?
2. When a researcher uses the grounded theory method of qualitative inquiry, the researcher may develop a framework or diagram as part of the findings of the study. Was a framework developed from the study findings?

Research Tradition

1. Identify the stated or implied research tradition upon which the study was based. In general, qualitative studies are founded in an interpretive paradigm and methods of naturalistic inquiry. A nurse appraising a study for which the research tradition was not stated can infer, for example, that the tradition was interpretive naturalistic inquiry. Naturalistic inquiry is a label that can be applied to most qualitative studies, because researchers using this approach collect data in real life, natural settings (Lincoln & Guba, 1985). The data are interpreted to describe participants' perspectives on the phenomenon being studied.
2. Provide a paraphrased description of the research tradition used. Refer back to Chapter 3 for descriptions of different qualitative research perspectives or traditions. Another source for this information is the Stanford Encyclopedia of Philosophy (*http://plato.stanford.edu/ contents.html*)
3. Were the methods used in the study consistent with the research tradition?

Sampling and Sample

Qualitative studies most often use purposeful sampling, also called purposive sampling. A researcher purposefully selects study participants who have experienced what the researcher is studying (Patton, 2004). For example, the researcher conducting a phenomenological study of chronic pain among cancer survivors will select subjects who are cancer survivors and have chronic pain. Characteristics that are used to decide if a person is an appropriate subject for a study are called inclusion criteria. Exclusion criteria are characteristics that indicate a person should not be included in a study, such as having mental illness or cognitive impairment. Chapter 9 provides more details on sampling in qualitative research.

1. Identify how subjects were selected.
2. At what sites were subjects recruited for the study? Did the sites for recruitment fit the sampling needs of the study?
3. What were the inclusion and exclusion criteria for the sample?
4. Were the selected subjects able to provide data relevant to the study purpose and research questions?
5. How many people participated in the study? Did any potential subjects refuse to participate? Did any of the participants start but not finish the study?

CRITICAL APPRAISAL GUIDELINES—cont'd

Data Collection

1. Qualitative researchers may use interviews, focus groups, or observations to gather data. How were data collected in this study?
2. What rationale did the author provide for using this data collection method?
3. Identify the time period for data collection of the study.
4. Describe the sequence of data collection events for a participant. For example, were data collected from one interview or a series of interviews? Were focus group participants provided an opportunity to provide additional data or review the preliminary conclusions of the researcher?

Protection of Human Participants

Qualitative studies tend to address areas of human life that are "sensitive" and require care in the way they are addressed by researchers (Cowles, 1988). For example, many of the topics studied by qualitative researchers are social or moral issues not talked about in common society. Imagine being a survivor of the Rwandan genocide and being asked to participate in a study about the health implications of being a survivor. Imagine having lost a child to a congenital heart defect and being asked to participate in a study of how the death of a child affects the parents. Researchers approaching persons about being in these studies would want to exercise additional caution and sensitivity. Qualitative topics may be personal or family issues that are seldom shared outside the family. The participants may feel embarrassment or shame at admitting that they or their family are involved in the topic being studied. They may fear that the researcher will talk to others about very private information they are sharing with the researcher. A qualitative report should provide clues that the researcher was aware of these concerns and addressed them appropriately.

1. Identify the benefits and risks of participation addressed by the authors. Were there benefits or risks the authors do not identify?
2. How were recruitment and consent techniques adjusted to accommodate the sensitivity of the subject matter and psychological distress of potential participants?
3. How were data collection and management techniques adapted in acknowledgment of participant sensitivity and vulnerability? For example, did the authors have a counselor or other resources available for participants who might become upset or disturbed by the interview?

Data Management and Analysis

1. Describe the data management and analysis methods used in the study.
2. Did the author discuss how the rigor of the process was assured? For example, does the author describe maintaining a paper trail of critical decisions that were made during the analysis of the data?
3. Analysis of qualitative data is influenced by the experiences and perspectives of those doing the analysis. What measures were used to minimize the effects of researcher bias? For example, did two researchers independently analyze the data and compare their analyses?
4. Did the data management and analysis methods fit the research purposes and data?

Continued

CRITICAL APPRAISAL GUIDELINES—cont'd

Findings

1. Did the findings address the purpose of the study?
2. Were the data sufficiently analyzed? Findings in a qualitative study are expected to be more than the words that participants said. The researcher is expected to identify themes or abstract concepts that emerged from the data.
3. Were the interpretations of data congruent with data collected?
4. Did the researcher address variations in the findings by relevant sample characteristics?

Discussion

1. Did the results offer new information about the target phenomenon?
2. Were the findings linked to findings in other studies or other relevant literatures?
3. Describe the clinical, policy, theoretical, and other significance of the findings. Does the author explore these applications?

Logic and Form of Findings

1. Were readers able to hear the voice of the participants and gain an understanding of the phenomenon studied?
2. Were elements of the research report easily found by readers?
3. Did the overall presentation of the study fit its purpose, method, and findings?
4. Was there a coherent logic to the presentation of findings?

Evaluation Summary

1. Do the findings provide a credible reflection of reality? If so, how can the findings be used in nursing practice?
2. What do the findings add to the current body of knowledge?
3. State the conclusion of the critical appraisal of the study.

CRITICAL APPRAISAL OF QUALITATIVE STUDY

This section of the chapter includes a qualitative study and a critical appraisal of that study. The study by Martsolf and Draucker (2008) on the legacy of childhood sexual abuse and family adversity is included in its entirety. This study is followed by a critical appraisal using the guidelines introduced in the previous section (Sandelowski & Barroso, 2007).

RESEARCH EXAMPLE OF A QUALITATIVE STUDY

Clinical Scholarship

The Legacy of Childhood Sexual Abuse and Family Adversity

Donna S. Martsolf, Claire Burke Draucker

Purpose: To describe the process by which childhood adversity influences the life course of survivors of childhood sexual abuse.

Design: A community-based, qualitative, grounded-theory design.

Methods: In this grounded theory study, data were drawn from open-ended interviews conducted as part of a larger study of women's and men's responses to sexual violence. The current study indicates the experiences of 48 female and 40 male survivors of childhood sexual abuse and family adversity. Data were analyzed using the constant comparison method.

Findings: Participants described a sense of inheriting a life of abuse and adversity. The process by which childhood adversity influences the life course of adult survivors of childhood sexual abuse is labeled Living the Family Legacy. The theory representing the process of Living the Family Legacy includes three major life patterns: (a) being stuck in the family legacy, (b) being plagued by the family legacy, and (c) rejecting the family legacy/creating a new one. Associated with these life patterns are three processes by which participants passed on a legacy to others, often their children: (a) passing on the family legacy, (b) taking a stab at passing on a new legacy, and (c) passing on a new legacy.

Conclusions: The legacy of abuse and adversity has a profound effect on the lives of survivors of childhood sexual abuse. There are several trajectories by which the influence of childhood adversity unfolds in the lives of adult survivors and by which the legacy is passed on to others.

Clinical Relevance: The model representing the theoretical process of Living the Family Legacy can be used by clinicians who work with survivors of childhood sexual abuse and childhood adversity, especially those who have parenting concerns.

[Key words: childhood sexual abuse, parenting, family adversity, grounded theory]

JOURNAL OF NURSING SCHOLARSHIP, 2008; 40:4, 333–340. ©2008 SIGMA THETA TAU INTERNATIONAL.

*   *   *

Childhood sexual abuse (CSA) is a prevalent social and public health problem. The American Medical Association (2003) defines CSA as "the engagement of a child in sexual activities for which the child is developmentally unprepared and cannot give consent" (p. 5). According to the World Health Organization (2002), CSA is a worldwide problem with 25% of girls and 8% of boys reporting experiencing sexual abuse before the age of 18. Because CSA often goes unreported, the actual incidence of CSA is thought to be much higher than that reported by governmental agencies (Russell & Bolen, 2000). For both women and men, a history of childhood sexual abuse is associated with a variety of short- and long-term psychological, social, behavioral, and health-related effects (Centers for Disease Control and Prevention, 2007; Dube et al., 2005).

Children who are sexually abused, whether the abuse is intra- or extra-familial, frequently grow up in adverse family environments. CSA often co-occurs with physical or emotional abuse or neglect; parental problems with substance abuse, mental illness, economic instability, or domestic violence; and maladaptive family functioning, such as low levels of cohesiveness and high levels of conflict (Dong et al., 2004; Gold, Hyman, & Andrés-Hyman, 2004; Higgins &

Donna S. Martsolf, RN, PhD. *Delta Xi*, Professor; **Claire Burke Draucker**, RN, PhD, *Delta Xi*, Distinguished Professor; both at College of Nursing, Kent State University, Kent, OH. This study is funded by the National Institute of Nursing Research [R01 NR08230–01 A1]; Claire Burke Draucker, Principal Investigator. Correspondence to Dr. Martsolf, College of Nursing, Kent State University, Kent, OH 44242–0001. E-mail: dmartsol@kent.edu
Accepted for publication June 8, 2008.

Continued

RESEARCH EXAMPLE OF A QUALITATIVE STUDY—cont'd

Legacy of Abuse

McCabe, 2003). Survivors of CSA often report that in their families the abuse was often minimized, denied, or blamed on the child (Dunlap, Golub, & Johnson, 2003).

The role of family dysfunction and other types of abuse as the cause of later negative outcomes in survivors of CSA has been debated. In some studies, pathogenic family variables have been shown to be better predictors of adult disturbance than are sexual abuse variables (Higgins & McCabe, 2003), whereas in other studies sexual abuse has been shown to be associated with negative long-term effects beyond those accounted for by family environment (Roesler & McKenzie, 1994). While the co-occurrence of multiple types of abuse seems to increase the risk of adult disturbance, the severity of abuse has been shown to be a stronger predictor of trauma symptoms in adults (Clemmons, Walsh, DiLillo, & Messman-Moore, 2007).

One area of functioning that is particularly likely to be affected by an adverse family environment is how survivors parent their children. Researchers have found that parenting problems of adult survivors of CSA include failure to establish clear generational boundaries, inadequate monitoring and supervision, and the use of harsh or inconsistent discipline (Banyard, Williams, & Siegel, 2003; DiLillo & Damashek, 2003). Experts warn, however, that the relationship among sexual abuse, childhood adversity, and parenting difficulties is complex and might be mediated by factors such as mental health problems, substance abuse, and domestic violence experienced by adult survivors (Banyard et al. 2003; Locke & Newcomb, 2004; Schuetze & Eiden, 2005).

While the influence of negative family characteristics on the later functioning of adult survivors of CSA has been examined, few studies (Dunlap et al., 2003) have explored how these characteristics shape the life course of survivors, especially from their own perspectives. Many researchers have attempted to isolate and measure types of childhood maltreatment and family characteristics to determine how they correlate with indices of adult psychopathology (DiLillo & Damashek, 2003). The complex processes by which the influences of adverse family experiences develop through adulthood have not been reported in-depth. The purpose of this study, therefore, is to describe the process by which childhood adversity influences the life course of adult survivors of CSA from their perspectives.

Methods

Data are drawn from an ongoing qualitative, community-based study aimed at developing a theoretical framework to describe, explain, or predict women's and men's responses to sexual violence. For the larger study, 121 women and men were recruited from several socioeconomically diverse communities in the metropolitan area of a mid-sized city in Midwestern United States. Participants were included in the larger study if they had expe-

rienced sexual violence at any time in their lives. Research associates placed announcements throughout the communities and networked with community leaders and residents, who then promoted the study in a variety of settings, including churches, community agencies, and neighborhood centers (Martsolf, Courey, Chapman, Draucker, & Mims, 2006). Interested individuals called a toll-free number and were screened by advanced-practice mental health nurses using a script of questions designed by the researchers to detect acute emotional distress that would make participation risky. Those who met inclusion criteria were scheduled for an interview if appropriate. Institutional review board approval was obtained and participants signed consent forms.

Advanced-practice psychiatric and mental health nurse research associates conducted open-ended, face-to-face interviews that lasted 1 to 2 hours. Participants were asked to describe (a) the sexual violence they had experienced, (b) how they managed following the violence, (c) how the violence affected their lives, and (d) how they healed, coped, or recovered from the violence. Participants were paid $35 for each interview to compensate for their time and transportation costs. Interviews were audiotaped and transcribed. Data were collected over a 17-month period from December 2004 to April 2006. Pseudonyms are used in this article to protect the identity of participants and others they discuss. Quotations are the verbatim words of the participants.

Grounded theory methods (Glaser & Strauss, 1967), which were focused on the complexities of people undergoing change and the influence of social interactions on outcomes (Benoliel, 1996), were used for both the larger and current study. The aim of grounded theory is to identify common psychosocial processes used by people who share a life challenge (Glaser & Strauss). The choice of grounded theory for the current study was based on the researchers' belief that the ways in which childhood adversity influence the life course of adult survivors of CSA are complex processes that change over time and are influenced by both psychological and social factors.

Sample

For this study, a subsample of participants was selected from the 121 participants of the larger study. Inclusion criteria for this study were having had (a) an experience of CSA (as defined above) and (b) a childhood family environment that was adverse. Adversity could include: (a) physical or emotional abuse or neglect; (b) domestic violence; (c) disturbed, chaotic, or non-nurturing family interactions; or (d) other indices of family dysfunction, including parental substance abuse, mental illness, or imprisonment.

Eighty-eight participants from the larger study met criteria for this study. The sample included 48 women and 40 men who experienced both CSA and family adversity. Ages ranged from 19 to 62 years. Thirty-eight participants were African American, 36 were Caucasian, 1 was Asian,

1 was Hispanic, 4 were more than one race, and 8 did not report race. Forty-eight of the participants reported an income under $10,000; 17 between $10,000 and $30,000; 10 between $30,000 and $50,000; 7 above $50,000; and 6 did not report income. Thirty-two participants had no children, 20 had one child, 12 had two children, 21 had more than two children (the most reported was eight); 3 did not report number of children.

Data Analysis

Data were analyzed by the research team using constant comparison techniques as described by Schreiber (2001). Constant comparison techniques involve comparing coded data with other data and with developing concepts through each of three levels of data analysis as described below. The theoretical constructs that serve as the basis for the theory presented in this article emerged as the team analyzed data for the larger study. Living the Family Legacy, therefore, is one of several theories that were developed from the data set of the larger project.

Three levels of coding were used to develop the theory for this study. First-level coding is a line-by-line examination of the data (Schreiber, 2001). During the first-level coding of transcripts for the larger study, the team noted that many participants, especially those whose sexual violence occurred during childhood, spoke as much—or more—about problems with how they were "raised" as they did about the sexual abuse itself. They described family environments characterized by parental maltreatment including harsh discipline, chaotic living situations, lack of nurturance, and lack of support for revealing, stopping, or healing from the abuse.

Because of the amount of data coded to parenting, the team determined that parenting was an emerging category. Second-level coding, the comparison of first-level codes with existing and new data (Schreiber, 2001), was conducted to create increasingly more abstract categories. As this process progressed, the team broadened the parenting category to create categories related to any adversity in the family-of-origin and its effects and began to hypothesize how these categories were related. The team determined that these categories were most applicable to those with CSA experiences, and thus these participants became the sample for the current study.

Third-level coding, the exploration of the relationship among categories, was conducted on selected transcripts of survivors of CSA to determine whether the hypotheses and the emerging theory were supported. Theoretical sampling principles (Draucker, Martsolf, Ross, & Rusk, 2007) guided selection of transcripts for third-level coding. Transcripts were selected that were information-rich (i.e., had much data related to the emerging theory), typical (i.e., were common manifestations of the theory), deviant (i.e., seemed to be inconsistent with the theory), extreme (i.e., had intense manifestations of the theory), and theoretically relevant (i.e., were illustrative of the construct of legacy). A close examination of these transcripts resulted in refinement of the theory. Grounded theory strategies of memo-ing (i.e., tracking analytic decisions), diagramming (i.e., depicting the proposed relationships among variables), and member checks (i.e., validating emerging constructs with subsequent participants) were used to enhance the credibility of the theory (Lincoln & Guba, 1985; Schreiber, 2001).

The Theory: Living the Family Legacy

The data showed that participants had a sense that they had inherited a life of adversity and abuse. They inherited this life not only from their parents or parent surrogates, but also from other family member—including ancestors whom they had never met. The inheritance included memories of traumatic events, vulnerabilities to further maltreatment, and ways of life that reflected those in their families-of-origin. The concept of a legacy was therefore used to indicate participants' sentiments that the inheritance came from several generations back, was something they carried with them to adulthood, and was something they could pass on to others, especially their children. The researchers therefore labeled the process by which childhood adversity influences the life course of adult survivors of CSA as Living the Family Legacy. A model depicting the process, which includes three life patterns and three ways of passing on a legacy, is shown in the **Figure.**

Inheriting the Legacy

Participants described an entire gamut of abuse and adverse experiences in their families-of-origin. The abuse was perpetrated by parents, stepparents, primary caretakers, grandparents, siblings, aunts, uncles, and cousins. Many participants had experienced several types of severe abuse. Stuart, a man who had experienced sexual abuse and beatings by his stepmother, said, "She'd lock me in cubbyholes, up in our attic, and sit in front of the door, to where I couldn't get out of it." Others described physical and emotional neglect; parental substance abuse, mental illness, imprisonment, absence, and domestic violence; and disturbed family interactions, such as rigid control of children's activities or a lot of conflict. For some, family life was chaotic. For others, the family environment was marked by a lack of supervision and absence of nurturance. Randy was a 38-year-old who had engaged in child prostitution, dealt drugs as a school-aged child, and was raped at age 14, all without his parents' awareness. He indicated that being ignored by his father caused him the most pain. He explained, "My father and me have talked collectively—you can count on this hand, and I'm almost 40 years old. We're just like strangers. I wanted what other kids had—a conversation."

Many participants indicated that memories of their painful childhood experiences would stay with them forever and left them particularly susceptible to ongoing maltreatment or victimization. Some engaged in sexual activities at

Continued

RESEARCH EXAMPLE OF A QUALITATIVE STUDY—cont'd

Legacy of Abuse

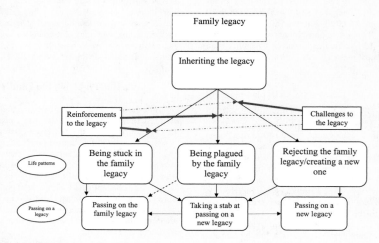

Figure. Living the family legacy.

an early age because they wanted "someone to love me," used drugs and alcohol to numb their pain, developed a poor sense of self because of how they were treated by their families, and failed to acquire the interpersonal skills or values they needed to form healthy relationships. Allison, a 25-year-old woman who experienced a lifetime of abuse, explained, "I don't get along with [others]. Being abused by my stepdad–like my conscience [sense of right and wrong] was taken away and maybe that made me more vulnerable." Some enacted the behaviors to which they had been subjected; several who had been molested by older family members, for example, in turn abused younger family members, often their siblings.

Although the participants' childhood legacy caused them much suffering, as children they often defended or guarded their family's way of life. Many indicated it was the only life they knew and assumed it to be normal. Despite being hurt by family members, participants often attempted to protect them from attack or observation by outsiders who might intervene. In their own minds, participants relieved their families of responsibility for the adversity by concluding that the maltreatment was deserved because the participants had been bad or had "asked for it." Participants had been afraid that if others were to become aware of "what was going on" in the household, the family would be torn apart or a family member would be punished, hurt, or taken away. Most did not tell others about the abuse or other family problems. When asked if he had told anyone about his childhood sexual abuse, Jerry, a 56-year-old man whose mother had abused drugs, responded, "Somebody outside the family? I don't know . . . . I guess that I just wanted to protect my family."

Reinforcements to the Legacy

When the participants were children, adults outside the family-of-origin often facilitated or enabled the abuse or failed to help the child with his or her family problems. We refer to these interactions as reinforcements to the legacy as the actions of the adults served to perpetuate the abuse and adversity. Some reinforcements were subtle, such as when an adult ignored signs and symptoms of abuse. Other reinforcements were more overt, such as when adults told participants that they were lying, punished them for revealing abuse, or ignored their cries for help. Sophie, a 62-year old woman, was asked if she ever told anyone about the many times she had been sexually abused. She responded, "I think I called the police one time. I was coming from . . . like the community center, and I called the police because a boy had tried to rape me and they told me I shouldn't have been out."

Challenges to the Legacy

Some adults outside the family-of-origin tried to confront the abuse and adversity. Participants indicated that substitute parents, extended family members, family friends, neighbors, teachers, coaches, professional counselors, or church members told them the abuse was wrong, attempted to stop the abuse, and provided positive experiences to counteract the family environment. We refer to these interactions as challenges to the legacy because the adult actions were in opposition to the abuse and adversity the participants usually experienced. Joanna, a 19-year old woman who had been sexually abused by her uncle and a neighbor and physically abused by her family, described her interaction with an older neighbor: "I told Miss Sandra. Well, I actually didn't have to tell her because she saw I was hurting. She was like . . . 'We gotta tell. We gotta tell, because it can't keep happening.'" Challenges such as this had not occurred often in the lives of the participants, however, and few adults were able to end the abuse or change family situations.

Life Patterns

Participants clearly believed that as adults the abuse and adversity they experienced in childhood continued to influence their behaviors, feelings, relationships, and plans for the future in profound ways. In the theory, the term "life patterns" is used to show all the facets of life that participants indicated were affected by their childhood adversity. The data revealed three life patterns of Living the Family Legacy.

Being stuck in the Family Legacy. Some participants described being stuck in the legacy as they continued to live with abuse and chaos similar to their early family life and saw few possibilities for living differently. As children, their family legacy had been rarely challenged and often reinforced. The participants went on to live adult lives marked by addictions, imprisonment, prostitution, poor health, family instability, and experiences with interpersonal violence, both as perpetrators and victims. Jackie, a 45-year old woman who had been molested by her father, talked about how she used drugs and drinking to escape the pain. She described her life as an adult: "At one time, I got into prostitution. Drugs. Sex. I would smoke crack and feel warm. Isn't that sad? I've heard a lot of people are abused and go that way."

Being plagued by the Family Legacy. Many participants indicated that they were functioning well "on the outside" but felt permanently bothered by the effects of their adverse childhood experiences. Unlike those who were stuck in the legacy, these participants did not endure ongoing violence and chaos in their lives, but nonetheless indicated that they were plagued by their legacies. As children, their family legacy had been rarely challenged or reinforced; often others had not noticed the problems in the family. This life pattern was marked with emotional pain, including sadness, depression, and anxiety; feelings of low self-worth; and lack of trust of others. Jackson, a 48-year-old man, had been molested for over a year by a neighbor when he was 9. He said, "You put it behind you . . . . You block it out . . . . My substitute was sports . . . . But it made me not want to trust people. I guess the biggest thing is trust. You just don't trust people."

Rejecting the Family Legacy and creating a new legacy. Some participants had rejected their family legacy and were creating a new one. Participants who described this pattern were most likely to have encountered others who challenged their family legacy. These participants were determined to find a new way to live their lives; refused to be mistreated by others, especially by partners; and vowed to create healthy families. Many had obtained professional help to resolve the issues stemming from childhood. They were particu-

larly concerned about finding ways to create lives free of abuse and to develop nurturing and supportive relationships. Christy, a 25-year-old woman who experienced sexual and emotional abuse as a child, discussed how she had rejected her family legacy and had learned to express love: "When you love somebody, you can do these things for somebody, like meaningful touch, just any kind of pat on the shoulder, or a hug . . . . You share . . . . I do it for my sister now."

Passing on a Legacy

It was in the context of these life patterns that participants talked about passing on a legacy to others. The legacy could be the family legacy of abuse and adversity or a new abuse-free legacy. The others to whom participants bequeathed the legacy were often their own children, although many talked about passing on a legacy to other children or to "future generations."

Passing on the Family Legacy. Some participants who were stuck with, and a few who were plagued by, their family legacy, described passing it on, typically to their children. These participants had created family environments that were strikingly similar to those of their childhood. Many raised children in homes in which mental illness, drug abuse, domestic violence, criminal activity, and economic instability were present. Some reported having been violent or neglectful toward their children, and several indicated that their children had experienced sexual abuse similar to their own. Abigail, a 45-year-old woman, explained,

> I didn't realize I was a parent until a few years ago. I knew I had kids, but to me it was never a responsibility. I left my kids with my sister and I went on my way, living my life.

Many participants who were stuck in the legacy decided not to have children because they were convinced they might abuse them. A few children of the participants had been removed from the home by protective services or raised by extended family members.

Taking a stab at passing on a new legacy. Many participants, especially those who were plagued by the legacy, wanted to nurture their children and protect them from abuse. Many "took a stab at" leaving a new legacy as they made sincere, but ineffective, attempts to parent differently than they had been parented.

Participants who took a stab at a new legacy tended to use such expressions as "I'll try to do better," "Hopefully it will be different," or "Maybe it won't happen to him [or her]." Some verbalized aspirations to protect their children from harm but did not take adequate measures to ensure their safety. Several expressed determination that the sexual abuse that happened to them would never happen to their children, only to later reveal that one or more of their children had, in fact, been sexually abused while in their care. Hilda, a 19-year-old woman who had experienced extensive abuse as a child, took a stab at a new legacy:

Continued

RESEARCH EXAMPLE OF A QUALITATIVE STUDY—cont'd

Legacy of Abuse

> My son, he is very, very, he's not bad, but he's a very good manip-
> ulator.... I try to do [things differently] with my son because my
> grandmother beat me. I didn't want to have no sense of discipline
> with him, [so] I put him in time out.

Yet, she followed this proclamation with an account about beating her son with a belt because he had damaged her friend's wood floor.

Passing on a New Legacy. Most of the participants who had rejected the family legacy and created a new legacy wanted to pass on the new legacy. Several told touching stories about absolutely refusing to hand down the legacy of abuse and adversity, especially to their children. Several were aware that the legacy was passed down from their grandparents, and participants vowed to "stop the cycle." They sought to leave a new legacy by protecting their children from violence, decreasing their children's vulnerability to violence by ensuring they felt loved and protected, and providing a nurturing and stable environment. Christy talked about how she protected her son from his father,

> They were all like ... doing drugs and stuff, and he would want
> me to bring [my son] over there ... and I told him, 'No, I'm not
> doing that.' I stopped living this lifestyle for my son and I'm not
> going to take him over there.

Several participants also talked about intervening in the lives of others' children as helping professionals, ministers, child advocates, or family friends and thereby make things better for "future generations." Many participants became part of the study to pass on a new legacy. They hoped their stories could stop abuse and improve the lives of vulnerable children.

Trajectories of Living the Family Legacy

The **Figure** shows common life trajectories of participants who lived the family legacy. The bold arrows indicate common paths (found in the transcripts of the majority of participants) and the dashed line arrows indicate paths that were found in the data, but were not as common. Reinforcements of the legacy, for example, were common for those who were stuck in the legacy, whereas challenges to the legacy were more common for those who rejected the legacy. Similarly, while some participants who were plagued by the legacy passed the family legacy on to their children, it was more typical that they took a stab at leaving a new legacy.

Although the two-dimensional model in the **Figure** indicates that the trajectories were orderly and progressive, many participants actually described life trajectories that were complex, cyclic, regressive, and iterative. The model, therefore, leaves open the possibility of any number of trajectories. While the model shows that one life pattern is often predominant, a survivor of childhood adversity might move from one life pattern to another. For example, one might progress from being stuck in the legacy to being plagued by the legacy. Similarly, a survivor might also move "back-

ward" in the model, from passing on a new legacy to being plagued by the legacy following a contentious interaction with a parent. Some might attempt a new legacy for one child, and leave a new legacy for another.

Discussion

The concept of family legacies is similar to other work appearing in healthcare literature. Boszormenyi-Nagy (1987) developed the construct of the intergenerational legacy, in which children assume obligations to their parents based on the burdens borne by parents in raising them. Plager (1999) examined how family legacies contribute to health-promoting habits in families with children of school age. Silverman, Baker, Cait, and Boerner (2002–2003) argued that children whose parents die might take on characteristics of the deceased parent to create a type of legacy. SmithBattle (2006) found that teen mothers refined, rejected, or modified family legacies of caregiving practices.

A major limitation of the current study is its retrospective design. Participants frequently recalled events that had occurred years ago, and their memories might have been diminished or distorted. Most participants, however, were able to recall their experiences in great detail, often beginning their stories with phrases such as, "I can remember it as if it were yesterday" or "I still remember to this day." In addition, the life narratives might have been affected by how the participants were functioning at the time of the interview. Those who were depressed, for example, would be likely to tell stories "through a negative lens." Nonetheless, the narratives were rich with descriptions of how the participants moved through life—from their own childhoods of adversity to their decision to participate in the interviews.

Transferability of these findings to other settings can be determined based on the description of the sample as provided above. Over half of these participants were of low socioeconomic status. However, the inclusion of almost equal numbers of women and men and of Caucasian and African American participants and the recruitment of participants in community settings allow for transfer of findings to a wide variety of settings.

These findings indicate several key points for nurses who provide care for survivors of CSA in any type of practice setting. In this sample, 45% of the participants were men. Thus, it is important for nurses to be aware that men experience CSA and that their narratives indicate that they often suffer lifelong social and emotional problems as a result. Both women and men in this sample shared life stories of childhood adversity and violation of generational boundaries that left them with difficulties with trusting others. Thus, nurses need to be especially careful in maintaining appropriate, clear professional boundaries with these clients and in fostering trust through use of supportive, gentle approaches (Draucker, 1999).

Legacy of Abuse

Attentive listening and empathic responses enhance the development of these trusted professional relationships (Courey, Martsolf, Draucker, & Strickland, 2008). Survivors of CSA who told adults about the abuse were often not believed and the abuse was minimized. Thus, it is critical that nurses to whom survivors disclose their experience of CSA respond empathically by assuring clients that they are believed and taken seriously. Because these survivors experienced childhood adversity that frequently included lack of parental involvement and direction in their lives, nurses should provide guidance for making health choices without taking away the client's autonomy (Courey et al., 2008).

Findings from this study indicate that nurses and other health professionals who work in mental-health settings with survivors of childhood adversity and sexual violence can be particularly helpful by providing challenges to the legacy of violence. The model shown in the **Figure** can be used as a tool to initiate conversations about the family legacy. Clients might trace their own trajectories on the model, thereby developing insights into how their histories contribute to their life patterns. When working with clients who are stuck in the family legacy, for example, clinicians can discuss what challenges would be needed for rejecting the family legacy. Those who are plagued by the family legacy might be especially amenable to therapeutic interventions because they suffer from the effects of their childhood, but do not experience the chaos or dysfunction of those who are stuck in the legacy. For clients who are parents, identifying their own life patterns and exploring their ways of passing on the legacy could open up discussion of new possibilities for parenting. Clients who are taking a stab at leaving a new legacy might be especially willing to try new parenting practices.

These findings indicate several avenues for further research. Studies designed to further explore relationships among adverse family environments, types of life patterns, and the ways of passing on a legacy could enhance refinements of the theory. Further development of the theory might lead to interventions that facilitate the rejection of family legacies of violence and adversity and enable clients to leave a new legacy for the next generation.

Conclusions

The processes by which childhood adversity influences the life course of adult survivors of CSA is best understood as Living the Family Legacy. Survivors of CSA described multiple trajectories that determined whether they passed on a legacy of abuse and adversity or left a new one. The trajectories are strongly influenced by others who either reinforce or challenge the family legacy. The model indicating the process of Living the Family Legacy can guide clinicians in initiating conversations about the influence of the family legacy on one's life pattern and one's parenting. The study

indicates numerous possibilities for further theorizing and research.

Clinical Resources

- https://www.who.int/topics/child_abuse/en/
- http://www.nlm.nih.gov/medlineplus/childsexual abuse.html
- http://www.childwelfare.gov/pubs/usermanuals/ sexabuse/sexabusef.cfm

---

References

American Medical Association. (2003). **Diagnostic and treatment guidelines on child sexual abuse.** Retrieved August 18, 2007, from http:/www.ama-assn.org/pub/upload/mm/386/childsexabuse.pdf

Banyard, V.L., Williams, L.M., & Siegel, J.A. (2003). The impact of complex trauma and depression on parenting: An exploration of mediating risk and protective factors. **Child Maltreatment,** 8(4), 334–349.

Benoliel, J.Q. (1996). Grounded theory and nursing knowledge. **Qualitative Health Research,** 6(3), 406–428.

Boszormenyi-Nagy, I. (1987). **Foundations of contextual therapy: Collected papers of Ivan Boszormenyi-Nagy, M.D.** New York: Brunner/Mazel.

Centers for Disease Control and Prevention, National Center for Injury Prevention and Control. (2007). **Sexual violence: Fact sheet.** Retrieved November 7, 2007, from http://www.cdc.gov/ncipc/factsheets/svfacts.htm

Clemmons, J.C., Walsh, K., DiLillo, D., & Messman-Moore, T.L. (2007). Unique and combined contributions of multiple child abuse types and abuse severity to adult trauma symptomology. **Child Maltreatment,** 12(2), 172–181.

Courey, T.J., Martsolf, D.S., Draucker, C.B., & Strickland, K.B. (2008). Hildegard Peplau's theory and the healthcare encounters of survivors of sexual violence. **Journal of the American Psychiatric Nurses Association,** 14(2), 136–143.

DiLillo, D., & Damashek, A. (2003). Parenting characteristics of women reporting a history of childhood sexual abuse. **Child Maltreatment,** 8(4), 319–333.

Dong, M., Anda, R.F., Felitti, V.J., Dube, S.R., Williamson, D.F., Thompson, T.J., et al. (2004). The interrelatedness of multiple forms of abuse, neglect, and household dysfunction. **Child Abuse & Neglect,** 28, 771–784.

Draucker, C.B. (1999). The psychotherapeutic needs of women who have been sexually assaulted. **Perspectives in Psychiatric Care,** 35(1), 18–28.

Draucker, C.B., Martsolf, D.S., Ross, R., & Rusk, T.B. (2007). Theoretical sampling and category in grounded theory. **Qualitative Health Research,** 17(1), 1137–1148.

Dube, S.R., Anda, R.F., Whitfield, C.L., Brown, D.W., Felitti, V.J., Dong, M., et al. (2005). Long-term consequences of childhood sexual abuse by gender of victim. **American Journal of Preventive Medicine,** 28(5), 430–438.

Dunlap, E., Golub, A., & Johnson, B.D. (2003). Girls' sexual development in the inner city: From compelled childhood sexual contact to sex-for-things exchanges. **Journal of Child Sexual Abuse,** 12(2), 73–96.

Glaser, B.G., & Strauss, A.L. (1967). **The discovery of grounded theory: Strategies for qualitative research.** Chicago: Aldine.

Gold, S.N., Hyman, S.M., & Andrés-Hyman, R.C. (2004). Family of origin environments in two clinical samples of survivors of intra-familial, extra-familial, and both types of sexual abuse. **Child Abuse & Neglect,** 28, 1199–1212.

Higgins, D.J., & McCabe, M.P. (2003). Maltreatment and family dysfunction in childhood and the subsequent adjustment of children and adults. **Journal of Family Violence,** 18(2), 107–120.

Lincoln, Y., & Guba, E. (1985). **Naturalistic inquiry.** Newbury Park, CA: Sage.

Continued

RESEARCH EXAMPLE OF A QUALITATIVE STUDY—cont'd

Legacy of Abuse

Locke, T.F., & Newcomb, M. (2004). Child maltreatment, parent alcohol- and drug-related problems, polydrug problems, and parenting practices: A test of gender differences and four theoretical perspectives. Journal of Family Psychology, 18(1), 120–134.

Martsolf, D.S., Courey, T.J., Chapman, T.R., Draucker, C.B., & Mims, B.L. (2006). Adaptive sampling: Recruiting a diverse community sample of survivors of sexual violence. Journal of Community Health Nursing, 23(3), 169–182.

Plager, K.A. (1999). Understanding family legacy in family health concerns. Journal of Family Nursing, 5(1), 51–71.

Roesler, T.A., & McKenzie, N. (1994). Effects of childhood trauma on psychological functioning in adults sexually abused as children. Journal of Nervous and Mental Disorders, 182, 145–150.

Russell, D.E.H., & Bolen, R.M. (2000). The epidemic of rape and child sexual abuse in the United States. Thousand Oaks, CA: Sage.

Schreiber, R.S. (2001). The "how to" of grounded theory: Avoiding the pitfalls. In R.S. Schreiber & P.N. Stern (Eds.), Using grounded theory in nursing (pp. 55–84). New York: Springer.

Schuetze, P., & Eiden, R.D. (2005). The relationship between sexual abuse during childhood and parenting outcomes: Modeling direct and indirect pathways. Child Abuse & Neglect, 29(6), 645–659.

Silverman, P.R., Baker, J., Cait, C., & Boerner, D. (2002–2003). The effects of negative legacies on the adjustment of parentally bereaved children and adolescents. OMEGA, 46, 335–352.

SmithBattle, L. (2006). Family legacies in shaping teen mothers' caregiving practices over 12 years. Qualitative Health Research, 16, 1129–1144.

World Health Organization. (2002). World report on violence and health. Geneva, Switzerland: Author.

Martsolf, D. S., & Draucker, C. B. (2008). The legacy of childhood sexual abuse and family adversity. *Journal of Nursing Scholarship*, *40*(4), 333-340.

EXAMPLE CRITICAL APPRAISAL OF A QUALITATIVE STUDY
Problem Statement

1. Identify the clinical problem that led to the study.

The clinical problem was childhood sexual abuse and family adversity. These experiences affect the children as they grow into adulthood and become parents themselves (Martsolf & Draucker, 2008). What was not known (research problem) were the perspectives of adults who experienced childhood sexual abuse and family adversity because these had "not been reported in-depth" (p. 448).

2. How did the authors establish the significance of the study?

The researchers convey the significance of the study with the statistic that 25% of girls and 8% of boys experience sexual abuse during childhood and that abuse frequently occurs concurrently with family adversity. The researchers indicated the study was significant because these experiences influence the parenting effectiveness of the children when they become adults.

Purpose and Research Questions

1. Identify the purpose of the study.

The purpose was clearly stated as "to describe the process by which childhood adversity influences the life course of adult survivors of CSA [childhood sexual abuse] from their perspectives" (Martsolf & Draucker, 2008, p. 448).

2. List research questions that the study was designed to answer.

The researchers did not explicitly identify the research questions. For grounded theory studies, one main research question may be appropriate. In this study, the main research question can be stated as a rephrase of the study purpose: Through what process does childhood adversity influence the life course of adult survivors of CSA? (Martsolf & Draucker, 2008, p. 448). The questions identified in the methods section are the interview questions, which guided data collection.

3. Were the purpose and research questions related to the problem?

The study purpose directly addressed the problem of sexual abuse and family adversity.

4. Were qualitative methods appropriate to answer the research questions?

Yes, the focus of the study was to better understand the perspective of adults who experienced childhood sexual abuse and family adversity. Perspectives of research participants can be explored appropriately by allowing their voices to be heard through a qualitative study.

Literature Review

1. Did the author cite quantitative and qualitative studies relevant to the focus of the study? What other types of literature did the author include?

The literature review for the study was included in the introductory paragraphs of the article. Of the references cited in the introduction, nine were reports of quantitative studies, one was a report of a qualitative study, and two were review articles. The researchers also cited three sources of publicly available statistics and definitions to establish the significance of the study.

2. Were the references current?

This article was accepted for publication in June 2008, so studies published after that date could not have been included. There is often a 2-year delay from submission to publication. In this article, the researchers reported part of the findings from a study funded by a grant that was awarded before December 2004 since this is when data collection started. This may explain why the majority of the articles cited in the literature review were published prior to 2003. The researchers did include two studies published after the study began. The prevalence of childhood sexual abuse was established using a source published by the World Health Organization (WHO) in 2002. A 2006 WHO report includes updated statistics that 20% of women and 5% to 10% of men have been affected by childhood sexual abuse (p. 20).

Continued

EXAMPLE CRITICAL APPRAISAL OF A QUALITATIVE STUDY—cont'd

3. Identify the disciplines of the authors of studies cited in this paper. Does it appear that the author searched databases outside of CINAHL for relevant studies?

The authors included nurses and other health professionals with specialties in community health, child psychology, and family nursing. The cited sources were published in journals from the fields of nursing, medicine, criminology, psychology, and sociology. Thus, the researchers appear to have searched databases outside of CINAHL.

4. Did the authors evaluate or indicate the weaknesses of the available studies?

The authors did not indicate the methodologies, limitations, or weaknesses of the studies they cited, other than the limitation that researchers had not studied the influence of the family adversity on adult development. Because the focus of the paper is the current study, the fact that the authors did not include this information is a minor issue and does not affect the quality of the current study.

5. Did the literature review include adequate information that built a logical argument? Did the authors provide enough evidence to support the verdict that the study is needed?

The researchers included reports of conflicting findings to provide a balanced view of the available evidence. Presenting a balanced view lent credibility to their argument. They established the significance of the problem and the gap in the literature that this study was designed to address.

Frame of Reference

1. Did the authors identify a specific perspective from which the study was developed? If so, what was it?

The researchers do not explicitly identify their frame of reference or the philosophical foundation for the study. The researchers describe their methods to include grounded theory, which is a frame of reference based in the philosophy of symbolic interactionism (Benzies & Allen, 2001). The major premise of symbolic interactionism is that a person's use of symbols reflects the meaning ascribed to the symbol by that person. Language is one of the symbols used by people in their interactions with each other that can be interpreted to extract meaning.

2. When a researcher uses the grounded theory method of qualitative inquiry, the researcher may develop a framework or diagram as part of the findings of the study. Was a framework developed from the study findings?

The researchers developed a framework from the findings that could guide researchers designing studies on this topic in the future. They provided a diagram to illustrate the themes and their interrelationships (p. 450).

Research Tradition

1. Identify the stated or implied research tradition upon which the study was based.

The study's methods were based on the framework and research tradition of grounded theory (Glaser & Strauss, 1967, as cited in Martsolf & Draucker, 2008). The researchers provided their rationale for this approach as being the fit of the purpose of grounded theory to their desire to better understand the "complex processes that change over time and are influenced by both psychological and social factors" (p. 448).

2. Provide a paraphrased description of the research tradition used.

The focus of grounded theory is to understand the processes of change from the perspectives of the persons who are changing. Reality for a person is created by the meaning given to the event by the person. Glaser and Strauss developed grounded theory as a framework and method over the course of several studies (Glaser, 1978). Part of the grounded theory method is generating a theory that further describes or explains the phenomenon being studied (Glaser, 1978). Grounded theory has become a research tradition used frequently by nurse researchers (Ghezeljeh & Emami, 2009).

3. Are the methods used in the study consistent with the research tradition?

The methods used in the study (interviews, analysis of transcripts) are consistent with grounded theory.

Sampling and Sample

1. Identify how subjects were selected.

The subjects were selected from the subjects of a larger study that focused on how persons had responded to sexual violence. The researchers do not identify the sampling method; however, it appears to be purposive or purposeful sampling (Patton, 2004).

2. At what sites were subjects recruited for the study? Did the sites for recruitment fit the sampling needs of the study?

The researchers conducted a community-based study. Subjects for the larger study were recruited from a variety of settings, such as churches and neighborhood centers, within one metropolitan area.

3. What were the inclusion and exclusion criteria for the sample?

The inclusion criteria were specifically stated by the researchers as being experience with childhood sexual abuse and growing up in an adverse family environment (Martsolf & Draucker, 2008, p. 448). The exclusion criterion must be inferred from the screening process. Persons at risk for acute emotional distress were excluded.

4. Were the selected subjects able to provide data relevant to the study purpose and research questions?

The subjects were selected from the larger sample to allow the researchers to address the research problem and study purpose.

5. How many people participated in the study? Did any potential subjects refuse to participate? Did any of the participants start but not finish the study?

The sample size was 88 persons. Because the subjects were selected from the sample for a larger study, no information was provided about the number of persons who were recruited but chose not to participate or the number who started but did not complete the study.

Data Collection

1. How were data collected in this study?

Data were collected through in-person interviews that lasted from 1 to 2 hours.

2. What rationale did the author provide for using this data collection method?

No rationale was provided for using interviews. The data collection method, however, is appropriate for qualitative studies (Munhall, 2007; Patton, 2004).

3. Identify the time period for data collection of the study.

The interviews were conducted from "December 2004 to April 2006" (p. 448).

4. Describe the sequence of data collection events for a participant.

Participants for the larger study were recruited from community settings. Each participant was interviewed one time. During the interview, the data collectors asked participants open-ended questions about their childhood experiences of sexual violence, the impact of these experiences on their lives when it occurred and into the present. The interviews lasted from 1 to 2 hours. Participants who were interviewed later during the data collection period may have been asked about constructs that emerged from previous interviews and the concurrent data analysis. This process of member checks increases the credibility of the researchers' interpretation of the participants' experiences.

Continued

EXAMPLE CRITICAL APPRAISAL OF A QUALITATIVE STUDY—cont'd

Protection of Human Participants

1. Identify the benefits and risks of participation addressed by the authors. Were there benefits or risks the authors do not identify?

The benefits of participation were not addressed by the authors. The participants may have benefited from talking about their childhood experiences with an advanced practice nurse with specialty training in active listening and counseling. The risk of participation was acute emotional distress, which can be inferred from the use of mental health specialists to screen participants and conduct the interviews. The researchers also acknowledged the risk of loss of confidentiality and decreased the risk by reporting the findings using pseudonyms.

2. How were recruitment and consent techniques adjusted to accommodate the sensitivity of the subject matter and psychological distress of potential participants?

Recruitment was done by announcements placed in the community. Persons identified themselves as potential participants by calling a toll-free number. This process protected the confidentiality of the participants. The process of screening by the trained professionals also minimized the risk of harm by excluding persons for whom participation might have caused undue psychological distress. The process for obtaining informed consent was not described.

3. How were data collection and management techniques adapted in acknowledgment of participant sensitivity and vulnerability?

The resources for addressing the potential emotional distress of the participants were incorporated into the data collection by having advanced practice nurses in psychiatry and mental health conduct the interviews.

Data Management and Analysis

1. Describe the data management and analysis methods used in the study.

Little information was provided about data management other than that interviews were audiotaped and transcribed. The process of data analysis was detailed. Constant comparison methods were used with three levels of coding. Line-by-line examination and coding of the data was the first step, followed by comparing codes from the first analysis to new data and reviewing all transcripts again. The third-level coding focused on relationships among the codes and resulted in an emerging theory.

2. Did the author discuss how the rigor of the process was assured? For example, did the author describe maintaining a paper trail of critical decisions that were made during the analysis of the data?

At the end of the data analysis section, the researchers indicated that they used memos, diagrams, and member checks to ensure the credibility of the analysis and subsequent findings. According to Beck (1993), validating the findings with participants, keeping field notes, and providing rich excerpts of the data are strategies for increasing the credibility of qualitative study findings.

3. What measures were used to minimize the effects of researcher bias? For example, did two researchers independently analyze the data and compare their analyses?

A team of researchers were involved in this study, creating the potential for individuals to independently analyze the transcripts with team discussion and comparisons of coding. The procedures for minimizing bias were not specifically described.

4. Did the data management and analysis methods fit the research purposes and data?

The use of transcripts and coding in three levels were congruent with the purpose of the study and grounded theory methods.

Findings

1. Did the findings address the purpose of the study?

The analysis of the data resulted in a diagram of the processes by which the lives of persons who experienced CSA were influenced by family adversity. The findings were congruent with the study's purpose.

2. Were the data sufficiently analyzed?

The data were analyzed into codes and the relationships among the codes were portrayed by a diagram (see Figure 12–4). The data were sufficiently analyzed.

3. Were the interpretations of data backed up by data collected?

The researchers provided their rationale for using the concept of legacy. Quotations from the participants were incorporated into the discussion of each concept to substantiate the concept. These quotations also allowed the perspectives and experiences of the participants to emerge.

4. Did the researcher address variations in the findings by relevant sample characteristics?

The researchers quoted the participants, identifying them by a pseudonym, age, and experiences with childhood sexual abuse. One variation that was noted was the participants who were unable to shed their family legacy often made a conscious decision not to have children.

Discussion

1. Did the results offer new information about the target phenomenon?

Because little research had been done describing how CSA and family adversity interact, the findings and the grounded theory provided new information.

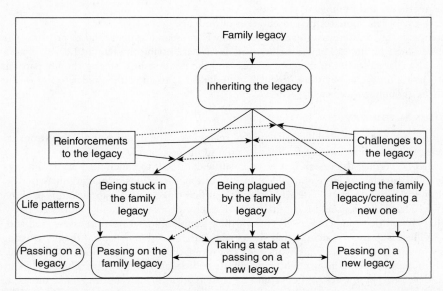

Figure 12–4. Living the family legacy. The researchers developed this model to describe the core process of the study and the related concepts. Martsolf, D. S., & Draucker, C. B. (2008). The legacy of childhood sexual abuse and family adversity. *Journal of Nursing Scholarship, 40*(4), 336.

Continued

EXAMPLE CRITICAL APPRAISAL OF A QUALITATIVE STUDY—cont'd

2. Were the findings linked to findings in other studies or other relevant literatures?

The researchers linked the study findings to the work of four authors who had written about family legacies. These authors were cited in the Discussion section.

3. Describe the clinical, policy, theoretical, and other significance of the findings. Did the author explore these applications?

The researchers directed the application of the findings toward nurses caring for persons who were CSA survivors. The theoretical significance of the findings was inferred from the development of the framework that can provide the foundation for future studies.

Logic and Form of Findings

1. Were readers able to hear the voice of the participants and gain an understanding of the phenomenon studied?

The quotations included in the report provided glimpses into the lives of survivors of CSA. The diagram of concepts and relationships has potential for being a solid theoretical foundation of future studies.

2. Were elements of the research report easily found by readers?

Headings were used that clearly identified the elements of the research report, such as sample and data analysis.

3. Did the overall presentation of the study fit its purpose, method, and findings?

The presentation of the results of a grounded theory study should culminate in the theoretical description. The authors of this research report provided a synthesized description that fit the purpose, methods, and findings of the study.

4. Was there a coherent logic to the presentation of findings?

The researchers' presentation was organized to follow the research process and to provide evidence to substantiate their findings. They identified and described "Living the Family Legacy" as the core process. The characteristics of the core process and the relationships among the life patterns and ways of passing on the legacy were gradually revealed so as to allow the reader to follow the researchers' thought processes.

Evaluation Summary

1. Do the findings provide a credible reflection of reality? Are the findings applicable (transferable) to other settings? If so, how can the findings be used in nursing practice?

The researchers described the research process in sufficient detail to conclude that the findings are credible. The sample was large and selected from different locations, providing increased transferability of the findings. The researchers identified three possible applications of the findings in practice. First, nurses should recognize that men have experienced sexual violence. The researchers noted that men comprised 45% of their sample. Nurses need to assess men and women for CSA. The researchers conclude that adults who experienced CSA have difficulty trusting others. Nurses who interact with CSA survivors need to express their belief that the CSA occurred and establish therapeutic relationships with appropriate professional boundaries. The family legacy diagram developed by the researchers could be used as a tool by advanced practice nurses and other healthcare providers in mental health settings to initiate discussions about the influences of CSA and family legacies.

2. What do the findings add to the current body of knowledge?

The Living the Family Legacy theory developed by Martsolf and Draucker (2008) provides a new perspective on the effects of CSA on survivors as they become adults and make decisions about their family legacy. This theory is a substantial contribution that provides a perspective that can be used to develop CSA interventions and future quantitative studies.

3. State the conclusion of the critical appraisal of the study.

The weaknesses of the study include limited information on how the data were managed and how team members worked together on the analysis of the data to minimize potential bias of one researcher. Another weakness of the study was the lack of information provided about potential participants who were approached but did not participate in the study. The inclusion of additional current literature in the background section would have strengthened the research report. The strengths of the study, however, outweigh the weaknesses of the study. The strengths are that Martsolf and Draucker (2008) clearly identified the significance of the clinical problem and provided sufficient literature support for the research problem. The sample size was large for a qualitative study. A major strength is that the grounded theory method was followed rigorously and a theoretical model was proposed. Using specialty nurses to screen and interview the participants was an unobtrusive way to reduce the risk of psychological distress of the participants. Martsolf and Draucker made a significant contribution to the understanding of the effects of CSA on survivors in adulthood.

KEY CONCEPTS

- An intellectual critical appraisal of research requires careful examination of all aspects of a study to judge its strengths, weaknesses, meaning, and significance.
- Research is critically appraised to broaden understanding, improve practice, and provide a background for conducting a study.
- All nurses, including students, practicing nurses, nurse administrators, nurse educators, and nurse researchers, need research critical appraisal expertise.
- The quantitative research critical appraisal process includes comprehension, comparison, analysis, and evaluation.
- The guideline for critical appraisal of qualitative studies includes assessing significance, rigor, the logic of the conclusions, and the congruence of methods to the research tradition.
- Example critical appraisals are provided for both a quantitative study and a qualitative study.

REFERENCES

Armstrong, D. J., Meenagh, G. K., Bickle, I., Lee, A. S. H., Curran, S., & Finch, M. B. (2007). Vitamin D deficiency is associated with anxiety and depression in fibromyalgia. *Clinical Rheumatology, 26*(4), 551-554.

Barbour, R. S., & Barbour, M. (2003). Evaluating and synthesizing qualitative research: The need to develop a distinctive approach. *Journal of Evaluation in Clinical Practice, 9*(2), 179-186.

Beck, C. T. (1993). Qualitative research: The evaluation of its credibility, fittingness, and auditability. *Western Journal of Nursing Research, 15*, 263.

Benzies, K. M., & Allen, M. N. (2001). Symbolic interactionism as a theoretical perspective for multiple method research. *Journal of Advanced Nursing, 33*(4), 541-547.

Berk, M., Sanders, K. M., Pasco, J. A., Jacka, F. N., Williams, L. J., Hayles, A. L., & Dodd, S. (2007). Vitamin D deficiency may play a role in depression. *Medical Hypotheses,* *69,* 1316-1319.

Brown, S. J. (2002). Focus on research methods. Nursing intervention studies: A descriptive analysis of issues important to clinicians. *Research in Nursing & Health,* *25*(4), 317-327.

Brown, S. J. (2009). *Evidence-based nursing: The research-practice connection.* Sudbury, MA: Jones & Bartlett.

Burns, N. (1989). Standards for qualitative research. *Nursing Science Quarterly,* *2*(1), 44-52.

Burns, N., & Grove, S. K. (2009). *The practice of nursing research: Appraisal, synthesis, and generation of evidence* (6th ed.). Philadelphia: Saunders.

Cesario, S., Morin, K., & Santa-Donato, A. (2002). Evaluating the level of evidence of qualitative research. *Journal of Obstetric, Gynecologic, and Neonatal Nursing,* *31*(6), 708-714.

Clissett, P. (2008). Evaluating qualitative research. *Journal of Orthopaedic Nursing,* *12*(2), 99-105.

Cohen, D. J., & Crabtree, B. F. (2008). Evaluative criteria for qualitative research in health care: Controversies and recommendations. *Annals of Family Medicine,* *6*(4), 331-339.

Cowles, K. V. (1988). Issues in qualitative research on sensitive topics. *Western Journal of Nursing Research,* *10*(2), 163-179.

Craig, J. V., & Smyth, R. L. (2007). *The evidence-based practice manual for nurses* (2nd ed.). Edinburgh: Churchill Livingstone.

Creswell, J. W. (2009). *Research design: Qualitative, quantitative and mixed methods approaches* (3rd ed.). Thousand Oaks, CA: Sage.

Cullum, N., Ciliska, D., Haynes, R. B., & Marks, S. (2008). *Evidence-based nursing: An introduction.* Oxford, UK: Blackwell.

DeKeyser, F. G., & Pugh, L. C. (1990). Assessment of reliability and validity of biochemical measures. *Nursing Research,* *39*(5), 314-317.

Duffy, M. E. (1988). Statistics: Friend or foe? *Nursing & Health Care,* *9*(2), 73-75.

Fossey, E., Harvey, C., McDermott, F., & Davidson, L. (2002). Understanding and evaluating qualitative research. *Australian and New Zealand Journal of Psychiatry,* *36,* 717-732.

Gaines, S. (2005). The saddest season. *Minneapolis Medicine,* *88,* 25-32.

Ghezeljeh, T. N., & Emami, A. (2009). Grounded theory: Methodology and philosophical perspective. *Nurse Researcher,* *17*(1), 15-23.

Glaser, B. G. (1978). *Theoretical sensitivity: Advances in the methodology of grounded theory.* Mills Valley, CA: The Sociology Press.

Grove, S. K. (2007). *Statistics for health care research: A practical workbook.* St. Louis: Saunders Elsevier.

Holick, M., & Jenkins, M. (2003). *The UV advantage.* New York: Ibooks.

Jorde, R., Waterloo, K., Salech, F., Haug, E., & Svartberg, J. (2006). Neuropsychological function in relation to serum parathyroid hormone and serum 25-hydroxyvitamin D levels: The Tromso study. *Journal of Neurology,* *253,* 464-470.

Kiraly, S., Kiraly, M., Hawe, R., & Makhami. N. (2006, January). Vitamin D as a neuroactive substance: Review. *Scientific World Journal,* *6,* 125-139.

Lincoln, Y. S., & Guba, E. G. (1985). *Naturalistic inquiry.* Thousand Oaks, CA: Sage.

Martsolf, D. S., & Draucker, C. B. (2008). The legacy of childhood sexual abuse and family adversity. *Journal of Nursing Scholarship,* *40*(4), 333-340.

Melnyk, B. M., & Fineout-Overholt, E. (2005). *Evidence-based practice in nursing & healthcare: A guide to best practice.* Philadelphia: Lippincott Williams & Wilkins.

Morse, J. M. (1991). Evaluating qualitative research. *Qualitative Health Research,* *1*(3), 283-286.

Munhall, P. L. (2007). *Nursing research: A qualitative perspective* (4th ed.). Sudbury, MA: Jones & Bartlett.

Munro, B. H. (2005). *Statistical methods for health care research* (5th ed.). Philadelphia: Lippincott Williams & Wilkins.

Nelson, A. M. (2008). Addressing the threat of evidence-based practice to qualitative inquiry through increasing attention to quality: A discussion paper. *International Journal of Nursing Studies,* *45*(7), 316-322.

Obradovic, D., Gronemeyer, H., Lutz, B., & Rein, T. (2006). Cross-talk of vitamin D and glucocorticoids in hippocampal cells. *Journal of Neurochemistry,* *96,* 500-509.

Olsen, D. P. (2003). Methods: HIPAA privacy regulations and nursing research. *Nursing Research,* *52*(5), 344-348.

Patton, M. Q. (2004). *Qualitative research & evaluation methods* (3rd ed.). Thousand Oaks, CA: Sage.

Pickler, R. H. (2007). Evaluating qualitative research studies. *Journal of Pediatric Health Care,* *21*(3), 195-197.

Roberts, W. D., & Stone, P. W. (2003). Ask an expert: How to choose and evaluate a research instrument. *Applied Nursing Research,* *16*(1), 70-72.

Robinson, J. H. (2001). Mastering research critique and statistical interpretation: Guidelines and golden rules. *Nurse Educator,* *26*(3), 136-141.

Sandelowski, M. (2008). Justifiying qualitative research. *Research in Nursing & Health,* *31,* 193-195.

Sandelowski, M., & Barroso, J. (2002). Reading qualitative studies. *International Journal of Qualitative Methods,* *1*(1), Article 5. Retrieved November 14, 2009, from *http://ejournals.library.ualberta.ca/index.php/IJQM/issue/view/385.*

Sandelowski, M., & Barroso, J. (2007). *Handbook for synthesizing qualitative research.* New York: Springer.

Santacroce, S. J., Maccarelli, L. M., & Grey, M. (2004). Methods: Intervention fidelity. *Nursing Research,* *53*(1), 63-66.

Shipowick, C. D., Moore, C. B., Corbett, C., & Bindler, R. (2009). Vitamin D and depressive symptoms in women during the winter: A pilot study. *Applied Nursing Research,* *22*(3), 221-225.

Sloan, D., & Kornstein, S. (2003). Gender differences in depression and response to antidepressant treatment. *Psychiatric Clinics of North America,* *26,* 581-594.

Stevens, K. R. (2005). Critically appraising knowledge for clinical decision making. In B. M. Melnyk & E. Fineout-Overholt. (2005). *Evidence-based practice in nursing & healthcare: A guide to best practice* (pp. 73-78). Philadelphia: Lippincott Williams & Wilkins.

Stige, B., Malterud, K., & Midtgarden, T. (2009). Toward an agenda for evaluation of qualitative research. *Qualitative Health Research, 19*(10), 1504-1516.

Whittemore, R. (2005). Combining evidence in nursing research: Methods and implications. *Nursing Research, 54*(1), 56-62.

Whittemore, R., Chase, S. K., & Mandle, C. L. (2001). Validity in qualitative research. *Qualitative Health Research, 11*(4), 522-537.

World Health Organization (2000). Setting the WHO agenda for mental health. *Bulletin of the World Health Organization, 78*(4), 500.

World Health Organization and the International Society for Prevention of Child Abuse and Neglect (2006). *Preventing child maltreatment: A guide to taking action and generating evidence.* Geneva, Switzerland: World Health Organization.

Building an Evidence-Based Nursing Practice

Chapter Overview

What Are the Barriers and Benefits to Evidence-Based Nursing Practice? 466

Barriers to Evidence-Based Nursing Practice 466

Benefits of Evidence-Based Nursing Practice 468

Searching for Evidence-Based Sources 469

Guidelines for Critically Appraising Research Syntheses 469

Critically Appraising Systematic Reviews of Research 469

Critically Appraising Meta-Analyses 471

Critically Appraising Integrative Reviews of Research 473

Evaluating Qualitative Syntheses of Research 475

Models to Promote Evidence-Based Practice in Nursing 477

Stetler Model of Research Utilization to Facilitate Evidence-Based Practice 477

Iowa Model of Evidence-Based Practice 480

Application of the Iowa Model of Evidence-Based Practice 482

Assemble, Critically Appraise, and Synthesize Research for Use in Practice 483

Sufficiency of the Research Base 486

Pilot the Change in Practice 487

Institute the Change in Practice 488

Monitor Outcomes 488

Developing Clinical Questions to Identify Evidence for Use in Practice 490

Implementing Evidence-Based Guidelines in Practice 492

History of the Development of Evidence-Based Guidelines 492

Evidence-Based Guideline Resources 494

Implementing the JNC 7 Evidence-Based Guideline in Practice 496

Introduction to Evidence-Based Practice Centers 499

Introduction to Translational Research 500

Learning Outcomes

After completing this chapter, you should be able to:

1. Identify the barriers and benefits of evidence-based practice in nursing.

2. Critically appraise systematic reviews, meta-analyses, integrative reviews, and qualitative syntheses (metasummaries and metasyntheses) of current research evidence.

3. Discuss models used to promote evidence-based practice in nursing, such as the Stetler Model of Research Utilization to Facilitate Evidence-Based Practice and Iowa Model of Evidence-Based Practice.

4. Apply the Iowa Model of Evidence-Based Practice in implementing evidence-based changes in your practice.

5. Use the PICO format to formulated clinical questions to identify evidence for use in practice.

6. Apply the Grove Model to implement national evidence-based guidelines in your practice.

7. Implement research-based protocols, algorithms, and policies and national evidence-based guidelines in your practice.

Key Terms

Algorithms, p. 471
Best research evidence,
   p. 465
Evidence-based guidelines,
   p. 492
Evidence-based practice
   (EBP), p. 465
Evidence-based practice
   centers, p. 499
Grove Model for
   Implementing Evidence-
   Based Guidelines in
   Practice, p. 496
Integrative review of
   research, p. 473

Iowa Model of Evidence-
   Based Practice,
   p. 480
Meta-analysis, p. 471
PICO format, p. 490
Qualitative research
   synthesis, p. 475
   Qualitative metasummary,
      p. 475
   Qualitative metasynthesis,
      p. 475
Research-based protocols,
   p. 482
Stetler Model of Research
   Utilization to Facilitate

Evidence-Based Practice,
   p. 477
Phase I: Preparation,
   p. 477
Phase II: Validation, p. 479
Phase III: Comparative
   evaluation, p. 479
Decision-making, p. 479
Phase IV: Translation/
   application, p. 480
Phase V: Evaluation,
   p. 480
Systematic review, p. 469
Translational research,
   p. 500

STUDY TOOLS

Go to your Companion CD for interactive review questions related to this chapter. Also, be sure to visit *http://evolve.elsevier.com/Burns/understanding* for additional review questions, critical appraisal activities, and more. For additional content review and practice in critically appraising and using research evidence in practice, go to Chapter 13 of the *Study Guide for Understanding Nursing Research*, 5th edition.

Research evidence has greatly expanded in the last 25 years with the conduct of numerous, quality nursing intervention studies that have been communicated by presentations, journal publications, and the Internet. The expectation of society is the delivery of quality, cost-effective nursing care to patients, families, and communities. To provide quality care, nurses must implement interventions based on the best research evidence available (Brown, 2009; Melnyk, Fineout-Overholt, Stillwell, & Williamson, 2010). Thus nurses and healthcare agencies are focused on delivering evidence-based health care to improve patient outcomes. Evidence-based practice (EBP) became a major focus for medicine in the 1980s and for nursing in the 1990s (Malloch & Porter-O'Grady, 2006; Sackett, Straus, Richardson, Rosenberg, & Haynes, 2000). However, research utilization or using research findings to improve practice has been a focus of nursing for decades (Stetler & Marram, 1976). With the implementation of EBP, there have been improved outcomes for patients, healthcare providers, and healthcare agencies (Craig & Smyth, 2007; Doran, 2003; Institute of Medicine, 2001; Melnyk et al., 2010; Pearson, Field, & Jordan, 2007). Evidence-based practice (EBP) is an important theme in this textbook and is defined as the conscientious integration of best research evidence with clinical expertise and patient values and needs in the delivery of quality, cost-effective health care (Craig & Smyth, 2007; Institute of Medicine, 2001; Sackett et al., 2000). Chapter 1 presented a model of EBP incorporating these ideas. Best research evidence comes from the conduct and synthesis of numerous, high-quality studies in a health-related area. Chapter 1 also introduced this concept of best research evidence and described the processes for synthesizing research evidence (systematic review, meta-analysis, integrative review, metasummary, and metasynthesis). This chapter builds on the previous

EBP discussions to provide you strategies for implementing best research evidence in your practice and moving the profession of nursing toward EBP. This chapter includes some of the barriers and benefits related to the development of an EBP in nursing. Guidelines are provided for you to critically appraise systematic reviews, meta-analyses, integrative reviews, metasummaries, and metasyntheses of research. It also introduces two nursing models developed to facilitate EBP by registered nurses (RNs) in healthcare agencies.

Expert researchers, clinicians, and consumers through government agencies, professional organizations, and healthcare agencies have developed an extensive number of evidence-based guidelines. Grove provides a model for reviewing the quality of these evidence-based guidelines and implementing them in practice. The chapter concludes with a discussion of the evidence-based practice centers and Institutional Clinical and Translational Science Awards that the United States (US) government has funded to expand the research evidence generated, synthesized, developed into evidence-based guidelines, and used in practice.

What Are the Barriers and Benefits to Evidence-Based Nursing Practice?

EBP is a goal for the nursing profession and for each practicing nurse. Currently, some of the nursing interventions are evidence based, or supported by research knowledge generated from several quality studies, but other areas of nursing practice require additional research. Some nurses readily use research-based interventions and others are slower to make changes in their practice based on current research (Melnyk et al., 2010). This section focuses on identifying the barriers and benefits of EBP to facilitate your use of research evidence in practice.

Barriers to Evidence-Based Nursing Practice

Barriers to the EBP movement have been both practical and conceptual. This section focuses on some of the barriers or constructive criticisms of EBP that need to be addressed as the nursing profession moves toward this goal. One of the barriers is that nursing lacks the research evidence for the implementation of an EBP in many areas. EBP requires synthesizing research evidence from randomized controlled trials (RCTs), and these types of studies are limited in nursing. However, the number of RCTs conducted to test nursing interventions has greatly increased in the last five years (Melnyk & Fineout-Overholt, 2005; Pearson et al., 2007).

Some of the systematic reviews and meta-analyses conducted in nursing indicate there is inadequate research evidence to support using certain nursing interventions in practice. Bolton, Donaldson, Rutledge, Bennett, and Brown (2007, p. 123S) conducted a critical appraisal of the "systematic/integrative reviews and meta-analyses on nursing interventions and patient outcomes in acute care settings." Their literature search covered 1999-2005 and produced 4000 systematic/integrative reviews and 500 meta-analyses covering seven topics selected by the authors: developmental care of neonates and infants, symptom management, eldercare, caregivers, pressure ulcer prevention/treatment, incontinence, and staffing. The authors recognized the need for additional research of selected nursing interventions but also noted that strong evidence existed "for the use of patient risk-assessment tools and interventions implemented by nurses to prevent patient harm" (Bolton et al., 2007, p. 123S). Thus you need to be able to critically appraise the systematic reviews, meta-analyses, and integrative reviews that have been conducted in nursing to determine the use of this evidence in your practice. Guidelines provided later in this chapter will assist you with this process.

Another criticism of the EBP movement is that the development of evidence-based guidelines has lead to a "cookbook" approach to nursing care. Nurses are expected to follow these guidelines in their practice as developed (Pearson et al., 2007). However, the definition of EBP indicates that it is the conscientious integration of best research evidence with clinical expertise and patient values and needs. Thus, RNs have a major role in determining how the best research evidence will be implemented in providing care to an individual patient and family. For example, an RN will use the national evidence-based guidelines for the assessment and education of patients with hypertension, the Joint National Committee on Prevention, Detection, Evaluation and Treatment of High Blood Pressure (JNC 7) and will also make clinical decisions based on the values and needs of individual patients. If you are caring for patients who are overweight, smoking, and/or not exercising, you would encourage them to make lifestyle changes to decrease their risk for major cardiovascular disease (CVD) (National Heart, Lung, and Blood Institute [NHLBI], 2003). You would also encourage patients to monitor their blood pressure in their homes to improve their knowledge of their health problem. If a patient refuses an intervention based on cultural or religious reasons, you would take these reasons into consideration in developing a nursing care plan for this patient. Evidence-based guidelines provide the gold standard for managing a particular health condition, but the nurse, physician, and patient individualize the plan to promote the best health outcomes (Brown, 2009; Melnyk et al., 2010; Sackett et al., 2000).

Another barrier is that the research evidence is generated based on population data and then is applied in practice to individual patients. In addition, there are difficulties in translating basic research knowledge generated in the lab with animals to human beings (Baumbusch, Kirkham, Khan, McDonald, Semeniuk, Tan, & Anderson, 2008; Chesla, 2008). Thus, more work is needed to facilitate the use of research evidence in caring for individual patients and families. The problem of translating research evidence into practice is not new and has been a concern for nurses, physicians, and healthcare administrators for several years. Recently a methodology has been developed called translational research to facilitate the application of research knowledge into practice settings. Translational research is a major initiative of the National Institutes of Health (NIH, 2008) and is discussed later in this chapter.

Another barrier is that some healthcare agencies and administrators do not provide the resources to support the implementation of EBP by nurses. Their lack of support might include the following: (1) not providing access to research journals and other sources of synthesized research findings and evidence-based guidelines, (2) limiting time to make research-based changes in practice, (3) limiting RNs authority to change patient care based on research findings, (4) providing minimal funds to support research-based changes for practice, and (5) providing few rewards for RNs delivering evidence-based care to patients and families. In addition, some nurses are barriers to EBP. They do not have the background to read research and do not see the value of implementing evidence-based interventions. Often this involves change and some are opposed to changing a policy or procedure that they have used for a long time. There is a need for both administrators and nurses to increase their focus on EBP (McCaughan, Thompson, Cullum, Sheldon, & Thompson, 2002; Parahoo, 2000; Pettengill, Gillies, & Clark, 1994; Retsas, 2000).

Benefits of Evidence-Based Nursing Practice

The benefits of EBP are improved outcomes for patients, providers, and healthcare agencies. The best research evidence has been synthesized in many areas by teams of expert researchers and clinicians to develop strong evidence-based guidelines for practice. These guidelines indicate the best treatment plan or gold standard for patient care in a selected area to promote quality health outcomes. Nurses and other healthcare providers have easy access to numerous evidence-based guidelines to assist them in making the best clinical decisions. These evidence-based guidelines are communicated by presentations and publications and are easily accessible online. These guidelines are extremely helpful to students, novice nurses, and experienced RNs to assist them in providing the best possible care (Brown, 2009; Kania-Lachance, Best, McDonah, & Ghosh, 2006). Nurses can access current evidence-based guidelines from a variety of websites maintained by government agencies, professional organizations, and EBP centers.

Many healthcare agencies are highly supportive of EBP because it promotes the delivery of quality, cost-effective care to patients and families and meets accreditation requirements. The Joint Commission on Accreditation of Healthcare Organizations (JCAHO) revised their accreditation criteria in 2002 to emphasize patient care quality achieved through EBP. Approximately 25% of the chief nursing officers (CNOs) identified movement toward evidence-based nursing practice as their number one priority (Nursing Executive Center, 2005).

Many CNOs and healthcare agencies are either trying to obtain or maintain magnet status that documents the excellence of nursing care in an agency. You can view the healthcare agencies that currently have magnet status online at the American Nurses Credentialing Center (ANCC) website at *http://www.nursecredentialing.org/Magnet/FindaMagnetFacility.aspx* (ANCC, 2009). The Magnet Status Program, provided through ANCC, recognizes evidence-based practice as a way to improve the quality of patient care and revitalize the nursing environment. Selection criteria for magnet status, which require healthcare agencies to promote the conduct of research and the use of research evidence in practice, are presented below. There is an emphasis on including practicing RNs in the research process and the implementation of EBP.

Force 6: Quality Care
Research and Evidence-Based Practice

22. Describe how current literature, appropriate to the practice setting, is available, disseminated, and used to change administrative and clinical practices.
23. Discuss the institution's policies and procedures that protect the rights of participants in research protocols. Include evidence of consistent nursing involvement in the governing body responsible for protection of human subjects in research.
24. Provide evidence that research consultants are actively involved in shaping nursing research infrastructure, capacity, and mentorship.
25. Provide a copy of the nursing budget or other sources of funding for the past year, the current year-to-date, and the future projection, highlighting the allocation and utilization of resources for nursing research.
26. Supply documentation of all nursing research activities that are ongoing, including internal validation studies, internal and external research, and participation in surveys completed within the past twelve (12) month period.

27. Provide evidence of education and mentoring activities that have effectively engaged staff nurses in research- and/or evidence-based practice activities.
28. Describe resources available to nursing staff to support participating in nursing research and nursing research utilization activities." (Nursing Executive Center, 2005, p. 15)

In working toward an EBP, nurses should embrace the benefits of EBP, use the evidence-based guidelines available, and support and/or participate in the research needed to determine the effectiveness of certain nursing interventions. The success of EBP depends on all involved in health care including nurses, physicians, administrators, and other healthcare professionals. You are encouraged to search a variety of resources to identify evidence for your practice.

Searching for Evidence-Based Sources

EBP requires searching a variety of databases and websites for the best research evidence for use in practice. You can identify research syntheses such as systematic reviews, meta-analyses, integrative reviews, metasummaries, and metasyntheses through searches of electronic databases, national library sites, evidence-based practice organizations, and professional organizations. Some of the key resources for EBP are in Table 13–1. Chapter 6 discusses the details for searching these resources. Once you have identified research syntheses, you needed to critically appraise these sources for relevant research evidence to use in your practice.

Guidelines for Critically Appraising Research Syntheses

Research evidence is synthesized using five different processes: systematic review, meta-analysis, integrative review, metasummary, and metasynthesis. These synthesis processes were introduced in Chapter 1 and the following section provides guidelines for critically appraising these synthesis processes to determine the status of knowledge for use in practice. Numerous research syntheses have been conducted in nursing and medicine and searching the sources in Table 13–1 will facilitate your identification of the research syntheses available. We encourage you to use the guidelines provided in this section to critically appraise these sources for relevant research knowledge to use in your practice.

Critically Appraising Systematic Reviews of Research

A **systematic review** is a structured, comprehensive synthesis of quantitative studies in a particular healthcare area to determine the best research evidence available for expert clinicians to use to promote an EBP. Systematic reviews are conducted to synthesis research evidence from numerous, high quality quantitative studies with similar methodologies, such as randomized clinical trial (RCT) (Craig & Smyth, 2007). Systematic reviews are often conducted by a team or panel of experts to provide the best research evidence for evidence-based guidelines. Guidelines are provided to assist you in critically appraising systematic reviews and the usefulness of the research evidence for your practice.

The critical appraise of a systematic review also needs to include an assessment of how current the review is. This leads to the question "How quickly do systematic reviews go out of date?" This question was investigated by Shojania, Sampson, Ansari, Ji, and Doucette (2007). These researchers conducted a survival analysis on 100 quantitative systematic reviews published from 1995 to 2005 "to estimate the average time to changes in evidence that is

Table 13-1	Evidence-Based Practice Resources
Resource	**Description**
Electronic Databases	
CINAHL (Cumulative Index to Nursing and Allied Health Literature)	CINAHL is an authoritative resource covering the English language journal literature for nursing and allied health. This database was developed in the United States (US) and includes sources published from 1982 forward.
MEDLINE (PubMed—National Library of Medicine)	Database developed by the National Library of Medicine in the United States and provides access to more than 11 million MEDLINE citations back to the mid-1960s and additional life science journals.
MEDLINE with MeSH	Database provides authoritative medical information on medicine, nursing, dentistry, veterinary medicine, the healthcare system, preclinical services, and more.
PsychINFO	Database that includes professional and academic literature for psychology and related disciplines from 1887 forward. This database was developed by the American Psychological Association.
CANCERLIT	Database of information on cancer that was developed by the US National Cancer Institute.
National Library Sites	
Cochrane Library	Provides high-quality evidence to inform people providing and receiving health care and those responsible for research, teaching, funding, and administration of health care at all levels. Included in the Cochrane Library is the Cochrane Collaboration that has many systematic reviews of research. The Cochrane Reviews are available at http://www.cochrane.org/reviews/
National Library of Health (NLH)	NLH is located in the United Kingdom (UK) and you can search for evidence-based sources using the following website: http://www.evidence.nhs.uk/
Evidence-Based Practice Organizations	
National Guideline Clearinghouse (NGC)	Agency for Healthcare Research and Quality developed the NGC to house the thousands of evidence-based guidelines that have been developed for use in clinical practice. The guidelines can be accessed online at http://www.guidelines.gov
National Institute for Health and Clinical Excellence (NICE)	NICE was organized in the UK to provide access to the evidence-based guidelines that have been developed; these guidelines can be accessed at http://nice.org.uk

sufficiently important to warrant updating systematic reviews" (Shojania et al., 2007, p. 224). They found the average time before a systematic review should be updated was 5.5 years. However, 23% of the reviews signaled a need for updating within two years and 15% needed updating within one year. Shojania et al. (2007) stressed that high-quality systematic reviews that were directly relevant to clinical practice require frequent updating to ensure they are current.

The Cochran Collaboration and library include extensive collections of systematic reviews and meta-analyses (http://www.cochrane.org/cochrane-reviews). A journal entitled *Medical Care Research & Review* includes a variety of research syntheses. Bolton et al. (2007) review introduced earlier identified 4000 systematic/integrative reviews that had been conducted in nursing. There are numerous nursing and medical systematic reviews of research

CRITICAL APPRAISAL GUIDELINES

Systematic Reviews

When critically appraising systemic reviews and the usefulness of the research evidence for your practice, consider the following questions:

1. Was the purpose [or objectives] of the review clearly stated?
2. Did the reviewers report a systematic and comprehensive search strategy to identify relevant studies?
3. Were inclusion and exclusion criteria for studies reported and were they appropriate (i.e., was selection bias avoided)?
4. Was the quality of included studies assessed appropriately?
5. Were the results of the included studies combined systematically and appropriately?
6. Were the conclusions supported by the data?

(Craig & Smyth, 2007, p. 194).

available and it is important for you to be able to critically appraise the quality of these reviews. Only quality, current systematic reviews provide the best research evidence to support protocols, algorithms, or policies for nursing practice. **Algorithms** are clinical decision-making trees or figures nurses use when implementing research evidence in practice. Chobanian et al. (2003) conducted an excellent systematic review to determine the best research evidence available for assessing, diagnosing, and managing hypertension. This systematic review, which included several meta-analyses and integrative reviews, was used to develop the JNC 7 evidence-based guideline for managing hypertension. This systematic review by Chobanian et al. in 2003 is critically appraised later in this chapter in the section entitled Implementing Evidence-Based Guidelines. The treatment of hypertension is presented as an algorithm.

Critically Appraising Meta-Analyses

Meta-analysis statistically pools the results from previous studies into a single quantitative analysis that provides the highest level of evidence for an intervention's efficacy (Conn & Rantz, 2003; Craig & Smyth, 2007). This approach allows the application of scientific criteria to factors such as sample size, level of significance, and variables examined. Through the use of meta-analysis, the following can be generated: (1) an extremely large, diverse sample that is more representative of the target population than the samples of the individual studies; (2) the determination of the overall significance of probability of pooled data from quality, confirmed studies; (3) the average effect size determined from several quality studies that indicates the efficacy of a treatment or intervention; and (4) the strength of relationships among the variables.

Meta-analyses make it possible to be objective rather than subjective in evaluating research findings for practice. The strongest evidence for using an intervention in practice comes from a meta-analysis of multiple, controlled studies. You can use the following guidelines to evaluate the quality of meta-analyses and to determine the usefulness of the research evidence in your practice (Craig & Smyth, 2007; Higgins & Green, 2008).

CRITICAL APPRAISAL GUDELINES

Meta-Analyses

When critically appraising and determining the quality of meta-analyses, consider the following questions:

1. Does the meta-analysis include a clearly expressed research problem and purpose?
2. Was a comprehensive search of the literature for eligible studies conducted?
3. Were the results of the studies statistically pooled?
4. Were the findings from the statistical results interpreted including examination of: (a) the benefit or harm of an intervention, (b) the effect size or strength of the intervention, (c) magnitude of relationships among study variables, (d) sensitivity and specificity of diagnostic tools, and/or (e) relative risk of an outcome in the treatment versus the control group (Craig & Smyth, 2007)?
5. The effect size for a relationship is the value of the r obtained through the Pearson Product Moment Correlation analysis. For example if the relationships between anxiety and depression is $r = 0.42$, the effect size (*ES*) is equal to 0.42 or the strength of the relationship. Thus: r = strength of the relationship = *ES* (Grove, 2007).
6. The *ES* for an intervention in a study is calculated using the following formula: Mean of the treatment ($M_{Tx\ Gr}$) or intervention group minus the mean of the comparison group ($M_{Comp\ Gr}$) divided by the standard deviation of the comparison group ($SD_{Comp\ Gr}$) (Grove, 2007).

$$\text{Formula Calculation of } ES: ES = (M_{Tx\ Gr} - M_{Comp\ Gr}) \div SD_{Comp\ Gr}$$

For example, a weight loss dietary intervention resulted in a mean weight loss of 4 pounds per month (*SD* = 5) for the treatment group and the comparison group had a mean weight loss of 1 pound per month (*SD* = 6).

$$\text{Example Calculation } ES: ES = (4 - 1) \div 6 = 3 \div 6 = 0.5$$

7. Were the findings from the meta-analysis clearly expressed with implications for clinical practice?

RESEARCH EXAMPLE Meta-Analysis

Banel and Hu (2009, p. 56) stated their objects were "to conduct a literature review and a meta-analysis to combine the results from several trials to estimate the effect of walnuts on blood lipids." The literature databases were searched to identify published clinical trials that compared a walnut-enhanced diet with a control diet. Thirteen studies met the inclusion criteria for the analysis and included a total sample of 365 subjects. The treatment groups in the 13 studies consumed diets supplemented with walnuts. The treatments in the different studies lasted from 4–24 weeks and provided 10% to 40% of the total calories consumed. A quantitative meta-analysis was conducted to determine the magnitude of the difference between the experimental and control groups in the selected studies. The treatment groups, who had a diet supplemented with walnuts, had significantly greater decreases in their total cholesterol and low density lipoprotein (LDL) cholesterol than the control groups. The high density lipoprotein (HDL) cholesterol and triglycerides were not significantly affected by the walnut supplements. Banel and Hu

(2009) concluded that the walnut-enriched diets significantly decreased the total and LDL cholesterol for the short term, but larger and longer-term clinical trials are needed to determine the effects of walnut consumption on cardiovascular risk and body weight.

CRITICAL APPRAISAL

The meta-analysis conducted by Banel and Hu (2009) included clearly stated objectives for the analysis. The search of the literature was guided by specific criteria and resulted in an adequate number of studies for the analyses. The total sample size achieved with the pooling of data from 13 studies was adequate but not large at $N = 365$. The results of the meta-analysis clearly identified the differences in cholesterol found between the treatment group consuming walnuts and the control group consuming a standard diet. The researchers' conclusions were consistent with the results and directions were provided for further research.

IMPLICATIONS FOR PRACTICE

Based on this meta-analysis, you might encourage your patients to supplement their diets with walnuts to decrease their total and LDL cholesterol. The sizes of these supplements need to be reasonable, approximately ½ to 1 cup depending on the percentage of dietary calories to be consumed in walnuts, to prevent weight gain. Additional research is needed to determine the long-term affects of the walnuts on cholesterol levels, cardiovascular risk, and weight.

Critically Appraising Integrative Reviews of Research

An integrative review of research includes the identification, analysis, and synthesis of research findings from independent quantitative and sometimes qualitative studies to determine the current knowledge (what is known and not known) in a particular area. An integrative review of research should be held to the same standards of clarity, rigor, and replication as primary research. You can use the following guidelines to critically appraise the quality of itegrative reviews of research.

In the past, most integrative reviews of research have included quantitative studies, but examining qualitative studies can also add some major contributions to the body of knowledge in a selected area. Dixon-Woods, Fitzpatrick, and Roberts (2001) identified the following contributions to integrative reviews by qualitative studies:

• Identify and refine the question of the review
• Identify the relevant outcomes of interest
• Identify the relevant types of participants and interventions
• Augment the data to be included in a quantitative synthesis
• Provide data for a non-numerical synthesis of research
• Highlight inadequacies in the methods used in quantitative studies
• Explain the findings of a quantitative synthesis
• Assist in the interpretation of the significance and applicability of the review
• Assist in making recommendations to practitioners and planners about implementing the conclusions in the review (Dixon-Woods et al., 2001, p. 126)

CRITICAL APPRAISAL GUIDELINES

Integrative Reviews of Research

When critically appraising integrative reviews of research, consider the following questions:

1. Were the purpose and scope of the integrative review clearly identified?
2. Were questions to be answered or hypotheses to be tested by the review identified?
3. Were criteria for inclusion and exclusion of studies in the review stated?
4. Was the literature search for relevant studies to include in the review described?
5. Was the adequacy of the number of studies included in the review discussed?
6. Did the authors develop a questionnaire or describe how they consistently gather information from quantitative and qualitative studies?
7. What criteria were used to evaluate the scientific quality of the studies?
8. Were the data from the studies analyzed in a systematic fashion?
9. Were the findings from the review expressed in a clear, concise, and complete manner (Dixon-Woods et al., 2001; Ganong, 1987; Gates, 2002; Stetler et al., 1998)?

RESEARCH EXAMPLE Integrative Review of Research

Putman-Casdorph and McCrone (2009, p. 34) conducted an integrative review of the literature

to determine the state of the science of COPD [chronic obstructive pulmonary disease], anxiety, and depression, and to identify nursing implications derived from these findings. ... A review of the literature was conducted using the PubMed and CINAHL databases targeting research studies and reviews from 2000 to the present and focusing on COPD, anxiety, and depression. Key words included in the search were *COPD, anxiety,* and *depression*. Seventy-five studies were initially identified. ... When seminal work was cited, studies occurring before 2000 were reviewed. ... A wide range of sample sizes, health status of subjects, and study specific aims was found. ... Sample sizes ranged from 6, in a small qualitative study, to 8387, in a large, multisite, quantitative study. Samples were recruited from inpatient, outpatient, and emergency department settings. Although some samples included both men and women, many studies were predominantly male.

The authors summarized studies in table format that included pharmacologic interventions, cognitive and behavioral interventions, and pulmonary rehabilitation. These tables included the study sample size, design/intervention, and outcomes.

Based on this integrative review of quantitative and qualitative studies, the authors concluded: The prevalence of anxiety and depression in patients with COPD is greater than in the general population. The literature supports the significant impact that anxiety and depression has on patients with COPD. Depression has been found to negatively affect exercise capacity, health perception/wellbeing, the use of inpatient and outpatient health services, and hospital stays. ... Both depression and anxiety have been found to negatively affect COPD treatment modalities, such as pulmonary rehabilitation and cigarette smoking-cessation efforts. ... There were discrepant results regarding the efficacy of pharmacologic interventions in the amelioration of anxiety, depression, respiratory symptoms, and physical comfort. ... Studies examining cognitive behavioral interventions in patients with COPD yielded mixed results. ... Pulmonary rehabilitation studies in patients with COPD and comorbid depression again produced mixed results. (Putman-Casdorph & McCrone, 2009, pp. 44-45)

CRITICAL APPRAISAL

Putman-Casdorph and McCrone (2009) conducted a rigorous integrative review of the quantitative and qualitative literature focused on COPD, anxiety, and depression. They provided a clear and specific description of their methods for searching the literature and the outcomes of their search. The studies focused on interventions were presented concisely and clearly in table format. The researchers summarized their findings from their literature review, and their conclusions were consistent with their findings. They also provided implications for practice and directions for future research.

IMPLICATIONS FOR PRACTICE

Putman-Casdorph and McCrone (2009, p. 45) indicated that:

> The analysis of the literature revealed several implications for practice. There is substantial evidence suggesting that anxiety and depression have an overall negative impact on the outcomes of patients with COPD. Depression and anxiety are largely overlooked, underdiagnosed, and undertreated. In light of the overall evidence regarding the prevalence and negative impact of anxiety and depression on patients, a routine assessment and screening for depression and anxiety in all patients diagnosed with COPD should be considered.

The researchers indicated that future research needed to include practical methods for improving provider and patient recognition of anxiety and depression. In addition, larger clinical trials are needed to determine the interventions that are most effective in managing COPD patients' depression and anxiety. Thus if you are working with COPD patients, this literature review encourages you to assess and screen them for depression and anxiety and report this information to ensure quality evidence-based care.

Evaluating Qualitative Syntheses of Research

Qualitative research synthesis is the process and product of systematically reviewing and formally integrating the findings from qualitative studies. Qualitative research synthesis includes two categories, qualitative metasummary and qualitative metasynthesis (Sandelowski & Barroso, 2007). Qualitative metasummary is the synthesis or summing of the findings across qualitative reports to determine the current knowledge in an area. Metasummary can be an end in itself to identify current knowledge or can provide a foundation for conducting qualitative metasynthesis. Qualitative metasynthesis provides a fully integrated, novel description or explanation of a target event or experience verses a summary view of that event or experience. Recently two noted qualitative researchers, Sandelowski and Barroso (2007), published the *Handbook for Synthesizing Qualitative Research* to facilitate the synthesis of qualitative studies. They identified the following criteria for determining the quality of qualitative research syntheses.

CRITICAL APPRAISAL GUIDELINES

Criteria for Evaluating Qualitative Research Syntheses
1. Did the authors conduct a systematic and comprehensive retrieval of the qualitative studies in a target area of inquiry?
2. Were qualitative and quantitative methods used systematically to analyze these reports?
3. Did the authors discuss the analysis and interpretation of the findings from the reports?
4. Were systematic and appropriately eclectic qualitative methods used to integrate the findings from these reports?
5. Were the findings from the qualitative synthesis clearly, concisely, and completely expressed (Sandelowski & Barroso, 2007)?

RESEARCH EXAMPLE Metasynthesis

Draucker, Martsolf, Ross, Cook, Stidham, and Mweemba (2009, p. 366) conducted a qualitative metasynthesis to identify the "essence of healing from sexual violence." The metasynthesis study was conducting using the procedures described by Sandelowski and Barroso (2007).

> The reports eligible for inclusion were of qualitative studies (a) conducted with participants of any race, ethnicity, nationality, or class conducted in the United States or Canada; (b) published in refereed venues prior to January 1, 2009; and (c) focused on adults' response to sexual violence of any type experienced at any point in the lifespan. We used the definition of sexual violence proposed by the CDC [Centers for Disease Control)]. (Draucker et al., 2009, p. 368)

The researchers appraised 82 articles using a 14-item reading guide developed by Sandelowski and Barroso (2007). The final sample included 55 reports from which the research team extracted 1897 statements related to healing from sexual violence. Of the 55 reports, 51 contributed to the final 514 edited statements. The 514 statements were reduced to 11 abstracted statements with effect sizes from 0.14 to 0.63. The statements and effect sizes were presented in a table in the article.

> Based on the findings from the 51 reports, four domains of healing were identified: (a) managing memories, (b) relating to important others, (c) seeking safety, and (d) reevaluating self. The ways of healing within each domain reflected the opposing responses. The dialectical process identified for each of the four domains include, respectively: (a) calling forth memories, (b) regulating relationships with others, (c) constructing an 'as-safe-as-possible' lifeworld, and (d) restoring a sense of self. These complex processes resulted in a new reality for the participants that was based on a greater sense of agency and provided a more satisfying life course. (Draucker et al., 2009, p. 366)

CRITICAL APPRAISAL

Draucker and colleagues (2009) conducted a high quality metasynthesis using the procedures of Sandelowski and Barroso (2007). The search and retrieval strategies for the relevant qualitative studies are clearly described. The process for critically appraising the studies to select the reports for analysis was conducted by the research team using set criteria. The results are both qualitative (11 statements related to healing) and quantitative (effect sizes for the 11 statements). Draucker et al. (2009) clearly and concisely presented their study findings and conclusions that seem to evolve from the study results.

IMPLICATIONS FOR PRACTICE

The study conclusions are expressed in the preceding example. Draucker et al. (2009, p. 376) identified the need for additional research and synthesis "to create an in-depth description of the factors that influence the process of healing and the trajectories that depict how healing changes over time." The researchers provided a clear description of the healing that takes place following sexual violence. They believe their metasynthesis study findings provide a basis to generate new treatment approaches to promote healing from sexual violence. They stress that these new approaches need to acknowledge the complexity of healing from sexual violence (Draucker et al., 2009).

Models to Promote Evidence-Based Practice in Nursing

EBP is a complex phenomenon that requires integration of best research evidence with clinical expertise and patient values and needs in the delivery of quality, cost-effective care. The two models that have been developed in nursing to promote EBP are the Stetler Model of Research Utilization to Facilitate EBP (Stetler, 2001) and the Iowa Model of Evidence-Based Practice to Promote Quality of Care (Titler et al., 2001). These two models are discussed in this section.

Stetler Model of Research Utilization to Facilitate Evidence-Based Practice

An initial model for research utilization in nursing was developed by Stetler and Marram in 1976 and expanded and refined by Stetler in 1994 and 2001 to promote EBP for nursing. The Stetler Model of Research Utilization to Facilitate Evidence-Based Practice (see Figure 13–1) provides a comprehensive framework to enhance the use of research evidence by nurses to facilitate an EBP. The research evidence can be used at the institutional or individual level. At the institutional level, study findings are synthesized and the knowledge generated is used to develop or refine policies, algorithms, procedures, protocols, or other formal programs implemented in the institution. Individual nurses, such as RNs, nurse practitioners, educators, and policymakers, summarize research and use the knowledge to influence educational programs, make practice decisions, and have an impact on political decision making. Stetler's model is included in this text to encourage the use of research evidence by individual nurses and healthcare institutions to facilitate the development of EBP. The five phases of the Stetler (2001) model are briefly described in the following sections: (1) preparation, (2) validation, (3) comparative evaluation/decision making, (4) translation/application, and (5) evaluation.

Phase I: Preparation

The intent of Stetler's (1994, 2001) model is to make using research evidence in practice a conscious, critical thinking process that is initiated by the user. Thus, Phase I: Preparation involves determining the purpose, focus, and potential outcomes of making an evidence-based change in a clinical agency. The agency priorities and other external and internal

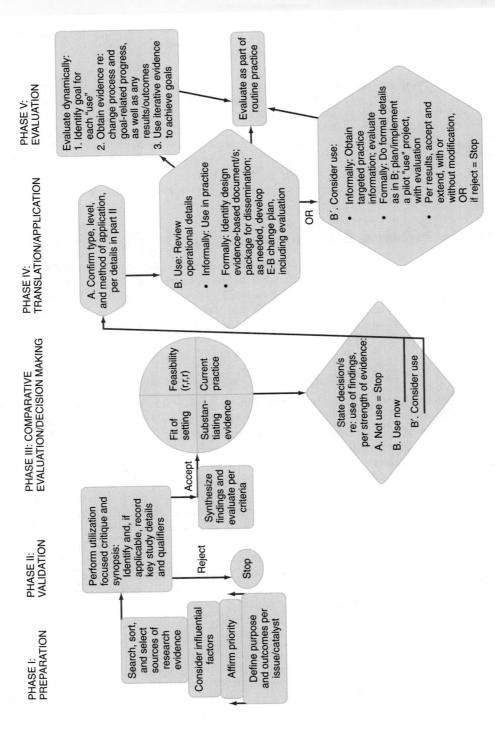

Figure 13–1. Stetler Model, Part I: Steps of research utilization to facilitate EBP. From Stetler, C. B. (2001). Updating the Stetler model of research utilization to facilitate evidence-based practice. *Nursing Outlook, 49*(6), 276.

factors that could be influenced by or could influence the proposed practice change need to be examined. Once the agency, individuals, or committee identify and approve the purpose of the evidence-based project, a detailed search of the literature is conducted to determine the strength of the evidence available for use in practice. The research literature might be reviewed to solve a difficult clinical, managerial, or educational problem; provide the basis for a policy, algorithm, or protocol; or prepare for an in-service program or other type of professional presentation.

Phase II: Validation

In Phase II: Validation, the research reports are critically appraised to determine their scientific soundness. If the studies are limited in number or are weak, or both, the findings and conclusions are considered inadequate for use in practice and the process stops. If a systematic review, meta-analysis, and/or integrative review have been conducted in the area where you want to make an evidence-based change, this greatly strengthens the quality of the research evidence. If the research knowledge base is strong in the selected area, the clinical agency must make a decision regarding the priority of using the evidence in practice.

Phase III: Comparative Evaluation/Decision Making

Phase III: Comparative Evaluation includes four parts: (1) substantiation of the evidence, (2) fit of the evidence with the healthcare setting, (3) feasibility of using research findings, and (4) concerns with current practice. Substantiating evidence is produced by replication, in which consistent, credible findings are obtained from several studies in similar practice settings. The studies generating the strongest research evidence are RCTs and meta-analyses of RCTs. However, quasi-experimental studies also provide extremely strong evidence for making a change in an agency. To determine the fit of the evidence in the clinical agency, examine the characteristics of the setting to determine the forces that will facilitate or inhibit implementation of the evidence-based change such as a policy, protocol, or algorithm for nursing practice. Stetler (2001) believes the feasibility of using research evidence in practice involves examining the three Rs related to making changes in practice: (1) potential risks, (2) resources needed, and (3) readiness of those involved. The final comparison involves determining whether the research information provides credible, empirical evidence for making changes in the current practice. Thus, the research evidence needs to document that an intervention increased the quality in current practice by solving practice problems and improving patient outcomes. By conducting phase III, you can assess the overall benefits and risks of using the research evidence in a practice setting. If the benefits are much greater than the risks for the organization or the individual nurse, or both, using the research based intervention in practice is feasible.

During the decision-making aspect of Phase III, three decisions are possible: (1) to use the research evidence, (2) to consider using the evidence, and (3) to not use the research evidence. The decision to use research knowledge in practice depends mainly on the strength of the evidence. Depending on the research knowledge to be used in practice, the individual RN, hospital unit, or agency might make this decision. Another decision might be to consider use of the available research evidence in practice. When a change is complex and involves multiple disciplines, additional time is often needed to determine how the evidence might be used and what measures will be taken to coordinate the involvement of different health professionals in the change. A final option might be to not use the research evidence in practice because the current evidence is not strong or the risks or costs of change in current practice are too high in comparison with the benefits (Stetler, 2001).

Phase IV: Translation/Application

Phase IV: Translation/Application involves planning for and actual use of the research evidence in practice. The translation phase involves determining exactly what knowledge will be used and how that knowledge will be applied to practice. The use of the research evidence can be cognitive, instrumental, or symbolic. With cognitive application, the research base is a means of modifying a way of thinking or one's appreciation of an issue (Stetler, 1994, 2001). Thus, cognitive application may improve the nurse's understanding of a situation, allow analysis of practice dynamics, or improve problem-solving skills for clinical problems. Instrumental application involves using research evidence to support the need for change in nursing interventions or practice protocols. Symbolic or political utilization occurs when information is used to support or change a current policy. The application phase includes the following steps for planned change: (1) assess the situation to be changed, (2) develop a plan for change, and (3) implement the plan. During the application phase, the protocols, policies, or algorithms developed with research knowledge are implemented in practice (Stetler, 1994, 2001). An agency may conduct a pilot project on a single hospital unit to implement the change in practice. The agency would then evaluate the results of this project to determine if the change should be extended throughout the healthcare agency.

Phase V: Evaluation

The final stage, Phase V: Evaluation, is to evaluate the impact of the research-based change on the healthcare agency, personnel, and patients. The evaluation process can include both formal and informal activities that are conducted by administrators, nurse clinicians, and other health professionals. Informal evaluations might include self-monitoring or discussions with patients, families, peers, and other professionals. Formal evaluations can include case studies, audits, quality assurance, and translational or outcomes research projects. The goal of Stetler's (2001) model is to increase the use of research evidence in nursing to facilitate EBP. This model provides detailed steps to encourage nurses to become change agents to make the necessary improvements in practice based on research evidence.

Iowa Model of Evidence-Based Practice

Nurses have been actively involved in conducting research, synthesizing research evidence, and developing evidence-based guidelines for practice. Thus, nurses have a strong commitment to EBP and can benefit from the direction provided by the Iowa model to expand their research-based practice. The Iowa Model of Evidence-Based Practice provides direction for the development of EBP in a clinical agency. This EBP model was initially developed by Titler and colleagues in 1994 and revised in 2001 (see Figure 13–2). In a healthcare agency, there are triggers that initiate the need for change and the focus should always be to make changes based on the best research evidence. These triggers can be problem focused and

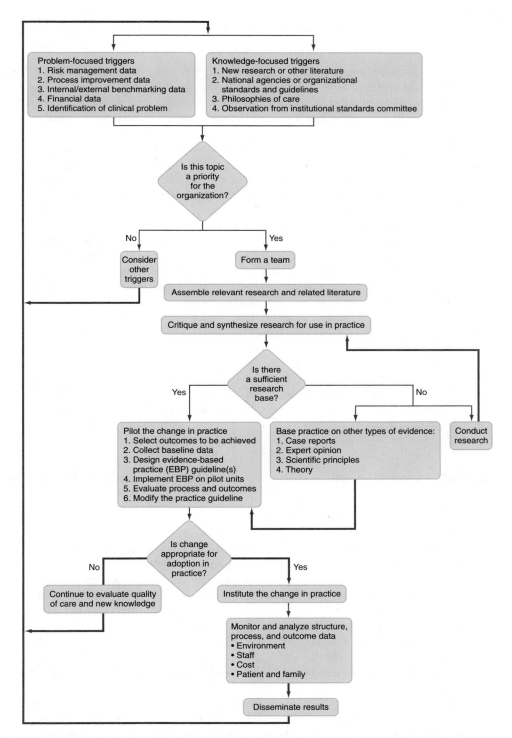

Figure 13–2. The Iowa Model of Evidence-Based Practice to Promote Quality Care. From Titler, M. G., Kleiber, C., Steelman, V. J., Rakel, B. A., Budreau, G., Everett, L. Q., et al. (2001). The Iowa model of evidence-based practice to promote quality care. *Critical Care Nursing Clinics of North America, 13*(4), 500.

evolve from risk management data, process improvement data, benchmarking data, financial data, and clinical problems. The triggers can also be knowledge focused, such as new research findings, change in national agencies or organizational standards and guidelines, expanded philosophy of care, or questions from the institutional standards' committee. The triggers are evaluated and prioritized based on the needs of the clinical agency. If a trigger is considered an agency priority, a group is formed to search for the best evidence to manage the clinical concern (Titler et al., 2001).

In some situations, the research evidence is inadequate to make changes in practice and additional studies are needed to strengthen the knowledge base. Sometimes the research evidence can be combined with other sources of knowledge (theories, scientific principles, expert opinion, and case reports) to provide fairly strong evidence for use in developing research-based protocols for practice (see Figure 13–2). **Research-based protocols** are structured guidelines for implementing nursing interventions in practice that are based on current research evidence. The strongest evidence comes from meta-analyses of several controlled clinical trials and systematic reviews that usually include meta-analyses, integrative reviews, and individual studies. Systematic reviews provide the best research evidence for developing evidence-based guidelines (see Figure 1–3 on p. 25). The research-based protocols or evidence-based guidelines would be pilot tested on a particular unit and then evaluated to determine the impact on patient care. If the outcomes are favorable from the pilot test, the change would be made in practice and monitored over time to determine its impact on the agency environment, staff, costs, and the patient and family (Titler et al., 2001). If an agency strongly supports the use of the Iowa model, implements patient care based on the best research evidence, and monitors changes in practice to ensure quality care, the agency is promoting EBP.

Application of the Iowa Model of Evidence-Based Practice

Preparing to use research evidence in practice raises some important questions. Which research findings are ready for use in clinical practice? What are the most effective strategies for implementing research-based protocols or evidence-based guidelines in a clinical agency? What are the outcomes from using the research evidence in practice? Do the risk management data, process improvement data, benchmarking data, or financial data support making the change in practice based on the research evidence? Is the research-based change proposed an agency priority? We suggest that effective strategies for using research evidence in practice will require a multifaceted approach that takes into consideration the evidence available, attitudes of the practicing nurses, the organization's philosophy, and national organizational standards and guidelines (Melnyk et al., 2010). In this section, the steps of the Iowa model (Titler et al., 2001) guide the use of a research-based intervention in a hospital to facilitate EBP. Research knowledge about the effects of heparin flush versus saline flush for irrigating peripheral intravenous (PIV) catheters is evaluated for use in nursing practice. This knowledge is used to develop a research-based protocol for making a change in practice, and outcome measures are identified for determining the effectiveness of this change in practice. Nurses making the switch from heparin flush to saline flush using a research-based protocol are providing evidence-based care (Craig & Smyth, 2007; Cullum, Ciliska, Haynes, & Marks, 2008; Pearson et al., 2007; Sackett et al., 2000).

Assemble, Critically Appraise, and Synthesize Research for Use in Practice

The body of nursing research must be assembled and evaluated for scientific merit and clinical relevance, and then the current findings need to be synthesized for use in practice (Conn & Rantz, 2003; Craig & Smyth, 2007; Gates, 2002). All types of research projects, including quantitative, qualitative, and outcomes studies, need to be evaluated when developing a research knowledge base for use in practice (Doran, 2003; Munhall, 2007).

Critical Appraisal for Scientific Merit

You determine the scientific merit of nursing studies by critically appraising the following aspects of a study: (1) the conceptualization and internal consistency, or the logical links of a study; (2) methodological rigor, or the strength of the design, sample, measurement methods, data collection process, and analysis techniques (Creswell, 2009); (3) generalizability of the findings, or the representativeness of the sample and setting; and (4) the number of replications (Burns & Grove, 2009; Craig & Smyth, 2007; Pearson et al., 2007). Chapter 12 presents the steps for critically appraising quantitative and qualitative studies to determine their scientific merit.

Evaluation of Clinical Relevance

The research-based knowledge might be used to solve practice problems, enhance clinical judgment, or measure phenomena in clinical practice. The research knowledge might be used on a single patient care unit, a hospital, or all hospitals in a corporation. Many settings will require a cost-benefit analysis to determine the impact of the proposed change on the clinical setting. A practitioner desiring to implement a research-based intervention must be able to assure the agency that the benefits of the intervention outweigh the cost in time, energy, and money and any real or potential risks. Nurses lag behind other disciplines in examining the cost of using new research-based interventions in practice. Stone, Curran, and Bakken (2002) provide different ways to analyze the costs for using an intervention in practice. Reading this source will assist you in analyzing costs for making changes in practice.

Synthesis of Research Evidence

The processes for synthesizing quantitative research evidence include systematic review, meta-analysis, and integrative review, which were described earlier in this chapter. The critical question you must address is, Is the evidence strong enough to support making a change in practice? For this evidence-based practice project, the objective is to determine the best research evidence available regarding the flushing of a PIV catheter for neonates, children, and adults. The literature was reviewed to determine which is the best flush solution, saline or heparin, for maintaining patency, increasing duration, and decreasing the incidence of phlebitis in PIV catheters. The following section includes a discussion of the research evidence available.

Extensive research was conducted with adults in the 1980s and 1990s to determine if there are significant differences in patency, duration, and incidence of phlebitis for PIV catheters irrigated with saline versus heparin flush. Goode et al. (1991) conducted a meta-analysis "to estimate the effects of heparin flush and saline flush solutions on maintaining patency, preventing phlebitis, and increasing duration of peripheral heparin locks [peripheral venous catheters]" (p. 324). The meta-analysis was conducted on 17 quality studies that are described in Table 13–2. Seven (41%) of the studies were RCTs and 10 (59%) were quasi-experimental (nonrandom) studies supporting the quality of the studies conducted. The total sample size of the 17 studies was 4153, and the settings of these studies were a variety of adult medical-surgical and critical care units. The small effect size values (most are less than 0.20) for clotting, phlebitis, and duration indicate that saline flush is as effective as heparin flush in maintaining PIV catheters. Goode et al. (1991) summarized current knowledge on the use of saline versus heparin flushes.

> "It can be concluded that saline is as effective as heparin in maintaining patency, preventing phlebitis, and increasing duration in peripheral heparin locks. Quality of care can be enhanced by using saline as the flush solution, thereby eliminating problems associated with anticoagulant effects and drug incompatibilities. In addition, an estimated yearly savings of $109,100,000 to $218,200,000 U.S. health care dollars could be attained" (Goode et al., 1991, p. 324).

In 2006, the American Society of Hospital Pharmacists (ASHP) published a Therapeutic Position Statement on the institutional use of 0.9% sodium chloride (saline) flush to maintain patency of PIV catheters, versus heparin flush. This is an example of an opinion published by a national organization based on research evidence. This type of evidence provides a basis for making a change in practice, but it is a much weaker form of evidence than the systematic review, meta-analysis, or individual RCTs (see Figure 1–3).

Additional research continued to be conducted regarding the best flush solution for PIV catheters. In 1998, Randolph, Cook, Gonzales, and Andrew published a systematic review and meta-analysis of randomized controlled trials to determine the effectiveness of saline versus heparin as a flush for peripheral venous and arterial catheters. These authors concluded that "flushing peripheral venous catheter locks between use with heparinized saline at 10 U/ml [units/milliliter] is no more beneficial than flushing with normal saline" (Randolph et al., 1998, p. 969). In 2000, the Intravenous Nursing Society (INS) published standards for the maintenance of PIV catheters.

Over the last decade research has been conducted to determine the effectiveness of heparin versus saline flush in PIV sites in children and neonates. Only a limited number of studies have been conducted and the results have been mixed. The Cochran Database included a systematic review of the effect of heparin in prolonging PIV catheter use in neonates, and Shah, Ng, and Sinha (2005) developed an abstract of the review:

> *Background:* Peripheral intravenous (PIV) catheters are widely used in modern medical practice. However, mechanical or infectious complications often necessitate their removal and/or replacement. Heparin has been shown to be effective in prolonging the patency of peripheral arterial catheters and central venous catheters, but may result in life threatening complications, especially in preterm neonates.
>
> *Objectives:* The primary objective was to determine the effectiveness of heparin versus placebo or no treatment on duration of PIV catheter patency, defined as number of hours of catheter use. The secondary objectives were to assess the effects of heparin on catheter blockage, phlebitis, or thrombophlebitis, catheter related sepsis, and complications including abnormality of coagulation profile, allergic reactions to heparin, heparin induced thrombocytopenia, intraventricular/intracranial hemorrhage and mortality.

Table 13-2   Studies Included in the Meta-Analysis

Study	N	Subjects	Assignment	Heparin Dose (U/cc)	Clotting Effect Size (d_c)	Phlebitis Effect Size (d_p)	Duration Effect Size (d_d)
Ashton et al, 1990	16 exp_c, 16 con_c; 13 exp_p, 14 con_p	Adult critical care	Random, double blind	10	0.3590	-0.1230	
Barrett & Lester, 1990	59 experimental, 50 control	Adult Med-Surg patients	Nonrandom double-blind crossover	10	-0.1068	-0.4718	
Craig & Anderson, 1991	129 exp. 145 con	Adult Med-Surg patients	Random double-blind crossover	10	0.0095	-0.0586	
Cyganski, Donahue, & Heaton, 1987	225 exp. 196 con	Adult Med-Surg patients	Nonrandom	100	0.2510		
Donham & Denning, 1987	8 exp_c, 4 con_c; 7 exp_p, 5 con_p	Adult critical care	Random, double blind	10	0.0000	0.0548	
Dunn & Lenihan, 1987	61 experimental 51 control	Adult patients	Nonrandom	50	-0.2057	-0.2258	
Epperson, 1984	138 exp, 120 con 138 exp, 154 con	Adult Med-Surg patients	Random, double blind	10 100			-0.1176 -0.1232
Garrelts et al., 1989	131 exp, 173 con	Adult Med-Surg patients	Random, double blind	10	-0.1773	0.1057	0.2753
Hamilton et al., 1988	137 exp, 170 con	Adult patients	Random, double blind	100	0.0850	-0.1819	-0.0604
Holford et al., 1977	39 experimental 140 control	Young adult volunteers	Nonrandom, double blind	3.3, 10, 16.5, 100, 132	0.6545		
Kasparek, Wenger, & Feldt, 1988	49 exp. 50 con	Adult Med patients	Random, double blind	10	0.3670	-0.5430	
Lombardi et al., 1988	34 experimental 40 control	Pediatric patients (4 wk to 18 yr)	Nonrandom, sequential, double blind	10		-0.2324	0.0000
Miracle et al., 1989	167 exp. 441 con	Adult Med-Surg patients	Nonrandom	100	-0.0042	-0.0977	
Shearer, 1987	87 exp, 73 con	Med-Surg patients	Nonrandom	10	-0.1170		
Spann, 1988	15 experimental 19 control	Adult telemetry step-down	Nonrandom, double blind	10	-0.3163	-0.3252	
Taylor et al., 1989	369 exp, 356 con	Adult Med-Surg patients	Nonrandom, time series	10	0.0308	0.0288	-0.1472
Tuten & Gueldner, 1991	43 exp, 71 con	Adult Med-Surg patients	Nonrandom	100	0.0000	0.1662	

From Goode, C.J., et al. (1991). A meta-analysis of effects of heparin flush and saline flush: Quality and cost implications. *Nursing Research, 40*(6), 325. Used with permission of Lippincott-Raven Publishers, Philadelphia.

Search Strategy: A literature search was performed using the following resources: MEDLINE (1966-February 2005); EMBASE (1980-February 2005); CINAHL (1982-February 2005); Cochrane Central Register of Controlled Trials (CENTRAL, The Cochrane Library, Issue 1, 2005); and abstracts from annual meetings of the Society for Pediatric Research, American Pediatric Society, and Pediatric Academic Societies that were published in Pediatric Research (1991-2004). No language restrictions were applied.

Selection Criteria: Randomized or quasi-randomized trials of heparin administered as flush or infusion versus placebo or no treatment were included. Studies which included a neonatal population and reported on at least one of the outcomes were included. ...

Main Results: Ten eligible studies were identified. Heparin was administered either as a flush solution, or as an additive to the total parenteral nutrition solution. Five studies reported data on the duration of use of the first catheter. Two of these studies found no statistically significant effect of heparin; two studies showed a statistically significant increase, and one study showed a statistically significant decrease in the duration of PIV catheter use in heparin group. The results were not combined for meta-analysis due to significant heterogeneity of the treatment effect ($p < 0.01$). In addition, there were marked differences between the studies in terms of the methodological quality, the dose, the timing, the route of administration of heparin, and the outcomes reported. From a limited number of studies, there were no significant difference between the heparin and the placebo/no treatment groups in the risks of infiltration, phlebitis, and intracranial hemorrhage.

Authors Conclusions: Implications for practice: The effect of heparin on the duration of peripheral intravenous catheter use varied across the studies. Because of clinical heterogeneity and heterogeneity in treatment effect, recommendations for heparin use in neonates with PIV catheters cannot be made. Implications for research: There are insufficient data concerning the effect of heparin for prolonging PIV catheter use in neonates. Further research on the effectiveness, the optimal dose, and safety of heparin is required. (Shah et al., 2005, Cochrane Database, online)

Sufficiency of the Research Base

The two meta-analyses of controlled clinical trials provide sound scientific evidence for making a change in practice from heparin flush to saline flush for irrigating PIV catheters or heparin locks in adults (Goode et al., 1991; Randolph et al., 1998). Clinical relevance is evident in that the use of saline to flush PIV catheters promotes quality outcomes for the patient (patent heparin lock, fewer problems with anticoagulant effects, and fewer drug incompatibilities); the nurse (decreased time to flush the catheter and no drug incompatibilities with saline); and the agency (extensive cost savings and quality patient care).

The research knowledge base is extremely strong for making the EBP change from heparin to saline flush to maintain the patency of PIV catheters in adults. This best research evidence continues to support the gold standard of using saline to flush PIV catheters in adults. Currently the Oncology Nursing Society included the flushing and maintenance of the PIV catheters in a national guideline (ONS, 2004). This guideline is titled *Access Device Guidelines: Recommendations for Nursing Practice and Education* and is available online at *http://www.guideline.gov/summary/summary.aspx?doc_id=8338&nbr=004666&string=access+AND+device+AND+guideline.*

However, there is need for additional research for the best flush (saline or heparin) to use for maintaining the patency of PIV catheters in neonates and children. The 2005 Cochrane systematic review clearly indicates that the research evidence is inadequate to implement in practice regarding the appropriate flush to use with PIV catheters in neonates. The areas for additional research were identified (Shah et al., 2005). More research is also needed to determine how often PIV catheters should be flushed in ambulatory settings (Campbell, Trojanowski, & Ackroyd-Stolarz, 2005). Thus, the evidence base for practice is adequate only for adults in the type of flush (saline) to use in irrigating PIV catheters in acute care settings (Goode et al., 1991, 1993; INS, 2000; Randolph et al., 1998). In addition, a national guideline exists to direct you in ensuring PIV catheters are correctly flushed and maintained in your practice setting (ONS, 2004).

Pilot the Change in Practice

The relative advantages of using saline are the improved quality of care and cost savings clearly documented in the research literature with standards developed to direct clinical practice (Goode et al., 1991, 1993; O'Grady et al., 2002; INS, 2000; Peterson & Kirchhoff, 1991; Randolph et al., 1998; Shoaf & Oliver, 1992). Table 13–3 summarizes the cost savings for different sizes of hospitals. You can determine the compatibility of the change by identifying the changes that will need to occur in your agency. What changes will the nurses have to make in irrigating PIV catheters with saline? What changes will have to occur in the pharmacy to provide the saline flush? Are the physicians aware of the research in this area? Are the physicians willing to order the use of saline to flush venous catheters?

The change in PIV catheter flush from heparin to saline has minimal complexity. The only thing changed is the flush, so no additional skills, expertise, or time is required by the nurse to make the change. Because saline flush, unlike heparin flush, is compatible with any drug that might be administered through the PIV catheter, the number of potential complications is decreased. The change might be started on one unit as a trial and then evaluated. Once the quality of care and cost savings are documented for nurses, physicians, and hospital administrators, the change will probably spread rapidly throughout the institution. Changing heparin flush to saline flush would be relatively simple to implement on a trial basis to demonstrate the positive outcomes for patients, nurses, and the healthcare agency.

The decision to use saline flush versus heparin flush as an irrigant requires institutional approval, physician approval, and approval of the nurses managing patients' PIV catheters. When a change requires institutional approval, decision making may be distributed through several levels of the organization. Thus, a decision at one level may lead to contact with

Table 13-3	Annual Cost Savings from Changing to Saline	
Study	**Cost Savings**	**Hospital**
Craig & Anderson, 1991	$40,000/yr	525-bed tertiary care hospital
Dunn & Lenihan, 1987	$19,000/yr	530-bed private hospital
Goode et al., 1991 (this study)	$38,000/yr	879-bed tertiary care hospital
Kasparek, Wenger, & Feldt, 1988	$19,000/yr	350-bed private hospital
Lombardi et al., 1988	$20,000–$25,000/yr	52-bed pediatric unit
Schustek, 1984	$20,000/yr	391-bed private hospital
Taylor et al., 1989	$30,000–$40,000/yr	216-bed private hospital

From Goode, C. J., et al. (1991). A meta-analysis of effects of heparin flush and saline flush: Quality and cost implications. *Nursing Research, 40*(6), 325. Used with permission of Lippincott-Raven Publishers, Philadelphia.

another official who must approve the action. In keeping with the guidelines of planned change, institutional changes are more likely to be effective if all those affected by the change have a voice in the decision. In your institution, who needs to approve the change? What steps do you need to take to get the change approved within your institution? Do the physicians support the change? Do the nurses on the units support the change? Who are the leaders in the institution and can you get them to support the change? Try to get the nurses to make a commitment and take a public stand to make the change because their commitment increases the probability that the change will be made. Contact the appropriate administrative people and physicians and detail the pros and cons of making the change to saline flush for irrigating PIV catheters. You need to clearly indicate to physicians and administrators that the change is based on extremely strong research evidence, provides extensive cost savings, and promotes quality patient care. Most physicians are positively influenced by research-based knowledge, and agencies will respond positively to cost savings and research-based decisions.

Institute the Change in Practice

Implementing a research-based change can be simple or complex, depending on the change. The change might be implemented as indicated in the research literature or may be modified to meet the agency's needs. In some cases, you may spend a long time in planning implementation of the change after the decision is made. In other cases, implementation can begin immediately. Usually, a great deal of support is necessary during initial implementation of a change. As with any new activity, unexpected events often occur. Contact with a person experienced in the change (a change agent) can facilitate the change process.

The change from heparin flush to saline flush will involve physicians ordering saline for flushing PIV catheters. You will need to speak with the physicians to gain their support for the change. You might convince some key physicians to support the change, and they will convince others to make the change. The pharmacy will have to package saline for use as a flush. The nurses will also be provided information about the change and the rationale for the change. It might be best to implement the change on one nursing unit and give the nurses on this unit an opportunity to design the protocol and plan for implementing the change. The nurses might develop a protocol similar to the one in Table 13–4, which is consistent with the ONS (2004) national guideline that includes flushing and maintenance of PIV catheters. The protocol must include referencing from the research literature to document that the intervention is evidence-based. The evidence-based protocol directs you in preparing for irrigating a PIV catheter, actually irrigating the catheter, and documenting your actions (see Table 13–4).

Monitor Outcomes

After an evidence-based change has been implemented in practice, nurses and other health professionals need to monitor appropriate outcomes to determine the effectiveness of the change. They need to document that the change improved quality of care, decreased the cost of care, saved nursing time, improved access to care, or any combination of these benefits. If the outcomes from the EBP change are positive, nurses, administrators, and physicians will often want to continue the change. Nurses usually seek feedback from those around

Table 13–4	Protocol for Flushing Peripheral Venous Catheters (PIV) in Adults in Acute Care Settings

1. Review the protocol for flushing of the PIV with normal saline (ASHP, 2006; Goode et al., 1991, 1993; ONS, 2004; Peterson & Kirchhoff, 1991; Randolph et al., 1998).
2. Wash hands: Good hand hygiene and standard precautions are used for insertion and IV maintenance. Wash hands before and after flushing the PIV catheter using antibacterial soap and water or antibacterial cleanser (Centers for Disease Control, 2002; O'Grady et al., 2002).
3. Evaluate the IPV catheter site every 8 hours for complications of phlebitis. Inspect catheter insertion site for erythema and palpate for tenderness, warmth, or a palpable cord (O'Grady et al., 2002; INS, 2000; ONS, 2004).
4. Put on gloves and cleanse the PIV catheter port with alcohol (Goode et al., 1991, 1993; INS, 2000; O'Grady et al., 2002).
5. Routinely flush intermittent devices with 3-5 ml of 0.9% sodium chloride solution or compatible solution with each use. Flush every 12 hours if frequency of use is >12 hours (ONS, 2004).
6. Routinely lock peripheral devices using the last 1-2 ml of normal saline flush solution. Lock the device using at least twice the volume capacity of the catheter plus the priming volume of add-on devices (e.g., extension tubing—commonly from 3 to 10 ml) (ONS, 2004).
7. Chart the date and time of the PIV catheter flushing and the appearance and patency of the catheter site (INS 2000; ONS, 2004).

References

American Society of Health Systems Pharmacists. (2006). ASHP therapeutic position statement on the institutional use of 0.9% sodium chloride injection to maintain patency of peripheral indewelling intermittent infusion devices. *American Journal of Health Systems Pharmacy*, 63(12), 1273-1275.

Center for Disease Control. (2002). Guideline for hand hygiene in health-care settings. *Morbidity and Mortality Weekly Report*, 51(RR-16), 1-45. Retrieved on August 17, 2009 from http://www.cdc.gov/mmwr/PDF/rr/rr5116.pdf.

Goode, C. J., Kleiber, C., Titler, M., Small, S., Rakel, B., Steelman, V. M., Walker, J. B., & Buckwalter, K. C. (1993). Improving practice through research: The case of heparin vs. saline for peripheral intermittent infusion devices. *Medical-Surgical Nursing*, 2(1), 23-27.

Goode, C. J., Titler, M., Rakel, B., Ones, D. S., Kleiber, C., Small, S., et al. (1991). A meta-analysis of effects of heparin flush and saline flush: Quality and cost implications. *Nursing Research*, 40(6), 324–330.

Intravenous Nursing Society (INS). (2000). Infusion nursing standards of practice. *Journal of Intravenous Nursing*, 23(Suppl 6), S53-54, S81-88.

O'Grady, N. P., Alexander, M., Dellinger, E. P., Gerberding, J. L., Heard, S. O., Maki, D. G., Masur, H., McCormick, R. D., Mermel, L. A., Pearson, M. L., Raad I. I., Randolph, A., & Weinstein, R. A. (2002). Guidelines for the prevention of intravascular catheter-related infections. *Morbidity and Mortality Weekly Report Recommendation Rep*, 9(51 RR-10), 1-29.

Oncology Nursing Society (ONS). (2004). *Access device guidelines: Recommendations for nursing practice and education*, 2nd ed. Pittsburgh (PA): Oncology Nursing Society (ONS). Retrieved on August 17, 2009 from http://www.guideline.gov/summary/summary.aspx?doc_id=8338&nbr=004666&string=access+AND+device+AND+guideline.

Peterson, F. Y., & Kirchhoff, K. T. (1991). Analysis of the research about heparinized versus nonheparinized intravascular lines. *Heart & Lung*, 20(6), 631-640.

Randolph, A. G., Cook, D. J., Gonzales, C. A., & Andrew, M. (1998). Benefits of heparin in peripheral venous and arterial catheters: Systematic review and meta-analysis of randomized controlled trials. *British Medical Journal*, 316(7136), 969–975.

them. Their peers' reactions to the change in nursing practice will influence continuation of the change.

You can confirm the effectiveness of the saline flush for PIV catheter irrigation by examining patient care outcomes and cost-benefit ratios. You can examine patient care outcomes by determining the number of clotting and phlebitis complications associated with PIV catheters one month before the EBP change and one month after the change. If no significant difference is seen, the use of saline flush is supported. You can calculate the cost savings for one month by determining the cost difference between heparin flush and saline flush. This cost difference can then be multiplied by the number of saline flushes conducted in one month. This cost savings can then be multiplied by 12 months and compared with the cost savings summarized in Table 13–3. Nurses should be given the opportunity to evaluate the change and indicate if it has saved nursing time and promoted quality care for management of their patients' PIV catheters. If positive patient and nurse outcomes and cost savings are demonstrated, the healthcare agency will support and extend the EBP of using saline flush for irrigating PIV catheters of adults. In addition, the agency will be following national guideline for the management of PIV catheters (ONS, 2004). If your healthcare agency is currently using saline flush for irrigating PIV catheters, be sure the agency protocols follow the national guidelines.

Developing Clinical Questions to Identify Evidence for Use in Practice

The Cochrane Collaboration, which was introduced earlier in this chapter, includes one of the most extensive collections of systematic reviews. To promote the development of quality reviews, the *Cochran Handbook for Systematic Reviews of Interventions* was published (Higgins & Green, 2008). A systematic review is initiated by a relevant clinical question that is formulated using the PICO format. **PICO format** includes the following elements:

P—Population or participants of interest
I—Intervention needed for practice
C—Comparisons of interventions to determine the best for practice
O—Outcomes needed for practice

You can use the PICO format to identify relevant studies, meta-analyses, and integrative reviews needed to develop a systematic review. Systematic reviews are often used as a basis for the development of guidelines for practice. Some publications include both systematic review and a guideline for practice. For example, Nicoll and Hesby (2002) developed a systematic review of the research literature focused on intramuscular (IM) injection techniques. This review provided the basis for their development of a clinical practice guideline entitled "Intramuscular Injection: Guidelines for Evidence-Based Technique." The goal of their systematic review and evidence-based guidelines was the "elimination of complications from IM injections" (Nicoll & Hesby, 2002, p. 152). The researchers summarized the medications routinely administered by the IM route with site recommendations in Table 13–5. This table includes the medication class, generic and brand names of the medication, and the recommended site and needle size for selected IM injections. The recommendations for sites and

Medication Class	Generic Name	Brand Names (Selected)[a]	Recommend Sites and Needle Size[b]
Antibiotics	Streptomycin sulfate	Streptomycin sulfate injection	Adults: ventrogluteal with 38 mm, 18- to 25-g needle
	Pencillin G benzathine Pencillin G procaine	Bicillin, Wycllin, Pfizerpen	Infants and young children: vastus lateralis with 16 to 25 mm, 22- to 25-g needle
Biologicals, including immune globulins, vaccines, and toxoids	Diptheria and tetanus toxoids adsorbed	DT (pediatric), Td (adult)	Adults: Deltoid with 25 to 38 mm, 22- to 25-g needle. Hepatitis B and rabies must be given in the
	Diptheria, tetanus, and acellular pertussis	Acel-Immune, Infanrix, Tripedia, Certiva	deltoid site. Immune globulin may be given in the deltoid (volumes of 2 mL or less) or VG
	Haemophilus influenzae type b conjugate	ActHIB	site (volumes of more than 2 mL).
	Haemophilus influenzae type b conjugate and hepatitis B (recombinant)	Comvax	Toddlers and older children: deltoid, if the muscle mass is adequate, with 16 to 32 mm,
	Hepatitis A vaccine, inactivated	Havrix, Vaqta	22- to 25-g needle
	Hepatitis B vaccine (recombinant)	Engerix-B, Recombivax HB	Infants, young children and those with inadequate muscle mass at the deltoid site: vastus lateralis
	Heptatitis B Immune Globuin (human)	BayHepB, Nabi-HB	with 22 to 25 mm, 22- to 27-g needle
	Hepatitis A inactivated and hepatitis B (recombinant)	Twinrix	
	Immune globulin for pre- and post-exposure prophylaxis for Hepatitis A infection		
	Influenza Virus Vaccine	Fluogen, FluShield, Fluvirin, Fluzone	
	Lyme disease vaccine	LYMErix	
	Pneumococcal vaccine, polyvalent	Prevnar	
	Rabies vaccine adsorbed	RabAvert	
	Rabies immune globulin (Human)		
	Rh°(D) immune globulin (human)	BayRhoD, MICRhoGAM, RhoGAM, WinRho SDF	
	Tetanus immune globulin (human)	BayTet	
	Tetanus toxoid adsorbed	Tetanus toxoid adsorbed purogenated	
Hormonal Agents	Medroxyprogesterone acetate	Depo-Provera	Adults: ventrogluteal with 38 mm, 18- to 25-g needle (these medications are typically not indicated for infants and young children)
	Chorionic gonadotropin	Novarel, Pregnyl	
	Menotropin	Humegon, Repronex	
	Testosterone enathanate	Delatestry	

[a]Selected brand names are included to be illustrative of products widely used in the US; in other countries in which the generic products are available (this is particularly true in the case of vaccines) they may go by different names. All brand names are copyrighted trademarks of their respective companies.

[b]Needle sizes are provided in metric lengths to conform to the international standard; for US readers, corresponding needle sizes in inches are as follows: 16 mm = 5/8"; 22 mm = 7/8"; 25 mm = 1"; 32 mm = 1¼"; 38 mm = 1½".

Nicoll, L. H., & Hesby, A. (2002). Intramuscular injection: An integrative research review and guideline for evidence-based practice. *Applied Nursing Research, 16*(2), p. 150.

needle size (length and gage) were for infants, toddlers, and adults. This is valuable research evidence for you to use when giving IM injection of a particular medication to patients of all ages in your practice. Table 13–6 presents the clinical practice guideline for giving IM injections using an evidence-based technique.

You can use the PICO format to determine the evidence-based delivery of an IM injection.

P—Population is adults needing influenza virus vaccine by IM injection. Confirm that the vaccine must be given by IM injection.

I—Intervention to deliver the right medication by the right route at the right site using the appropriate needle size (length and gauge).

C—Comparison of interventions reveals: Influenza virus vaccine should be given to adults in the deltoid site with 25- to 38-mm, 22- to 25-gauge needles (see Table 13–5). The evidence-based technique for giving the IM injection is in Table 13–6.

O—Outcome desired is an IM injection of vaccine without complications.

You can use Tables 13–5 and 13–6 to ensure that you give IM injections using the best research evidence available. You can then share this evidence with others in clinics, hospitals, or rehabilitation centers to promote EBP for the delivery of IM injections.

Implementing Evidence-Based Guidelines in Practice

EBP of nursing has expanded extensively over the last 10 years. Research knowledge is generated every day that needs to be critically appraised and synthesized to determine the best evidence for use in practice (Brown, 2009; Craig & Smyth, 2007; Melnyk & Fineout-Overholt, 2005). The best research evidence has been synthesized by a panel of experts into evidence-based guidelines that provide current, comprehensive directions for using research in practice. This section of the chapter discusses the development of evidence-based guidelines and provides a model for using evidenced-based guidelines in practice. The evidence-based guideline for assessment, diagnosis, and management of hypertension is provided as an example (Chobanian et al., 2003).

History of the Development of Evidence-Based Guidelines

Since the 1980s, the Agency for Healthcare Research and Quality (AHRQ) has had a major role in the identification of health topics and the development of evidence-based guidelines for these topics (see *http://www.ahrq.gov/*). The initial guidelines developed by the AHRQ in the late 1980s and early 1990s were often done by a panel or team of experts. The AHRQ solicited panel members, who were usually nationally recognized researchers in the topic area or expert clinicians, such as physicians, nurses, pharmacists, and social workers. They also sought healthcare administrators, policy developers, economists, government representatives, and consumers. The group designated the scope of the guidelines and conducted extensive reviews of the literature including relevant systematic reviews, meta-analyses, integrative reviews of research, individual studies, and theories.

These experts synthesized the best research evidence available to develop recommendations for practice. Most of the evidence-based guidelines included meta-analyses, integrative

Table 13-6	Clinical Practice Guideline

Intramuscular Injection Guidelines for Evidence-Based Technique

Patient Population: Infants, toddlers, children, and adults receiving medication by the IM route for curative or prophylactic purposes.

Objective: Administration of medication to maximize its therapeutic effect for the patient and minimize or eliminate patient injury and discomfort associated with the procedure.

Key Points: "An injection should only be given if it is necessary—and each injection that is given must be safe" (WHO, 1998).

Justification for IM injection. Consider:
- Medication characteristics including formulation, onset and intensity of effect, and duration of effect.[*]
- Patient characteristics including compliance, uncooperativeness, reluctance, or inability to take medication via another route.[*]

Site selection. Site is the single most consistent factor associated with complications and injury. Consider:

Age of patient:
- Infants: vastus lateralis is the preferred site[*]
- Toddlers and children: vastus lateralis or deltoid[*]
- Adults: ventrogluteal or deltoid[*]

Medication type
- Biologicals (including immune globulins, vaccines, and toxoids): vastus lateralis (infants and young children); deltoid in older children and adults[*]
- Hepatitis B and rabies must be given in the deltoid; injection in other sites decreases the immunogenicity of the medication[*]
- Depot formulations: ventrogluteal site[*]
- Medications that are known to be irritating, viscous or in oily solutions should be administered at the ventrogluteal site[*]

Medication volume
- Small volumes of medication (2 mL or less) may be given in the deltoid site[*]
- Large volumes of medication (2-5 mL) should be given in the ventrogluteal site
  Always use bony landmarks to properly identify the site[*]

Preparation of the medication. Consider:

Equipment

Needle length corresponds to the site of injection and age of patient according to the following guidelines:
- Vastus lateralis: 16 mm to 25 mm[2][*]
- Deltoid (children): 16 mm to 32 mm[*]
- Deltoid (adults): 25 mm to 38 mm[*]
- Ventrogluteal (adults): 38 mm[*]

   Needle gauge: often dependent on needle length. In general, most biologicals and medications in aqueous solutions can be administered with a 20-25 gauge needle; medications in oil-based solutions require 18- to 25-gauge needles[†]
   Always use a new, sterile syringe and needle for every injection.[*]

Use a filter needle to withdraw medication from a glass ampule[*] or rubber-topped vial.[§]

With a filter needle, change needle before injection[*]

Use the markings on the syringe barrel to determine the correct dose[*]
   Do not include an air bubble in the syringe[*]

Patient preparation and positioning. Consider site of injection:
- Deltoid: patient may sit or stand.[†] A child may be held in an adult's lap.[*]
- Ventrogluteal: patient may stand, sit, or lay laterally or supine[*]
- Vastus lateralis: infants and young children may lay supine or be held in an adult's lap[*]
- Remove clothing at the site for adequate visualization and palpation of bony landmarks[†]
- Position patient to relax the muscle[*]

Injection procedure.
- Cleanse the site with alcohol and allow to dry[†]
- Insert needle into the muscle using a smooth, steady motion[†]
- Research on two alternate techniques to reduce pain at the moment of injection is inconclusive at this time, but warrants further study[†,§]
- Aspirate for 5 to 10 seconds[*]
- Inject slowly at a rate of 10 sec/mL[†]
- After injection, wait 10 seconds before withdrawing the needle[†]
- Withdraw needle slowly, apply gentle pressure with a dry sponge[†]

Postinjection.
- Assess site for complications, both immediately and 2 to 4 hours later, if possible (A)
- Instruct patient regarding assessment, self-management of minor reactions, and when to report more serious problems[*]
- Properly and promptly dispose of all equipment[*]

Note. Needle sizes are provided in metric lengths to conform to the international standard; for US readers, corresponding needle sizes in "are as follows: 16 mm = 5/8"; 22 mm = 7/8"; 25 mm = 1'; 32 mm = 1¼" ; 38 mm = 1½" .

Criteria for grading of the evidence:

[*]Empirical data from published research reports, recommendations of established advisory panels, and generally accepted scientific principles.

[†]Surveys, reviews, consensus among clinicians, and expert opinion.

[‡]Published case reports.

[§]Anecdotal evidence and letters.

Nicoll, L. H., & Hesby, A. (2002). Intramuscular injection: An integrative research review and guideline for evidence-based practice. *Applied Nursing Research, 16*(2), p. 159.

reviews, and multiple individual studies. They examined guidelines for their usefulness in clinical practice, their impact on health policy, and their cost-effectiveness (Stone et al., 2002). Often consultants, other researchers, and additional expert clinicians reviewed the guidelines and provided input. Based on the experts' critical appraisal, the AHRQ guidelines were revised and packaged for distribution to healthcare professionals. Some of the first guidelines focuses on the following healthcare problems: (1) acute pain management in infants, children, and adolescents; (2) prediction and prevention of pressure ulcers in adults; (3) urinary incontinence in adults; (4) management of functional impairments with cataracts, (5) detection, diagnosis, and treatment of depression; (6) screening, diagnosis, management, and counseling about sickle cell disease; (7) management of cancer pain; (8) diagnosis and treatment of heart failure; (9) low back problems; and (10) otitis media diagnosis and management in children.

Evidence-Based Guideline Resources

Currently the guideline development process ranges from a very structured process like the one just discussed to a less structured process in which a guideline might be developed by a healthcare organization, healthcare plan, or professional organization. AHRQ initiated the National Guideline Clearinghouse (NGC) in 1998 to store the evidence-based guidelines. Initially the NGC had 200 guidelines but now the collection has expanded to more than 2400 clinical practice guidelines from numerous professional organizations, healthcare agencies, healthcare plans, and other groups in the United States and other countries. The NGC (2009) is a publicly available database of evidence-based guidelines and related documents. It provides Internet users with free online access to guidelines at *http://www.guideline.gov*. The NGC is updated weekly with new content that the AHRQ produces in partnership with the American Medical Association (AMA) and the American Association of Health Plans (AAHP) (now the American's Health Insurance Plans). The key components of the NGC and its user friendly resources are on the AHRQ website at *http://www.guideline.gov/about/about.aspx*. Some of the critical information on the NGC is provided in the following so you will be able to know what is available and how to access the NGC resources.

Key components of NGC include:

- Structured abstracts (summaries) about the guideline and its development.
- Links to full-text guidelines, where available, and/or ordering information for print copies.
- Palm-based *PDA Downloads* of the Complete NGC Summary for all guidelines represented in the database.
- A *Guideline Comparison* utility that gives users the ability to generate side-by-side comparisons for any combination of two or more guidelines.
- Unique guideline comparisons called *Guideline Syntheses* prepared by NGC staff, compare guidelines covering similar topics, highlighting areas of similarity and difference. NGC Guideline Syntheses often provide a comparison of guidelines developed in different countries, providing insight into commonalities and differences in international health practices.
- An electronic forum, *NGC-L* for exchanging information on clinical practice guidelines, their development, implementation, and use.
- An *Annotated Bibliography* database where users can search for citations for publications and resources about guidelines, including guideline development and methodology, structure, evaluation, and implementation

Other user-friendly features include the following:

- *What's New* enables users to see what guidelines have been added each week and includes an index of all guidelines in NGC.
- *NGC Update Service* is a weekly electronic mailing of new and updated guidelines posted to the NGC Website.
- *Detailed Search* enables users to create very specific search queries based on the various attributes found in the *NGC Classification Scheme.*
- *NGC Browse* permits users to scan for guidelines available on the NGC site by disease/ condition, treatment/intervention, or developing organization.
- *PDA/Palm List* provides users with information regarding the availability of full-text guidelines and/or companion documents available through the guideline developer, that can be downloaded for the handheld computer (Personal Digital Assistant [PDA], Palm, etc.).
- *AHRQ Evidence Reports/Technical Assessments* list provides users with links to the Summaries and Full-Text Reports for evidence reports and technology assessments produced under the Agency for Healthcare Research and Quality (AHRQ) Evidence-based Practice Center (EPC) Program. Access the list of EPC Reports, with links to summaries and/or full-text publications.
- *Glossary* provides definitions of terms used in the standardized abstracts (summaries).

(About the NGC, 2009, *http://www.guideline.gov/about/about.aspx*)

The NGC provides varied audiences with an easy-to-use mechanism for obtaining objective, detailed information on clinical practice guidelines. Audiences that might use the NGC guidelines include individual nurses, physicians, and other clinicians; healthcare organizations; educational institutions; professional healthcare organizations; and state and local government agencies.

The NGC also provides a list of the guidelines that are in the process of being developed or revised at the following website: *http://www.guideline.gov/browse/workqueue.aspx*. In addition to the evidence-based guidelines, the AHRQ has developed many tools to assess the quality of care that is provided by the evidence-based guidelines. You can search the AHRQ Website (*http://www.innovations.ahrq.gov/qualitytools/*) for an appropriate tool to evaluate care in a clinical agency (AHRQ, 2009).

There are also a variety of professional organizations, healthcare agencies, universities, and other groups that provide evidence-based guidelines for practice. Some of these websites are identified in the following:

- Academic Center for Evidence-Based Nursing: *http://www.acestar.uthscsa.edu*
- Association of Women's Health, Obstetric, and Neonatal Nurse: *http://awhonn.org*
- Centre for Health Evidence.net: *http://www.cche.net/*
- CMA InfoBase: *http://mdm.ca/cpgsnew/cpgs/index.asp*
- Guidelines Advisory Committee: *http://www.gacguidelines.ca*
- Guidelines International Network: *http://www.G-I-N.net*
- Health Services/Technology Assessment Text (HSTAT): *http://hstat.nlm.nih.gov*
- HerbMed: Evidence-Based Herbal Database, 1998, Alternative Medicine Foundation: *http://www.herbmed.org*
- National Association of Neonatal Nurses: *http://www.nann.org*
- National Institute for Clinical Excellence (NICE): *http://www.nice.org.uk/catcg2.asp?c=20034*

- Oncology Nursing Society: *http://www.ons.org*
- U.S. Preventive Services Task Force: *http://ahrq.gov/clinic/uspstfab.htm*

Implementing the JNC 7 Evidence-Based Guideline in Practice

Evidence-based guidelines have become the standards for providing care to patients in the United States and other nations. A few nurses have participated on committees that have developed these evidence-based guidelines, and many nurses are using these guidelines in their practices. The text provides an evidence-based guideline for the assessment, diagnosis, and management of high blood pressure as an example. This guideline was developed from the seventh report of the Joint National Committee on Prevention, Detection, Evaluation, and Treatment of High Blood Pressure (JNC 7) and was published in the *Journal of the American Medical Association* (Chobanian et al., 2003). The National Heart, Lung, and Blood Institute (NHLBI) within the National Institutes of Health (NIH) of Department of Health and Human Services (DHHS) developed educational materials to communicate the specifics of this guideline to promote its use by healthcare providers. The JNC 1 guideline was initiated in 1976 and revised over the years with the JNC 7 being published in 2003. The JNC 7 guideline is currently under revision with the JNC 8 expected to be available for public review and comment in March, 2010, with the expected release of the guideline in Summer 2010 (NHLBI, 2009; *http://www.nhlbi.nih.gov/guidelines/hypertension/jnc8/index.htm*).

The JNC 7 is the most current practice guideline for hypertension and is presented in Figure 13–3. This guideline provides clinicians with direction for the following: (1) classification of blood pressure as normal, prehypertension, hypertension stage 1, and hypertension stage 2; (2) conduct of a diagnostic workup of hypertension; (3) assessment of the major cardiovascular disease risk factors; (4) assessment of the identification of causes of hypertension; and (5) treatment of hypertension. An algorithm provides direction for the selection of the most appropriate treatment method(s) for each patient diagnosed with hypertension (NHLBI, 2003).

Registered nurses need to assess the usefulness and quality of each evidence-based guideline before they implement it in their practice. Figure 13–4 provides the **Grove Model for Implementing Evidence-Based Guidelines in Practice** to assist you in critically appraising national evidence-based guidelines. In this model, nurses identify a practice problem, search for the best research evidence to manage the problem in their practice, and note that an evidence-based guideline has been developed. The nurse needs to assess the quality and usefulness of the guideline before it is used in practice, and that involves examining the following: (1) the authors of the guideline, (2) significance of the healthcare problem, (3) strength of the research evidence, (4) the link to national standards, and (5) cost-effectiveness of using the guideline in practice. The quality of the JNC 7 guideline is critically appraised using the four criteria identified in the Grove Model (see Figure 13–4). The authors of the JNC 7 guideline were expert researchers, clinicians (medical doctors), policy developers, health care administrators, and the National High Blood Pressure Education Program Coordinating Committee. These individuals and committee have the expertise to develop an evidenced-based guideline for hypertension.

Hypertension is a significant health care problem because it affects approximately 50 million individuals in the United States and approximately 1 billion individuals worldwide. ... Hypertension is the most common primary diagnosis in the United States with 35 million office

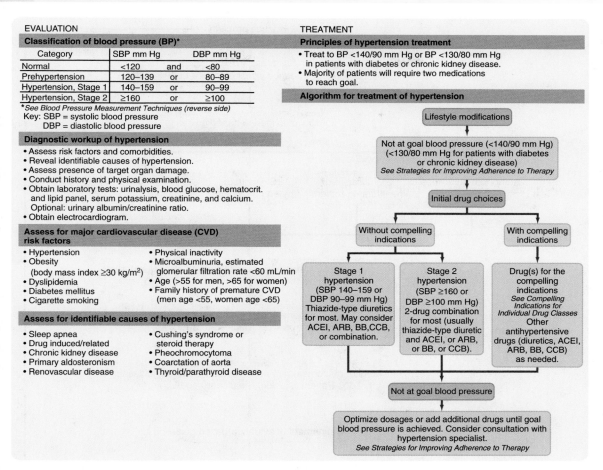

Figure 13–3. Reference card from the seventh report of the Joint National Committee on Prevention, Detection, Evaluation, and Treatment of High Blood Pressure [JNC 7]. From U.S. Department of Health and Human Services, National Institutes of Health, National Heart, Lung, and Blood Institute (2003). Reference Card from the Seventh Report of the Joint National Committee on Prevention, Detection, Evaluation, and Treatment of High Blood Pressure. Bethesda, MD: NIH Publication No. 03-5231. Retrieved August 3, 2009, from *www.nhlbi.nih.gov/guidelines/hypertension/jnc7card. htm.*

visits as the primary diagnosis. ... Recent clinical trials have demonstrated that effective BP [blood pressure] control can be achieved in most patients with hypertension, but the majority will require 2 or more antihypertensive drugs. (Chobanian et al., 2003, p. 2562)

The research evidence for the development of the JNC 7 guideline was extremely strong. The JNC 7 report included 81 references; 9 (11%) of the references were meta-analyses and 35 (43%) were randomized controlled trials (experimental studies). Thus, 44 (54%) sources contained extremely strong research evidence. The other references were strong and included retrospective analyses or case-controlled studies, prospective or cohort studies, cross-sectioned surveys or prevalence studies, and clinical intervention studies (nonrandom)

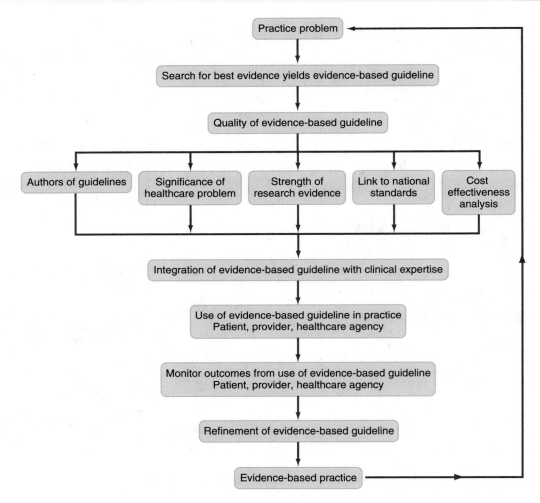

Figure 13–4. Grove Model for Implementing Evidence-Based Guidelines in Practice.

(Chobanian et al., 2003). The JNC 7 provides the national standard for the assessment, diagnosis, and treatment of hypertension. The recommendations from the JNC 7 are supported by DHHS and disseminated through NIH publication no. 03-5231. Use of the JNC 7 guideline in practice is cost-effective because the clinical trials have shown that "antihypertensive therapy has been associated with 35% to 40% mean reductions in stroke incidence; 20% to 25% in myocardial infarction [MI]; and more than 50% in HF [heart failure]" (Chobanian et al., 2003, p. 2562).

The next step is for RNs to use the JNC 7 guideline in their practice to classify patients' blood pressures and assess their major cardiovascular disease (CVD) risk factors (see Figure 13–3). Nurses can use this information to educate patients about their blood pressure and encourage them to make lifestyle changes (weight loss, no added salt in diet, and exercise program) to decrease their CVD risks. Nurses also need to examine the outcomes for the patient, nurse, physician, and healthcare agency. The outcomes would be recorded in the patients' charts and possibly in a database and would include the following: (1) blood pressure readings for patients; (2) incidence of diagnosis of hypertension based on the JNC 7 guidelines; (3) appropriateness of the treatments implemented to manage hypertension; and (4) the incidence of stroke, myocardial infarction (MI), and heart failure (HF) over 5, 10, 15, and 20 years. The healthcare agency outcomes include the access to care by patients with hypertension, patient satisfaction with care, and the cost related to diagnosis and treatment of hypertension and the complications of stroke, MI, and HF. The AHRQ (2009) has developed a website of quality tools to measure healthcare outcomes at *http://www.innovations.ahrq. gov/qualitytools/*. The JNC 7 guideline will be refined in 2010 based on clinical outcomes, outcome studies, and new controlled clinical trials. The use of this evidence-based guideline and additional guidelines promote an EBP for nurses (see Figure 13–4).

Introduction to Evidence-Based Practice Centers

In 1997, the AHRQ launched its initiative to promote evidence-based practice by establishing 12 Evidence-Based Practice Centers in the United States and Canada. The **Evidence-Based Practice Centers** (EPCs) develop evidence reports and technology assessments on

> topics relevant to clinical, social science/behavioral, economic, and other health care organization and delivery issues–specifically those that are common, expensive, and/or significant for the Medicare and Medicaid populations. With this program, AHRQ became a "science partner" with private and public organizations in their efforts to improve the quality, effectiveness, and appropriateness of health care by synthesizing the evidence and facilitating the translation of evidence-based research findings. Topics are nominated by non-federal partners such as professional societies, health plans, insurers, employers, and patient groups. (AHRQ, 2008, *http://www.ahrq.gov/clinic/epc/*)

Under the EPC Program, the AHRQ awards five-year contracts to institutions to serve as EPCs. The EPCs review all relevant scientific literature on clinical, behavioral, and organization and financing topics to produce evidence reports and technology assessments. These reports are used for informing and developing coverage decisions, quality measures, educational materials and tools, guidelines, and research agendas. The EPCs also conduct research on methodology of systematic reviews. AHRQ developed the following criteria as the basis for selecting a topic to be managed by an EPC:

- High incidence or prevalence in the general population and in special populations, including women, racial and ethnic minorities, pediatric and elderly populations, and those of low socioeconomic status.
- Significance for the needs of the Medicare, Medicaid, and other Federal health programs.
- High costs associated with a condition, procedure, treatment, or technology, whether due to the number of people needing care, high unit cost of care, or high indirect costs.
- Controversy or uncertainty about the effectiveness or relative effectiveness of available clinical strategies or technologies.
- Impact potential for informing and improving patient or provider decision making.

- Impact potential for reducing clinically significant variations in the prevention, diagnosis, treatment, or management of a disease or condition; in the use of a procedure or technology; or in the health outcomes achieved.
- Availability of scientific data to support the systematic review and analysis of the topic.
- Submission of the nominating organization's plan to incorporate the report into its managerial or policy decision making, as defined above.
- Submission of the nominating organization's plan to disseminate derivative products to its members and plan to measure members' use of these products, and the resultant impact of such use on clinical practice. (AHRQ, 2008; *http://www.ahrq.gov/clinic/epc/*)

The AHRQ Web site provides the names of the EPCs and the focus of each center (http://www.ahrq.gov/clinic/epc/epcenters.htm). This site also provides a link to the evidence-based reports produced by these centers. These EPCs have had an important role in the development of evidence-based guidelines over the last decade and will continue to make significant contributions to EBP in the future. They are also involved in the development of measurement tools to examine the outcomes from EBP.

Introduction to Translational Research

Some of the barriers to EBP have resulted in the development of a new type of research to improve the translation of research knowledge to practice. The new research methodology is called transitional research that is being supported by the NIH (2008). **Translational research** is an evolving concept that is defined by the NIH as the translation of basic scientific discoveries into practical applications. Basic research discoveries from the laboratory setting need to be tested in studies with humans. In addition, the outcomes from human clinical trials need to be adopted and maintained in clinical practice. Translational research is being encouraged by both medicine and nursing to increase the implementation of evidence-based interventions in practice and to determine if these interventions are effective in producing the outcomes desired in clinical practice (Chesla, 2008; NIH, 2008).

NIH wanted to encourage researchers to conduct translational research and developed the Clinical and Translational Science Awards (CTSA) Consortium in October 2006. The consortium started with 12 centers located throughout the nation and expanded to 39 centers in April of 2009. The program is projected to be fully implemented in 2012 with about 60 institutions involved in the clinical and translational science. The CTSA has developed a website to enhance communication and encourage sharing of information related to translational research projects at *http://www.ctsaweb.org/*.

The CTSA Consortium is mainly focused on expanding the translation of medical research to practice. Titler (2004, p. S1) defined transitional research for the nursing profession as the: "Scientific investigation of methods, interventions, and variables that influence adoption of evidence-based practices (EBPs) by individuals and organizations to improve clinical and operational decision making in health care. This includes testing the effect of interventions on promoting and sustaining the adoption of EBPs." Baumbusch et al. (2008) developed a collaborative model for knowledge translation between research and practice in clinical settings. As you search the literature for relevant research syntheses and studies you will note that translation studies are being published in nursing. For example, Whittemore, Melkus, Wagner, Dziura, Northrup, and Grey (2009) conducted a translation study to promote the transfer of a Diabetic Prevention Program to primary care. These types of studies will assist you in translating research findings to your practice and determining the impact of EBP on patients' health. However, national funding is needed to expand the conduct of transitional research in nursing.

We hope that the content in this chapter increases your understanding of EBP, the critical appraisal of research syntheses, the application of EBP models, and the implementation of EBP guidelines. We encourage you to take an active role in moving nursing toward an EBP that improves outcomes for patients, healthcare professionals, and healthcare agencies.

KEY CONCEPTS

- Evidence-based practice (EBP) is the conscientious integration of best research evidence with clinical expertise and patient values and needs in the delivery of quality, cost-effective health care.
- Best research evidence is produced by the conduct and synthesis of numerous, high-quality studies in a health-related area.
- The barriers and benefits for EBP were described. The benefits of EBP is that the standards for hospital accreditation by the Joint Commission support EBP as does the Magnet Hospital Program managed by the American Nurses' Credentialing Center.
- Guidelines are provided to critically appraise research syntheses (systematic reviews, meta-analyses, integrative reviews, metasummaries, and metasyntheses). The quality of these research syntheses determines the best research evidence in a selected area and the quality of the research evidence available for practice.
- Two models have been developed to promote EBP in nursing: the Stetler Model of Research Utilization to Facilitate EBP (Stetler, 2001) and the Iowa Model of Evidence-Based Practice to Promote Quality of Care (Titler et al., 2001).
- The phases of the revised Stetler model are (1) preparation, (2) validation, (3) comparative evaluation/decision making, (4) translation/application, and (5) evaluation.
- The Iowa Model of Evidence-Based Practice provides guidelines for implementing patient care based on the best research evidence and monitoring changes in practice to ensure quality care. The Iowa model is used to direct the implementation of an EBP protocol for using saline flush to irrigate intravenous catheters in adults.
- A format developed to promote implementation of the best research evidence in practice is PICO (population, intervention, comparison of interventions, and outcomes). The PICO format was used to demonstrate the evidence-based delivery of IM injections by nurses.
- Resources for identifying evidence-based guidelines are provided. The evidence-based guideline for assessment, diagnosis, and treatment of hypertension was provided as an example.
- The Grove Model for Implementing Evidence-Based Guidelines in Practice is provided to assist nurses in determining the quality of evidence-based guidelines and the steps for using these guidelines in practice.
- An excellent source for evidence-based guidelines is the National Guideline Clearinghouse that was initiated by the Agency for Healthcare Research and Quality (AHRQ) in 1998.

- Evidence-based practice centers (EPCs), created by the AHRQ in 1997, have had an important role in the conduct of research, development of systematic reviews, and formulation of evidence-based guidelines in selected practice areas.
- The new research methodology called translational research is being supported by the National Institutes of Health (NIH) to increase the translation of research findings into practice. To encourage researchers to conduct transitional research, the NIH developed the Clinical and Translational Science Awards (CTSA) Consortium in October 2006.

REFERENCES

Agency for Healthcare Research and Quality. (2009). *Quality tools*. Washington, DC: Author. Retrieved August 4, 2009, from *http://www.innovations.ahrq.gov/qualitytools/*.

Agency for Healthcare Research and Quality. (2008). *Evidence-based practice centers: Overview*. AHRQ Publication No. 03-P006. Rockville, MD. Retrieved August 4, 2009, from *http://www.ahrq.gov/clinic/epc/*.

American Nurses Credentialing Center (2009). *Find a magnet organization*. Silver Springs, MD: Author, a subsidiary of American Nurses Association. Retrieved August 1, 2009, from *http://www.nursecredentialing.org/Magnet/FindaMagnetFacility.aspx*.

American Society of Health Systems Pharmacists. (2006). ASHP therapeutic position statement on the institutional use of 0.9% sodium chloride injection to maintain patency of peripheral indwelling intermittent infusion devices. *American Journal of Health Systems Pharmacy, 63*(12), 1273-1275.

Ashton, J., Gibson, V., & Summers, S. (1990). Effects of heparin versus saline solution on intermittent infusion device irrigation. *Heart & Lung, 19*(6), 608-612.

Banel, D. K., & Hu, F. B. (2009). Effects of walnut consumption on blood lipids and other cardiovascular risk factors: A meta-analysis and systematic review. *American Journal of Clinical Nutrition, 90*(1), 56-63.

Barrett, P. J., & Lester, R. L. (1990). Heparin versus saline flush solutions in a small community hospital. *Hospital Pharmacy, 25*(2), 115-118.

Baumbusch, J. L., Kirkham, S. R., Khan, K. B., McDonald, H., Semeniuk, P., Tan, E., & Anderson, J. M. (2008). Pursuing common agendas: A collaborative model for knowledge translation between research and practice in clinical settings. *Research in Nursing & Health, 31*(2), 130-140.

Bolton, L. B., Donaldson, N. E., Rutledge, D. N., Bennett, C., & Brown, D. S. (2007). The impact of nursing interventions: Overview of effective interventions, outcomes, measures, and priorities for future research. *Medical Care Research & Review, 64*(2), Supplement 123S-143S.

Brown, S. J. (2009). *Evidence-based nursing: The research-practice connection*. Sudbury, MA: Jones & Bartlett.

Burns, N., & Grove, S. K. (2009). *The practice of nursing research: Appraisal, synthesis, and generation of evidence* (6th ed.). Philadelphia: Saunders.

Campbell, S. G., Trojanowski, J., & Ackroyd-Stolarz, S. A. (2005). How often should peripheral intravenous cathe-

ters in ambulatory patients be flushed? *Journal of Infusion Nursing, 28*(6), 399-408.

Centers for Disease Control. (2002). Guideline for hand hygiene in health-care settings. *Morbidity and Mortality Weekly Report, 51*(RR-16), 1-45. Retrieved on August 17, 2009 from *http://www.cdc.gov/mmwr/PDF/rr/rr5116.pdf*.

Chesla, C. A. (2008). Translational research: Essential contributions from interpretive nursing science. *Research in Nursing & Health, 31*(4), 381-390.

Chobanian, A. V., Bakris, G. L., Black, H. R., Cushman, W. C., Green, L. A., Izzo, J. L., et al. (2003). The seventh report of the Joint National Committee on Prevention, Detection, Evaluation, and Treatment of high blood pressure: The JNC 7 report. *Journal of the American Medical Association, 289*(19), 2560-2572.

Conn, V. S., & Rantz, M. J. (2003). Research methods: Managing primary study quality in meta-analyses. *Research in Nursing & Health, 26*(4), 322-333.

Craig, F. D., & Anderson, S. R. (1991). *A comparison of normal saline versus heparinized normal saline in the maintenance of intermittent infusion devices*. Unpublished manuscript.

Craig, J. V., & Smyth, R. L. (2007). *The evidence-based practice manual for nurses* (2nd ed.). Edinburgh: Churchill Livingstone.

Creswell, J. W. (2009). *Research design: Qualitative, quantitative and mixed methods approaches* (3rd ed.). Thousand Oaks, CA: Sage.

Cullum, N., Ciliska, D., Haynes, R. B., & Marks, S. (2008). *Evidence-based nursing: An introduction*. Oxford, UK: Blackwell.

Cyganski, J. M., Donahue, J. M., & Heaton, J. S. (1987). The case for the heparin flush. *American Journal of Nursing, 86*(6), 796-797.

Dixon-Woods, M., Fitzpatrick, R., & Roberts, K. (2001). Including qualitative research in systematic reviews: Opportunities and problems. *Journal of Evaluation in Clinical Practice, 7*(2), 125-133.

Donham, J., & Denning, V. (1987). Heparin vs. saline in maintaining patency in intermittent infusion devices: Pilot study. *Kansas Nurse, 62*(11), 6-7.

Doran, D. M. (2003). *Nursing-sensitive outcomes: State of the science*. Sudbury, MA: Jones & Bartlett.

Draucker, C. B., Martsolf, D. S., Ross, R., Cook, C. B., Stidham, A. W., & Mweemba, P. (2009). The essence of healing from sexual violence: A qualitative metasynthesis. *Research in Nursing & Health, 32*(4), 366-378.

Dunn, D. L., & Lenihan, S. F. (1987). The case for the saline flush. *American Journal of Nursing, 87*(6), 798-799.

Epperson, E. L. (1984). Efficacy of 0.9% sodium chloride injection with and without heparin for maintaining indwelling intermittent injection sites. *Clinical Pharmacy, 3*(6), 626-629.

Ganong, L. H. (1987). Integrative reviews of nursing research. *Research in Nursing & Health, 10*(1), 1-11.

Garrelts, J., LaRocca, J., Ast, D., Smith, D. F., & Sweet, D. E. (1989). Comparison of heparin and 0.9% sodium chloride injection in the maintenance of indwelling intermittent I.V. devices. *Clinical Pharmacy, 8*(1), 34-39.

Gates, S. (2002). Review of methodology of quantitative reviews using meta-analysis in ecology. *Journal of Animal Ecology, 71*(4), 547-557.

Goode, C. J., Kleiber, C., Titler, M., Small, S., Rakel, B., Steelman, V. M., Walker, J. B., & Buckwalter, K. C. (1993). Improving practice through research: the case of heparin vs. saline for peripheral intermittent infusion devices. *Medical-Surgical Nursing, 2*(1), 23-27.

Goode, C. J., Titler, M., Rakel, B., Ones, D. S., Kleiber, C., Small, S., et al. (1991). A meta-analysis of effects of heparin flush and saline flush: Quality and cost implications. *Nursing Research, 40*(6), 324-330.

Grove, S. K. (2007). *Statistics for health care research: A practical workbook.* Philadelphia: Saunders Elsevier.

Hamilton, R. A., Plis, J. M., Clay, C., & Sylvan, L. (1988). Heparin sodium versus 0.9% sodium chloride injection for maintaining patency of indwelling intermittent infusion devices. *Clinical Pharmacy, 7*(6), 439-443.

Higgins, J. P., & Green, S. (2008). *Cochrane handbook for systematic reviews of interventions: Cochrane book series.* West Sussex, UK: The Cochrane Collaboration and John Wiley & Sons.

Holford, N. H., Vozeh, S., Coates, P., Porvell, J. R., Thiercelin, J. F., & Upton, R. (1977). More on heparin lock [Letter]. *New England Journal of Medicine, 296*(22), 1300-1301.

Institute of Medicine. (2001). *Crossing the quality chasm: A new health system for the 21st century.* Washington, DC: National Academy Press.

Intravenous Nursing Society (INS). (2000). Infusion nursing standards of practice. *Journal of Intravenous Nursing, 23*(Suppl 6), S53-54, S81-88.

Kania-Lachance, D. M., Best, P. J., McDonah, M. R., & Ghosh, A. K. (2006). Evidence-based practice and the nurse practitioner. *The Nurse Practitioner, 31*(10), 46-54.

Kasparek, A., Wenger, J., & Feldt, R. (1988). *Comparison of normal versus heparinized saline for flushing or intermittent intravenous infusion devices (pp. 1-18).* Unpublished manuscript. Cedar Rapids, IA: Mercy Medical Center.

Lombardi, T. P., Gunderson, B., Zammett, L. O., Walters, J. K., & Morris, B. A. (1988). Efficacy of 0.9% sodium chloride injection with or without heparin sodium for maintaining patency of intravenous catheters in children. *Clinical Pharmacy, 7*(11), 832-836.

Malloch, K., & Porter-O'Grady, T. (2006). *Introduction to evidence-based practice in nursing and health care.* Sudbury, MA: Jones & Bartlett.

McCaughan, D., Thompson, C., Cullum, N., Sheldon, T. A., & Thompson, D. R. (2002). Issues and innovations in nursing practice: Acute care nurses' perceptions of barriers to using research information in clinical decision-making. *Journal of Advanced Nursing, 39*(1), 46-60.

Melnyk, B. M., & Fineout-Overholt, E. (2005). *Evidence-based practice in nursing & healthcare: A guide to best practice.* Philadelphia: Lippincott Williams & Wilkins.

Melnyk, B. M., Fineout-Overholt, E., Stillwell, S. B., & Williamson, K. M. (2010). The seven steps of evidence-based practice. *American Journal of Nursing, 110*(1), 51-53.

Miracle, V., Fangman, B., Kayrouz, P., Kederis, K., & Pursell, L. (1989). Normal saline vs. heparin lock flush solution: One institution's findings. *Kentucky Nurse, 37*(4), 1, 6-7.

Munhall, P. L. (2007). *Nursing research: A qualitative perspective* (4th ed.). Sudbury, MA: Jones & Bartlett.

National Guideline Clearinghouse (2009). *About the National Guideline Clearinghouse.* Washington, DC: Agency for Healthcare Research and Quality. Retrieved August 4, 2009, from *http://www.guideline.gov/about/about.aspx.*

National Heart, Lung, and Blood Institute. (2003). *The seventh report of the Joint National Committee on prevention, detection, evaluation, and treatment of high blood pressure: The JNC 7 report.* Bethesda, MD: National Institutes of Health. Retrieved August 4, 2009 from *www.nhlbi.nih.gov/guidelines/hypertension.*

National Heart, Lung, and Blood Institute. (2009). *The eighth report of the Joint National Committee on prevention, detection, evaluation, and treatment of high blood pressure (JNC 8).* Bethesda, MD: National Institutes of Health. Retrieved August 4, 2009 from *http://www.nhlbi.nih.gov/guidelines/hypertension/jnc8/index.htm.*

National Institutes of Health (NIH) (2008). *NIH roadmap for medical research: Translational research.* Bethesda, Maryland: Author. Retrieved August 4, 2009 from *http://nihroadmap.nih.gov/clinicalresearch/overview-translational.asp.*

Nicoll, L. H., & Hesby, A. (2002). Intramuscular injection: An integrative research review and guideline for evidence-based practice. *Applied Nursing Research, 16*(2), 149-162.

Nursing Executive Center (2005). *Evidence-based nursing practice: Instilling rigor into clinical practice.* Washington, DC: The Advisory Board Company.

O'Grady, N. P., Alexander, M., Dellinger, E. P., Gerberding, J. L., Heard, S. O., Maki, D. G., Masur, H., McCormick, R. D., Mermel, L. A., Pearson, M. L., Raad I. I., Randolph, A., & Weinstein, R. A. (2002). Guidelines for the prevention of intravascular catheter-related infections. *Morbidity and Mortality Weekly Report Recommendation Rep, 9*(51 RR-10), 1-29.

Oncology Nursing Society (ONS). (2004). *Access device guidelines: Recommendations for nursing practice and education,* 2nd ed. Pittsburgh (PA): Oncology Nursing Society (ONS). Retrieved on August 17, 2009 from *http://www.guideline.gov/summary/summary.aspx?doc_id=8338&nbr=004666&string=access+AND+device+AND+guideline.*

Parahoo, K. (2000). Barriers to, and facilitators of, research utilization among nurses in Northern Ireland. *Journal of Advanced Nursing, 31*(1), 89-98.

Pearson, A., Field, J., & Jordan, Z. (2007). *Evidence-based clinical practice in nursing and health care: Assimilating research, experience, and expertise.* Oxford, UK: Blackwell Publishing.

Peterson, F. Y., & Kirchhoff, K. T. (1991). Analysis of the research about heparinized versus nonheparinized intravascular lines. *Heart & Lung, 20*(6), 631-640.

Pettengill, M. M., Gillies, D. A., & Clark, C. C. (1994). Factors encouraging and discouraging the use of nursing research findings. *Image—Journal of Nursing Scholarship, 26*(2), 143-147.

Putman-Casdorph, H., & McCrone, S. (2009). Chronic obstructive pulmonary disease, anxiety, and depression: State of the science. *Heart & Lung, 38*(1), 34-47.

Randolph, A. G., Cook, D. J., Gonzales, C. A., & Andrew, M. (1998). Benefits of heparin in peripheral venous and arterial catheters: Systematic review and meta-analysis of randomized controlled trials. *British Medical Journal, 316*(7136), 969-975.

Retsas, A. (2000). Barriers to using research evidence in nursing practice. *Journal of Advanced Nursing, 31*(3), 599-606.

Sackett, D. L., Straus, S. E., Richardson, W. S., Rosenberg, W., & Haynes, R. B. (2000). *Evidence-based medicine: How to practice & teach EBM* (2nd ed.). London: Churchill Livingstone.

Sandelowski, M., & Barroso, J. (2007). *Handbook for synthesizing qualitative research.* New York: Springer.

Schustek, M. (1984). A cost-effective approach to PRN device maintenance...the change from heparin to saline. *Journal of the National Intravenous Therapy Association, 7*(6), 527.

Shah, P. S., Ng, E., & Sinha, A. K. (2005). Heparin for prolonging peripheral intravenous catheter use in neonates. *Cochrane Database of Systematic Reviews* (Online), Cochrane AN: DOI: 10.1002/14651858.CD002774.pub2.

Shearer, J. (1987). Normal saline flush versus dilute heparin flush. *National Intravenous Therapy Association, 10*(6), 425-427.

Shoaf, J., & Oliver, S. (1992). Efficacy of normal saline injection with and without heparin for maintaining intermittent intravenous site. *Applied Nursing Research, 5*(1), 9-12.

Shojania, K. G., Sampson, M., Ansari, M. T., Ji, J., & Doucette, S. (2007). How quickly do systematic reviews go out of date? Survival analysis. *Annals of Internal Medicine, 147*(4), 224-234.

Spann, J. M. (1988). Efficacy of two flush solutions to maintain catheter patency in heparin locks. *Dissertation Abstracts, 28*(1), 1337125, 1-58. *Dissertation Abstracts International, 42*(4), 1394B (University Microfilms No. 8120152).

Stetler, C. B. (1994). Refinement of the Stetler/Marram model for application of research findings to practice. *Nursing Outlook, 42*(1), 15-25.

Stetler, C. B. (2001). Updating the Stetler Model of Research Utilization to facilitate evidence-based practice. *Nursing Outlook, 49*(6), 272-279.

Stetler, C. B., & Marram, G. (1976). Evaluating research findings for applicability in practice. *Nursing Outlook, 24*(9), 559-563.

Stetler, C. B., Morsi, D., Rucki, S., Broughton, S., Corrigan, B., Fitzgerald, J., et al. (1998). Utilization-focused integrative reviews in a nursing service. *Applied Nursing Research, 11*(4), 195-206.

Stone, P. W., Curran, C. R., & Bakken, S. (2002). Economic evidence for evidence-based practice. *Journal of Nursing Scholarship, 34*(3), 277-282.

Taylor, N., Hutchison, E., Milliken, W., & Larson, E. (1989). Comparison of normal versus heparinized saline for flushing infusion devices. *Journal of Nursing Quality Assurance, 3*(4), 49-55.

Titler, M. G. (2004). Overview of the U.S. invitational conference "Advancing Quality Care Through Translation Research." *Worldviews on Evidence-Based Nursing, 1*(1), S1-S5.

Titler, M. G., Kleiber, C., Steelman, V. J., Rakel, B. A., Budreau, G., Everett, L. Q., et al. (1994). Research-based practice to promote the quality of care. *Nursing Research, 43*(5), 307-313.

Titler, M. G., Kleiber, C., Steelman, V. J., Rakel, B. A., Budreau, G., Everett, L. Q., et al. (2001). The Iowa Model of Evidence-Based Practice to promote quality care. *Critical Care Nursing Clinics of North America, 13*(4), 497-509.

Tuten, S. H., & Gueldner, S. H. (1991). Efficacy of sodium chloride versus dilute heparin for maintenance of peripheral intermittent intravenous devices. *Applied Nursing Research, 4*(2), 63-71.

Whittemore, R., Melkus, G., Wagner, J., Dziura, J., Northrup, V., & Grey, M. (2009). Translating the diabetes prevention program to primary care: A pilot study. *Nursing Research, 58*(1), 2-12.

14

Introduction to Outcomes Research

Chapter Overview

**The Theoretical Basis of Outcomes
   Research** 508
   Donabedian's Theory of Quality Health
   Care 508
   Implications for Practice 520
**Outcomes Research and Nursing
   Practice** 522

The American Nurses Association's "Nursing's
   Safety & Quality Initiative" 522
   Nursing-Sensitive Patient Outcomes 526
**Disseminating Outcomes of Research
   Findings** 529

Learning Outcomes

After completing this chapter, you should be able to:

1. Discriminate between traditional quantitative research and outcomes research.
2. Explain the theoretical basis of outcomes research.

3. Explain the importance of outcomes research on nursing practice.

Key Terms

Cost, p. 519
Health, p. 508
Outcomes research, p. 507

Out-of-pocket costs, p. 519
Quality, p. 508

Standard of care, p. 511
Structures of care, p. 520

STUDY TOOLS

Be sure to visit *http://evolve.elsevier.com/Burns/understanding* for additional examples and self-tests. Also, a review of this chapter's concepts and practice exercises can be found in Chapter 14 of the Study Guide for *Understanding Nursing Research: Building an Evidence-Based Practice*, 5th edition.

Outcomes research focuses on the end results of patient care. The purpose of an outcome study is to appraise quality. The end results being examined may not be those commonly discussed in nursing studies: the outcomes of your care for a particular patient. The outcomes of interest in outcomes research might be the outcomes of all of the patients in your unit, of all patients with a certain healthcare problem in your hospital or the outcomes in a large number of hospitals. The outcomes studied are not the outcomes that occur for each patient, but rather the desired outcomes for all such patients: what should be occurring if excellent care is being provided. Standards of care, critical pathways, and care maps have been developed to define these desired outcomes. These outcomes may be studied in relation to the number of nurses on a unit, the educational level of the nurses, the management strategies of the supervisor or hospital administrator, or the size of the hospital in relation to number of beds, number of patients, types of units provided, etc. A study might examine the quality of the same care provided in hospitals, home healthcare agencies, and nursing homes.

The American Nurses Association (ANA) is in the forefront of this research, which is critically important to the practice of nursing. Many hospitals are participating with ANA in collecting the data needed to examine outcomes. The Magnet program uses information from this area of research in designating Magnet hospitals. Much of the work of developing critical pathways, care maps, and related forms designed to improve quality of outcomes (for groups of patients) emerged from outcome studies.

Outcomes research is very different than the other types of research addressed in this text. It is more complex. The designs are different and the researchers are often from a mix of disciplines, such as economics and public health, as well as nursing. The studies use a unique theoretical framework that focuses on health outcomes.

The outcomes studies being conducted at this time do not examine patient care at the individual nurse/individual patient level, as occurs in many nursing studies. Rather, a study might examine, for example, all of the nursing care provided to patients in a particular intensive care unit. Some of the questions researchers might ask in a study include the following:

- What are the end results of patients' care (all care provided by all care providers)?
- What effect does nursing care (all care by all nurses) have on the end results of a patient's care?
- Are there some nursing acts that have no effects at all on outcomes or that actually cause harm?
- Can we measure and thus identify the end results of nursing care?
- How do we distinguish care provided by nurses from care provided by other professionals in examining patient outcomes?
- When do we measure the effects of care (end results): immediately after the care, when the patient is discharged, or much later?

We are expected to demonstrate that the care we provide is effective. This "we" is not just one nurse, but rather all nurses caring for patients in a particular system of care.

We must know and be able to justify our costs (the costs of nurses providing care) within a particular health care system, particularly if we are negotiating for more nurses or better educated nurses. We justify our costs based on the need to maintain or improve the outcomes of the patients for whom we care. We work for a system; thus, it is systems that we must study and systems we must influence. The system we study might be units, hospitals, or types of units or hospitals providing a specific type of care.

To help you understand this type of research, and use the results to influence the quality of nursing care and improve patient care in areas in which you choose to practice, this chapter provides a brief explanation of the theoretical basis of outcomes research, discusses the current foci for outcomes research, describes the use of outcomes research to examine and improve nursing practice, and provides example nursing outcome studies.

The Theoretical Basis of Outcomes Research

The theorist Avedis Donabedian (1976, 1978, 1980, 1982, 1987) proposed a theory of quality health care and provided a process of evaluating it. Donabedian's theory dominates outcomes research. Other theories of outcomes have been developed, but we will limit our discussion to Donabedian's theory.

Donabedian's Theory of Quality Health Care

Quality is the major concept of Donabedian's Theory of Quality Health Care, although he never defines this concept (Mark, 1995). The cube shown in Figure 14–1 helps explain the elements of quality health care. The three dimensions of the cube are health, subjects of care, and providers of care. The concept of health has many aspects; three are shown on the cube: physical-physiological function, psychological function, and social function. Donabedian (1987, p. 4) proposes that "the manner in which we conceive of health and of our responsibility for it, makes a fundamental difference to the concept of quality and, as a result, to the methods that we use to assess and assure the quality of care."

Loegering, Reiter, and Gambone (1994) modified Donabedian's levels to include the patient, family, and community as providers of care as well as recipients of care. They suggest that access to care is one dimension of the provision of care by the community. Figure 14–2 illustrates their modifications.

Donabedian (1987) identifies three focuses of evaluation in appraising quality: structure (nursing units, hospitals, home health agencies, etc.), process (of how care is provided, such as a practice style or standard of care), and outcome (end results). These are described in the section that follows.

Evaluating Outcomes

The goal of outcomes research is the evaluation of the quality of outcomes as defined by Donabedian. Donabedian's theory requires that outcomes be clearly linked with the process that caused the outcome. This requires that the process be clearly defined. The providers of

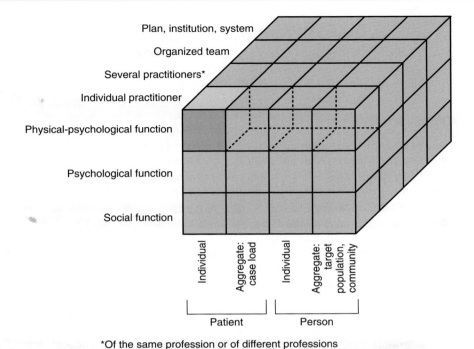

Figure 14–1. Level and scope of concern as factors in the definition of quality. From Donabedian, A. (1987). Some basic issues in evaluating the quality of health care. In L. T. Rinke (Ed.), *Outcome measures in home care* (vol. 1, pp. 3-28). New York: National League of Nursing.

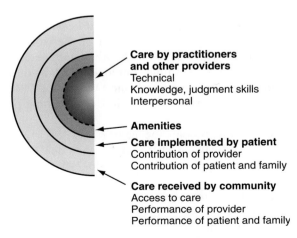

Care by practitioners and other providers
Technical
Knowledge, judgment skills
Interpersonal

Amenities

Care implemented by patient
Contribution of provider
Contribution of patient and family

Care received by community
Access to care
Performance of provider
Performance of patient and family

Figure 14–2. Various levels at which the quality of health care can be assessed. From Donabedian, A. (1988). The quality of care: How can it be assessed? *Journal of the American Medical Association, 260*(12), 1744. Copyright 1988, American Medical Association.

care (the nurses) may say what is achievable, but the subjects of care (the patients) must say what is desirable. The outcomes must be relevant to the goals of the healthcare professionals, the healthcare system, and society.

Outcomes are time dependent. Some outcomes may not be apparent for a long period after the process that is claimed to cause them, whereas others may be apparent immediately. Some outcomes are temporary and others are permanent. Thus, the selection of an appropriate time frame for measuring the selected outcomes must be established. If one is studying the incidence of bladder infection after a catheter is inserted during a hospitalization, the time period for the outcome might be a few weeks or months after discharge (sometimes no one discovers that the patient has a bladder infection for some time after the hospitalization. During this time, the bladder infection becomes chronic and may require months to treat. This is not only costly but slows the recovery of the patient, thus lowering his or her quality of life. If one is studying recovery after a stroke, or a particular approach to care after a stroke, the time period for measuring the outcome could be several years.

Finally, in outcomes research one must determine the place and degree of responsibility for the outcomes observed. A specific outcome often is influenced by multiple factors and various health professionals. Patient factors, such as compliance, predisposition to disease, age, propensity to use resources, high-risk behaviors (e.g., smoking), and lifestyle, also must be taken into account (Lewis, 1995). Environmental factors such as air quality, public policies related to smoking, and occupational hazards also must be included. Responsibility for outcomes may be distributed among providers, patients, employers, insurers, and the community. To identify relevant outcomes, determine a set of closely related outcomes specific to the condition for which care is being provided. Critical pathways and care maps may be useful in defining related outcomes.

Evaluating Process

Understanding the process of care sufficiently to study it must begin with much careful reflection, dialogue, and observation. In nursing, we are just beginning to study the processes of care. It is not just what happens at the patient bedside, but all of the actions that a nurse takes on behalf of the patients and on behalf of the work of the unit of practice. It also involves the interactions with other nurses, other staff, and institutional management.

Clinical management has multiple components. Many of these components have not yet been clearly defined or tested. Bergmark and Oscarsson (1991, pp. 139-140) suggest the following questions as important to consider in the evaluating process:

(1) "What constitutes the 'therapeutic agent'?"
(2) "Do practitioners actually *do* what they say they do?"
(3) "Do practitioners always know what they do?"

Current outcomes studies are using process variables that are easy to identify. Answers to questions such as those posed by Bergmark and Oscarsson are more difficult to define. Observation, interviews, and the use of qualitative research methodologies will be needed to answer such questions.

Three components of process of particular interest to Donabedian are standards of care, practice styles, and costs of care.

Standards of Care

A standard of care is a norm by which quality of care is judged. Clinical guidelines, critical paths, and care maps define standards of care. A practitioner has legitimate responsibility to apply available knowledge in the management of a dysfunctional state to accomplish the following:

1. The identification or diagnosis of the dysfunction
2. The decision whether to intervene
3. The choice of intervention objectives
4. The choice of methods and techniques to achieve the objectives
5. The skillful execution of the selected techniques

Judging the Quality of Care

1. Clinical guidelines. The Agency for Healthcare Research and Quality (AHRQ) establishes norms on which the validity of clinical management can be judged.
2. Care maps. Clinical professionals expert in a specific field of care develop care maps by which the quality of care can be judged.
3. Clinical judgment. Analysis of the process of making diagnoses and therapeutic decisions is critical to the evaluation of the quality of care.

Perme and Chandrashekor (2009) have developed an Early Mobility and Walking Program for patients in intensive care units with the goal of developing a standard of care. In this study, clinical judgment was considered to have occurred when the nurse determined which phase of the program a patient had met (see Tables 14–1, 14–2, and 14–3). The program is particularly targeted at patients receiving mechanical ventilation. The program consists of 4 phases. "Each phase includes guidelines on positioning, therapeutic exercises, transfers, walking reeducation, and duration and frequency of mobility sessions. Additionally, the criteria for progressing to the next phase are provided" (p. 212).

Standards of care have been developed for only a few aspects of nursing care. In the effort to define standards of care, preliminary efforts have been made to define various degrees of quality of care. This understanding will come from many carefully planned nursing research programs to observe existing care and identify varying degrees of quality. Then the researchers must determine what caused the care to vary and why. Then they can identify the process of care that results in the best quality. Understanding different levels of quality of care will hopefully enable us to develop standards of care. Standards of care will enable nurses, units, hospitals and other healthcare facilities to document in more detail the care provided, and to be held accountable for providing defined standards of care. In the example above, Perme and Chandrashekor (2009) developed guidelines for early mobility and walking of intensive care patients receiving mechanical ventilation. Phases of progression were defined. With further studies, additional knowledge that defines quality of care can be acquired, enabling the development of standards of care.

Practice Styles

The style of practice is another dimension of the process of care that influences quality. Initially studies of practice styles focused on physicians. Then a few studies of practice styles

Table 14–1	Early Mobility and Walking Program for Patients in Intensive Care Units			
Description	Patients in an acute phase with multiple medical problems, condition unstable at times, unable to fully participate with therapy. Also includes patients without significant medical problems but with profound weakness, limited activity tolerance, and/or inability to walk.	Patients in an acute/subacute phase with multiple medical problems, condition stable most of the time, able to participate better with activities. Patients still weak but able to stand; also have limited tolerance for activity.	Patients in an acute/subacute phase, with multiple medical problems or resolving medical problems, able to participate actively in therapy. Patients still weak but able to tolerate increased levels of activity.	Patients in a subacute phase who have been weaned from mechanical ventilation, able to participate actively in therapy. Patients working toward functional independence and hospital discharge.
General criteria for progressing to next phase	Patient follows commands. Hemodynamic status is stable.* Oxygenation acceptable. Patient stands with walker and tolerates prewalking activities, including –full standing posture –weight shifting on legs.	Patient follows commands. Hemodynamic status is stable.* Oxygenation acceptable. Patient transfers to chair with walker and assistance. Patient safely tolerates walking reeducation with walker and assistance for limited distances.	Patient follows commands. Hemodynamic status is stable.* Oxygenation acceptable. Patient tolerates progressive walking program and increased levels of activity.	
Ultimate goals	Have patient sit at edge of bed unsupported or with minimal assistance. Initiate standing activities with walker and assistance. Initiate prewalking activities if appropriate.	Initiate transfer training with walker. Initiate walking reeducation with walker.	Initiate independent transfer training with walker. Provide progressive walking reeducation.	Promote progressive transfers and walking independence. Promote independence of patient and patient's family members with exercises and mobility program.

*Acceptable limits for stable hemodynamic status are heart rate <110/min at rest, mean arterial blood pressure between 60 and 110 mm Hg, and fraction of inspired oxygen <0.6. Supplemental oxygen is usually titrated to maintain saturations >88% with activity. Exceptions are determined by the physician on an individual basis.

(From Perme & Chandrashekor (2009). Early mobility and walking program for patients in intensive care unites: Creating a standard of care. *American Journal of Critical Care, 18*(3), 212-221.)

of nurses began to appear in the literature (Bircumshaw & Chapman, 1988; Fullerton, Hollenbach, & Wingard, 1996). Now practice styles of nurses are being examined in terms of the setting in which they work. Following are some examples of these studies.

Schmalenberg and Kramer (2007) studied types of intensive care units with the healthiest, most productive work environments. They used a tool based on the 6 standards essential to a healthy work environment, which are aligned to the Essentials of Magnetism processes. They found that intensive care unit structures provided support for processes and relationships that led to job satisfaction among nurses and quality care for patients. The questionnaire used in this study could be used to identify intensive care units with poor structures for purposes of improving both work conditions and quality of patient care.

Table 14–2 Mobility Interventions

Intervention	Phase			
	1	2	3	4
Education	Instruction of patient and patient's family members on the importance of positioning, exercise program, and early mobility.	Same as phase 1, plus instructions on –proper use of walker –safety during transfers –importance of gradual increase in time sitting out of bed	Same as phase 2, plus instructions on –importance of progressive mobilization –safety issues during transfers and walking	Discharge planning. Family training on bed mobility, transfers, and walking. Safety issues during transfers and walking. Home exercise and activity program with guidelines for progression and self-monitoring.
Positioning	Focus on preventing pressure ulcers, especially on heels and sacrum. Recommendations for appropriate program for patients with orthopedic and/or neurological deficits.	Same as phase 1.	Not a concern if patients tolerate several hours out of bed, unless orthopedic and/or neurological deficits still present.	Not a concern unless orthopedic and/or neurological deficits still present.
Bed mobility training	Turning side to side Scooting/bridging Supine <–> sitting Sitting on side of the bed associated with –leg exercises –breathing exercises –balance/coordination exercises for trunk control –self-care activities –unsupported sitting	Same as phase 1.	Gradual withdrawal of assistance. Initiation of training to promote patient's independence.	Focus on training to promote independence. Family training on selected issues as appropriate.
Transfer training	Transfer out of bed only to stretcher chair with total assistance. Initiation of sit to stand with walker and assistance as appropriate.	Transfers training to using walker and assistance to –bedside chair –bedside commode –stretcher chair (to facilitate safe transfers back to bed).	Gradual withdrawal of assistance during transfers to chair and bedside commode with nursing staff and/or family assistance.	Promotion of independence during transfers with or without assistive device. Family training if appropriate.
Walking program	Patients not ambulatory. Focus on attempts to stand with walker and prewalking activities.	Initiation of walking reeducation with walker and assistance (see Table 14–4).	Walking reeducation with focus on gradual increase in distance and endurance. Gradual withdrawal of assistive device if appropriate (see Table 14–4).	Gradual withdrawal of assistive device if appropriate. Gait reeducation on different surfaces as needed, including stairs, curb, ramp, carpet. (Some patients may benefit from wheelchair mobility training if still unable to walk.)

Continued

Table 14-2	Mobility Interventions—cont'd			
	Phase			
Intervention	1	2	3	4
Exercises	Inclusion of one or a combination of –passive range of motion –active assisted range of motion –stretching –resistance exercise on leg press, light weights (1-5 lb [0.45-2.25 kg]), and/or exercise band –breathing exercises (deep breathing, coughing, incentive spirometer).	Same as phase 1.	Same as phase 1.	More intense strengthening and endurance exercises as appropriate, including –arm ergometry –treadmill –stationary bike –leg press –stairs training –inspiratory muscle training.
Duration of mobility sessions	15-30 minutes as tolerated.	15-45 minutes as tolerated.	30-60 minutes as tolerated.	30-60 minutes as tolerated.
Frequency of mobility sessions	Once daily 1-7 days per week. Twice daily as needed. (Patients may still have ongoing medical problems that can affect availability for therapy or ability to tolerate activity.)	Once daily 5-7 days per week. Twice daily as needed.	Once daily 5-7 days per week. Twice daily as needed.	Once daily 5-7 days per week. Twice daily as needed.

(From Perme & Chandrashekor (2009). Early mobility and walking program for patients in intensive care units: Creating a standard of care. *American Journal of Critical Care, 18*(3), 212-221.)

Cohen-Mansfield and Parpura-Gill (2008) explored practice style in the nursing home. "This paper describes a nomenclature for components of care based on previous findings and observations during several studies in nursing homes. Examining staff and institutional components, we seek to operationalize those aspects of the nursing home practice style that can be improved" (p. 376). Staff conduct was operationalized in terms of knowledge, practice style proficiency, flexibility and individuality of care, and communication. Institutional conduct was operationalized as staff support, resources, and flexibility/rigidity of policies (see Tables 14–4, 14–5, and 14–6). Note that the tables illustrate a very negative practice style and a very negative environment within which to practice. In addition, it is clear that the staff have little or no education to prepare them for their practice and no source of information available if they were to seek it. The authors continue to work in this area of study. How do they move from this depressive scenario to developing a standard of care for nursing homes? Can a standard of care that is developed be used by certifying agencies to require improvements in the care or otherwise improve the care in nursing homes?

Stroke rehabilitation is a focus of interest related to practice styles. Teasell, Meyer, McClure, Pan, Murie-Fernandez, Foley, and Salter (2009) say there is a revolution underway internationally in stroke rehabilitation. According to these authors,

Table 14-3	Guidelines for Walking Reeducation in the Intensive Care Unit

1. Safety precautions
   a. A nurse must be present to assist with tubes and arterial and venous catheters that can temporarily be disconnected or need to come with the patient.
   b. Patients must be connected to portable telemetry equipment to monitor heart rate, rhythm, blood pressure, and oxygen saturation if walking away from the bedside.
   c. All equipment needed for therapy session must be readily available and all catheters/tubes must be secured.
   d. A gait belt must be used for all transfers and walking reeducation activities.
   e. Patient must be followed with a wheelchair to allow resting periods and safe return to bedside if needed.
   f. Full oxygen tank must be available.
   g. Adequate staff assistance must be available to ensure patient's safety
2. Changes in respiratory rate, oxygen saturation, heart rate, heart rhythm, respiratory pattern, blood pressure, and complaints of fatigue by the patient should be evaluated throughout walking reeducation activity.
3. For patients dependent on mechanical ventilation—A decision must be made to determine if the patient is to participate in the walking program with ventilation provided by a portable ventilator, tracheostomy collar, or manual resuscitation bag (a great opportunity to talk to physicians and gather additional information about the patient's medical condition)—Endotracheal or tracheotomy tubes must be secured— An effective communication strategy must be established because patients with artificial airways are unable to talk, except for patients with a tracheostomy collar, who can tolerate the use of a Passy-Muir valve during activities—A respiratory therapist must be present to disconnect the mechanical ventilator and equip the patient with a portable ventilator, tracheostomy collar, or manual resuscitation bag; the respiratory therapist is also responsible for making any ventilator changes ordered by the physician during physical therapy sessions; the respiratory therapist must be available throughout the walking training session and should reestablish mechanical ventilation at the appropriate settings after physical therapy.—As a general rule, if the ventilator settings exceed the parameters described in the following, the patient should not be removed from the ventilator to ambulate; exceptions can be made, however, when the patient's condition has been thoroughly assessed and specific orders have been written by the physician a. Pressure support = 20 cm H_2O b. Synchronized intermittent mandatory ventilation with rate >18 c. Fraction of inspired oxygen >0.7 d. Positive end-expiratory pressure >10 cm H_2O e. Any evidence of decompensation with interruption of mechanical ventilation.
4. The activity should be terminated if any of the following develop:
   a. Oxygen saturation <88% on supplemental oxygen during activity, unless otherwise specified by the physician
   b. Hypotension associated with dizziness, fainting, and/or diaphoresis
   c. Heart rate greater than maximum heart rate
   d. Change in heart rhythm
   e. Change in breathing pattern with an increase in accessory muscle use, paradoxical pattern, nasal flaring, or an appearance of facial distress
   f. Extreme fatigue or severe intolerable dyspnea with respiratory rate greater than baseline by >20/min
   g. Significant chest pain
   h. Excessive pallor or flushing of skin
   i. Request of patient to stop

(From Perme, C., & Chandrashekor, R. (2009). Early mobility and walking program for patients in intensive care units: Creating a standard of care. *American Journal of Critical Care, 18,* (3), 212-221.)

Table 14-4	Practice Style Components Nomenclature

STAFF
Understanding and knowledge
General knowledge
Knowledge of skills
  Preparing the care process based on human factors principles
  Process of care
  Communication: importance of communication, how dementia affects communication, what to say, cultural and
    educational differences
  Individualization of care
Assessment of etiology
Quality vs. technically good care

Practice proficiency
Respect
Compassion
Maximizing comfort
Maximizing contentment

Flexibility, autonomy, and individualized care
Timing of care
Alternatives of care
Individualization of care
Resident involvement, control, and autonomy
Family involvement

Communication
Receipt: Hearing, listening, understanding, encouraging, valuing
Delivery: Failure to communicate, manner of communication, tailoring the communication to fit the residents' abilities

INSTITUTION
Staff
Support: Psychological support, mentoring and professional support
Empowerment to problem solve
  Respect
  Inclusion in decision making and communication processes
  Promoting innovation in care

Resources
Staff
Materials: Shortage of needed supplies, of materials to engage residents, of materials expected to be in a home, resource
  planning
Environment: Design and upkeep can affect the ability to provide care and to receive and deliver communication; it also
  affects comfort

Policies: rigidity vs. flexibility
Timing of care
Task assignment and responsibility
Alternatives of care and environment
Resident involvement, control, and autonomy
Family involvement

From Cohen-Mansfield, J., & Parpura-Gill, A. (2008). Practice style in the nursing home: Dimensions for assessment and quality improvement. *International Journal of Geriatric Psychiatry 23*, 376-386.

Table 14-5	Example of Knowledge Domains in which Staff Members Have Deficits in Knowledge or Appreciation of the Importance of the Domain
Domain	Examples
Skills: Task procedures	Preparing all materials needed for a specific care activity including materials that the caregiver needs as well as the resident (e.g., preparing a clear way to wheel the person from the bathroom rather than having to stop and open and close doors, preparing all showering supplies as well as laying out clothing for resident). Bathing methodology, such as knowing which part of the body should be washed first during bathing or showering so as to minimize discomfort to the bathed person.
The importance of the *process* of care (how care is provided rather than simply its provision)	When dressing a resident, what choices should be offered? What should caregivers ask the resident to do and in what manner? What should they simply do themselves for the resident? How long should they wait between a verbal prompt and actually assisting the resident? The importance of positive communication.
Communication	Knowledge regarding the importance of communication and surveillance of resident. Caregivers often devalue the resident's need to communicate and ability to communicate. Interaction during care is a potent skill that is often lacking (Cohen-Mansfield et al., 2006) Understanding of ways in which dementia affects communication abilities of a person and how to adjust staff communications with the person with dementia. Knowing what to say. Staff members often do not know what they should say as they are washing residents (Rasin, Barrick, & Leeman, 2004) or when a resident complains. Understanding of differences in cultural and educational backgrounds between residents and staff.
Individualization of care based on resident needs, preferences, functional, sensory, and cognitive abilities	When staff members witness a successful intervention, they tend to apply it to other residents, regardless of their level of functioning or interest. Individualization of care is most often applied to ADLs that take into account the residents; functional status, but individualization often neglects the person's preferences and needs, especially if the resident is more severely cognitively impaired and cannot communicate effectively.
Understanding of etiology of mood and behavior	Inappropriate use of a medical model when a psychosocial one or a more comprehensive examination would be more useful for promoting quality care. For example, a behavior is often perceived as an indication for psychoactive medication, thereby eliminating the need to assess other potential causes such as pain, hunger, or environmental triggers. Staff members describe the reason for a problem behavior as agitation—a tautological explanation. *Agitation* as a symptom and a diagnosis is used very liberally by staff members, without further characterization of behaviors. Staff members see certain problem behaviors as personal affronts rather than attempting to understand the reasons for the behavior. Residents who prefer a different type/timing/help with care are labeled as resistive to care. A resistant behavior is frequently attributed to the character of the resident rather than to the care process.
Discriminating between quality care and technically good care	Staff members have difficulty understanding the relative importance of certain aspects of care vs. allowing the resident to live life in a more enjoyable manner. For example, a very old and frail resident is denied his or her favorite food because the resident is on a low-fat diet; or a person is forbidden to walk for fear of falling.

From Cohen-Mansfield, J., & Parpura-Gill, A. (2008). Practice style in the nursing home: Dimensions for assessment and quality improvement. *International Journal of Geriatric Psychiatry 23*, 376-386.

Table 14-6	**Communication Receipt Deficits: Domains and Examples**
Communication not heard	The unit is so short-staffed that there is no one in the corridor for a long period of time, let alone in the residents' rooms. Residents may cry or call for help with no caregiver around to notice. When staff members are around, they are so involved in the performance of the task itself that they do not hear the communication. We observed this phenomenon during training of staff members, when we repeated the residents' words back to the staff members and they had literally not heard the requests.
Communication is ignored	When nursing staff members do not know how to interpret verbal or nonverbal communication by a resident (such as a repeated request for help), when they do not know how to respond to it, or when they do not have the resources to address it, they sometimes simply ignore it. The majority of verbal agitation is ignored (Cohen-Mansfield et al., 1992) and characterized as nonsense or a behavior problem. If communication is repetitive, or when attempts to alleviate the problem are unsuccessful, the communication is frequently characterized as meaningless, and the staff members become habituated to it. Many behaviors that express pain are also ignored. Over time, staff members can become so accustomed to what they perceive as inappropriate behaviors—even extreme behaviors such as screaming—that they may stop noticing them. Even when communication is understood, if it is not specific enough, it is often not acted upon. For example, a resident who complains about pain, but is unable to point to a painful part of the body, may go untreated.
Communication is not understood	Although the decline in the ability to communicate is characteristic of dementia, persons with dementia still convey important messages. At times staff members can infer the message from circumstances. For example, one resident complained that the bench on which she sat was wet from the rain. The caregiver had to infer that she had wet herself and was cold and needed to change her clothes.
Communication is discouraged	Residents and family members sometimes feel that if they raise issues the resident will suffer from negative repercussions, or that they will disturb the staff member. Similarly, staff members are often uncomfortable questioning family's requests in fear of jeopardizing their relationship with the family (Hertzberg & Ekman, 2000).
Communication is devalued or discounted	Because a resident has dementia, staff members at times assume that she does not know what she is saying, and therefore her preferences are ignored. Often staff members' perceptions are used as a standard to which residents' statements and requests are compared, resulting in invalidation of the residents' point of view. The residents' point of view is not understood. One resident asked to go to the bathroom and was told to urinate in the diaper. One resident told a staff member that he was cold, and was told in response that it was not cold. The caregiver may not be cold because she is running around, or because she is less prone to feeling cold. The resident, however, may indeed feel cold. A resident complained that she was thirsty, but was only allowed thickened liquids to avoid choking, despite the fact that these liquids did not address her thirst.

From Cohen-Mansfield, J. & Parpura-Gill, A. (2008). Practice style in the nursing home: Dimensions for assessment and quality improvement. *International Journal of Geriatric Psychiatry 23*, 376-386.

this revolution involves a return to some fundamental principles of stroke rehabilitation with a focus on getting patients to their home environment. Rehabilitation clinicians will function more as an interdisciplinary team, with greater overlapping of roles and improved integration of care. The incorporation of new technologies will have an increasingly important impact, but new technologies alone will not be enough. (p. 44)

Comparing different stroke rehabilitation systems from various countries provides important information. Comparisons are made of various systems using the categories of structure, processes, and outcomes of care. Following are categories of Structures of Care, Processes of Care, and Outcomes of Care as used for research in stroke rehabilitation.

STRUCTURES OF CARE
- Specialized interdisciplinary stroke rehabilitation units
- Outpatient programs

PROCESSES OF CARE
- Time to admission
- Intensity of therapy
- Task-specific therapy
- Discharge planning

Differences in these processes of care have been shown through research to result in significant differences in outcomes. When structures and processes of care reflect best evidence, better outcomes are achieved. The studies focus on three outcomes: optimizing brain reorganization, maximizing neurological recovery, and returning the patient to his or her home environment. Outcomes are measured with the Barthel index (BI). The best outcomes are achieved on interdisciplinary stroke units. However, a continuum of care from the time of the stroke through return to the home environment is important. An effective outpatient program after the patient goes home is also important.

Costs of Care

A third dimension of the examination of quality of care is **cost**. Maintaining a specified level of quality of care necessarily has cost consequences. Providing more and better care is likely to increase costs, but also is likely to produce savings. Economic benefits can be obtained by preventing illness, preventing complications, maintaining a higher quality of life, or prolonging productive life.

A related issue is who bears the costs of care. Some measures purported to reduce costs have instead simply shifted costs to another party. For example, in certain instances a hospital can reduce its costs by discharging a particular type of patient earlier, but total costs will increase if necessary community-based health care increases and raises costs above those incurred by keeping the patient hospitalized longer. In this case, the third-party provider may experience higher costs. In many cases, the costs are shifted from the healthcare system to the family as **out-of-pocket costs**. Studies examining changes in costs of care must consider total costs, including out-of-pocket costs.

Harris and Shannon (2008) conducted a study of an innovative enterostomal therapy (ET) nurse model of community wound care delivery. Their purpose was to examine the role and impact of ET nursing in Canada. They performed a "retrospective analysis of the cost-effectiveness and benefits of ET nurse-driven resources for the treatment of acute and chronic wounds in the community" (p. 169). The study involved data from four community nursing agencies and one specialty company owned and operated by ET nurses.

> Three hundred sixty chronic wounds and 54 acute surgical wound charts were audited. Involvement of a registered nurse (RN) with ET or advanced wound ostomy skills (AWOS) and a hybrid group that includes interventions developed by an ET nurse and followed by general visiting nurses that could include both RNs and registered practical nurses is an expected reduction in healing times of 45 days and an expected cost difference of $5927.00

per chronic wound treated. Conclusions: The greater the involvement both directly and indirectly of an ET/AWOS in the management of wounds, the greater the savings and the shorter the healing times. The analyses included methods to evaluate healing outcomes, nursing costs, and cost effectiveness.

Implications for Practice

Nursing practice is affected by decisions of institutions to change policies regarding the number of nurses or type of nurses assigned to particular types of patient care. The institution may hire more of a particularly educated nurse or more nurses. This will affect the budget of the institution by increasing costs, but these costs (of higher educated nurses) may be justifiable because healing of wounds may occur in less time, the patient can be discharged sooner, thus providing space to admit another patient. The institution will then gain a better reputation in the community for healing wounds more rapidly, thus getting an increase in referrals, and thus increasing their overall income. Insurance companies will like this improvement also because it lowers their cost and they will increase their support of that institution for referral.

Evaluating Structure

Structures of care are the elements of organization and administration that guide the processes of care. The first step in evaluating structure is to identify and describe the elements of the structure. Examples of such elements are leadership, tolerance of innovativeness, organizational hierarchy, decision-making processes, distribution of power, financial management, and administrative decision-making processes. In the following study, two structures are studied: closed model health maintenance organizations and Veterans Affairs medical clinics.

> Nurse case management has been shown to improve the quality of diabetes care in closed model health maintenance organizations and Veterans Affairs medical clinics. A randomized controlled trial of a similar intervention within Health Texas Provider Network, a fee-for-service primary care network in North Texas, demonstrated no benefit in processes of care or clinical outcomes for Medicare diabetes patients. To investigate whether the case management model impacted the cost of diabetes care from the Medicare perspective, we compared the average payments and charges incurred between intervention arms: claims-based audit and feedback; claims- and medical-record-based audit and feedback; and claims- and medical-record-based audit and feedback plus a practice-based diabetes resource nurse. Following adjustment for baseline differences between groups, no significant differences were observed. Thus, within this setting, it appears the nurse case management model produced no improvement in either clinical quality or costs associated with diabetes from a Medicare perspective (Herrin, Cangialose, Nicewander, & Ballard, 2007, p. 328).

Although randomized controlled trials are not generally used in outcome studies, cost analyses are, as well as analyses to examine differences in clinical quality by comparing two different models of care. However, in this case, neither approach showed a difference in care or costs.

EXAMPLE: NURSING OUTCOMES STUDY

Organizational effects on patient satisfaction in hospital medical-surgical units

Abstract

Objective: The purpose of this study was to examine the relationships among hospital context, nursing unit structure, and patient characteristics and patients' satisfaction with nursing care in hospitals.

Background: Although patient satisfaction has been widely researched, our understanding of the relationship between hospital context and nursing unit structure and their impact on patient satisfaction is limited.

Methods: The data source for this study was the Outcomes Research in Nursing Administration Project, a multisite organizational study conducted to investigate relationships among nurse staffing, organizational context and structure, and patient outcomes. The sample for this study was 2720 patients and 3718 RNs in 286 medical-surgical units in 146 hospitals.

Results: Greater availability of nursing unit support services and higher levels of work engagement were associated with higher levels of patient satisfaction. Older age, better health status, and better symptom management were also associated with higher levels of patient satisfaction.

Conclusions: Organizational factors in hospitals and nursing units, particularly support services on the nursing unit and mechanisms that foster nurses' work engagement and effective symptom management, are important influences on patient satisfaction (Bacon & Mark, 2009, abstract, p. 220).

CRITICAL APPRAISAL

Bacon and Mark (2009) conducted a small outcomes study that illustrates the characteristics of a typical outcomes study. Data were obtained from the Outcomes Research in Nursing Administration Project, which collects and stores outcomes data from a variety of hospitals for a variety of analysis purposes. This project analyzed data from medical surgical units in multiple hospitals for the purpose of examining the relationships between hospital context, nursing unit structure, patient characteristics, and patients' satisfaction with nursing care in hospitals. The findings indicate that when nursing unit support services are more available, levels of work engagement are higher and patient satisfaction is higher. Higher levels of patient satisfaction were found in older patients who had a better health status and better symptom management.

IMPLICATIONS FOR PRACTICE

Typical of outcome studies, these findings cannot be applied to individual patients, or even individual hospitals. They cannot be applied to the nursing practice of an individual nurse. The study is examining the end results of patient care, using patient satisfaction as a measurement of an end result. The quality of the patient care is reflected in patient satisfaction. The findings are important in examining the effects of hospital context, nursing unit structure, and patient characteristics on patient satisfaction. Why is this information important? How could we use such information? How is it important to nursing practice or patient care? Nurses have been trying for a very long time to persuade hospital administrators of the importance of resources such as nursing unit structure and nursing unit support services to how well they

Continued

IMPLICATIONS FOR PRACTICE—cont'd

can practice nursing. The structure of a nursing unit strongly effects how well a nurse can care for patients. There are a number of structural impediments that can slow down the work of the nurse, as can the storage of supplies for nursing practice. When nursing unit support services are inadequate, which could mean slow, inadequate, perhaps hostile, nurses often cannot get the services they need to provide patient care, at least in a timely manner or a pleasant way. Under poor conditions, nurses are not satisfied and neither are the patients being cared for by the nurses, and this will be reflected in patient evaluations. One would hope that hospital management personnel would look at this information and consider changing unit structures, and improving hospital unit services with the intent of improving the environment in which nurses practice and the satisfaction of patients with the care being provided by the nurses. This information can also be used by nurses who can take the initiative to join together to approach hospital administration with the purpose of proposing changes to improve the environment in which they work for the purpose of improving nursing practice.

Outcomes Research and Nursing Practice

Outcome studies provide rich opportunities to build a stronger scientific underpinning for nursing practice (Maas & Delaney, 2004; Rettig, 1991): "Nursing needs to be able to explain the impact of care provided by its practitioners through measures of outcomes of patient care that reflect nursing practice" (Moritz, 1991, p. 113).

The American Nurses Association's "Nursing's Safety & Quality Initiative"

In the late 1980s and early 1990s, hospitals were confronted with managed care requirements to reduce costs. To accomplish this goal, hospitals across the country reduced their nursing staff and replaced them with unlicensed personnel having very little training for their assignments. Managed care dictated earlier patient discharges, resulting in hospitalized patients who were sicker and required complex care. Nurses repeatedly complained that patient care was inadequate and that patients were experiencing complications and dying needlessly because of the inadequate staffing of RNs. However, nursing had little concrete evidence of these statements. Many nurses left nursing practice or changed to community areas of nursing practice. The RNs remaining in hospital practice tended to be new graduates who were placed in positions of responsibility without adequate experience. Assignment loads became increasingly difficult. Nurses tended to leave the hospital after 2 years, and more new graduates replaced them. A shortage of nurses, already in place, was exacerbated by this situation. Recruitment of new students became increasingly difficult as greater numbers of news items discussed the problems.

In 1994 the ANA, in collaboration with the American Academy of Nursing Expert Panel on Quality Health Care (Mitchell, Ferketich, Jennings, & American Academy of Nursing Expert Panel on Quality Health Care, 1998), launched an initiative to identify indicators of quality nursing practice, and to collect and analyze data using these indicators across the United States. The goal was to identify or develop nursing-sensitive quality measures. Donabedian's theory was used as the framework for the project. The committee conducted an extensive literature review, expert panel discussions, and focus group interviews to identify nursing care indicators relevant to nursing care quality in acute care, based on Donabedian's theory or established evidence of a strong link to nursing care quality. The indicators that were being used by the American Nurses Association in 2010 (the most recent list publicly available at the time of publication of this text) are listed in Table 14–7.

When these indicators began to be studied in 1994, ANA entered a new area of research and asked questions that had not previously been studied. No one knew what indicators were sensitive to the nursing care provided to patients or what relationships existed between nursing inputs and patient outcomes. They had to persuade hospitals to participate in the study at a time when hospitals had a severe case of "data paranoia" (fear of providing data to anyone outside the hospital because of how third parties might interpret the data). Every hospital had a different way of measuring the indicators selected by ANA. Persuading them to change to a standardized measure of the indicators for consistency across hospitals was a major endeavor (Jennings, Loan, DePaul, Brosch, & Hildreth, 2001; Rowell, 2001). Nurse researchers and cooperating hospitals instituted the mechanisms required for data collection and began multiple pilot studies. These pilot studies identified multiple obstacles to the project. They learned that not only must the indicators be measured consistently, but that data collection must be standardized. As studies continued, indicators were amplified and continue to be tested. As this testing continued, further alterations in the indicators occurred (Anonymous, 1997; Campbell-Heider, Krainovich-Miller, King, Sedhom, & Malinski, 1998; Jennings et al., 2001).

The ANA proposed that all hospitals collect and report on the nursing-sensitive quality indicators. The ANA worked to ensure that these indicators were included in data collected by accrediting organizations and by the federal government, and that the data be shared with key groups. The ANA also encouraged state nurses' associations to lobby state legislatures to include the nursing-sensitive quality indicators into regulations or state law.

In 1998, the ANA provided funding to develop a national database to house data collected using nursing-sensitive quality indicators. This database, named The National Database of Nursing Quality Indicators (NDNQI), a program of the National Center for Nursing Quality, is still funded by the ANA. The database is housed at the University of Kansas Medical Center Research Institute (KUMCRI) and of the University of Kansas School of Nursing. In 2001, data from nursing-sensitive quality indicators were being collected from more than 120 hospitals in 24 states across the United States. By 2005, that number had increased to 767 hospitals in the 50 states and the District of Columbia. In 2010, the number of participating hospitals had increased to 1500. The National Center for Nursing Quality analyzes the data quarterly and provides feedback reports to all participating hospitals. Confidential benchmarking reports are provided to allow hospitals to compare their results with those of other hospitals (Rowell, 2001; Patton, 2009). You may reach the National Center for Nursing Quality at http://www.nursingworld.org/MainMenuCategories/ThePracticeofProfessionalNursing/PatientSafetyQuality.aspx for current information on Nursing Quality.

In 1997, the ANA appointed members of an Advisory Committee on Community-Based Non-Acute Care Indicators to identify the first core set of indictors for non-acute care settings. Some of the members of this committee had helped develop the Acute Care Indicators, giving the committee some continuity of the work. The committee began by selecting a theoretical base for its work: Evans and Stoddart's (1990) determinants of health model and also Donabedian's model of quality. As its work progressed, the committee chose to

Table 14-7	American Nurses Association National Database of Nursing Quality Indicators (NDNQI)

NDNQI Indicators

Indicator	Sub-indicator	Measure(s)
1. Nursing Hours per Patient Day[1,2]	a. Registered Nurses (RN) b. Licensed Practical/Vocational Nurses (LPN/LVN) c. Unlicensed Assistive Personnel (UAP)	Structure
2. Patient Falls[1,2]		Process & Outcome
3. Patient Falls with Injury[1,2]	a. Injury Level	Process & Outcome
4. Pediatric Pain Assessment, Intervention, Reassessment (AIR) Cycle		Process
5. Pediatric Peripheral Intravenous Infiltration Rate		Outcome
6. Pressure Ulcer Prevalence[1]	a. Community Acquired b. Hospital Acquired c. Unit Acquired	Process & Outcome
7. Psychiatric Physical/Sexual Assault Rate		Outcome
8. Restraint Prevalence[2]		Outcome
9. RN Education/Certification		Structure
10. RN Satisfaction Survey Options[1,3]	a. Job Satisfaction Scales b. Job Satisfaction Scales Short Form c. Practice Environment Scale (PES)[2]	Process & Outcome
11. Skill Mix: Percent of total nursing hours supplied by[1,2]	a. RN b. LPN/LVN c. UAP d. % of total nursing hours supplied by Agency Staff	Structure
12. Voluntary Nurse Turnover[2]		Structure
13. Nurse Vacancy Rate		Structure
14. Nosocomial Infections (Pending for 2007) a. Urinary catheter-associated urinary tract infection (UTI)[2] b. Central line catheter associated bloodstream infection (CABSI)[1,2] c. Ventilator-associated pneumonia (VAP)[2]		Outcome

[1]Original ANA Nursing-Sensitive Indicator.

[2]NQF Endorsed Nursing-Sensitive Indicator.

[3]The RN Survey is annual, whereas the other indicators are quarterly.

synthesize a model to guide the identification and testing of indicators (Figure 14–3). The committee followed the acute care group's process in selecting the indicators. A hired contractor conducted the literature review, whereas the committee conducted focus groups and interviews with key stakeholders such as consumers of care, registered nurses, policy makers, regulators, payers, facility administrators, and purchasers. The initial development was limited to 10 indicators, but these have since been expanded (see Table 14–7). These indicators are included in the Magnet criteria. The committee requested that all nurses and nursing organizations join with the ANA to continue to expand this work (Head, Maas, & Johnson,

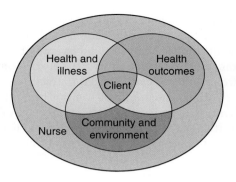

Figure 14–3. Model used to guide identification and testing of community-based non-acute care indicators by the American Nurses Association (ANA) Advisory Committee (1997). In Sawyer, L. M., Berkowitz, B., Haber, J. E., Larrabee, J. H., Marino, B. L., Martin, K. S., et al. Expanding American Nurses Association Nursing Quality Indicators to community-based practices. *Outcomes Management, 6*(2), p. 53.

2003; Nakrem, Vinsnes, Harkless, Paulsen, & Seim, (2009); Sawyer et al., 2002, Swan, Lang, & McGinley, 2004). (For current information on the ANA's Safety & Quality Initiative, visit the following web site: *http://nursingworld.org/quality*.) The current list of indicators continues to increase and change as more research is conducted and more hospitals are agreeing to participate in the collection of data.

A number of studies on the effects of nursing staff mix on patient outcomes have been published (Blegen, Goode, & Reed, 1998; Buerhaus & Needleman, 2000; Cho, Ketefian, Barkauskas, & Smith, 2003; Hall, et al., 2001; Houser, 2000; Huston, 1997; Needleman, Buerhaus, Mattke, Steward, & Zelevinsky, 2002a,b; Seago, Williamson, & Atwood, 2006; Upenieks, Kotlerman, Akhavan, Esser, & Ngo, 2007; Yang, 2003). These studies reveal a significant effect of staffing mix on patient outcomes.

Needleman et al. (2002a,b), used discharge and staffing data from 799 hospitals in 11 states to estimate nurse staffing levels for RNs, LPN/LVNs, and aides, as well as the frequency of a wide range of complications developed by patients during their hospital stay. The data cover 6 million patients discharged from hospitals in 1997. These investigators found that low levels of RN staffing among a hospital's nurses were associated with high rates of serious complications, such as pneumonia, upper gastrointestinal bleeding, shock, and cardiac arrest, including deaths among patients with these three complications, as well as sepsis or deep vein thrombosis. These complications occurred 3% to 9% more often in hospitals with lower levels of RN staffing.

Sochalski (2001), after a review of studies on staff mix, cautions that

> … missing from these studies is a more thorough explanation of *how* nurse staffing affects patient outcomes. That is, does increasing staffing levels and/or skill mix, under any circumstances, yield better outcomes, or are the effects of staffing titrated by other features in the practice environment that influence nursing's ability to deliver the quality of care that results in better patient outcomes? Trying to establish minimum staffing ratios in the absence of clear information on just how staffing levels affect outcomes may result in ratios that overestimate or underestimate what is really needed to improve patient care. Furthermore, if the effect of staffing on patient outcomes can only be fully achieved in the presence of other features in the practice environment, then it will be the presence or absence of these features and not solely staffing levels that will produce the desired patient results. Without a clear understanding of the circumstances under which staffing affects outcomes, we lack the capacity to improve patient outcomes if efforts are directed only at changing staffing levels. (p. 11)

Standing, Anthony, and Hertz (2001) conducted a triangulated study of outcomes after delegation to unlicensed assistive personnel (UAP), funded by the National Council of State Boards of Nursing. This report describes the qualitative analysis of interviews of RNs who described a delegation with a positive outcome and a delegation with a negative outcome. Negative outcomes after delegation ranged from family or client upsets, to fractures or other injuries, to death. In some cases, the UAP performed activities that had not been delegated to them. Negative outcomes were most frequently because the UAP did not receive or follow directions or adhere to established policy. Positive outcomes included enhanced client well-being, as indicated by increased socialization and other measures, prevention of poor client outcomes, and enhanced unit functioning.

These seminal studies have stimulated a number of important studies examining the issue of practice outcomes and their relationship to nurse staffing levels. The references later in this chapter will provide a sense of the growth of the body of knowledge in this area of concern.

Nursing-Sensitive Patient Outcomes

Donabedian (1976) states that a clear link must be established between an outcome and the process that resulted in the outcome. Thus, selecting a nursing-sensitive outcome requires a clear explanation of the process that led to that outcome. The process that needs to be defined is likely to be a complex combination of nursing acts, acts of other professionals, organizational acts, and patient characteristics and behaviors. Nursing acts are not clearly defined and are inconsistent across nurses and institutions. Few studies have attempted to describe a particular nursing process, much less link it to outcomes.

Stetler, Morsi, and Burns (2000) have worked to develop a comprehensive, in-depth profile of nursing-sensitive outcomes of hospital nursing care at the unit level and to use the information in routine quality monitoring. They used a prevention framework based on the work of Stetler and DeZell (1989). The framework describes the nurse's role in preventing complications in a nosocomial hospital environment; treatment consequences; a patient's health status, disease state, or evolving condition; and the patient's inability to care for herself or himself safely. From a safety perspective, the framework classifies outcomes as positive or negative. Outcomes are further classified in terms of preventability, impact, severity, and a holistic view of patient safety. Positive behaviors protect or rescue patients from potential or actual negative events. These actions are categorized as (1) detection/reporting, (2) detection/prevention, and (3) facilitation of resolution/prevention.

Other work has included development of a model of nursing effectiveness to use as a framework in studies of patient outcomes. Irvine, Sidani, and Hall (1998) have developed The Nursing Role Effectiveness Model (Figure 14–4) to guide the examination and explanation of the links between nursing processes and patient outcomes. The model is based on Donabedian's theory of quality care. Roles are defined as

> … positions in organizations that have attached to them a set of expected behaviors. Professional roles are complex because they consist of components that are based on normative expectations concerning standards of practice that have been established by external regulatory bodies and secondly, on normative expectations that have evolved over time that are unique to the organization. (p. 59)

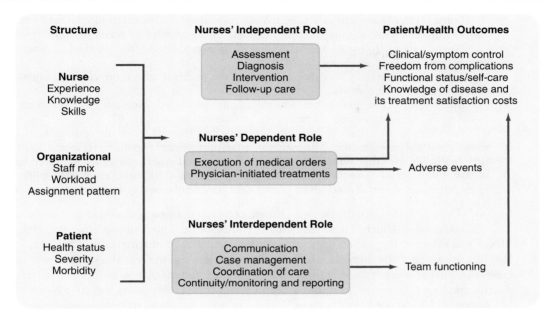

Figure 14–4. The Nursing Role Effectiveness Model. From Irvine, D., Sidani, S., & Hall, L. M. (1998). Linking outcomes to nurses' roles in health care. *Nursing Economics, 16*(2), 59.

The Nursing Role Effectiveness Model has three major components: structure, the nurses' role, and patient/health outcomes. Structure has three subcomponents: nurse, organization, and patient. Nurse variables that influence quality of nursing care include factors such as experience level, knowledge, and skill level. Organizational components that can affect quality of nursing care include staff mix, workload, and assignment patterns. Patient characteristics that can affect quality of care include health status, severity, and morbidity. Nurses' role has three subcomponents: nurses' independent role, nurses' dependent role, and nurses' interdependent role. Independent role functions include assessment, diagnosis, nurse initiated interventions, and follow-up care. The patient/health outcomes of the independent role are clinical/symptom control, freedom from complications, functional status/self-care, knowledge of disease and its treatment, satisfaction, and costs. The dependent role functions include execution of medical orders and physician-initiated treatments. It is the dependent role functions that can lead to patient/health outcomes of adverse events. Interdependent role functions include communication, case management, coordination of care, and continuity/monitoring and reporting. The interdependent role results in team functioning and affects the patient/health outcomes of the independent role.

The Propositions of The Nursing Role Effectiveness Model were stated as follows (Irvine, et al., 1998):

> Nursing's capacity to engage effectively in the independent, dependent, and interdependent role functions is influenced by individual nurse variables, patient variables, and organizational structure variables. (p. 61)

Nurses' interdependent role function depends upon the nurse's ability to communicate and articulate her/his opinion to other members of the health care team. (p. 61)

Nurse, patient, and system structural variables have a direct effect on clinical, functional, satisfaction, and cost outcomes. (p. 61)

Nurses' independent role function can have a direct effect on clinical, functional, satisfaction, and cost outcomes. (p. 61)

Medication errors and other adverse events associated with nurses' dependent role function can ultimately affect all categories of patient outcome. (p. 62)

Nursing's interdependent role function can affect the quality of interprofessional communication and coordination. The nature of inter-professional communication and coordination can influence other important patient outcomes and costs such as risk-adjusted length of stay, risk-adjusted mortality rates, excess home care costs following discharge, unplanned visits to the physician or emergency department, and unplanned re-hospitalization. (p. 62)

In 2002, Doran, Sidani, Keatings, and Doidge conducted an empirical test of The Nursing Role Effectiveness Model. These investigators found that The Nursing Role Effectiveness Model was effective in guiding the evaluation of outcomes of nursing care. They noted that "for the most part the hypothesized relationships among the variables were supported. However, further work is needed to develop an understanding of how nurses engage in their coordinating role functions and how we can measure these role activities" (p. 30).

Gazarian (2008) used the Nursing Role Effectiveness Model to examine nurse decision making and the prevention of adverse events, using a qualitative design. The study used the cognitive task analysis method of the Critical Decision Method. According to Gazarian (2008),

the nurses in this study operated from a perspective of maintaining patient safety while balancing organization expectations. Examination of these decision situations demonstrated the complexity of clinical practice and the many factors that affect nurse's ability to identify and interrupt adverse events. This study demonstrated that the patient's experience of illness, severity of illness and trends over time are useful in identifying risk of clinical deterioration. Teamwork and flexibility was evident among the unit nursing staff and across disciplines. When team members knew and trusted each other, they were better positioned to share decision making and adapt to rapidly changing conditions. Lastly this study demonstrated the importance of knowledge management as an organization resource. The Nursing Role Effectiveness model highlights decision making as an independent role of the nurse.

Redekopp (2007) used the Nursing Role Effectiveness Model to examine relationships of professional nurse characteristics and nurse staffing to adverse patient outcomes. Redekopp found no significant relationships among nurse characteristics, nurse staffing and adverse patient outcomes.

Tarlier (2006) studied nursing practice, continuity of care, and maternal-infant health outcomes in a remote First Nations community. The ethnographic study was designed to study nurses' primary care practice, continuity of patient care, and clinical health outcomes. Relational, informational, and management continuity were explored as well as clinical health outcomes. Two selected health indicator conditions: (a) prenatal care and (b) infant care were followed through the first year. This allowed the researcher to explore nurses' practice and examine continuity at the individual level and to relate the findings to continuity and fragmentation at the community and population levels. Four overarching themes emerged from analysis and interpretation of the data: (a) nurses' work, influenced by a broader context of inequity and marginalization, occurred at the margins of mainstream nursing practice, (b) health outcomes and continuity of care were characterized by fragmentation, (c) nurse-patient encounters were suggestive of relational disengagement and (d) dissonance existed between perceptions of health care and demonstrated health outcomes.

It appears that the Nursing Role Effectiveness Model will be important in the future in building a body of knowledge related to nursing effectiveness. Studies are supporting the propositions of the theory. Of particular interest are the statements of the theory related to independent role of the nurse in decision-making. For example, the role of the nurse in identifying the risk of deterioration of the patient is very important. Decisions of the nurse in complex patient care situations have been shown to be critical elements of independent nursing practice Gazarian (2008).

Disseminating Outcomes of Research Findings

Including plans for the dissemination of findings as a component of a program of research is a new idea within nursing if the process of dissemination is considered to be more than publishing the results in professional journals. The costs associated with dissemination are not included in funding for nursing studies beyond those of publication of the research findings. Strategies for the dissemination of research findings tend to be performed by groups other than the original researchers. The transfer of knowledge from nurse researchers to nurse clinicians has been, for the most part, ineffective.

Nursing, as a discipline, has not yet addressed the various constituencies for nursing research knowledge. A research team conducting a program of outcomes research must identify its constituencies. These should include (1) the clinicians, who will apply the knowledge to practice, (2) the public, members of which may make healthcare decisions on the basis of the information, (3) healthcare institutions, which must evaluate care in their facilities on the basis of the information, (4) health policy makers, who or which may set standards on the basis of the information, and (5) researchers, who may use the information in designing new studies. Disseminating information to these various constituencies through presentations at meetings and publications in a wide diversity of journals and magazines, as well as release of the information to the news media, requires careful planning. Mattson and Donovan (1994) suggest that dissemination involves strategies for debunking myths, addressing issues related to feasibility, communicating effectively, and identifying opinion leaders.

KEY CONCEPTS

- Outcomes research was developed to examine the end results of patient care.
- The scientific approaches used in outcomes studies differ in some important ways from those used in traditional research.
- The theory on which outcomes research is based was developed by Donabedian (1987). Quality is the overriding construct of the theory. The three major concepts of the theory are health, subjects of care, and providers of care.
- The goal of outcomes research is the evaluation of outcomes as defined by Donabedian, whose theory requires that identified outcomes be clearly linked with the process that caused the outcome.

- Outcomes research programs are complex and may consist of multiple studies using a variety of designs whose findings must be merged in the process of forming conclusions.
- The researcher must consider the measure's sensitivity to change and the magnitude of change that can be detected.
- Statistical approaches used in outcomes studies include new approaches to examining measurement reliability, strategies to analyze change, and the analysis of improvement.
- Strategies must be developed in nursing to disseminate the findings from outcomes studies to the various constituencies needing the information.

REFERENCES

Anonymous. (1997). A report on the implementation of a nursing report card for acute care settings executive summary—January 1997. *New Mexico Nurse*, 42(2), 11.

Bacon, C. T., & Mark, B. (2009). Organizational effects on patient satisfaction in hospital medical-surgical units. *Journal of Nursing Administration*, 39(5), 220-227.

Bergmark, A., & Oscarsson, L. (1991). Does anybody really know what they are doing? Some comments related to methodology of treatment service research. *British Journal of Addiction*, 86(2), 139-142.

Bircumshaw, D., & Chapman, C. M. (1988). A study to compare the practice style of graduate and non-graduate nurses and midwives: The pilot study. *Journal of Advanced Nursing*, 13(5), 605-614.

Blegen, M. A., Goode, C. J., & Reed, L. (1998). Nurse staffing and patient outcomes. *Nursing Research*, 47(1), 43-50.

Buerhaus, P. I., & Needleman, J. (2000). Policy implications of research on nurse staffing and quality of patient care. *Policy, Politics, & Nursing Practice*, 1(1), 5-15.

Campbell-Heider, N., Krainovich-Miller, B., King, K. B., Sedhom, L., & Malinski, V. (1998). Empowering staff nurses to participate in the American Nurses Association's call for quality indicators research. *Journal of the New York State Nurses' Association*, 29(3/4), 21-27.

Cho, S., Ketefian, S., Barkauskas, V. H., & Smith, D. G. (2003). The effects of nurse staffing on adverse events, morbidity, mortality, and medical costs. *Nursing Research*, 52(2), 71-79.

Cohen-Mansfield, J., & Werner, P. (1992). The Social Environment of the Agitated Nursing Home Resident. *International Journal of Geriatric Psychiatry*, 7(11), 789-798.

Cohen-Mansfield, J., Lipson, S., & Horton, D. (2006). Medical decision-making in the nursing home. *Journal of Gerontological Nursing*, 32(12), 14-21.

Cohen-Mansfield, J., & Parpura-Gill, A. (2008). Practice style in the nursing home: Dimensions for assessment and quality improvement. *International Journal of Geriatric Psychiatry*, 23, 376-386.

Donabedian, A. (1976). *Benefits in medical care programs*. Cambridge: Harvard University Press.

Donabedian, A. (1978). *Needed research in quality assessment and monitoring*. Hyattsville, MD: U.S. Department of Health, Education, and Welfare, Public Health Service, National Center for Health Services Research: NCHSR Office of Scientific and Technical Information. [Available from National Technical Information Service, Springfield, VA.]

Donabedian, A. (1980). *Explorations in quality assessment and monitoring*. Ann Arbor, MI: Health Administration Press.

Donabedian, A. (1982). *The criteria and standards of quality*. Ann Arbor, MI: Health Administration Press.

Donabedian, A. (1987). Some basic issues in evaluating the quality of health care. In L. T. Rinke (Ed.), Outcome measures in home care (*vol. I*, pp. 3-28). New York: National League for Nursing. [Original work published 1976.]

Donabedian, A. (1988). The quality of care: How can it be accessed? *Journal of the American Medical Association*, 260(12), 1744.

Doran, D. I., Sidani, S., Keatings, M., & Doidge, D. (2002). An empirical test of the Nursing Role Effectiveness Model. *Journal of Advanced Nursing*, 38(1), 29-39.

Evans, R. G., & Stoddart, G. L. (1990). Producing health, consuming health care. *Social Science and Medicine*, 31(12), 1347-1363.

Fullerton, J. T., Hollenbach, K. A., & Wingard, D. L. (1996). Research exchange. Practice styles: A comparison of obstetricians and nurse-midwives. *Journal of Nurse-Midwifery*, 41(3), 243-250.

Gazarian, P. K. (2008). *Nurse decision making and the prevention of adverse events*. Unpublished doctoral dissertation, University of Massachusetts Amherst.

Hall, L. M., Doran, D. I., Baker, G. R., Pink, G., Sidani, S., O'Brien, P., et al. (2001). A study of the impact of nursing staff mix models & organizational change strategies on patient, system & caregiver outcomes. Available at: *http://www.nursing.utoronto.ca/lmcgillishall/research/nsmos%20summary%20report.pdf*.

Harris, C., & Shannon, R. (2008). An innovative enterostomal therapy nurse model of community wound care delivery: a retrospective cost-effectiveness analysis. *Journal of Wound, Ostomy & Continence Nursing*, 35(2), 169-183.

Head, B. J., Maas, M., & Johnson, M. (2003). Validity and community-health-nursing sensitivity of six outcomes for community health nursing with older clients. *Public Health Nursing*, 25(5), 385-398.

Herrin, J., Cangialose, C. B., Nicewander, D., & Ballard, D. J. (2007). Cost and effects of performance feedback and nurse case management for Medicare beneficiaries with diabetes: A randomized controlled trial. *Disease Management*, 10(6), 328-336.

Hertzberg, A., & Ekman, S. (2000). We, Not Them and Us! Views on the relationships and interactions between staff and relatives of older people permanently living in nursing homes. *Journal of Advanced Nursing, 31*(3), 614-622.

Houser, J. L. (2000). *A model for evaluating the context of nursing care delivery. Unpublished doctoral dissertation.* Greeley, CO: University of Northern Colorado.

Huston, C. L. (1997). *The replacement of registered nurses by unlicensed assistive personnel: the impact on three process/outcome indicators of quality.* Unpublished doctoral dissertation: University of Southern California.

Irvine, D., Sidani, S., & Hall, L. M. (1998). Linking outcomes to nurses' roles in health care. *Nursing Economics, 16*(2), 58-64, 87.

Jennings, B. M., Loan, L. A., DePaul, D., Brosch, L. R., & Hildreth, P. (2001). Lessons learned while collecting ANA indicator data. *Journal of Nursing Administration, 31*(3), 121-129.

Lewis, B. E. (1995). HMO outcomes research: Lessons from the field. *Journal of Ambulatory Care Management, 18*(1), 47-55.

Loegering, L., Reiter, R. C., & Gambone, J. C. (1994). Measuring the quality of health care. *Clinical Obstetrics and Gynecology, 37*(1), 122-136.

Maas, M. L., & Delaney, C. (2004). Nursing process outcome linkage research: Issues, current status, and health policy implications. *Medical Care, 42*(2), Supplement II, 40-48.

Mark, B. A. (1995). The black box of patient outcomes research. *The Journal of Nursing Scholarship, 27*(1), 42.

Mattson, M. E., & Donovan, D. M. (1994). Clinical applications: The transition from research to practice. *Journal of Studies on Alcohol, 12*(Suppl), 163-166.

Mitchell, P. H., Ferketich, S., Jennings, B. M., & American Academy of Nursing Expert Panel on Quality Health Care. (1998). Quality health outcomes model. *The Journal of Nursing Scholarship, 30*(1), 43-46.

Moritz, P. (1991). Innovative nursing practice models and patient outcomes. *Nursing Outlook, 39*(3), 111-114.

Nakrem, S., Vinsnes, A.G., Harkless, G. E., Paulsen, B., & Seim, A. (2009). Nursing Sensitive Quality Indicators for Nursing Home Care: International Review of literature, policy and practice. *International Journal of Nursing Studies, 46* (6): 848-857.

Needleman, J., Buerhaus, P., Mattke, S., Stewart, M., & Zelevinsky, K. (2002a). Nurse staffing and quality of care in hospitals in the United States. *Policy, Politics, & Nursing Practice, 3*(4), 306-308.

Needleman, J., Buerhaus, Pl., Mattke, S., Steward, M., & Zelevinsky, K. (2002b). Nurse-staffing levels and the quality of care in hospitals. *The New England Journal of Medicine, 346*(22), 1715-1722.

Patton, R. M. (2009). From your ANA President: Anatomy lesson 101. *American Nurse Today, 4*(8), 14.

Perme, C., & Chandrashekor, R. (2009). Early mobility and walking program for patients in intensive care units: Creating a standard of care. *American Journal of Critical Care, 18*(3), 212-221.

Rasin, J., Barrick, A. L., & Leeman, J. (2004). Effect of person-centered showering and the towel bath on bathing associated aggression, agitation, and discomfort in nursing home residents with dementia: A randomized controlled trial. *American Journal of Nusing, 104*(3), 30-32, 34.

Rettig, R. (1991). History, development and importance to nursing of outcomes research. *Journal of Nursing Quality Assurance, 5*(2), 13-17.

Redekopp, M. A. (2007). *Relationships of professional nurse characteristics and nurse staffing to adverse patient outcomes.* Unpublished doctoral dissertation. University of Wisconsin-Milwaukee.

Rowell, P. (2001). Lessons learned while collecting ANA indicator data: The American Nurses Association responds. *Journal of Nursing Administration, 31*(3), 130-131.

Sawyer, L. M., Berkowitz, B., Haber, J. E., Larrabee, J. H., Marino, B. L., Martin, K. S., et al. (2002). Expanding American Nurses Association Nursing Quality Indicators to community-based practices. *Outcomes Management, 6*(2), 53-61.

Schmalenberg, C., & Kramer, M. (2007). Types of intensive care units with the healthiest, most productive work environments. *American Journal of Critical Care, 16*(5), 458-468.

Seago, J. A., Williamson, A., & Atwood, C. (2006). Longitudinal analyses of nursing staffing and patient outcomes: More about failure to rescue. *Journal of Nursing Administration, 36*(1), 13-21.

Sochalski, J. (2001). Quality of care, nurse staffing, and patient outcomes. *Policy, Politics, & Nursing Practice, 2*(1), 9-18.

Standing, T., Anthony, M. K., & Hertz, J. E. (2001). Nurses' narratives of outcomes after delegation to unlicensed assistive personnel. *Outcomes Management for Nursing Practice, 5*(1), 18-23.

Stetler, C., Morsi, D., & Burns, M. (2000). Physical and emotional patient safety: A different look at nursing-sensitive outcomes. *Outcomes Management for Nursing Practice, 4*(4), 159-166.

Stetler, C., & DeZell, A. D. (1989). In M. L. Etheredge (Ed.), *Collaborative care: Nursing case management* (pp. 67-77). Chicago: American Hospital Association.

Swan, B. A., Lang, N. M., & McGinley, A. M. (2004). Access to quality health care: Links between evidence, nursing language and informatics. *Nursing Economics, 22*(6), 325-332.

Tarlier, D. S. (2006). *Nursing practice, continuity of care, and maternal-infant health outcomes in a remote First Nations community.* Unpublished doctoral dissertation, University of British Columbia (Canada).

Teasell, R., Meyer, M. J., McClure, A., Pan, C., Murie-Fernandez, M., Foley, N., & Salter, K. (2009). Stroke rehabilitation: an international perspective. *Topics in Stroke Rehabilitation, 16*(1), 44-57.

Upenieks, W., Kotlerman, J., Akhavan, J., Esser, J., & Ngo, M. J. (2007). Assessing nursing staffing ratios: Variability in workload intensity. *Policy, Politics, and Nursing Practice, 8*(1), 7-19.

Yang, K. (2003). Relationships between nurse staffing and patient outcomes. *Journal of Nursing Research, 11*(3), 148-157.

GLOSSARY

A

Abstract (adjective) Expressed without reference to any specific instance.

Abstract (noun) Clear, concise summary of a study, usually limited to 100 to 250 words.

Abstract thinking Thinking that is oriented toward the development of an idea, without application to or association with a particular instance; independent of time and space. Abstract thinkers tend to look for meaning, patterns, relationships, and philosophical implications. (*Compare* Concrete thinking.)

Academic library Library located within an institution of higher learning; contains numerous research reports in journals and books.

Acceptance rate The number or percentage of the subjects who agree to participate in a study. The percentage is calculated by dividing the number of subjects agreeing to participate by the number of subjects approached. For example, for a study in which 100 subjects are approached and 90 agree to participate, the acceptance rate is 90%: $90 \div 100 = 0.90 \times 100\% = 90\%$.

Accessible population Portion of the target population to which the researcher has reasonable access.

Accidental sampling *See* Convenience sampling.

Accuracy Addresses the extent to which the instrument measures what it is supposed to in a study. Comparable to validity.

Accuracy of a screening test Screening tests or tests used to confirm a diagnosis are evaluated in terms of their ability to correctly assess the presence or absence of a disease or condition as compared with a gold standard.

Adoption Full acceptance and implementation of an innovation in practice.

Algorithm Decision tree that provides a set of rules for solving a particular practice problem. Its development usually is based on research evidence and theoretical knowledge.

Alpha (α) Cutoff point used to determine whether the samples being tested are members of the same population or of different populations; alpha commonly is set at 0.05, 0.01, or 0.001.

Alternate forms reliability Degree of equivalence of two versions of the same paper-and-pencil instrument.

Analysis of covariance (ANCOVA) Statistical procedure in which a regression analysis is carried out before performing ANOVA; designed to reduce the variance within groups by partialing out the variance due to a confounding variable.

Analysis of variance (ANOVA) Statistical test used to examine differences among two or more groups by comparing the variability between groups with the variability within each group.

Analysis phase Phase of research that involves a critical appraisal of the logical links connecting one study element with another.

Analyzing research reports Critical thinking skill that involves determining the value of a study by breaking the contents of a study report into parts and examining the parts for accuracy, completeness, uniqueness of information, and organization.

Anonymity Conditions in which the subject's identity cannot be linked, even by the researcher, with his or her individual responses.

Applied (practical) research Scientific investigations conducted to generate knowledge that will directly influence clinical practice.

Assent to participate in research A child's affirmative agreement to participate in research.

Associative hypothesis Hypothesis that identifies variables that occur or exist together in the real world, such that when one variable changes, the other changes.

Assumptions Statements taken for granted or considered true, even though they have not been scientifically tested.

Authority Person with expertise and power who is able to influence the opinions and behavior of others.

Autonomous agents Prospective subjects who are informed about a proposed study and who can voluntarily choose whether to participate.

B

Background for a problem Briefly identifies what we know about the problem area in a research study.

Basic (pure) research Scientific investigations for the pursuit of "knowledge for knowledge's sake" or for the pleasure of learning and finding truth.

Benchmarking Process of measuring outcomes from a healthcare agency for comparison with identified national standards.

Beneficence, principle of Principle that encourages the researcher to do good and "above all, do no harm."

Benefit-risk ratio Ratio considered by researchers and reviewers of research as they weigh potential benefits (positive outcomes) and risks (negative outcomes) of a study; used to promote the conduct of ethical research.

Best research evidence Produced by the conduct and synthesis of numerous, high-quality studies in a health-related area. The best research evidence is generated in the areas of health promotion; illness prevention; and the assessment, diagnosis, and management of acute and chronic illnesses.

Between-group variance A source of variation of the group means around the grand mean.

Bias Influence or action in a study that distorts the findings or slants them away from the true or expected.

Bibliographical database Compilation of citations.

Bimodal distribution Describes a data set in which two modes exist.

Bivariate analysis Statistical procedure in which the summary values from either two groups of the same variable or two variables within a group are compared.

Bivariate correlation Measure of the extent of the linear relationship between two variables.

Borrowing Appropriation and use of knowledge from other disciplines to guide nursing practice.

Bracketing Qualitative research technique of suspending or setting aside what is known about an experience being studied.

Breach of confidentiality Accidental or direct action that allows an unauthorized person to have access to raw study data.

C

Case study In-depth analysis and systematic description of one patient or a group of similar patients to promote understanding of nursing interventions.

Case study design Intensive exploration of a single unit of study, such as a person, family, group, community, or institution.

Causal hypothesis Hypothesis that states the relationship between two variables, in which one variable (independent variable) is thought to cause or determine the presence of the other variable (dependent variable).

Causality Relationship that includes three conditions: (1) there must be a strong correlation between the proposed cause and effect, (2) the proposed cause must precede the effect in time, and (3) the cause must be present whenever the effect occurs.

Chi-square test of independence Used to analyze nominal data to determine significant differences between observed frequencies within the data and frequencies that were expected.

Citation Information necessary to locate a reference. Citation for a journal article includes the author's name, year of publication, title, journal name, volume number, issue number, and page numbers.

Clinical expertise A practitioner's knowledge, skills, and past experience in accurately assessing, diagnosing, and managing an individual patient's health needs.

Clinical importance Measure related to the practical relevance of the findings of a study.

Cluster sampling Sampling in which a frame is developed that includes a list of all the states, cities, institutions, or organizations (clusters) that could be used in a study; a randomized sample is drawn from this list.

Coding Way of indexing or identifying categories in qualitative data.

Coefficient of determination (R^2) Computed from a matrix of correlation coefficients and provides important information on multi-colinearity. This value indicates the degree of linear dependencies among the variables.

Coercion Overt threat of harm or excessive reward intentionally presented by one person to another in order to obtain compliance; an example is offering prospective subjects a large sum of money to participate in a dangerous research project.

Coefficient of multiple determination Statistical technique that involves the use of multiple independent variables to predict one dependent variable and is represented by R^2 statistic.

Comparative descriptive design Design used to describe differences in variables in two or more groups in a natural setting.

Comparison group The group of subjects in a study not receiving a treatment when nonrandom methods are used for sample selection. There are four types of comparison groups: (a) groups that receive no treatment, (b) groups that receive a placebo treatment, (c) groups that receive standard or usual health care, and (d) groups that receive a second experimental treatment or a different treatment dose for comparison with the first experimental treatment.

Comparison phase Phase or step of a critical appraisal in which the reader compares the ideal for each step of the research process with the real steps in a study.

Complete review Type of institutional review process for studies with risks that are greater than minimal. The review of a study is extensive or complete by an institutional review board.

Complex hypothesis Hypothesis that predicts the relationship (associative or causal) among three or more variables; thus, the hypothesis can include two (or more) independent and/or two (or more) dependent variables.

Complex search Search that combines two or more concepts or synonyms in one search. The concepts selected for search may be based on the results of previous searches.

Comprehending research reports Critical thinking process used in reading a research report, in which the focus is on understanding the major concepts and the logical flow of ideas within a study.

Comprehension phase Step of a critical appraisal during which the reader gains understanding of the terms in a research report; identifies the study elements; and grasps the nature, significance, and meaning of these elements.

Concept Term that abstractly describes and names an object or phenomenon, thus providing it with a separate identity or meaning.

Conceptual definition Definition that provides a variable or concept with connotative (abstract, comprehensive, theoretical) meaning; established through concept analysis, concept derivation, or concept synthesis.

Conceptual model Set of highly abstract, related constructs that broadly explains phenomena of interest, expresses assumptions, and reflects a philosophical stance.

Conclusions Syntheses and clarifications of the meanings of study findings.

Concrete thinking Thinking that is oriented to and limited by tangible things or events observed and experienced in reality. (*Compare* Abstract thinking.)

Confidentiality Management of private data in research in such a way that only the researcher knows the subjects' identities and can link them with their responses.

Confirmatory analysis Analysis performed to confirm expectations regarding data that are expressed as hypotheses, questions, or objectives.

Confounding variables Variables that cannot be controlled; they may be recognized before the study is initiated or may not be recognized until the study is in process.

Consent form Written form, tape recording, or videotape used to document a subject's agreement to participate in a study.

Construct validity Measure of how well the conceptual and operational definitions of variables match each other; determine whether the instrument measures the theoretical construct it purports to measure.

Constructs Concepts at very high levels of abstraction that have general meanings.

Content-related validity Extent to which the method of measurement includes all the major elements relevant to the construct being measured.

Control Writing of a prescription to produce the desired outcomes in practice. In research, the imposing of rules by the researcher to decrease the possibility of error and increase the probability that the study's findings are an accurate reflection of reality.

Control group The group of elements or subjects not exposed to the experimental treatment in a study in which the sample is randomly selected.

Convenience sampling Including subjects in the study who happened to be in the right place at the right time, with addition of available subjects until the desired sample size is reached. Also referred to as "accidental sampling."

Correlational research Systematic investigation of relationships between two or more variables to explain the nature of relationships in the world; does not examine cause and effect.

Covered entity Public or private entity that processes or facilitates the processing of health information.

Covert data collection Data collection that occurs without subjects' knowledge or awareness.

Critical appraisal of research Examination of the strengths, weaknesses, meaning, and significance of nursing studies using four steps: comprehension, comparison, analysis, and evaluation.

Current sources Sources published within five years prior to acceptance of a respective manuscript for publication.

D

Data Information that is collected during a study.

Data analysis Technique used to reduce, organize, and give meaning to data.

Data-based literature Consists of research reports, both published reports in journals and books and unpublished reports such as theses and dissertations.

Data collection Identification of subjects and the precise, systematic gathering of information (data) relevant to the research purpose or the specific objectives, questions, or hypotheses of a study.

Data use agreement Agreement that limits how the data set with health information may be used and how it will be protected in research.

Deception Misinforming subjects for research purposes. After a study is completed, subjects must be debriefed or informed of the true purpose and outcomes of a study so that areas of deception are clarified.

Decision theory Theory based on assumptions associated with the theoretical normal curve; used in testing for differences between groups, with the expectation that all of the groups are members of the same population. The expectation is expressed as a null hypothesis, and the level of significance (alpha) is often set at 0.05 before data collection.

Deductive reasoning Reasoning from the general to the specific or from a general premise to a particular situation.

Degrees of freedom (df) The freedom of a score's value to vary, given the values of other existing scores and the established sum of these scores ($df = N - 1$).

Demographic variables Characteristics or attributes of subjects that are collected to describe the sample.

Dependent groups Subjects or observations selected for data collection that are in some way related to the selection of other subjects or observations. For example, when subjects in the control group are matched for age or gender with the subjects in the experimental group, these groups are dependent groups.

Dependent (response or outcome) variable The response, behavior, or outcome that is predicted or explained in research; changes in the dependent variable are presumed to be caused by the independent variable.

Description Identification of the characteristics of nursing phenomena, or of the relationships among these phenomena.

Descriptive correlational design Design used to describe variables and examine relationships that exist in a situation.

Descriptive design Design used to identify a phenomenon of interest, identify variables within the phenomenon, develop conceptual and operational definitions of variables, and describe variables.

Descriptive research Research that provides an accurate portrayal or account of characteristics of a particular person, event, or group in real-life situations; research that is conducted to discover new meaning, describe what exists, determine the frequency with which something occurs, and categorize information.

Descriptive statistics Statistics that allow the researcher to organize the data in ways that give meaning and facilitate insight; examples are frequency distributions and measures of central tendency and dispersion.

Design Blueprint for conducting a study; maximizes control over factors that could interfere with the validity of the findings.

Diminished autonomy Condition of subjects whose ability to give informed consent voluntarily is decreased because of legal or mental incompetence, terminal illness, or confinement to an institution.

Direct measures Concrete variables that can be measured objectively with a specific measurement strategy, such as using a scale to measure weight.

Directional hypothesis Hypothesis stating the specific nature of the interaction or relationship between two or more variables.

Discomfort and harm Phrase used to describe the degree of risk for a subject participating in a study. These levels of risk include no anticipated effects, temporary discomfort, unusual levels of temporary discomfort, risk of permanent damage, or certainty of permanent damage.

Dissertation An extensive, usually original research project that is completed by a doctoral student as part of the requirements for a doctoral degree.

E

Effect size The degree to which the phenomenon studied is present in the population or to which the null hypothesis is false.

Electronic journals Journals that are published and available on the Internet.

Element of a study A person (subject), event, behavior, or any other single unit of a study.

Eligibility criteria *See* Sampling criteria.

Embodied The belief that the person is a self within a body.

Emic approach Anthropological research approach to studying behaviors from within a culture.

Empirical generalizations Statements that have been repeatedly tested through research and have not been disproved (scientific theories have empirical generalizations).

Environmental variables Types of extraneous variables composing the setting in which a study is conducted.

Error in physiological measures Error caused by environmental factors, variations in operation of equipment, machine instability and calibration, or misinterpreted electrical signals.

Ethical principles Principles of respect for persons, beneficence, and justice that are relevant to the conduct of research.

Ethnographic research Qualitative research methodology for investigating cultures. The research involves collection, description, and analysis of data to develop a theory of cultural behavior.

Ethnonursing research Type of research that emerged from Leininger's Theory of Transcultural Nursing; focuses mainly on observing and documenting interactions with people to determine how daily life conditions and patterns influence human care, health, and nursing care practices.

Etic approach Anthropological research approach to studying behavior from outside the culture and examining similarities and differences across cultures.

Evaluation phase Step of a critical appraisal in which the reader examines the meaning and significance of a study according to set criteria and compares it with previous studies conducted in the area.

Evidence-based guidelines Patient care guidelines that are based on synthesized research findings from meta-analyses, integrative reviews of research, and extensive clinical trials; supported by consensus from recognized national experts; and affirmed by outcomes obtained by clinicians.

Evidence-based practice (EBP) The conscientious integration of best research evidence with clinical expertise and patients values and needs in the delivery of high-quality, cost-effective health care.

Evidence-based practice centers (EPCs) Centers established in 1997 to develop evidence reports and technology assessments on topics relevant to clinical, social science/behavioral, economic, and other healthcare organization and delivery issues-specifically those that are common, expensive, and/or significant for the Medicare and Medicaid population.

Evidence for best practices Synthesis of research findings to determine the best empirical knowledge to guide care delivery in a discipline.

Evidence of validity from contrasting groups Tested by identifying groups that are expected (or known) to have contrasting scores on the instrument.

Evidence of validity from convergence Determined when a relatively new instrument is compared with an existing instrument(s) that measures the same construct. Both instruments are administered to a sample concurrently and results are evaluated using correlational analyses. If the measures are highly positively correlated, the validity of each instrument is strengthened.

Evidence of validity from divergence Correlational procedures performed with the measures of two opposite concepts. If the divergent measure (despair scale) is negatively correlational with the other instrument (hope scale), validity for each of the instruments is strengthened.

Exclusion sample criteria Sampling criteria or characteristics that can cause a person or element to be excluded from the target population.

Exempt from review Designation given to studies that have no apparent risks for the research subjects and thus are designated as exempt by an institutional review board.

Existence statement Declaration that a given concept or relationship exists.

Expedited review Institutional review process for studies that have some risks, but the risks are minimal or no greater than those ordinarily encountered in daily life or during the performance of routine physical or psychological examinations.

Experiment Procedure in which subjects are randomized into groups, data are collected, and statistical analyses are conducted to support a premise.

Experimental design Design that provides the greatest amount of control possible in order to examine causality more closely.

Experimental group Group of subjects receiving the experimental treatment.

Experimental research Objective, systematic, controlled investigation to examine probability and causality among selected variables for the purpose of predicting and controlling phenomena.

Explained variance Variation in values that is explained by the relationship between the two variables.

Explanation Clarification of relationships among variables and identification of reasons why certain events occur.

Exploratory analysis Examining the data descriptively to become as familiar as possible with it.

Extraneous variables Variables that exist in all studies and can affect the measurement of study variables and the relationships among these variables.

F

Fabrication in research A form of scientific misconduct in research that involves making up results and recording or reporting them.

Factor A category of several closely related variables that are considered together.

Factor analysis Analysis that examines interrelationships among large numbers of variables and disentangles those relationships to identify clusters of variables that are most closely linked. Two types of factor analysis are exploratory and confirmatory.

Falsification of research A type of scientific misconduct that involves manipulating research materials, equipment, or processes, or changing or omitting data or results, such that the research is not accurately represented in the research record.

Feasibility of a study Suitability of a study; determined by examining the time and money commitment; the researcher's expertise; availability of subjects, facility, and equipment; cooperation of others; and the study's ethical considerations.

Field notes Notes recorded by the researcher while an observation is taking place.

Findings The translated and interpreted results from a study.

Focus groups Measurement strategy where groups are assembled to obtain the participants' perceptions in focused areas in settings that are permissive and nonthreatening in a qualitative study.

Framework Abstract, logical structure of meaning, such as a portion of a theory, that guides the development of the study, is tested in the study, and enables the researcher to link the findings to nursing's body of knowledge.

Frequency distribution Statistical procedure that lists all possible measures of a variable and tallies each datum on the listing.

Full-text databases Internet resource that provides full text and list of citations of journal articles for a specific topic.

G

Generalization Extension of the implications of the findings from the sample or situation that was studied to a larger population or situation.

Gestalt Organization of knowledge about a particular phenomenon into a cluster of linked ideas; the clustering and interrelatedness enhance the meaning of the ideas.

Grant Proposal developed to seek research funding from private or public institutions.

Grounded Theory that has its roots in the qualitative data from which it was derived.

Grounded theory research Inductive research technique based on symbolic interaction theory; conducted to discover the problems that exist in a social scene and the process that persons involved use to handle them; involves formulation, testing, and redevelopment of propositions until a theory is developed.

Grouped frequency distribution Means of grouping continuous measures of data into categories.

Grove Model for Implementing Evidence-Based Guidelines in Practice In this model, nurses identify a practice problem, search for the best research evidence to manage the problem in their practice, and use an evidence-based guideline to manage the problem.

H

Health Concept including many aspects, including physical-physiological function, psychological function, and social function.

Health Insurance Portability and Accountability Act (HIPAA) Federal regulations implemented in 2003 to protect an individual person's health information. The HIPAA Privacy Rule affects not only the healthcare environment but also the research conducted in this environment.

Heterogeneous sample A sample in which subjects have a broad range of values being studied, which increases the representativeness of the sample and the ability to generalize from the accessible population to the target population.

Highly controlled setting Artificially constructed environment that is developed for the sole purpose of conducting research, such as a laboratory, research or experimental center, or test unit.

Historical research Narrative description or analysis of events that occurred in the remote or recent past.

Homogeneous sample Sample in which subjects' scores on selected measurement methods in a study are similar, resulting in a limited or narrow distribution or spread of scores.

Human rights Claims and demands that have been justified in the eyes of an individual person or by the consensus of a group of people and are protected in research.

Hypothesis Formal statement of the expected relationship between two or more variables in a specified population.

I

Implications for nursing The meaning of research conclusions for the body of knowledge, theory, and practice.

Implicit framework Rudimentary ideas for the framework of a theory or portions of a theory expressed in an introduction or in a literature review in which linkages among variables found in previous studies are discussed.

Inclusion sample criteria Those sampling criteria or characteristics that the subject or element must possess to be considered part of the target population.

Independent groups Study groups chosen so that the selection of one subject is unrelated to the selection of other subjects. For example, if subjects are randomly assigned to a treatment group or a comparison group, the groups are independent.

Independent (treatment or experimental) variable Treatment or experimental activity that is manipulated or varied by the researcher to cause an effect on the dependent variable.

Index Library resource that can be used to identify journal articles and other publications relevant to a topic.

Indirect measures Methods used with abstract concepts that are not measured directly; rather, indicators or attributes of the concepts are used to represent the abstraction and are measured in the study.

Individually identifiable health information (IIHI) "… any information, including demographic information collected from an individual that is created or received by healthcare provider, health plan, or healthcare clearinghouse; and related to past, present, or future physical or mental health condition of an individual, the provision of health care to an individual, or the past, present, or future payment for the provision of health care to an individual, and identifies the individual; or with respect to which there is a reasonable basis to believe that the information can be used to identify the individual" (U.S. Department of Health and Human Services, 2003, *45 CFR*, Section 160.103).

Inductive reasoning Reasoning from the specific to the general, in which particular instances are observed and then combined into a larger whole or general statement.

Inference Generalization from a specific case to a general truth, from a part to the whole, from the concrete to the abstract, or from the known to the unknown.

Informed consent Agreement by a prospective subject to participate voluntarily in a study after he or she has assimilated essential information about the study.

Institutional review Process of examining studies for ethical concerns by a committee of peers.

Institutional review board (IRB) A committee that reviews research to ensure that the investigator is conducting the research ethically.

Instrumentation Component of measurement in which specific rules are applied to develop a measurement device or instrument.

Integrative review of the literature Rigorous analysis and synthesis of results from independent quantitative and qualitative studies and theoretical and methodological literature to determine the current knowledge (what is known and not known) for a particular concept, measurement methods, or practice topic.

Integrative review of research Review conducted to identify, analyze, and synthesize the results from independent studies to determine the current knowledge (what is known and not known) in a particular area.

Intellectual critical appraisal of a study Careful examination of all aspects of a study to judge the strengths, weaknesses, meaning, and significance of the study based on previous research experience and knowledge of the topic.

Interlibrary loan department Department that locates books and articles in other libraries and provides the sources within a designated time.

Interpretation of research outcomes Process in which researchers examine the results from data analysis, form conclusions, consider the implications for nursing, explore the significance of the findings, generalize the findings, and suggest further studies.

Interval-scale measurement Use of interval scales or methods of measurement with equal numerical distances between intervals of the scale; follows the rules of mutually exclusive categories, exhaustive categories, and rank ordering, such as temperature.

Intervention Treatment or independent variable that is manipulated during the conduct of a study to produce an effect on the dependent or outcome variables.

Interview Structured or unstructured oral communication between the researcher and the subject, during which information is obtained for a study.

Intraproject sampling Additional sampling that is done during data collection and analysis to promote the development of quality study findings.

Intuition Insight or understanding of a situation or an event as a whole that usually cannot be logically explained.

Invasion of privacy Sharing private information with others without a person's knowledge or against his or her will.

Iowa Model of Evidence-Based Practice Provides direction for the development of EBP in a clinical agency. In a healthcare agency, there are triggers that initiate the need for change and the focus should always be to make changes based on the best research evidence.

J

Justice, principle of Ethical principle stating that human subjects should be treated fairly.

K

Keywords Major concepts or variables of a research problem or topic that are used to begin a search of a database.

Knowledge Information that is acquired in a variety of ways, is expected to be an accurate reflection of reality, and is incorporated and used to direct a person's actions.

L

Landmark studies Major projects generating knowledge that influence a discipline and sometimes society in general.

Level of significance *See* Alpha (α).

Levels of measurement Organized set of rules for assigning numbers to objects so that a hierarchy in measurement from low to high is established. The levels of measurement are nominal, ordinal, interval, and ratio.

Levels of statistical significance Probability level at which the results of statistical analysis are judged to indicate a statistically significant difference between the groups. The level of significance for most nursing studies is 0.05.

Library resources Library personnel, interlibrary loan department, circulation department, reference department, audiovisual department, computer search department, and photocopy services.

Library sources Sources for research, including journals, books, monographs, master's theses, doctoral dissertations, government documents, and other publications of research findings.

Limitations Theoretical and methodological restrictions in a study that may decrease the generalizability of the findings.

Line of best fit Best reflection of the values on the scatterplot.

Linking Activity that moves a computer user from one website to another.

Literature review Summary of theoretical and empirical sources to generate a picture of what is known and not known about a particular problem.

Logic A science in which valid ways of relating ideas are used to promote human understanding; includes abstract and concrete thinking and logistic, inductive, and deductive reasoning.

Logistic reasoning Reasoning used to break the whole into parts that can be carefully examined, as can the relationships among the parts.

M

Manipulation Moving around or controlling a specific attribute (such as movement) of, as in the manipulation of a treatment.

Mean The value obtained by summing all the scores and dividing the total by the number of scores being summed.

Measurement Process of assigning numbers to objects, events, or situations in accordance with some rule.

Measurement error Difference between what exists in reality and what is measured by a research instrument.

Measures of central tendency Statistical procedures (mode, median, and mean) for determining the center of a distribution of scores.

Measures of dispersion Statistical procedures (range, difference scores, sum of squares, variance, and standard deviation) for examining how scores vary or are dispersed around the mean.

Median Score at the exact center of the ungrouped frequency distribution.

Mentorship Intense form of role modeling in which an expert nurse serves as a teacher, sponsor, guide, exemplar, and counselor for a novice nurse.

Meta-analysis Performing statistical analyses to integrate and synthesize findings from completed studies to determine what is known and not known about a particular research area.

Metasummary Synthesis of multiple primary qualitative studies to develop a description of current knowledge in an area.

Metasynthesis Synthesis of qualitative research involving the critical analysis of primary qualitative studies and synthesis of findings into a new theory or framework for the topic of interest.

Methodological limitations Restrictions in the study design that limit the credibility of the findings and the population to which the findings can be generalized.

Middle-range theories Theories that are relatively concrete and specific in focus and include a limited number of concepts and propositions. These theories are tested by empirical research.

Minimal risk Research subject's risk of harm anticipated in the proposed study that is not greater, considering probability and magnitude, than that ordinarily encountered in daily life or during the performance of routine physical or psychological examinations.

Mixed results Study results that include both significant and nonsignificant findings.

Mode Numerical value or score that occurs with the greatest frequency in a distribution but does not necessarily indicate the center of the data set.

Monographs Sources that usually are written once, such as books, booklets of conference proceedings, or pamphlets, and may be updated with a new edition.

Mortality rate, sample The percentage of subjects who drop out of a study before its completion, creating a threat to the internal validity of the study. Also referred to as attrition rate.

Multicausality Recognition that a number of interrelated variables can cause a particular effect.

Multiple regression Extension of simple linear regression; more than one independent variable is analyzed.

N

Natural (field) setting Uncontrolled, real-life setting where research is conducted, such as subjects' homes, work sites, and schools.

Necessary relationship Relationship in which one variable or concept must occur for the second variable or concept to occur.

Negative relationship Relationship in which one variable or concept changes (its value increases or decreases), and the other variable or concept changes in the opposite direction.

Network (or snowball) sampling Sampling technique that takes advantage of social networks and the fact that friends tend to have characteristics in common; subjects meeting the sample criteria are asked to assist in locating others with similar characteristics.

Networking Process of developing channels of communication among people with common interests.

Nominal-scale measurement Lowest level of measurement used when data can be organized into categories that are exclusive and exhaustive, but the categories cannot be compared, such as gender, race, marital status, and nursing diagnoses.

Nondirectional hypothesis Hypothesis that states that a relationship exists but does not predict the exact nature of the relationship.

Nonequivalent control group designs Designs in which the control group is not selected by random means, such as the one-group posttest-only design, the posttest-only design with nonequivalent groups, and the one-group pretest-posttest design.

Nonprobability sampling Sampling in which not every element of the population has an opportunity for selection, such as convenience sampling, quota sampling, purposive sampling, and network sampling.

Nonsignificant results Results that are negative or contrary to the researcher's hypotheses; the results may accurately reflect reality or may be caused by study weaknesses.

Nontherapeutic research Research conducted to generate knowledge for a discipline; the results might benefit future patients but will probably not benefit the research subjects.

Normal curve Symmetrical, unimodal, bell-shaped curve that is a theoretical distribution of all possible scores; no real distribution exactly fits the normal curve.

Null (statistical) hypothesis Hypothesis stating that no relationship exists between the variables being studied; a hypothesis used for statistical testing and for interpreting statistical outcomes.

Nuremberg code Ethical code of conduct to guide investigators in conducting research ethically.

Nursing process Subset of the problem-solving process. Steps include assessment, diagnosis, plan, implementation, evaluation, and modification.

Nursing research Scientific process that validates and refines existing knowledge and generates knowledge that directly and indirectly influences clinical nursing practice.

O

Observability Extent to which the results of an innovation are visible to others.

Observational measurement Use of structured and unstructured observation to measure study variables.

One-tailed test of significance Analysis used with directional hypotheses, in which extreme statistical values of interest are thought to occur in a single tail of the normal curve.

Open context Condition that requires deconstructing a sedimented view, allowing the researcher to see the depth and complexity within the phenomenon being examined in qualitative research.

Open-ended interview Interview with a defined focus but no fixed sequence of questions. The questions addressed may change as the researcher gains insight from previous interviews and observations and respondents are encouraged to raise important issues not addressed by the researcher.

Operational definition Description of how variables or concepts will be measured or manipulated in a study.

Opportunity costs Costs related to loss of opportunity for financial or other growth experiences by the patient, family member, or others.

Out-of-pocket costs Expenses incurred by the patient or family or both that are not reimbursable by the insurance company.

Ordinal-scale measurement Measurement yielding data that can be ranked, but the intervals between the ranked data are not necessarily equal, such as levels of coping.

Outcomes research Important scientific methodology that was developed to examine the end results of patient care. The strategies used in outcomes research are a departure from the traditional scientific endeavors and incorporate evaluation research, epidemiology, and economic theory perspectives.

Outliers Extreme scores or values due to inherent variability, errors of measurement or execution, or error in identifying the variables important in explaining the nature of the phenomenon under study.

P

Parallel forms reliability *See* Alternate forms reliability.

Parameter Measure or numerical value of a population.

Paraphrasing Clearly and concisely restating the ideas of an author in the researcher's own words.

Partially controlled setting Environment that is manipulated or modified in some way by the researcher.

Participants Subjects in qualitative studies who participate cooperatively in the study with the researcher.

Pearson product-moment correlation Parametric test used to determine relationships among variables.

Peer reviewed Term that refers to publications for which scholars familiar with the topic of the research read the report and validate its accuracy and the appropriateness of the methodology used in the study.

Percentage distributions Percentage of the sample whose scores fall into a specific group and the number of scores in that group.

Periodicals Literature sources such as journals that are published over time and are numbered sequentially for the years published.

Permission to participate in research The agreement of parent(s) or guardian to the participation of their child or ward in research.

Personal experience Knowledge gained through participation in rather than observation of an event, situation, or circumstance. Benner (1984) described five levels of experience in the development of clinical knowledge and expertise: (1) novice, (2) advanced beginner, (3) competent, (4) proficient, and (5) expert.

Phenomenology A philosophy and a group of research methods congruent with the philosophy.

Phenomenon (*plural:* phenomena) An occurrence or a circumstance that is observed, something that impresses the observer as extraordinary, or a thing that appears to and is constructed by the mind.

Philosophical stance Specific philosophical view held by an individual person or group of persons.

Philosophies Rational, intellectual explorations of truths; principles of being, knowledge, or conduct.

PICO format Format used to formulate a relevant clinical question for a systematic review. Elements include: **P**opulation or participants of interest; **I**ntervention needed for practice; **C**omparisons of interventions to determine the best for practice; and **O**utcomes needed for practice.

Pilot study Smaller version of a proposed study conducted to develop and refine the methodology, such as the treatment, instruments, or data collection process to be used in the larger study.

Plagiarism A type of scientific misconduct with appropriation of another person's ideas, processes, results, or words without giving appropriate credit, including those obtained through confidential review of others' research proposals and manuscripts.

Population All elements (people, objects, events, or substances) that meet the sample criteria for inclusion in a study; sometimes referred to as a target population.

Population-based studies Important type of outcomes research that involves studying health conditions in the context of the community rather than the context of the medical system.

Positive relationship Relationship in which one variable changes (its value increases or decreases) and the second variable changes in the same direction.

Posthoc analyses Statistical techniques performed in studies with more than two groups to determine which groups are significantly different. For example, ANOVA may indicate significant differences among three groups, but the posthoc analyses indicate specifically which groups are different.

Power Probability that a statistical test will detect a significant difference or relationship that exists; power analysis is used to determine the power of a study.

Power analysis Technique used to determine the risk of a Type II error so that the study can be modified to decrease the risk if necessary.

Practice theories Very specific theories that are developed to explain a particular element of practice. These theories can be generated through research and also tested by research.

Precision Accuracy with which the population parameters have been estimated within a study; also used to describe the degree of consistency or reproducibility of measurements with physiologic instruments.

Prediction Estimation of the probability of a specific outcome in a given situation that can be achieved through research.

Predictive correlational design Design developed to predict the value of one variable based on values obtained for other variables; an approach to examining causal relationships between variables.

Premise Proposition or statement of the proposed relationship between two or more concepts.

Primary source Source whose author originated or is responsible for generating the ideas published.

Principle of beneficence Ethical principle that encourages researchers to do good and "above all, do no harm."

Privacy Freedom to determine the time, extent, and general circumstances under which private information will be shared with or withheld from others.

Probability Chance that a given event will occur in a situation; addresses the relative rather than the absolute causality of events.

Probability sampling Random sampling technique in which every member (element) of the population has a probability higher than zero of being selected for the sample; examples include simple random sampling, stratified random sampling, cluster sampling, and systematic sampling.

Probability theory Theory addressing statistical analysis from the perspective of the extent of a relationship or the probability of accurately predicting an event.

Probes Queries made by the researcher to obtain more information from the participant about a particular question.

Problem-solving process Systematic identification of a problem, determination of goals related to the problem, identification of possible approaches to achieve those goals, implementation of selected approaches, and evaluation of goal achievement.

Problem statement Statement that concludes the discussion of a problem and indicates the gap in the knowledge needed for practice. The problem statement usually provides a basis for the study purpose.

Process Purpose, series of actions, and goal.

Proposition Abstract statements that further clarify the relationship between two concepts in theories.

Public library Library that serves the needs of the community in which it is located; usually contains few research reports.

Purposive sampling Judgmental or selective sampling that involves the conscious selection by the researcher of certain subjects or elements to include in a study. This sampling strategy is used most frequently in qualitative research.

Q

Q-plots Displays of scores or data in a distribution by quartile for exploratory data analysis.

Q-sort Exploratory data analysis technique for comparative rating, in which a subject sorts cards with statements into designated piles (usually 7 to 10 piles in the distribution of a normal curve) that might range from best to worst.

Qualitative research Systematic, subjective methodological approach used to describe life experiences and give them meaning.

Qualitative research synthesis Process and product of systematically reviewing and formally integrating the findings from qualitative studies (Sandelowski & Barroso, 2007).

Quality of care Outcome examined in the conduct of outcomes research.

Quantitative research Formal, objective, systematic process used to describe variables, test relationships between them, and examine cause-and-effect interactions among variables.

Quantitative research process Conceptualizing, planning, implementing, and communicating the findings of a quantitative research project.

Quasi-experimental designs Types of designs developed to determine the effectiveness of interventions in quantitative quasi-experimental studies.

Quasi-experimental research Type of quantitative research conducted to explain relationships, clarify why certain events happen, and examine causality between selected independent and dependent variables.

Questionnaire Printed self-report form designed to elicit information that can be obtained through written or verbal responses of the subject.

Quota sampling Convenience sampling technique with an added strategy to ensure the inclusion of subjects who are likely to be underrepresented in the convenience sample, such as women, minority groups, and undereducated persons.

R

Random assignment Procedure used to assign subjects randomly to treatment or control groups; subjects have an equal probability of being assigned to either group.

Random error Error that causes individual subjects' observed scores to vary haphazardly around their true scores.

Random sampling Technique in which every member (element) of the population has a probability higher than zero for being selected for a sample, which increases the sample's representativeness of the target population.

Random variation The expected difference in values that occurs when the researcher examines different subjects from the same sample.

Randomized clinical trial Classic means of examining the effects of various treatments in which the effects of a treatment are examined by comparing the treatment group with the non-treatment group.

Recommendations for further study Suggestions provided by a study's researcher for ways to design a better study next time. Recommendations can include replications or repeating the design with a different or larger sample, using different measurement methods, or testing a new treatment.

Rating scale Scale that lists an ordered series of categories of a variable and is assumed to be based on an underlying continuum.

Reading research reports Process used to learn about research studies; skills used include skimming, comprehending, and analyzing the content of the report.

Reasoning Processing and organizing ideas to reach conclusions; types of reasoning include problematic, operational, dialectic, and logistic.

Refereed journal Journal that uses referees or expert reviewers to determine whether a manuscript will be accepted for publication.

Referencing Comparing a subject's score against a standard; used in norm-referenced and criterion-referenced testing.

Reflexive thought Process in which a qualitative researcher explores personal feelings and experiences that may influence the study and integrates this understanding into the study.

Refusal rate The percentage of subjects who declined to participate in the study. The study should include their rationale for not participating. The refusal rate is calculated by dividing the number refusing to participate by the number of potential subjects approached. For example, if 100 subjects are approached and 15 refuse to participate, the refusal rate is $15 \div 100 = 0.15 \times 100\% = 15\%$.

Regression analysis Statistical procedure used to predict the value of one variable using known values of one or more other variables.

Relational statement Declaration that a relationship of some kind exists between two or more concepts.

Relative advantage Extent to which an innovation is perceived to be better than current practice.

Relevant sources Sources that are pertinent or highly important in providing the in-depth knowledge needed to make changes in practice or to study a selected problem.

Relevant studies Those investigations or studies that have a specific focus on in a researcher's area of interest.

Reliability Extent to which an instrument consistently measures a concept; three types of reliability are stability, equivalence, and homogeneity.

Reliability testing Measure of the amount of random error in the measurement technique.

Replication studies Studies that are reproduced or repeated to determine whether similar findings will be obtained.

Representative sample Sample that is like the population it is supposed to represent in as many ways as possible.

Representativeness Degree to which the sample, accessible population, and target population are alike.

Research Diligent, systematic inquiry or investigation to validate and refine existing knowledge and generate new knowledge.

Research-based protocol Document providing clearly developed steps for implementing a treatment or intervention in practice that is based on findings from studies.

Research design Blueprint for conducting a study; maximizes control over factors that could interfere with the validity of the findings; guides the planning and implementation of a study in a way that is most likely to achieve the intended goal.

Research evidence Knowledge generated from the synthesis of research findings from several quality studies.

Research hypothesis Alternative hypothesis to the null hypothesis; states that a relationship exists between two or more variables.

Research misconduct *See* Scientific misconduct.

Research objective Clear, concise, declarative statement expressed to direct a study; focuses on identifying and describing variables and relationships among variables.

Research outcomes Conclusions of findings, generalization of findings, implications of findings for nursing, and suggestions for further study presented in the discussion section of the research report.

Research problem An area of concern in which there is a gap in the knowledge base needed for nursing practice. Research is conducted to generate essential knowledge to address the practice concern, with the ultimate goal of providing evidence-based practice.

Research process Process that requires an understanding of a unique language and involves rigorous application of a variety of research methods.

Research proposal Written plan that identifies the major elements of a study, such as the problem, purpose, and framework, and outlines the methods that will be used to conduct the study.

Research purpose Concise, clear statement of the specific goal or aim of the study. The purpose is generated from the problem.

Research question Concise interrogative statement developed to direct a study; focuses on describing variables, examining relationships among variables, and determining the differences between two or more groups.

Research report Report summarizing the major elements of a study and identifying the contributions of that study to nursing knowledge.

Research topic Concept or broad problem area that provides the basis for generating numerous questions and research problems.

Research tradition A program of research that is important for building a body of knowledge related to the phenomena explained by a particular conceptual model.

Research utilization Process of communicating and using empirical or research-generated knowledge to affect or change the existing practices in the healthcare system.

Research variables or concepts The qualities, properties, or characteristics identified in the research purpose and objectives that are observed or measured in a study.

Researcher-participant relationships Relationships between the researcher and the individual subjects being studied in qualitative research.

Respect for persons, principle of Principle indicating that each person has the right to self-determination and the freedom to participate or not participate in research.

Results Outcomes from data analysis that are generated for each research objective, question, or hypothesis; results can be mixed, nonsignificant, significant and not predicted, significant and predicted, or unexpected.

Review of literature Summary of current theoretical and empirical sources to generate a picture of what is known and not known about a particular problem.

Review of relevant research literature Review of current studies conducted to generate what is known and not known about a problem and to determine whether the knowledge is ready for use in practice.

Rigor Excellence in research; attained through the use of discipline, scrupulous adherence to detail, and strict accuracy.

Role modeling Process of teaching less experienced professionals by demonstrating model behavior.

S

Sample Subset of the population that is selected for a study.

Sample attrition Withdrawal or loss of subjects from a study that can be expressed as a number of subjects withdrawing or a percentage. The percentage is the sample attrition rate and it is best if researchers include both the number of subjects withdrawing and the attrition rate.

Sample characteristics Demographic data analyzed to provide a picture of the sample.

Sample mortality or attrition rate Number of subjects who withdraw from or who are lost during a study. The attrition rate is calculated by dividing the number of subjects lost to the study by the sample size or 10 subjects lost ÷ by 100 sample size = 0.10 × 100% = 10% sample mortality or attrition rate.

Sample retention Number of subjects who remain in and complete a study.

Sample size Number of subjects, events, behaviors, or situations that are examined in a study.

Sampling Process of selecting a group of people, events, behaviors, or other elements that are representative of the population being studied.

Sampling criteria List of the characteristics essential for inclusion or exclusion in the target population.

Sampling distribution Table of statistical values (such as the mean) of many samples obtained from the same population.

Sampling error Difference between a sample statistic used to estimate a population parameter and the actual but unknown value of the parameter.

Sampling frame List of every member of the population; the sampling criteria are used to define membership in the population.

Sampling method Strategies used to obtain a sample, including probability and nonprobability sampling techniques; also called a sampling plan.

Saturation of data Phenomenon that occurs when additional sampling provides no new information, or there is redundancy of previously collected data. Sample size in a qualitative study is determined when saturation of data occurs.

Scale Self-report form of measurement composed of several items thought to measure the construct being studied; the subject responds to each item on the continuum or scale provided.

Scatterplot Diagram or figure showing the dispersion of scores on a variable from a study, or depicting the relationship of scores on one variable with scores on another variable. A scatterplot has two scales: horizontal (X-axis) and vertical (Y-axis).

Science Coherent body of knowledge composed of research findings, tested theories, scientific principles, and laws for a discipline.

Scientific community Cohesive group of scholars within a discipline who create new research ideas and develop innovative methodologies to conduct research.

Scientific method Approach to research comprising all procedures that scientists have used, currently use, or may use in the future to pursue knowledge; examples include quantitative research, qualitative research, outcomes research, and triangulation.

Scientific misconduct Intentional deviation from practices commonly accepted within the scientific community for proposing, conducting, or reporting research. May include fabrication, falsification, or plagiarism; does not include honest errors or honest differences in interpretation or judgment of data.

Scientific theory Theory that has been repeatedly tested through research with valid and reliable methods of measuring each concept and relational statement.

Search field Areas of research topics that are searched to identify relevant sources.

Secondary source Source whose author summarizes or quotes content from primary sources.

Sedimented view View from the perspective of a specific frame of reference, world view, or theory that gives a sense of certainty, security, and control.

Semi-structured interview Interview fixed set of questions and no fixed responses.

Sensitivity of physiological measures Amount of change of a parameter that can be measured precisely.

Setting Location for conducting research; can be natural, partially controlled, or highly controlled.

Significance of a research problem Indicates the importance of the problem to nursing and health care and to the health of individuals, families, and communities.

Significant and unpredicted results Results that are opposite of those predicted by the researcher and indicate that flaws are present in the logic of both the researcher and the theory being tested.

Significant results Results that agree with those identified by the researcher.

Simple hypothesis Hypothesis stating the relationship (associative or causal) between two variables.

Simple random sampling Random selection of elements from the sampling frame for inclusion in a study.

Situated Belief that the person is shaped by the language, culture, history, purposes, and values of his or her world and is constrained by that shaping in the ability to establish meanings.

Skewness Absence of symmetry in the curve formed by the distribution of scores; distribution can be positively or negatively skewed.

Skimming research reports Quickly reviewing a source to gain a broad overview of the content by reading the title, the author's name, the abstract or introduction, headings, one or two sentences under each heading, and the discussion section.

Small area analyses Geographical analyses used to examine variations in health status, health services, patterns of care, or patterns of use by geographical area.

Social system Set of interrelated persons (e.g., the nurses on a specific hospital unit, in one hospital, or in a corporation of hospitals) engaged in joint problem solving to accomplish a common goal or outcome.

Special library Library that contains a collection of material on a specific topic or specialty area.

Split-half reliability Technique used to determine the homogeneity of an instrument's items, in which the items are split in half and a correlational procedure is performed between the two halves.

Stability Type of measurement reliability that is concerned with the consistency of repeated measures; usually referred to as test-retest reliability.

Standard deviation Measure of dispersion that is calculated by taking the square root of the variance.

Standardized mortality ratio (SMR) The observed number of deaths divided by the expected number of deaths and multiplied by 100. SMR is regarded as a measure of the relative risk of the studied group to die of a particular condition.

Standardized scores Scores used to express deviations from the mean (difference scores) in terms of standard deviation units, such as Z-scores, in which the mean is 0 and the standard deviation is 1.

Standard of care A norm on which quality of care is judged.

Statements Express claims that compute to a theory; theories include existence and relational statements.

Statistic Numerical value obtained from a sample; it is used to estimate the parameters of a population.

Statistical conclusion validity Extent to which the conclusions about relationships and differences drawn from statistical analyses reflect reality.

Statistical regression Movement or regression of extreme scores toward the mean in studies using a pretest-posttest design.

Statistical significance Extent to which the results are probably not due to chance.

Stem-and-leaf display Type of exploratory data analysis in which scores are visually presented to obtain insights.

Stetler Model of Research Utilization to Facilitate Evidence-Based Practice An initial model for research utilization in nursing to promote evidence-based practice for nursing. Provides a comprehensive framework to enhance the use of research evidence by nurses to facilitate an EBP.

Stratification Design strategy used to distribute subjects evenly throughout the sample.

Stratified random sampling Technique used when the researcher knows some of the variables in the population that are critical to achieving representativeness; the sample is divided into strata or groups using these identified variables.

Structural equation modeling Analysis technique designed to test theories.

Structured interview Interview in which strategies are used that give the researcher increasing control over the content. An example is a questionnaire with structured responses.

Structured observation Clear identification of what is to be observed and precise definition of how the observations are to be made, recorded, and coded.

Structures of care The elements of organization and administration that guide the processes of care.

Subjects Individuals participating in a study (those being studied).

Substantive theory Theory recognized within a discipline as useful for explaining important phenomena.

Substitutable relationship Relationship in which a similar concept can be substituted for the first concept and the second concept will occur relatively unchanged.

Sufficient relationship Relationship in which, when the first variable or concept occurs, the second will occur, regardless of the presence or absence of other factors.

Summary statistics *See* Descriptive statistics.

Surfing the Web Following the links (underlined or highlighted names) on one website to reveal other websites.

Survey design Design used to describe a phenomenon by collecting data using questionnaires or personal interviews.

Survival analysis Set of techniques designed to analyze repeated measures from a given time (e.g., beginning of the study, onset of a disease, beginning of a treatment) until a certain attribute (e.g., death, treatment failure, recurrence of the phenomenon) occurs.

Symbolic interaction theory Explores how people define reality and how their beliefs are related to their actions.

Symmetrical This is a term used to describe the normal curve where both sides of the curve are mirror images of each other.

Symmetrical relationship Relationship in which, if A occurs or changes, B will occur or change, and if B occurs or changes, A will occur or change (A ↔ B).

Symmetry plot Exploratory data analysis technique designed to determine the presence of skewness in the data.

Synthesis of sources Clustering and interrelating ideas from several sources to form a gestalt or a new, complete picture of what is known and not known in an area.

Systematic bias *See* Systematic variation.

Systematic error Measurement error that is not random but occurs consistently in the same direction, such as a scale that inaccurately weighs subjects at 3 pounds heavier than their actual weight.

Systematic extension replication Constructive replication performed under distinctly new conditions, in which the researchers conducting the replication do not follow the design or methods of the original researchers; rather, the second investigative team begins with a similar problem statement but formulates new means to verify the first investigator's findings.

Systematic review Structured, comprehensive synthesis of quantitative and outcomes studies in a particular healthcare area to determine the best research evidence available for expert clinicians to use to promote evidence-based practice.

Systematic review of research Narrowly focused synthesis of the findings from quantitative studies focused on a particular practice intervention or problem.

Systematic sampling Selecting every *k*th individual from an ordered list of all members of a population, using a randomly selected starting point.

Systematic variation Phenomenon that occurs when the selected subjects' measurement values vary in some way from those of the population.

T

Tails Extremes of the normal curve where the significant statistical values fall.

Target population Population determined by the sampling criteria.

Tendency statement Deterministic relationship that describes what always happens if there are no interfering conditions.

Tentative theory Theory that is newly proposed, has had minimal exposure to critique by scholars in the discipline, and has undergone little testing.

Testable hypothesis Hypothesis containing variables that can be measured or manipulated in the real world.

Test-retest reliability Determination of the stability or consistency of a measurement technique by correlating the scores obtained from repeated measures.

Text analysis Analysis of changes or patterns in a particular event being studied based on written descriptions of historical events, letters, and documents.

Theoretical connectedness Theoretical schema developed from a qualitative study; is clearly expressed, logically consistent, reflective of the data, and compatible with nursing's knowledge base.

Theoretical limitations Weaknesses in the study framework and conceptual and operational definitions that restrict the abstract generalization of the findings.

Theoretical literature Concept analyses, maps, theories, and conceptual frameworks that support a selected research problem and purpose.

Theoretical sampling Sampling in which data are gathered from any individual subject or group that can provide relevant information for theory generation.

Theory Integrated set of defined concepts, existence statements, and relational statements that present a view of a phenomenon and can be used to describe, explain, predict, and control that phenomenon.

Therapeutic research Research that provides a patient with an opportunity to receive an experimental treatment that might have beneficial results.

Thesis Research project completed by a graduate student as part of the requirements for a master's degree

Time-dimensional designs Designs used to examine the sequence and patterns of change, growth, or trends across time.

Time lag Time span between the generation of new knowledge through research and the use of this knowledge in practice.

Time-series analysis Technique designed to analyze changes in a variable across time and thus uncover patterns in the data.

Total variance The combination of the within-group variance and the between-group variance.

Traditions Truths or beliefs that are based on customs and past trends.

Transcriptions Written records created from audio recordings.

Translational research Evolving concept that is defined by the NIH as the translation of basic scientific discoveries into practical applications.

Trend designs Designs used to examine changes in the general population in relation to a particular phenomenon.

Trial and error Approach with unknown outcomes used in an uncertain situation when other sources of knowledge are unavailable.

Trialability Extent to which the results of an individual or agency allow an idea to be tried out on a limited basis, with the option of returning to previous practices.

Triangulation Use of two or more theories, methods, data sources, investigators, or analysis methods in a study.

True score Score that would be obtained if no measurement error occurred (but there is always some measurement error).

t-test Parametric analysis technique used to determine significant differences between measures of two samples.

Two-tailed test of significance Analysis technique used for a nondirectional hypothesis when the researcher assumes that an extreme score can occur in either tail of the normal curve.

Type I error Error that occurs when the researcher concludes that the samples tested are from different populations (a significant difference exists between groups) when, in fact, the samples are from the same population (no significant difference exists between groups); the null hypothesis is rejected when it is true.

Type II error Error that occurs when the researcher concludes that no significant difference exists between the samples examined when, in fact, a difference exists; the null hypothesis is regarded as true when it is false.

U

Unexpected results Study results that indicate relationships between variables or differences among groups that were not hypothesized and not predicted from the framework being used.

Unexplained variance Part of the variation between or among two or more variables that is the result of things other than the relationship.

Ungrouped frequency distribution Means of identifying and displaying all numerical values obtained for a particular variable from the subjects studied.

Ungrouped frequency distribution Categorical data in the form of a table that is developed to display all numerical values obtained for a particular variable.

Unstructured interview Interview that is initiated with a broad question; subjects usually are encouraged to elaborate further on particular dimensions of a topic and often control the content of the interview.

Unstructured observation Spontaneous observation and recording of what is seen; planning is minimal.

Utilization of research findings Use of knowledge generated through research to guide nursing practice.

V

Validity Extent to which an instrument accurately reflects the abstract construct (or concept) being examined.

Variables Qualities, properties, or characteristics of persons, things, or situations that change or vary and are manipulated or measured in research.

Variance Measure of dispersion, where the larger the variance, the larger the dispersion of scores. Variance is calculated as one of the steps in determining standard deviation.

Variance analysis Outcomes research strategy to track individual and group variance from a specific critical pathway. The goal is to decrease preventable variance in process, thus helping patients and their families achieve optimal outcomes.

Verification of information When researchers are able to further confirm hunches, relationships, or theoretical models.

Virus, computer Program developed to alter and destroy information stored in a computer.

Visual analog scale A 100-mm line, with right angle stops at either end, on which subjects are asked to record their response to a study variable.

Voluntary consent Decision made by a prospective subject, of his or her own volition, without coercion or any undue influence, to participate in a research study.

Wald-Wolfowitz runs test Nonparametric analysis technique used to determine differences between two populations.

Wilcoxon matched-pairs signed-ranks test Nonparametric analysis of changes that occur in pretest-posttest measures or matched-pairs measures.

Within-group variance Source of variation that reflects the individual scores in a group that vary from the group mean.

World Wide Web (www) An information service for access to Internet resources by content rather than file names.

X **axis** The horizontal scale of a scatterplot.

Y **axis** The vertical scale of a scatterplot.

Z

Z-score Standardized score of the normal curve that is equivalent to the standard deviation of the normal curve.

INDEX

A

AAALAC. *See* American Association for Accreditation of Laboratory Animal Care
AACN. *See* American Association Colleges of Nursing
Abstracts
    as adjective, describing theories, 228
    of database articles, 213
    definition and example of research report, 55, 56b-57b
Academic Center for Evidence-Based Nursing, website, 495
Academic libraries, 208
Academic Search Premier, keeping written search records in, 212t
Acceptance rates, of subjects, 295-296
Accessible populations
    definition of, 290-291
    representativeness, 294-298
Accidental sampling. *See* Convenience sampling
Accuracy
    of physiological measures, 338-339
    and precision, in quantitative research, 39
Acquired immunodeficiency syndrome (AIDS), history of emphasis on, 13-14
Administration, and nursing research, 4
ADN. *See* Associate Degree in Nursing
"Advanced beginner" stage, of nursing experience, 17-18
Advances in Nursing Science, 11t, 12, 54
Advisory Committee on Community-Based Non-Acute Care Indicators, 523-525, 524t
African American women, blood pressure in, 6, 7f
Age, as demographic variable, 182, 183t
Agency for Health Care Policy and Research (AHCPR)
    on outcomes research, 11t, 14
    research priorities and current missions, 157
Agency for Healthcare Research and Quality (AHRQ), 11t, 14-15, 157
    developing evidence-based guidelines, 26
    publishing integrative reviews, 221-222
AHCPR. *See* Agency for Health Care Policy and Research
AHRQ. *See* Agency for Healthcare Research and Quality
AIDS. *See* Acquired immunodeficiency syndrome
Ajzen's theory, 155-156, 156f
Algorithms, 470-471
Alpha (α), discussion of, 377
American Association Colleges of Nursing (AACN)
    grants from, 158
    on nursing research, 11t, 15, 27-28
American Association for Accreditation of Laboratory Animal Care (AAALAC), 140
American Journal of Nursing, history of, 11t, 12

American Nurses Association (ANA)
    on nursing research, 11t, 12, 27-28
    "Nursing Safety & Quality Initiative," and outcomes research, 522-526
    nursing-sensitive quality indicators, 523
American Organization of Nurse Executives (AONE), addressing research priorities, 157
American Psychological Association (APA), format for recording references, 219-220
American Society of Hospital Pharmacists (ASHP), 484
ANA. *See* American Nurses Association
Analyses. *See also* Data analysis
    of research reports, 60
Analysis of covariance (ANCOVA)
    definition of, 408
    uses for, 408
Analysis of variance (ANOVA)
    definition of, 406
    interpreting results of, 406
    research example, 406b-408b
Analysis phase
    of critique process, 425
    in summary research example, 440-441
Analytic Techniques for Qualitative Metasynthesis, 442
ANCOVA. *See* Analysis of covariance
Animals, ethics of research use of, 139-140
Annual Review of Nursing Research, 11t, 13
    integrative reviews in, 221-222
Anonymity, definition of, 117
ANOVA. *See* Analysis of variance
Anthropology, and ethnographic research, 79-80
AONE. *See* American Organization of Nurse Executives
APA. *See* American Psychological Association
Applied Nursing Research, 54
Applied Nursing Research and Nursing Science Quarterly, 11t, 13
Applied research
    definition of, 37
    example of, 38b
ASHP. *See* American Society of Hospital Pharmacists
Assent forms, sample, 113t
Assessments, step of nursing process, 41t, 42
Associate Degree in Nursing (ADN)
    career retention of, 304b
    job satisfaction of, 304b
    job satisfaction research example, using quantitative methods, 148-149
Association of Women's Health, Obstetric, and Neonatal Nurse, website, 495
Associative hypotheses
    versus causal, 167-171
    critique of, 168-169
    definition of, 167

Assumptions
  definition an examples of, in quantitative study, 43f, 48
  definition of conceptual model, 228-229
Authority, definition of, 16
Authors, database searching by, 211
Autonomous agents, definition of, 110
Autonomy, diminished, and informed consent competence, 111, 114

B

Bachelor of Science Degree in Nursing (BSN)
  career retention of, 304b
  job satisfaction of, 304b
  job satisfaction research example, using quantitative methods, 148-149
  roles of, in nursing research, 27-28, 27f
Barroso, Dr. Julie, 442
Basic research
  definition of, 36
  example of, 37b
Bathing, research concerning, 348b-349b
Behavioral research, ethical conduct in, 103-104
Belmont Report, 107-108
Benchmarking, definition of, 222
Beneficence, principle of, 107-108, 118-119
Benefit-risk ratios
  research example of, 136b-137b
  of study, 134-137
    definition of, 134
    diagram illustrating, 135f
Benefits, risks and, informed consent competence and, 124
Best research evidence, 4-5, 5f, 22-26, 465-466
Bias
  definition of, 254
  protection against, 256
  in research design, 254-255
Bibliographic databases, 210
Biobehavioral factors, related to immunocompetence, history of emphasis on, 13-14
Biological Research for Nursing, 11t, 15
Biomedical research, ethical conduct in, 103-104
Bivariate correlation, 394-395
Blood pressure
  in African American women, 6, 7f
  classification of, with nursing interventions, 5-6, 6t
  as physiological measure, 338
Bonferroni procedures, 406
Borrowing, in nursing, 16-17
Bracketing, definition and purpose of, 96
Breach of confidentiality, 117-118, 125
BSN. *See* Bachelor of Science Degree in Nursing

C

Cancer, unethical research in, at Jewish Chronic Disease Hospital, 107
CANCERLIT, evidence-based practice resource, 470t
Cardiovascular diseases, and smoking risk, 5-6, 6t

Care Management Mission, of Agency for Health Care Policy and Research, 157
Caring
  conceptual *versus* denotative definition of, 231
  as phenomenon, 228
Case studies
  definition of, 12
  design of, 262-264
Case study designs
  definition of, 262
  research examples, 263b
Casual hypotheses
  versus associative, 167-171
  critique of, 170
  definition of, 170-171
Causality
  definition of, 253
  in research design, 253
  testing
    in experimental designs, 276-281, 277f
    in quasi-experimental designs, 270-276, 275f
  using statistics to examine, 401-408
Center for Epidemiologic Studies Depression (CES-D) Scale, 358-360, 359f
Center for Nursing Scholarship, 208
Centre for Health Evidence, website, 495
CES-D. *See* Center for Epidemiologic Studies Depression Scale
CFR. *See Code of Federal Regulations*
Child sexual abuse, research example concerning, 44b
Children
  assent form for, 113t
  ethical laws concerning, 111-112, 112t
  informed consent for, 112t
  legal issues concerning, 111-112, 112t
  sexual abuse of, research example concerning, 44b-45b, 45, 46f, 47-49, 50f, 51-52, 53b
Chi-square test of independence
  interpreting results, 402
  purpose of, 401-402
  research example of, 402b-403b
Chronic illnesses, history of emphasis on living with, 13-14
CINAHL. *See* Cumulative Index to Nursing and Allied Health Literature
Citations
  accessing on-line, 210-212
  definition of, 190
  print *versus* on-line full-text format, 220
  search fields, 217
Clinical and Translational Science Awards (CTSA), 500
Clinical expertise, 5
Clinical importance, statistical, 410-411
Clinical journals, focus on research articles, 55t
Clinical nursing
  grounded theory research example, 78b-79b
  important theories in, 227
Clinical Nursing Research, 13
Clinical Nursing Research: An International Journal, 54
Clinical practice guidelines, 493t
Clinical questions, development of, 490-492, 491t, 493t
Clinical relevance, evaluation of, 483

Clinical research, history of, 10, 12-13
Clinical significance, of study outcomes, 410-411
Clinical trials, designs and examples of, 280b-281b
Cluster sampling, as probability sampling method, 302-303
Clustering, of sources, 220-221
CMA InfoBase, website, 495
Cochran Handbook for Systematic Review of Interventions, 490
Cochrane Collaboration, 11t
  publishing integrative reviews, 221-222
Cochrane Library
  evidence-based practice resource, 470t
  keeping written search records in, 212t
  source for evidence-based guidelines, 26
Code of Federal Regulations (CFR), 108, 109t
Coding, method of, 94-95
Coefficient of multiple determination, 399
Coercion, 110
Cognitive impairments
  competency issues with, 113-114
  history of emphasis on, 13-14
Comas
  competency issues with, 113-114
  legal issues concerning, 113-114
Comfort Theory, 237-238
Community-based nursing models, history of emphasis on, 13-14
Comparative descriptive designs
  definition of, 260-262
  diagram illustrating, 260f
  research example, 261b
Comparison and analysis, phase of critique process, 425
  guidelines for, 425, 426b-427b
Comparison groups
  in design mapping, 284-285
  and representativeness, 298
Comparison phase
  of critique process, 425
  in summary research example, 440-441
"Competent" stage, of nursing experience, 17-18
Complete reviews, by institutional review boards, 133
Complex hypotheses
  definition of, 172-173
  versus simple hypotheses, 172-173
Complex searches, method of performing, 213-214, 214f
Comprehension
  in informed consent information, 123
  phase
    of critique process, 422
    guidelines for, 423b-424b
    in summary research example, 433-439
  of research reports, 60
Computers. *See also* Databases; Websites
  accessing on-line databases via, 210-213
  in libraries, 209
  locating relevant literature on, 213-220
Concepts
  at basic element of theory, 230
  definition of, 230
  extracting from research framework, 240

Conceptual definitions
  bias protection and, 256
  case study examples of, 64, 67, 181b-182b
  description of, 231
  extracting from research framework, 240
  of variables, 47, 47b, 178-180
Conceptual frameworks, of theories, 238-239
Conceptual maps
  definition of, 233
  example of, 247f
Conceptual models
  function of, 228-230
  nursing research traditions, 246-248
  research example of frameworks, 246-248
Conclusions
  in reasoning, 18-19
  from statistical outcomes, 412-415
Concrete, as descriptive term, *versus* abstract, 228
Conduct and Utilization of Research in Nursing (CURN), history of, 11t, 13
Confidentiality
  breaches of, 117
  definition of, 117
  rights to, 117-118
Confirmatory analyses, during data analysis process, 375
Consent. *See also* Informed consent
  from research subjects, 52
Consent forms, elements of informed, 123, 124f, 125-128, 127f
Consent process, Nuremberg Code and, 104-105, 105t
Consistency, maintaining in data collection, 362
Constructs, defining in theory, 230
Control groups
  in design mapping, 284-285
  in experimental research, 35-36
  terminology of, 298
Controls
  definition of, in quantitative research, 39-41, 39t
  maintaining in data collection, 362
  nursing research definition of, 9-10
  in research design, 255
Convenience sampling, as nonprobability sampling method, 299t, 305-306
Correlation coefficients
  from Pearson product-moment analysis, 395
  testing significance of, 396
Correlation studies, framework and theory development in, 242-244
Correlational analyses, to examine relationships, 394-395
Correlational designs
  algorithm for determining type of, 264f
  critique of, 266b-267b, 269b
  descriptive, 264-266, 265f
  model testing, 264f, 268-270, 268f
  predictive, 264f, 266-268, 266f
  purpose of, 264-270
Correlational research
  control levels in, 39-40, 39t
  definition of, 35
  examples of, 148, 149t-150t
  introduction and classification of, 20-21, 21t

Correlational research *(continued)*
  Pearson, Karl, on, 34
  problems and purpose of, 44, 149
Cost, Organization, and Socio-Economics Mission, of
     Agency for Health Care Policy and Research, 157
Costs
  of care, and quality, 519-520
  Donabedian's theory of quality and, 519-520
  of health care, 4-5, 9-10, 19, 21-22
  of research studies, 158-159
Covered entities, definition of, 114-115
Covert data collection, 110
Critical appraisal of quantitative studies, 419
Critical appraisal of research, 28
Critical pathway tool, 220
Critical thinking, to generate theory, 232
Critique guidelines
  for adequacy of sample, in quantitative studies, 311b
  of conceptual model-theory frameworks, 248
  data analysis and sample, 373
  for examining research ethics, 136-137
  for experimental interventions, 282b-284b
  for measurement error, 336b
  for rating scales, 355b
  for reliability and validity, of measurement instruments,
    336b
  for sample adequacy, 319b
  for self-determination, 120-122
  for study designs, 256b
  for study frameworks, 233-235
Critiques. *See also* Critiquing
  literature review, 193-208
  of research, elements of, 3
Critiquing
  basic research, 37
  of comparative descriptive designs, 261b
  experimental study, 68
  guidelines for frameworks, 240b
  informed consent process, 128-129
  of institutional review boards, 136-137
  middle range theories, 241
  operational and conceptual definitions, 178b-180b
  of problem and purpose feasibility, 158-159
  published literature reviews, 193-208
  qualitative problems, purpose, and aims, 162b-163b
  quantitative problems, purpose, and objectives, 160b-161b
  quasi-experimental designs, 273b-274b
  questions, 164b-166b
  randomized clinical trials, 281b
  sample of literature review, 195-208
CTSA. *See* Clinical and Translational Science Awards
Cultures, ethnographic research and, 79-80, 84-85
Cumulative frequency table, 384t
Cumulative Index to Nursing and Allied Health Literature
    (CINAHL)
  evidence-based practice resource, 470t
  keeping written search records in, 212t
  linking, 217
  search fields available for, 216-217
  searching tips for, 194, 213-220
  website information, 211

CURN. *See* Conduct and Utilization of Research in
  Nursing
Current sources, definition of, 191-192

D

Data. *See also* Data collection
  analysis stages, 94-97
  collection in qualitative research, 85-90
  identifying private personal, 114-117
  management in qualitative research, 93-94
  reliability and validity, 48
  tasks for collecting, 362-366
Data analysis
  process of, 372-375
  in qualitative research, 94-97
  research design and, 49
  techniques, 310-312
Data collection
  definition and examples, of quantitative, 43f, 52
  in historical research, 86
  measurement strategies and
    interviews, 350-352
    observational measurements, 348-349
    physiological measurements, 345-347
    questionnaires, 353-354
    scales, 355-361
  measurements and
    measurement theory concepts, 328-338
    nursing measurement strategies, 345-361
    precision and accuracy, 338-340
    process of, 361-366, 363f
  methods in qualitative research, 85-90
    case studies, 92
    focus groups, 87-88
    interviews, 85-87
    life story construction, 91-92
    observation, 88-90
    story collection, 90-91
    text as source, 90
  in problem-solving, nursing and research processes,
    41t
  procedures in randomized clinical trials, 280-281
  process of, 361-366, 363f
    example of form, 363f
    serendipity, 366
    tasks, 362-366
  research design and, 49
  research example, 364b-366b
  role of nurses in, 27f
  tasks
    maintaining consistency, 362
    maintaining controls, 362
    protecting study integrity, 364-366
    recruiting subjects, 362
    solving problems, 366
Data use agreements, 116-117
Data-based literature
  components of, 190-191
  in literature reviews, 222

Databases
    keywords, 211-212
    locating relevant literature, 213-220
    search fields, 216-217
    selecting and searching, 210-211
    written search records of, 212t
Deception
    definition of, 110
    self-determination and, 110
Decision theory, discussion of, 377-378
Decision-making, in Stetler Model of Research
        Utilization to Facilitate Evidence-Based Practice,
        479-480
Declaration of Helsinki, 105-106
Deductive reasoning, definition and example of, 19
Degrees of freedom (df), concept of, 383
De-identification, of protected health information,
        115-116
Demographic variables
    clinical characteristics in sample and, 183t
    definition of, 182
Department of Health, Education, and Welfare (DHEW),
        on human research subject protection, 107
Department of Health and Human Services, US (DHHS).
    See Department of Health and Human Services
Department of Health and Human Services (DHHS)
    description of, 15
    focus on research subject protection, 107-109
    guidelines for IIHI, 115
    HIPAA Privacy Rule and, 108-109
    on informed consent, 122-123
    Protection of Human Subjects Regulation, 108
Dependent groups, 392
Dependent variables
    case study example of, 63, 67
    definition of, 176
    in predictive correlational designs, 265f, 266-268
    in quasi-experimental research, 270-276, 271f-272f,
        273b-274b, 275f
Descriptions, nursing research definition of, 7-8
Descriptive correlational designs, 264-266, 265f
Descriptive designs
    algorithm for determining type of, 258f
    comparative, 260-262, 260f
    definition of, 256
    diagram of typical, 259f
    in nursing studies, 256-264
    research example and critique, 259b-260b
Descriptive mode, within grounded theory research,
        78-79
Descriptive phenomenology, 244-245
Descriptive research
    control levels in, 39-40, 39t
    data analysis techniques, 52-53
    definition of, 34-35
    examples of, 148, 149t-150t
    introduction and classification of, 20-21, 21t
    problems and purposes in, 44, 148
Descriptive statistics
    definition of, 383
    results, 389

Designs
    algorithm for determining type of, 257f
    case studies, 262-264
    comparative descriptive, 260-262
    concepts important to, 253-256
        bias, 254-255
        causality, 253
        control, 255
        critique guidelines, 256b
        manipulation, 255-256
        multicausality, 254
        probability, 254
    correlational, 264-270, 264f
    definition of, 253
    descriptive, 256-264
    descriptive correlational, 264-266, 265f
    mapping, 284-285
    model testing, 268-270, 268f
    predictive correlational, 266-268, 266f
    purpose of, 253
    for quantitative studies, 252-287
        defining experimental interventions, 282-284
        design mapping, 284-285
        important design concepts, 253-256
        nursing study designs, 256-270
        replication studies, 285
        testing causality, 270-281
    random clinical trials, 280-281
DHEW. See Department of Health, Education, and
        Welfare
DHHS. See Department of Health and Human Services
Diagnoses
    as demographic variable, 182, 183t
    step of nursing process, 41t, 42
Diagnostic tests
    likelihood ratios, 344
    quality determination of, 341-344
    sensitivity of, 341-342, 341t
    specificity of, 341t, 342-344
Diet, Florence Nightingale's work on, 10-12
Diminished autonomy, 111-114
Direct measures, definition of, 328
Directional hypotheses
    definition of, 174
    versus nondirectional hypotheses, 173-174
Discomfort and harm
    definition and categories of, 118-119
    rights to protection against, 118-120
Discovery mode, within grounded theory research, 78-79
"Discussion" section
    abstract components of, 56t
    case study examples of, 65, 68
    of research reports, 52, 59
Dispersion, measures of, 387
Dissertation, definition of, 190-191
Doctorate degree, roles of, in nursing research, 27-28, 27f
Documentation
    of database searches, 212t
    of informed consent, 125-128, 127f
Dogpile, 219
Donabedian, Avedis, 508

Donabedian's Theory of Quality Health Care
  assessment of, 508, 509f
  defining quality, 508, 509f
  evaluating outcomes, 508-510
  evaluating process, 510-520
  evaluating structure, 520
  levels of quality, 509f
  nursing-sensitive patient outcomes, 526-529
  in outcomes research, 508-520, 509f
Dunnett's test, 406

E

EBP. *See* Evidence-based practice
EBSCOhost, 211
Education
  as demographic variable, 182, 183t
  history of nursing, 10, 11t
  nursing, 4
  research participation according to, 27f
Effect sizes, definition of statistical, 382-383
Electronic journals, searching tips, 217-218
Electronic resources, on-line access to, 211
Elements, definition of population/study, 290-291
Eligibility criteria, definition of, in sampling theory,
    291-293
Emergent fit mode, within grounded theory research,
    78-79
Emic approach, to anthropological research, 80
Empirical generalizations, 413
Empirical knowledge, 4-7, 9, 13, 19, 22
Empirical sources, 190
EndNote, 212
Environmental variables, definition of, 177
EPCs. *See* Evidence-Based Practice Centers
Ethical codes, historical events influencing,
    104-109
Ethical issues
  concerning research sources, 222
  concerning research with neonates, 111
Ethical principle of justice, rights to fair treatment and,
    118
Ethical principles, defining three important,
    107-108
Ethics
  benefits *versus* risks, 159
  critique guidelines for reviewing, 136-137, 136b
  federal regulations on, 108-109, 109t
  Office of Research Integrity, 138-139
Ethnic origins, as demographic variable, 182, 183t
Ethnographic research
  examples of, 151, 152t-153t
  literature review purpose in, 193t
  problems and purposes in, 153
  researcher-participant relationships in, 84-85
Ethnographical research, introduction and classification of,
    21, 21t
Ethnography, definition of, 79-80
Ethnonursing research, description of, 80-81
Etic approach, to anthropological research, 80

Evaluation phase
  of critique process, 427
    guidelines for, 427, 428b
  in summary research example, 441-442
Evaluations
  in problem-solving, nursing and research process, 41t,
    42
  step of nursing process, 41t, 42
  when appraising quality, 508
Evidence, strength of research, 25f
Evidence-based guidelines
  definition of, 26
  development of, 26, 492-494
  implementation of, 492-499
  JNC 7 implementation in, 496-499, 497f
  resources, 494-496
  websites, 26
Evidence-Based Nursing journal, 221-222
Evidence-based practice (EBP)
  barriers to, 466-467
  benefits of, 468-469
  best research evidence and, 4-5
  blood pressure
    in African American women, 6, 7f
    classification of with nursing interventions for, 5-6, 6t
  clinical expertise and, 5
  definition of, 465-466
  elements of, 5f
  as goal for nursing, 4-5
  guidelines, movement toward and, 11t, 14. *See also*
      Evidence-based guidelines
  importance of research to, 5-6
  models to promote, 477-482
    Iowa Model of Evidence-Based Practice, 480-482,
        481f
    Stetler Model of Research Utilization to Facilitate
        Evidence-Based Practice, 477-480, 478f
  research priorities for developing, 156-157
  role of replication studies in, 285
  searching sources, 469, 470t
Evidence-Based Practice Centers (EPCs), 499-500
Evolve website
  additional grounded theory research on, 79
  on ethnographic research, 81
  on phenomenological research, 77
Exclusion sampling criteria, 291
Exempt from review, 131, 131t
Existence statements, within theories, 231
Expedited reviews, 131-132, 132t
Experience, levels of personal, 17-18
Experimental designs
  algorithm to determine type of, 277f
  case study example of, 67
  definition of, 276
  illustration of classical, 278f
  pretest-posttest, 276-280, 278f
Experimental interventions, 282-284
Experimental research
  case study example of, 66b-68b
  control levels in, 39-40, 39t
  essential elements of, 270

Experimental research *(continued)*
   examples of, 148, 149t-150t
   introduction and classification of, 20-21, 21t
   mapping the design, 284-285
   problems and purposes of, 35-36, 44, 151
   studies, framework and theory development in, 242-244
   testing causality in, 276, 277f, 280-281
   tips for reading reports on, 54-60
   variables in, 177, 181-182
Experiments, definition of research, 33
"Expert" stage, of nursing experience, 17-18
Explained variances, 395
Explanation, nursing research definition of, 8-9
Exploratory analysis, during data analysis process, 374
Extraneous variables
   and control, in quantitative research, 40
   definition of, 177

F

F statistics, 406
Fabrication
   of data, 103
   definition of research, 137
FACES Pain Scale, 356f
Factor analysis, 397-398
Factors, 397-398
Fair treatment, right to, 118
False negative, 341
False positive, 341
Falsification
   of data, 103
   definition of research, 137
FDA. *See* US Food and Drug Administration
Federal regulations, for human subject protection, 108-109
Fetuses
   ethical laws concerning, 111, 113
   legal issues concerning, 113, 132t
Field settings, 40-41
Financial outcomes, element of outcomes research, 21-22
Findings
   research example illustrating, 411b-412b
   statistical, 410
Fisher, Ronald, 34
Food and Drug Administration, US (FDA)
   on human subject protection, 108
   informed consent and, 122-123
Forging. *See* Plagiarism
Frameworks
   based on middle range theories, 240-242
   case study example of experimental, 66
   conceptual maps, 247f
   of conceptual nursing models, 246-248
   definition and example of study, in quantitative research process, 45, 46f
   definition of, 238-239
   derived from qualitative studies, 244-245
   including conceptual nursing models, 246-248
   middle range theories used as, 235-237, 236t
   for physiological studies, 113

Frameworks *(continued)*
   practice research example, 62-63, 63f
   in qualitative research, 74, 78-79, 244-245
   section in quantitative reports, 192
   understanding theory and research, 226-251
Fraud, in research, 103, 137-139
Frequency distributions
   common graphic displays of, 386f
   definition of, 384
   display of, 384
   grouped, 384, 385t
   ungrouped, 384, 384t
Full-text databases, 210-211
Functional maintenance, element of outcomes research, 21-22

G

Gender, as demographic variable, 182, 183t
General propositions, hierarchy within theories, 232, 232t
Generalizations
   definition of, 48
   interferences and, 378
   in sampling theory, 291
   of statistical study findings, 413
Gestalt, 74-75
Goals, of research studies, 44
Goal-setting, in problem-solving, nursing and research processes, 41t, 42
Gold standard, 341
Graphs, displaying frequency distribution, 386f
Grounded theory research
   definition and example of, 77-78, 78b-79b
   development of, 77-78
   examples of, 151, 152t-153t
   introduction and classification of, 21, 21t
   literature review purpose in, 193t
   nursing knowledge and, 78-79
   problems and purposes in, 151-153
   theory development in, 244-245
   using theoretical sampling, 316-317
Grouped frequency distributions
   common graphic displays of, 386f
   definition of, 384
Groups, grounded theory research and, 77-78
Grove Model for Implementing Evidence-Based Guidelines in Practice, 496-497, 498f
Guided imagery, smoking cessation and, 155
Guidelines Advisory Committee, website, 495
Guidelines International Network, website, 495

H

Handbook for Synthesizing Qualitative Research, 442, 475
Harm, discomfort and, rights to protection against, 118-120
HCFA. *See* Health Care Finance Administration
Health, concept of, 508, 509f
Health care costs. *See* Costs

Health Care Finance Administration (HCFA), on outcomes research, 14
Health care services, nursing research and, 6-7
Health information, disclosure authorization, 126-128, 127f
Health Insurance Portability and Accountability Act (HIPAA)
  development of, 108
  influence on institutional review boards, 133, 134t
  Privacy Rule
    authorization for uses and disclosures, 126-128, 127f
    clarification of, 108, 109t
    expansion of, 114-115
Health Services/Technology Assessment Text (HSTAT), website, 495
Healthy People 2000, 11t
Healthy People 2010, 11t, 15
Heart rate, as physiological measure, 338
Heideggerian phenomenology, 96
HerbMed: Evidence-Based Herbal Database, website, 495
Hermeneutics, description of, 76-77
Heterogeneous samples, 291
Highly controlled settings, 41, 322-323
Highly sensitive test, 342
Highly specific test, 342
Hinshaw, Dr. Ada Sue, 13-14
HIPAA. *See* Health Insurance Portability and Accountability Act
Historical research
  definition and example of, 81-83
  determining sources for, 82b-83b
  examples of, 151, 152t-153t
  introduction and classification of, 21, 21t
  literature review purpose in, 193t
  problems and purposes in, 153-154
History
  ethical code development and, 104-109
  of nursing research, 10-15, 11t
  philosophical orientation of, 82
H$_o$. *See* Null hypotheses
Homogenous samples, 291
HSD. *See* Tukey's Honestly Significantly Different test
HSTAT. *See* Health Services/Technology Assessment Text
Human immunodeficiency virus (HIV), history of emphasis on, 13-14
Human rights
  definition of, 110
  protecting, 110-122
Human subjects. *See* Subjects
Hypotheses
  associative *versus* causal, 167-171
  definition of, 167
  description and example of, 43f, 46-47
  development of, from descriptive designs, 257-260
  Fisher, Ronald, on, 34
  hierarchy within theories, 232
  purpose of, in research studies, 145-146
  research, 43f, 46-47
  types of, 167-175

Hypothesis testing
  case study examples of, 63
  discussion of, 377-378

I

ICUs. *See* Intensive care units
IIHI. *See* Individually identifiable health information
Immunizations, child positioning for, 38b
Implementation
  in problem-solving, nursing and research processes, 41t, 42
  step of nursing process, 41t, 42
Implications, considering, of scientific research, 413-414
Implicit frameworks, definition of, 239
Inclusion sampling criteria, definition of, in sampling theory, 291
Income, as demographic variable, 182, 183t
Independent groups, 392
Independent variables
  case study examples of, 64-65, 67
  definition of, 176
  in predictive correlational designs, 266-268, 266f
  in quasi-experimental research, 256b, 271f-272f, 275f
Indicators
  of measurement concepts, 328-329
  quality, for community-based non-acute care, 522-523, 524t
  for quality of care, 522-526
Indirect measures, of concepts, 328-329
Individually identifiable health information (IIHI), definition of, 114-115
Inductive reasoning, definition and example of, 18-19
Inference, reasoning behind, 378
Inferential research, data analysis techniques, 52-53
Information, on-line access to, 210
Informed consent
  definition of, 122
  documentation of, 125-128, 127f
  four elements of, 122
    competence, 124
    comprehension, 123
    essential information, 122-123, 124f
    voluntary consent, 125
  guide to obtaining, 135f
  research example, 129b
  waiving of, 125
INS. *See* Intravenous Nursing Society
Institutional review
  definition of, 130
  influence of HIPAA Privacy Rule on, 133, 134t
  levels of, 131-133
  research exempted from, 131-132, 131t-132t
Institutional review boards (IRBs)
  to examine ethical aspects of studies, 103
  influence of HIPAA Privacy Rule on, 133, 134t
  levels of review, 131-133

Institutions, research on prisoners in, ethics of, 114
Integrative reviews
    of qualitative studies, contributions of, 24
    of research
        critically appraising, 473
        definition of, 24, 220, 473
        research example, 474b-475b
Integrative reviews of literature
    characteristics of, 23t
    to determine evidence for practice, 23t, 24
Integrity, protecting study, in data collection,
        364-366
Intellectual research critiques
    critique guidelines of, 420b
    examining elements of, 419-421
    guidelines for, 420b
    roles of nurses in conducting, 421
    steps for, 420t
Intensive care units (ICUs), 154, 154t
Interlibrary loan departments, 208
International Journal of Nursing Studies, 11t, 12
Internet, search of, 218-219
Interpretations
    of analysis of variance, 406
    of chi-square results, 402
    process of, of types of results, 408-411
    of qualitative research, 97
    of statistical outcomes, 408-411
        conclusions, 412-415
        findings, 410
        further study suggestions, 415
        generalized findings, 413
        implications, 413-414
        significance, 410
Interval levels, of measurements, 51
Interval-scale measurements, description and example of,
        330, 336b-338b
Intervention mode, within grounded theory research,
        78-79
Intervention theories
    example of, 238
    purpose of, 237-238
Interventions
    definition of, 282
    experimental, 282-284
    history of emphasis on HIV/AIDS, 13-14
    research example of, 283b
Interviews
    critiquing, 351b
    definition of, 350
    in qualitative research, 85-87
    research examples of, 351b-352b
    transcribing, 93
Intravenous Nursing Society (INS), 484
"Introduction" sections
    abstract components, 56t, 57-58
    building new research from, 155
    in literature reviews, 222
    of research report, 57-58
Intuition, definition of, 18
Invasion of privacy, 114

Iowa Model of Evidence-Based Practice, 480-482, 481f
    application of, 482-490
        assemble, critically appraise, and synthesize research,
            483-486
        institute change in practice, 488, 489t
        monitor outcomes, 488-490
        pilot change in practice, 487-488, 487t
        sufficiency of research base, 486-487
IRBs. *See* Institutional review boards

J

Jewish Chronic Disease Hospital Study, 107, 110, 118
JNC 7. *See* Joint National Committee on Prevention,
        Detection, Evaluation, and Treatment of High
        Blood Pressure
Job classification, as demographic variable, 182
Joint National Committee on Prevention, Detection,
        Evaluation, and Treatment of High Blood Pressure
        (JNC 7), implementation of, 496-499, 497f
Journal of Nursing Measurement, 11t, 13
Journal of Nursing Scholarship, 11t, 54
Journal of the American Medical Association, 496
Journals
    electronic, 217-218
    increase in number, 189
    list of clinical and research, 55t
    on-line access to, 210
    search fields, 216-217
    web addresses for nursing, 218
Justice, principle of, definition of, 107-108

K

Keywords, selecting, 211-212
Knowledge
    acquiring through nursing research, 19-22
    authority and, 16
    definition of, 15
    factors to consider, in research problems and purposes,
        155-157
    gaps and research, 146-148
    historical research and, 81-82
    literature review providing, 189-190
    methods of acquiring, 15-19

L

Laboratory animals, humane use of, 139-140
Landmark studies, 194
Leininger's Theory of Transcultural Nursing, 80-81
Levels of significance. *See also* Alpha
    discussion of, 377-378
    normal curve and, 379-380
Libraries, 208-209, 209t
Library sources, 209
Likelihood ratios (LR), 344
Likert scale, 357-360

Limitations, definition and examples of, in quantitative study, 43f, 48
Line of best fit, definition and illustration of, 398-399, 399f
Linking, description of, 217
Literature reviews, 188-225
  case study example of experimental, 66
  clarifying evidence for best practices, 220-222
  critique guidelines and sample, 193-208
    in qualitative research, 202-208, 202b-208b
    in quantitative research, 195-202, 195b-201b
  definition and example of, in quantitative research process, 43f, 44-45, 45b
  integrative, 220-222
  practice research example, 62
  procedure for performing, 208
  in published studies, 189-193
  purpose of, 189
    in qualitative research, 192-193, 193t
    in quantitative research, 192
  search fields, 216-217
  sections, building new research from, 155
  sources included in, 190-192
  writing outline for, 222
Logical positivism, 20
Low sensitivity test, 342
Low specificity test, 342
LR. *See* Likelihood ratios

M

Manipulation, 255-256
Marital status, as demographic variable, 182, 183t
Master of science degree in nursing (MSN), roles of, in nursing research, 27-28, 27f
Mead, George Herbert, on symbolic interaction theory, 77-78
Mean, definition of, 387
Measurement errors, critique guidelines for, 336b-338b
Measurement theory, concepts of, 328-338
  direct measures, 328-329
  errors, 331-332
  levels of, 329-331
  reliability, 332-334
  validity, 334-338
Measurements
  data collection and
    measurement theory concepts, 328-338
    nursing measurement strategies, 345-361
    precision and accuracy, 338-340
    process of, 361-366, 363f
  definition and examples of, in quantitative study, 43f, 51
  in design mapping, 284
  directness of, 328-329
  errors, 331-332
  interval-scale, 330
  levels of, 329-331
  methods and levels of, 51
  nominal-scale, 329-330
  ordinal-scale, 330
  purpose of, 327

Measurements (*continued*)
  ratio-scale, 330-331
  research design and, 49
  sensitivity, 310
  strategies in nursing
    interviews, 350-352
    observational measurements, 348-349
    physiological measurements, 345-347
    questionnaires, 353-354
    scales, 355-361
Measures of central tendency, 385-387, 386f
  definition of, 385
Measures of dispersion, 387-389
Mechanical ventilation, research on prolonged, 14b
Medians
  definition of, 385-387
  in measures of central tendency, 385-387
Medical Care Research & Review, 470-471
MEDLINE. *See* PubMed National Library of Medicine
Mentally impaired persons
  competency issues with, 113-114
  legal issues concerning, 113-114
Mentorship, 18
Meta-analysis
  benchmarking and, 222
  characteristics of, 23t
  critically appraising, 471
  definition of, 471
  research example, 472b-473b
  of research literature, 23t, 24
  studies included in, 485t
Metasummaries
  characteristics of, 23t
  of qualitative research, 24
Metasynthesis
  characteristics of, 23t
  of qualitative research, 24
  research example, 476b-477b
Methodological limitations, definition and example of, 48
"Methods" section
  abstract components of, 56t
  determining research resources, 159
  of research report, 58
Middle range theories
  description and basis for, 235
  frameworks based on, 240-242
  list of current framework, 236t
"Minimal risks," definition of, 131-132
Minors, legal issues concerning, 111-112, 112t
Misconduct. *See* Scientific misconduct
Mixed results, 409-410
Model testing designs
  definition of, 268-270
  diagrams illustrating, 268f
  research example, 269b
Modes
  definition of, 385
  in measures of central tendency, 385
Modification, step of nursing process, 41t, 42
Money. *See* Costs
Monographs, definition of, 190

Morbidity data, gathered by Florence Nightingale, 10-12
Mortality data, gathered by Florence Nightingale, 10-12
MSN. *See* Master of science degree in nursing
Multicausality, 254
Multiple regression, 398-399

N

National Association of Neonatal Nurses
    source for evidence-based guidelines, 26
    website, 495
National Center for Nursing Research (NCNR), 11t, 13-14
National Commission for the Protection of Human Subjects, of Biomedical and Behavioral Research, 107-108
National Database of Nursing Quality Indicators (NDNQI), 523, 524t
National Guideline Clearinghouse (NGC)
    of Agency for Healthcare Research and Quality, 494-495
    as evidence-based guidelines source, 26
    evidence-based practice resource, 470t
    resources, 494-495
National Institute for Clinical Excellence (NICE)
    evidence-based practice resource, 470t
    website, 495
National Institute for Nursing Research (NINR)
    addressing research priorities, 157
    federal grants from, 158
    history of, 11t, 13-14
    mission of, 14-15
National Library of Health (NLH), evidence-based practice resource, 470t
National Library of Medicine, website information, 211
National Research Act, 107-108, 130
Natural settings, 40-41, 321
Nazi Medical Experiments, 104, 118, 120
NCNR. *See* National Center for Nursing Research
NDNQI. *See* National Database of Nursing Quality Indicators
Negative likelihood ratio, 344
Negative relationships, 395
Neonates
    definition of, 111
    ethical conduct of research with, 111
    legal issues concerning, 111, 112t
    viable *versus* nonviable, 111
Network sampling, description and example of, 314-316, 315b-316b
Newman-Keuls' test, 406
NGC. *See* National Guideline Clearinghouse
NICE. *See* National Institute for Clinical Excellence
Nightingale, Florence, role in nursing research, 10-12, 11t
NINR. *See* National Institute for Nursing Research
NLH. *See* National Library of Health
Nominal levels, of measurements, 51
Nominal-scale measurements
    categories, 329-330
    definition of, 329-330

Nondirectional hypotheses
    definition of, 173-174
    versus directional hypotheses, 173-174
Nonprobability sampling methods
    convenience sampling, 299t, 305-306
    versus probability sampling methods, 299t
    quota sampling, 299t, 307
Nonsignificant results, 409
Nontherapeutic research
    benefits/risks ratios in, 134-137
    definition of, 105
    guide to informed consent, for children, 112t
    versus therapeutic research, 112t
Normal curves, significance and illustration of, 379-380, 379f
"Novice" stage, of nursing experience, 17-18
NRS. *See* Numeric Rating Scale
Null hypotheses (H_o)
    definition of, 174
    versus research hypotheses, 174-175
Numeric Rating Scale (NRS), 356f
Nuremberg Code, 104-105, 105t, 120
Nurses
    characteristics and roles of, nursing research and, 4
    importance of nursing research to, 4
    role in intellectual research critiques, 421
    staffing mix, 523-526, 524t
Nursing
    education, 4
    educational degree levels of, 27-28, 27f
    ethnography and, 80-81
    grounded theory research example, 78-79
    knowledge. *See* Knowledge
    levels of experience, 17-18
    measurement strategies in, 345-361
        interviews, 350-352
        observational measurements, 348-349
        physiological measurements, 345-347
        questionnaires, 353-354
        scales, 355-361
    outcomes research and, 522-529
    research knowledge and, 155
    role effectiveness model, 526, 527f
    theories guiding practices, 227
    web addresses for journals of, 218
Nursing interventions. *See* Interventions
Nursing journals. *See* Journals
Nursing process
    comparison to problem-solving, 41t, 42
    definition of, 42
    description and components of, 41t, 42
    versus research process, 42-43
Nursing research
    from 1900s through 1970s, 12-13
    from 1980 and 1990s, 13-14
    acquiring knowledge through, 19-22
    addressing priorities in, 156-157
    characteristics and roles of, 4
    classification system for, 21t
    critique guidelines for, 158-159
    definition of, 7f

Nursing research *(continued)*
  designs for
    comparative descriptive designs, 260-262
    correlational designs, 264-270
    descriptive designs, 256-264
  ethical conduct in, 103
  frameworks, 238-240
  goals for twenty-first century, 14-15
  history of, 10-15, 11t
  informed consent and, 122-129
  landmark studies in, 194
  participation levels, according to education, 27f
  role of nurses in, 10-15
  statistics
    data analysis process, 372-375
    descriptive statistics, 383-389
    to examine causality, 401-408
    to examine relationships, 394-398
    interpreting statistical outcomes, 408-415
    judging statistical suitability, 392
    to predict, 398-399
    reasoning behind, 376-383
Nursing Research, 54, 62
  history of, 11t, 12
Nursing Role Effectiveness Model, 526, 527f
Nursing Science Quarterly, 11t, 13
Nursing sensitive patient outcomes, outcomes research
    and, 526-529

Obesity, as health risk, 6t
Objectives, purpose of, in research studies, 145-146
Observational measurements, definition of, 348
Observations
  in design mapping, 284
  in qualitative research, 88-90
  structured *versus* unstructured, 348
Office of Research Integrity (ORI), 137-139
Office of Scientific Integrity Review (OSIR),
  137-138
Oncology Nursing Society, website, 496
One-tailed test of significance, 12, 381f
On-line full-text versions, of citation format, 220
Operational definitions
  bias protection and, 256
  case study examples of, 64
  examples of, 178b-180b
  of variables, 47, 47b, 178-180
Ordinal levels, of measurements, 51
Ordinal-scale measurements, description and example of,
  330
Orem's Theory of Self-Care, 229
ORI. *See* Office of Research Integrity
OSIR. *See* Office of Scientific Integrity Review
Outcomes
  benefits/risks ratio and, 135f
  examples of common, 154
  predictions and, 9
  research design and, 49

Outcomes research
  disseminating findings, 529
  essential elements of, 21-22
  focus of, 507
  history of, 382
  integration with evidence-based practice, 3
  nursing practice and, 522-529
    American Nurses Association's "Nursing Safety &
      Quality Initiative," 522-526
    nursing sensitive patient outcomes, 526-529
  problems and purposes in, 154, 154t
  theoretical basis of, Donabedian's Theory of Quality
    Health Care, 508-520, 509f
Outliers, 374
OVID, 211, 215

Pain
  grounded theory research on, 78b-79b
  measuring chronic, 38b
Paraphrasing, description of, 220
Partially controlled settings, 40-41, 322
Participants, in qualitative research, 84
Patient responses, element of outcomes research, 21-22
Patient satisfaction, element of outcomes research, 21-22
Patient's rights, ethics and hospital research, 114
Pearson, Karl, on statistical approaches to variables, 34
Pearson product-moment correlation, 53b, 394-396
Peer reviewed literature, 190-191, 191t
Percentage distributions, definition of, 385
Percents, examples of, 53b
Periodicals, description of, 190
Personal experience, acquiring knowledge through, 17-18
Phase I: Preparation, in Stetler Model of Research
  Utilization to Facilitate Evidence-Based Practice,
  477-479, 478f
Phase II: Validation, in Stetler Model of Research
  Utilization to Facilitate Evidence-Based Practice,
  478f, 479
Phase III: Comparative Evaluation/Decision Making, in
  Stetler Model of Research Utilization to Facilitate
  Evidence-Based Practice, 478f, 479-480
Phase IV: Translation/Application, in Stetler Model of
  Research Utilization to Facilitate Evidence-Based
  Practice, 478f, 480
Phase V: Evaluation, in Stetler Model of Research
  Utilization to Facilitate Evidence-Based Practice,
  478f, 480
Phenomena
  definition of, 228
  descriptive designs and, 257-260
Phenomenological research
  definition and example of, 75-76, 76b-77b
  examples of, 151, 152t-153t
  introduction and classification of, 21, 21t
  literature review purpose in, 193t
Phenomenology, 75-76
PHI. *See* Protected health information
Philosophical stance, in conceptual models, 229

Philosophies, definition of, 229
PHS. *See* Public Health Service
Physical inactivity, as health risk, 6t
Physiological measurements
    accuracy of, 338-339
    approaches to obtaining, 345-347
    error in, 339-340
    precision of, 339
    research examples of, 340b
PICO format, 490
Pie charts, illustration of, 386f
Pilot studies, definition and reasons for, 49
Plagiarism
    of data, 103
    definition of research, 137
Planning, step of nursing process, 41t, 42
Plans
    in problem-solving, nursing and research processes, 41t,
        42
    research design and, 49
Plots, structure of, 389f
Policy on Humane Care and Use of Laboratory Animals,
    by Public Health Service, 140
Populations
    definition and examples of, in quantitative study,
        43f, 51
    definition of, 51, 290-291
    purpose of, in research studies, 145-146
    research design and, 49
    samples and, 288-325
        key concepts, 323-324
        nonprobability quantitative sampling methods,
            305-307
        probability sampling methods, 298-304
        representativeness, 294-298
        research settings, 321-323
        sample size in qualitative studies, 317-320
        sample size in quantitative studies, 308-312
        sampling in qualitative research, 312-317
        sampling theory, 290-293
Positive likelihood ratio, 344
Positive relationships, 395
Post-doctorate degree, roles of, in nursing research,
    27-28, 27f
Posthoc analyses, during data analysis process, 375
Posttest-only designs, 271, 272f
Power, 308
    definition of, in statistics, 382-383
Power analysis, of sample size, 308
Practical research. *See* Applied research
Practice
    institute change in, 488, 489t
    pilot change in, 487-488, 487t
Practice theories, *versus* middle range theories,
    237-238
Precision
    definition of, in quantitative research, 39
    of physiological measures, 339
Predictions, nursing research definition of, 9
Predictive correlational designs, 266-268, 266f
Pregnancy, defining, 113

Pregnant women
    ethical laws concerning, 111, 113
    legal issues concerning, 113
Premise, definition of, 19
Pretest and posttest designs
    with comparison group, 271, 271f
    in experimental design, 276-280, 278f
Pretest-posttest control group design, 278f
Preventive Services Task Force, US, website, 496
Primary sources
    critique of, 197b-201b, 205b-208b
    definition of, 191-192
    of historical data, 82b-83b
Principle of beneficence, 107-108, 118-119
Principle of justice, definition of, 107-108
Principle of respect for persons, 107-108
Print version, of citation format, 220
Privacy
    definition of, 114
    identifying private personal data, 114-117
Privacy Rule, of Health Insurance Portability and
        Accountability Act
    authorization for uses and disclosures, 126-128, 127f
    clarification of, 108, 109t
    expansion of, 114-115
Probability
    versus nonprobability sampling methods, 299t
    normal curve and, 379-380
    of relative *versus* absolute causality, 254
Probability sampling, methods of, 298-304
    cluster sampling, 302-303
    simple random sampling, 299-301
    stratified random sampling, 301-302
    systematic sampling, 303-304
Probability theory, in statistics, 376-377
Problem definition, in problem-solving, nursing and
        research processes, 41t
Problems. *See* Research problems
Problem-solving processes
    comparison to nursing and research processes, 41t, 42
    solving data collection issues, 366
"Procedures" section, in research reports, 52
Processes
    evaluating in Donabedian's Theory, 510-520
    of research, 41-42
Professional standards review organizations (PSROs), 14
"Proficient" stage, of nursing experience, 17-18
Propositions
    definition of, 19
    example of critiquing and extracting, 232
    general *versus* specific, within theories, 232
    research example of, 232t
Protected health information (PHI), 115-116
PSROs. *See* Professional standards review organizations
PsychINFO, evidence-based practice resource, 470t
Public Health Service (PHS), Policy on Humane Care and
        Use of Laboratory Animals, 140
Public libraries, 208
PubMed National Library of Medicine (MEDLINE)
    evidence-based practice resource, 470t
    keeping written research records in, 212t

PubMed National Library of Medicine (MEDLINE) *(continued)*
    with MeSH, evidence-based practice resource, 470t
    website information, 211
Pure research. *See* Basic research
Purposes. *See* Research purposes

Q

Qualitative analysis, research example of, 95b
Qualitative Health Research, 11t, 13
Qualitative metasummary, 475
Qualitative metasynthesis, 475
Qualitative Nursing Research, 54
Qualitative research
    approaches to, 75-83
        ethnographic research, 79-81
        grounded theory research, 77-79
        historical research, 81-83
        phenomenological research, 75-77
        questions and sources, 82-83
    characteristics *versus* quantitative, 20t
    critical appraisal process, 442
        guidelines for, 443-446
        literature review, 443
        research example of, 446-454
    critique process, 442
    data analysis stages of, 94-97
    data management, 93-94
    definition of, 73
    definition of process, 20
    frameworks in, 244-245
    history of, 13
    integrative reviews of, 23t, 24
    introduction to, 19-21, 72-100
    metasummaries and metasynthesis of, 24
    methodology of, 83-85
        participant selection, 40
        researcher-participant relationships, 84-85
    probability *versus* nonprobability sampling methods in,
        299t
    problems and purposes in types of, 151-154, 152t-153t
    purpose of literature review in, 192-193
    research objectives in, 161-163, 162b-163b
    rigor in, 75
    types and classification of, 21, 21t
Qualitative research synthesis, 475
Qualitative studies, frameworks derived from, 244-245
Quality, evidence for practice and, 22
Quality of care
    assessment of, 508, 509f
    costs and, 519-520
    element of outcomes research, 21-22
    indicators, 522-523, 524t
    levels and scopes of concern, 509f
    standards, 511
Quantitative research
    characteristics *versus* qualitative, 20t
    concept and conceptual definition extraction, 231
    data analysis process in, 372-375

Quantitative research *(continued)*
    definition of process, 20, 34
    designs, 252-287
        defining experimental interventions, 282-284
        design mapping, 284-285
        important design concepts, 253-256
        nursing study designs, 256-270
        replication studies, 285
        testing causality, 270-281
    framework critique guidelines, 240b
    frameworks in, 238-240
    identifying problems and purposes in, 148-151, 149t-150t
    introduction to, 19-21
    key concepts concerning, 68-69
    probability *versus* nonprobability sampling methods in,
        299t
    process
        definition of, 43
        steps of, 5f, 21-22
    purpose of literature review in, 192
    research objectives in, 160-161
    rigor and control in, 39-41, 39t
    tips for reading reports, 59-60
    types and classification of, 21, 21t, 34-36
Quantitative studies
    clarifying research designs for, 252-287
        defining experimental interventions, 282-284
        design mapping, 284-285
        important design concepts, 253-256
        nursing study designs, 256-270
        replication studies, 285
        testing causality, 270-281
    critical appraisal of, 428
        research example, 428b-442b
    sample size in
        adequacy of, 308, 311b
        critique guidelines, 311b
        data analysis techniques, 310-312
        effect size, 308-309
        measurement sensitivity, 310
        number of variables, 310
        types of, 309
    summary example of report, 428b-442b
Quasi-experimental designs
    algorithm for determining types of, 275f
    definition of, 270
    testing causality in, 270-276, 273b-274b, 275f
Quasi-experimental research
    control levels in, 39-40, 39t
    examples of, 148, 149t-150t
    framework and theory development in, 242-244
    introduction and classification of, 20-21, 21t
    mapping the design, 284-285
    problems and purposes of, 35, 44, 151
    testing causality in, 270-276, 273b-274b, 275f
    tips for reading reports on, 59-60
    variables in, 181-182
Questionnaires
    critique guidelines, 353b
    definition of, 353
    example of research, 354b

Questions
   evolution of research, 163-166
   purpose of, in research studies, 145-146
   sources for qualitative research and, 82-83
Quota sampling, as nonprobability sampling method, 299t, 307

R

R. *See* Regression coefficient
Race, as demographic variable, 182, 183t
Random error, in measurement, 331-332
Random numbers table, 300t
Random sampling, purpose of, 298
Random variation, definition of, 294
Randomized clinical trials, 280-281
   description and example of, 280b-281b
Randomized controlled trials (RCTs), 466
Range
   calculation of, 385t, 387
   definition of, 387
Rating scales
   definition of, 355
   example of, 355-357, 356f
Ratio levels, of measurements, 51
Ratio-scale measurements, description and example of, 330-331
RCTs. *See* Randomized controlled trials
Reading research reports, *versus* skimming or comprehending, 60
Reasoning, behind statistics, 376-383
Reasoning process
   deductive, 19
   definition of, 18-19
   inductive, 18-19
   in qualitative research, 73-74
Reasons Model, 269b
Record keeping. *See also* Documentation
   of database searches, 212t
Recruiting, of subjects, 362
Reference management software, 212-213
References, recording of, 219-220
"References" section, of research reports, 59
Reflexive thoughts, 95
Refusal rates
   example of, 295-296
   of subjects, 295-296
Registered nurses (RNs), job satisfaction research example using quantitative methods, 148-149
Regression analysis
   definition of, 398-399
   outcomes of, 399
   research example of, 399b-401b
Regression coefficient (R), 399
Relational statements, function of, within theories, 231-232
Relationships, using statistics to examine, 394-398
Relevant studies, definition of, 189-190
Reliability
   definition of, 332
   example of, 336b-338b

Reliability *(continued)*
   of measurement techniques, 51, 333-334
   testing measurement, during data analysis process, 374
Reliability testing, 332-334
Replications studies, role in evidence-based practice, 285
Representativeness
   definition of, 294
   evaluation of, 294-298
Research. *See also* Basic research
   benefits/risks ratios in, 134-137
   for building evidence-based practice, 464-504
   critiques, guidelines, 158-159
   definition of, 4
   disclosure authorization, 126-128, 127f
   ethics
      of animal use in, 139-140
      scientific misconduct, 137-139
   experimentation and, 33
   identifying priorities in, 156-157
   informed consent and, 122-129
   institutional review boards, 130-133
   integrative review of, 4, 163-165
   judging statistical suitability, 392
   literature review, 188-225
   objectives, questions and hypotheses, 43f, 46-47
   populations and samples, 288-325
      key concepts, 323-324
      nonprobability quantitative sampling methods, 305-307
      probability sampling methods, 298-304
      representativeness, 294-298
      research settings, 321-323
      sample size in qualitative research, 312-317
      sample size in qualitative studies, 317-320
      sample size in quantitative studies, 308-312
      sampling theory, 290-293
   settings, 40-41
   statistics
      data analysis process, 372-375
      descriptive statistics, 383-389
      to examine causality, 401-408
      to examine relationships, 394-398
      interpreting statistical outcomes, 408-415
      judging statistical suitability, 392
      to predict, 398-399
      reasoning behind, 376-383
   strength of evidence, 25f
   synthesis of findings, to determine evidence for practice, 22-24
   systematic reviews of, 23-24, 23t
Research base, sufficiency of, 486-487
Research designs
   algorithm for determining type of, 257f
   case studies, 262-264
   comparative descriptive, 260-262
   concepts important to, 253-256
      bias, 254-255
      causality, 253
      control, 255
      critique guidelines, 256b
      manipulation, 263b

Research designs *(continued)*
    multicausality, 254
    probability, 261b
  correlational, 264-270
  definition and examples of, in quantitative study, 43f, 49-50, 50f
  definition of, 253
  descriptive, 256-264
  descriptive correlational, 264-266, 265f
  Fisher, Ronald, on, 34
  mapping, 284-285
  model testing, 268-270, 268f
  predictive correlational, 266-268, 266f
  purpose of, 266
  for quantitative studies, 252-287
    defining experimental interventions, 282-284
    design mapping, 284-285
    important design concepts, 253-256
    nursing study designs, 256-270
    replication studies, 285
    testing causality, 270-281
  random clinical trials, 280-281
Research evidence, synthesis of, 483-486
Research hypotheses
  definition of, 175
    in qualitative research process, 43f, 46-47
  versus null, 174-175
Research in Nursing & Health, 11t, 12-13, 54
Research objectives
  definition and example of study, in quantitative research process, 43f, 46-47
  definition of, 160-161
  evolution of, 159-175
  example of critiquing, 160b-163b
Research outcomes. *See also* Outcomes research
  definition and examples of, in quantitative study, 43f, 53
  interpretation of, 53
Research problems
  critiquing guidelines, 158-159
  definition of, 146-148
    in quantitative research process, 156f, 159-175
  determining significance of, 155-157
  examples of critiquing, 160b-166b
  in outcomes research, 154, 154t
  purpose of, 145-146
  qualitative examples of, 151-154, 152t-153t
  quantitative examples of, 148-151, 149t-150t
  research example, 44b, 62, 66
Research process
  comparison to nursing, 41t, 42-43
  definition of, 42
  pilot studies, 49
  steps of
    case study example of, 62-63
    case study of experimental study, 66b-68b
Research purposes
  case study example of experimental, 66
  critiquing guidelines, 158-159
  definition of
    identification of and, 102, 146-151
    in quantitative research process, 43f, 44

Research purposes *(continued)*
  determining significance of, 155-157
  examples of critiquing, 160b-166b
  in outcomes research, 154, 154t
  qualitative examples of, 151-154, 152t-153t
  quantitative examples of, 148-151, 149t-150t
  research example, 44b, 62, 66
Research questions
  critiquing, 164b-166b
  definition of, 163-165
    in quantitative research process, 43f, 46-47
  practice research example, 61b
Research reports
  abstracts, 55, 56b-57b
  analyzing, 60
  comprehension of, 60
  contents of, 55-59
  critique of, 28
  definition of, 54
  discussion, 59
  functions of, 54
  introduction, 57-58
  methods, 58
  nursing review methods, 23t
  reading *versus* skimming, 60
  references, 59
  results, 58
  sections of, 55, 56t
  sources of, 54
  tips for reading, 54, 59-60
Research settings. *See* Settings
Research studies, judging statistical suitability, 392
Research syntheses, critical appraisal guidelines for, 469-475
Research traditions, definition and example of, 246-248
Research-based protocols, 482
Researcher-participant relationships, in qualitative research, 84-85
Researchers, expertise of, 158
Resources, historical research, 82b-83b
Respect, principle of, 107-108, 110
Respect for persons, principle of, 107-108
Results
  of analysis of variance, 406
  causality, 401-408
  research example illustrating, 411b-412b
  types of, 409-410
"Results" section
  abstract components of, 56t
  case study example of, 65, 68
  of research reports, 53, 58
Review of literature. *See* Literature reviews
Right to Privacy, 114-117
Rights
  to confidentiality and anonymity, 117-118
  to fair treatment, 118
  to protection from discomfort and harm, 118-120
Rigor
  definition of, in quantitative research, 39
  in qualitative research, 75

Risks
  balancing with benefits, Nuremberg Code and, 104-105
  versus benefits, informed consent and, 112t
  benefits and, informed consent competence and, 124
  benefits ratio and, 134-137, 135f
  defining minimal, 131-132
  permanent damage of, to subjects, 118-120
  studying health, 8
  temporary discomfort and, 119
RNs. *See* Registered nurses
Role modeling, learning through, 18
Roper, William, on outcome research, 14

S

Sample attrition
  definition of, 296
  example of, 296
Sample characteristics, definition and examples of, 182
Sample sizes
  in qualitative studies, 81, 317-320
  in quantitative studies, 308-312
    adequacy of, 308, 311b
    critique guidelines, 311b
    data analysis techniques, 310-312
    effect size, 308-309
    measurement sensitivity, 310
    number of variables, 310
    types of, 309
Samples
  case study example of, 64, 67
  definition of, 51
    in quantitative study, 43f, 51
    in sampling theory, 34-35
  describing in data analysis process, 373
  populations and, 288-325
    key concepts, 323-324
    nonprobability quantitative sampling methods, 305-307
    probability sampling methods, 298-304
    representativeness, 294-298
    research settings, 321-323
    sample size in qualitative studies, 317-320
    sample size in quantitative studies, 308-312
    sampling size in qualitative research, 312-317
    sampling theory, 290-293
Sampling
  definition of
    process, 40
    in sampling theory, 290
  in qualitative research, 312-317
    network sampling, 314-316
    purposive sampling, 313-314
    theoretical sampling, 316-317
Sampling criteria, definition of, in sampling theory, 291
Sampling frames, 298
Sampling methods, probability *versus* nonprobability, 299t
Sampling plans, 298
  definition of, in sampling theory, 290

Sampling theories
  elements and populations, 290-291
  eligibility criteria, 291-293
  introduction to, 290
Sandelowski, Dr. Margarete, 442
Sanitation, Florence Nightingale's work on, 10-12
Saturation of information, 317-318
Scales
  definition of, 355
  Likert, 357-360
  rating, 355-357, 356f
  visual analogue, 360-361
Scatterplots
  definition of, 389
  illustration of, 389f-390f
  overlay with best-fit line, 399f
Scheffe's test, 406
Scholarly Inquiry for Nursing Practice, 11t
Scholarly Inquiry for Nursing Practice: An International Journal, 54, 421
Scientific merit, critical appraisal for, 483
Scientific misconduct, understanding, 137-138
Scientific rigor. *See* Rigor
Screening tests
  accuracy of, 341
  likelihood ratios, 344
  outcomes of, 341
  quality determination of, 341-344
  sensitivity of, 341-342, 341t
  specificity of, 341t, 342-344
SCUs. *See* Special care units
Search engines, 210-211
  variances in, 218-219
Search fields, list of common, 216-217
Searches
  limiting of, 214-215
  list of fields of, 216-217
  locating relevant literature, 213-220
Secondary sources
  critique of, 197b-201b, 205b-208b
  definition of, 191-192
  of historical data, 82b-83b
Self-determination
  critique of, 120-122
  rights to, 110-114
  violation of, 110
Sensitivity, research example of, 342b-344b
Serendipity, 366
Settings
  case study example of experimental, 67
  definition of, 40-41, 321
  description and types of, 39t, 40-41, 321
  highly controlled settings, 41, 322-323
  natural settings, 40-41, 321
  partially controlled settings, 40-41, 322
Sexual abuse, of children, research example concerning, 44b-45b, 45, 46f, 47-49, 47b, 50f, 51-52, 53b
Sigma Theta Tau Journal, description of, 11t, 12-13, 158
Significance
  clinical, 410-411
  exploring findings, 410

Significant and predicted results, 409
Significant and unpredicted results, 409
Simple hypotheses
    versus complex hypotheses, 172-173
    critique of, 172-173
    definition of, 172-173
Simple random sampling, as probability sampling method,
    299-301
Skimming, a research report, 60
Smoking
    as health risk, 6t
    lung damage and, as correlational research example,
        35
"Snowball sampling." See Network sampling
Solutions, in problem-solving, nursing, and research
    processes, 41t
Sources
    electronic, 210-211
    identifying relevant research, 210-213
    on-line access to, 210
    primary and secondary historical, 82b-83b
Special care units (SCUs), 154, 154t
Special libraries, 208
Specific propositions
    example of critiquing and extracting, 232, 232t
    hierarchy within theories, 232, 232t
Specificity, research example of, 342b-344b
Staffing mix, studies concerning, 523-526, 524t
Standard deviation
    calculation example, 385t, 388
    definition of, 388
    examples of, 53b
    normal curve and, 379-380
Standardized scores, 388
Standards of care
    definition of, 511
    evaluating in Donabedian's Theory, 511
Starvation, Florence Nightingale's work on, 10-12
Statements
    extracting from published studies, 231
    within theories, definition of, 231
Statistical analysis
    Fisher, Ronald, on, 34
    outcomes of
        conclusions, 412-415
        findings, 410
        further study suggestions, 415
        generalized findings, 413
        implications, 413-414
        importance, 410-411
Statistical hypothesis, definition of, 174
Statistical outcomes, interpretation of, 408-411
    conclusions, 412-415
    findings, 410
    further study suggestions, 415
    generalized findings, 413
    implications, 413-414
    importance, 410-411
Statistical significance, 377-378
Statistical suitability, 392
Statistical tests, algorithm for choosing, 393f

Statistics, understanding in research
    data analysis process, 372-375
    descriptive, 383-389
    to examine causality, 401-408
    to examine relationships, 394-398
    interpreting outcomes, 408-411
    judging suitability, 392
    to predict, 398-399
    reasoning behind, 376-383
Steps of Research Utilization to Facilitate Evidence-Based
        Practice, 11t
Stetler Model of Research Utilization to Facilitate
        Evidence-Based Practice, 477-480, 478f
    Phase I: Preparation, 477-479, 478f
    Phase II: Validation, 478f, 479
    Phase III: Comparative Evaluation/Decision Making,
        478f, 479-480
    Phase IV: Translation/Application, 478f, 480
    Phase V: Evaluation, 478f, 480
Stratification, 301
Stratified random sampling, as probability sampling
        method, 301-302
Structures of care, definition of, 520
Subjects. See also Participants
    animals as, 139-140
    characteristics of, ungrouped frequency of, 384t
    definition of population, 290-291
    informed consent, 122-129
    with mental or cognitive impairments, 113-114
    mentally or legally competent, 111
    protection of
        with DHEW regulations, 107
        human rights and, 110-122
        Nuremberg Code and, 104-105
    recruiting of, 362
    self-determination rights of, 110
    terminally ill, ethical considerations, 114
    unethical events involving, regulations, 107
"Summary" section, of literature review, 222
Summated scales, 355
Symbolic interaction theory, 77-78
Symmetrical, definition of, 394-395
Synthesis of sources, 220-221, 221t
Syphilis, studied in African Americans, in unethical
        Tuskegee study, 106
Systematic bias. See Systematic variation
Systematic error, in measurement, 332
Systematic reviews
    characteristics of, 23t
    critically appraising, 469-471
    definition of, 469
    of research, focus and steps of, 23-24
Systematic sampling, as probability sampling method,
        303-304
Systematic variation, definition of, 295

T

Tailedness, of normal curves, 380-381
Tails, 380-381

Target populations
    definition of, 290-291
    representativeness, 294-298
Temporary discomfort, 119
Terminally ill subjects, ethical considerations, 114
Testable hypotheses, definition of, 175
Text, as qualitative data source, 90
Theoretical limitations, definition and example of, 48
Theoretical literature, 190-191
Theoretical sampling, description and example of, 316-317
Theories
    assumptions and, 48
    conceptual models, 228-230
    definition of, 45, 228
    Donabedian's, 508-520
    elements of, 230-235
        concept, 230-231
        conceptual map, 233-235
        rational statements, 231-232
    frameworks, 238-240
    generated by problems and purposes, 155, 156f
    generating and refining, in basic research, 36
    importance of, in guiding nursing practice, 227
    middle range, 235-237, 236t
    testing and development of, 155-156, 156f
Theory of health promotion behavior, 236t
Theory of mother-infant attachment, 236t
Theory of planned behavior, 155-156, 156f
Theory of uncertainty in illness, 236t
Therapeutic research
    benefits/risks ratios in, 134-137
    definition of, 105
    guide to informed consent, for children, 112t-113t
    versus nontherapeutic research, 112t
Thesis, definition of, 190-191
Total variances, 406
Traditions, definition of nursing, 16
Transcripts, of interviews, 76-77, 93
Translational research, 500-501
Treatment, in design mapping, 284
Trial and error approach, to acquiring knowledge, 17
True measure, 331
True negative, 341
True positive, 341
True score, 331
T-tests
    interpreting results of, 404
    purpose of, 404
    research example of, 404b-405b
Tukey's Honestly Significantly Different (HSD) test, 406
Tuskegee Syphilis Study, 106, 118, 120
Two-tailed test of significance, 380-381
Type I errors, in decision theory, 381-382, 382f
Type II errors, description of, 381-382

U
UAP. See Unlicensed assistive personnel
Unconscious patients, legal issues concerning, 111
Unethical research, historical events surrounding, 104-109

Unexpected results, 410
Unexplained variances, 395
Ungrouped frequency distributions
    definition of, 384
    subject characteristics example, 384t
Unlicensed assistive personnel (UAP), 524t, 526

V
Validity
    definition of, 334-335
    example of, 336b-338b
    of instruments, 334-338
    of measurement, 51
    and quasi-experimental design, 271
    uncontrolled threats to, in experimental design, 278f
Variability. See Measures of dispersion
Variables
    case study examples of, 63, 67
    causality and, 253
    correlational design, 264
    critique guidelines, 178b
    critique of framework, 240b
    definition of, 176
        in quantitative study, 43f, 47
        in theory, 230
    description of, in different hypotheses, 167-175
    within descriptive designs, 256
    in different research types, 34-36
    extraneous, 177
    independent and dependent, 176
    purpose of, in research studies, 145-146
    in quasi-experimental research, 270-276, 271f-272f,
        273b-274b
    research, 176-177
    types of, 176-177
    ungrouped frequency distribution, 384, 384t
Variances
    calculation of, 384t, 387-388
    definition of, 387-388
    unexplained versus explained, 395
VAS. See Visual analogue scale
Ventilation, Florence Nightingale's work on, 10-12
Visual analogue scale (VAS), 360-361
Voluntary consent, 125

W
Water, purity of, Florence Nightingale's work on, 10-12
Watson's theory of caring, 72
Web addresses, for nursing journals, 218
Websites
    for additional grounded theory research, 79
    on Belmont Report, 107-108
    for Cochrane Collaboration, 221-222
    concerning Declaration of Helsinki, 105-106
    databases available on, 211
    on ethical principles, 107-108
    for HIPAA Privacy Rule, 109

Websites *(continued)*
  identifying research priorities, 156-157
  information on ethnographic studies, 81
  on institutional review, 130
  for National Institute of Nursing Research, 11t, 15
  for nursing journals, 218
  for Office of Research Integrity, 138-139
  for phenomenological studies, 77
  for reference management software, 212-213
  storing addresses, 219
Weight, as physiological measures, 338
Western Journal of Nursing Research, 11t, 12-13, 54, 421
Willowbrook Study, 106, 118
Within-group variances, 406
World Wide Web. *See also* Websites
  searching, 218-219
Worldviews on Evidence-Based Nursing, 11t, 15

Writing, literature review, 222
Written search records, 212t

X

X axis, 389, 389f

Y

Y axis, 389, 389f
Yakson, 283b

Z

Z-scores, 388